OXYGEN TRANSPORT
TO TISSUE — III

ADVANCES IN EXPERIMENTAL MEDICINE AND BIOLOGY

Recent Volumes in this Series

OXYGEN TRANSPORT
TO TISSUE — III

Edited by

I. A. Silver
University of Bristol
Bristol, England

M. Erecińska
University of Pennsylvania
Philadelphia, Pennsylvania

and

H. I. Bicher
Roswell Park Memorial Institute
Buffalo, New York

SPRINGER SCIENCE+BUSINESS MEDIA, LLC

Library of Congress Cataloging in Publication Data

International Symposium on Oxygen Transport to Tissue, 3rd, Churchill College, 1977.
Oxygen transport to tissue, III.

Bibliography: p.
1. Oxygen transport (Physiology)—Congresses. 2. Oximetry—Congresses. 3. Oxygen in the body—Congresses. I. Silver, I. A. II. Erecińska, M. III. Bicher, Haim I. IV. Title. [DNLM: 1. Oxygen—Blood—Congresses. 2. Oxygen consumption—Congresses. 3. Biological Transport—Congresses. W3 IN931BB 3d 1977/QV312 I613 1977o]
QP99.3.09I54 1977   599'.01'2   77-17140

ISBN 978-1-4684-8892-0   ISBN 978-1-4684-8890-6 (eBook)
DOI 10.1007/978-1-4684-8890-6

Proceedings of the Third International Symposium
on Oxygen Transport to Tissue held at Churchill College,
Cambridge, England, July 4-7, 1977

© 1978 Springer Science+Business Media New York
Originally published by Plenum Press, New York in 1978
Softcover reprint of the hardcover 1st edition 1978

INTERNATIONAL SOCIETY
OF
OXYGEN TRANSPORT TO TISSUE

President   — Dr. I.A. Silver
                         Bristol, England

President Elect   — Dr. J. Strauss
                         Miami, Florida, U.S.A.

Past President   — Dr. B. Chance
                         Philadelphia, Pennsylvania, U.S.A.

Secretary   — Dr. H.I. Bicher
                         Buffalo, New York, U.S.A.

Treasurer   — Dr. D.W. Lübbers
                         Dortmund, Federal Republic of Germany

Members of the International Committee

Dr. D.F. Bruley, Terre Haute, Indiana, U.S.A.
Dr. J. Ditzel, Aarlborg, Denmark
Dr. R.E. Forster, Philadelphia, Pennsylvania, U.S.A.
Dr. J. Grote, Mainz, Federal Republic of Germany
Dr. J. H. Halsey, Birmingham, Alabama, U.S.A.
Dr. C.R. Honig, Rochester, New York, U.S.A.
Dr. F.F. Jöbsis, Durham, North Carolina, U.S.A.
Dr. M. Kessler, Dortmund, Federal Republic of Germany
Dr. A.G.B. Kovách, Budapest, Hungary
Dr. F. Kreuzer, Nijmegen, Netherlands
Dr. I.S. Longmuir, Raleigh, North Carolina, U.S.A.
Dr. M. Mochizuki, Yamagata, Japan
Dr. D.D. Reneau, Ruston, Louisiana, U.S.A.
Dr. G. Thews, Mainz, Federal Republic of Germany
Dr. W.J. Whalen, Cleveland, Ohio, U.S.A.

Preface

This volume contains the papers which were presented at the Third International Symposium on Oxygen Transport to Tissue together with the discussions at the end of each Session. The meeting was held at Churchill College, Cambridge from July 4th-7th 1977.

Our special thanks are due to Mrs. Valerie Jeal and Mr. Charles Drown of the Department of Pathology, Bristol, who were invaluable in ensuring the smooth running of the meeting and the preparation of this book. We are very grateful to Dr. Marian Silver for proof-reading and helping to disentangle the "discussion". We would also express our thanks for the general help received from Janet and Fiona Silver and Steven James and our appreciation of the cheerful assistance of Miss Sadie Williams in putting the finishing touches to the manuscript.

August,1977

I.A. Silver
M. Erecińska
H.I. Bicher

Contents

Session 3 – MODEL SYSTEMS

Session 9 — TISSUE PO$_2$ AND CELL FUNCTION

Oxygen Electrodes
and
Blood Monitoring Devices

THE BITUMEN PO$_2$ ELECTRODE - A NEW METHOD TO MANUFACTURE PO$_2$ NEEDLE ELECTRODES

H. Acker, D. Sylvester, E. Dufau and H. Durst

Max-Planck-Institut für Systemphysiologie

46 Dortmund, West Germany

The development of needle electrodes has allowed the measurement of various parameters in the tissue of different organs such as nervous activity, microflow, ion activities, and oxygen partial pressure. To investigate the interdependence and mutual influence of these parameters, simultaneous recorders with multi-channel electrodes may be used. Different methods have been employed to use one of the channels for the polarographic measurements of oxygen or hydrogen. Silver (1976) centrifuges an organic liquid compound of palladium and gold into the channel. Tsacopoulos and Lehmenkühler (in press) introduce an etched platinum wire into the channel of the microelectrodes and fix it with wax. In the following report we would like to present a further method that allows the use of one channel of a 2 channel glass electrode for polarographic measurement.

Figure 1 demonstrates the general procedure. A two-channel Theta glass electrode (Neumann, Munich) is drawn to a tip diameter of 3 μm. A 25 μm platinum wire is etched to a diameter of less than 1 μm according to the method developed by Baumgärtl and Lübbers (1973). Then the platinum wire is inserted into a glass capillary. One channel of the microelectrode and the glass capillary are filled with Bitumen Mexphalt 80 (Deutsche Shell AG) dissolved in benzine. Bitumen is a high-ohmic material ($<10^{12}$ Ω) with a consistency which may vary from brittleness to viscousness; the consistency of Mexaphalt 80 is viscous.

When dissolved in benzine the material easily flows into glass tips of diameters down to 0.2 μm. After being filled with bitumen, the glass capillary containing the platinum wire is introduced into

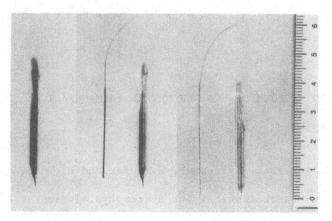

Fig. 1. Three preparation-steps of the bitumen-PO_2 electrode.
        From left to right: Pulled two-channel electrode and
        etched platinum wire shielded in a glass capillary;
        bitumen two-channel-electrode and glass capillary; glass
        capillary and platinum wire inserted in one channel of the
        two-channel electrode.

the glass microelectrode.   The platinum wire is inserted up to the
tip under the microscope and then both glass capillary and platinum
wire are glued to the back end of the glass electrode.   Benzine is
vacuum-evaporated (10^{-2} Torr) from the bitumen material for three
days.   Then the original consistency of bitumen is reestablished
so that the platinum wire is kept in the glass tip.   In addition,
bitumen electrically insulates the platinum wire because of its
high resistance and, as a third effect, it makes the tip of the
glass electrode rigid and so facilitates the penetration through
connective tissues.   The free channel can be filled with magnesium
acetate and used for simultaneous DC measurement.

    Figure 2 shows the tip of the microelectrode.   The channel
filled with bitumen can be seen distinctly, in contrast to the
platinum wire which is scarcely recognizable because of the optical
density of the bitumen material.   The polarographic measurement
is performed with a Knick nanoamperemeter (Knick, Berlin, Type 22/
23) using the polarizing voltage described by Baumgärtl and
Lübbers (1973).   Apart from DC registration, the second channel
serves as a reference for the polarizing voltage as described by
Lehmenkühler et al (1975).

    Figure 3 shows the recording circuit employed.   The DC
potential is measured with the amplifier, V 1, and conducted to
the difference amplifier, V 4.   V2 serves as a buffer for the
source of the polarization voltage of the PO_2 electrode.

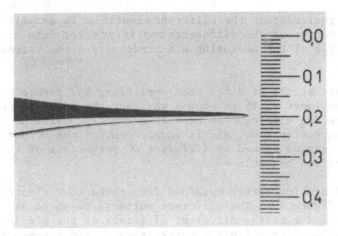

Fig. 2. Tip of the bitumen PO$_2$ electrode. The bitumen-filled
   channel and the bitumen-free channel can be clearly
   seen (0.1 – 0.2 = 100 μm).

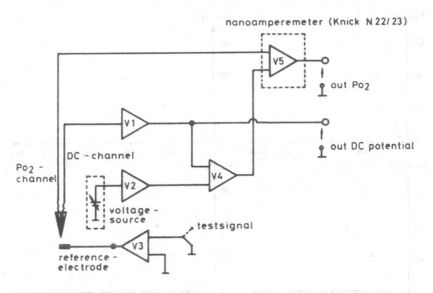

Fig. 3. Electronic device for simultaneous measurement of PO$_2$
   and bioelectrical activity included in the usual
   polarographic circuit.

Its output signal reaches the difference amplifier V4 as well.   In
this way the output of the difference amplifier takes into account
the DC potential of the measuring electrode versus the reference
electrode.

The output signal of difference amplifier, V4, regulates the
voltage at the input of V5 in such a way that the polarization
voltage of the PO_2 electrode is kept at a constant value as compared
to the reference electrode, and is independent of the DC potential.
Thus current changes caused by different DC potentials of the object
to be measured can be excluded.

Four calibration curves obtained from these four electrodes
are shown in Figure 4.   The different currents measured at a PO_2
of 120 mmHg are due to the different diameters of the platinum
wires and, perhaps, to different thicknesses of the bitumen layers
at the platinum tips.   All of the extrapolated nitrogen values are
in the picoampere range which indicates the satisfactory insulation
of the platinum wires by bitumen.   So far, a period of observation
of three weeks has been possible and during that time the bitumen

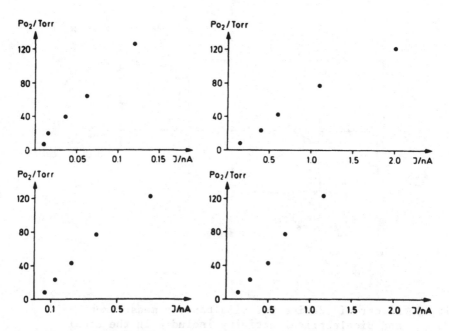

Fig. 4.   Four different calibration curves of four different
           bitumen-PO_2 electrodes.   X-axis: current in nanoampere.
           Y-axis: oxygen pressure in Torr.

Figure 5 shows a simultaneous measurement of DC and tissue PO_2 performed in the muscle in the back of the cat's neck. The muscle is covered with Ringer's solution. When the microelectrode goes through Ringer's solution, a PO_2 decrease caused by the oxygen consumption of the muscle is found without DC change. When the electrode penetrates the muscle, the DC level changes, but PO_2 remains constant. When the electrode is withdrawn from the tissue, the fall of the DC level to zero indicates that the electrode is no longer in the tissue but has reached Ringer's solution. The PO_2 electrode records the initial values.

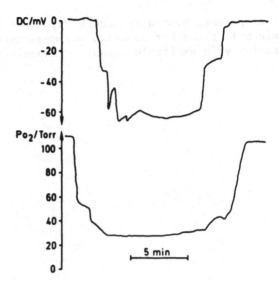

material prevented the entrance of water into the tip of the microelectrode and, thus, the incidence of electrical short-circuits of the platinum wires.

In summary it can be said that it is possible to use one channel of a two-channel glass electrode as a PO_2 electrode by equipping it with a bitumen-insulated platinum wire.

REFERENCES

Baumgärtl, A. and Lübbers, D.W. (1973) In 'Oxygen Supply. Theoretical and practical aspects of oxygen supply and micro-circulation of tissue', p. 130 (eds. Kessler, M. et al). Urban & Schwarzenberg, Munich.

Lehmenkühler, A., Caspers, H. and Speckmann, E.-J. (1975) In 'Oxygen transport to tissue II' (eds. Reneau, D. and Thews, G.) Adv. Exper. Med. & Biol. 75, p.3. Plenum Press, New York & London.

Silver, I.A. (1976) In 'Ion and Enzyme Electrodes in Biology and Medicine' p. 119 (eds. Clark, L.C. et al). Urban and Schwarzenberg, Munich.

Tsacopoules, M. and Lehmenkühler, A.   A double barrelled Pt-microelectrode for simultaneous measurement of PO_2 and bioelectrical activity in excitable tissue.   Experientia (in press).

A WORKING EQUATION FOR OXYGEN SENSING DISK ELECTRODES

T.E. Tang, R.E. Barr, V.G. Murphy and A.W. Hahn

John M. Dalton Research Center, University of
Missouri-Columbia, Mo. 65201 USA

For more than 35 years, noble metal electrodes have been
employed to measure oxygen partial pressure in biological fluids
and other media. Anyone who has attempted to use these types
of electrodes is well aware of the instability and drift attendant
to them. While a great deal of material can be found in the
electrochemical and analytical chemical literature regarding the
catalytic interaction of noble metal surfaces with oxygen, this
literature usually pertains to large surfaces, non isotonic media
and/or rotating ring-disc systems. Comparatively little has been
published concerning the interaction between oxygen and noble
metal surfaces for electrode sizes employed in biological applications.

Work in our laboratories has been aimed at developing oxygen
microelectrodes with long term stability. There are two characteristics that must be addressed in such an effort: poisoning and
aging (1). For the purposes of this paper, poisoning will refer
to those interactions with the electrode surface that cause rapid
changes in response characteristics. Aging will refer to the
comparatively slow change in response characteristics, which seem
to occur even in the "cleanest" media. In any systematic study,
an attempt must be made to separately address these two phenomena.
It is clear that if one does not understand the aging phenomenon,
little can be done to achieve long term stability. The progress
we have made in this regard is the subject of this paper.

According to Forbes and Lynn (2), there are two principal
pathways involved in the catalytic reduction of oxygen at a
noble metal surface. These are shown in Fig. 1. In this and following figures and text, superscripts b, s and a will refer to

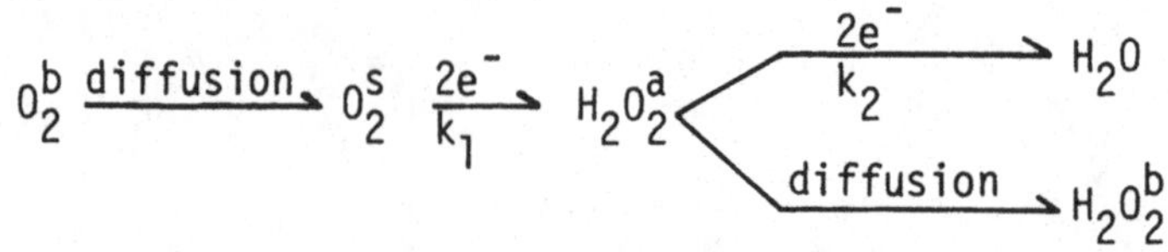

$$O_2^b \xrightarrow{\text{diffusion}} O_2^s \xrightarrow[k_1]{2e^-} H_2O_2^a \begin{cases} \xrightarrow[k_2]{2e^-} H_2O \\ \\ \xrightarrow{\text{diffusion}} H_2O_2^b \end{cases}$$

Fig. 1. The oxygen reduction process at a cathodically
         polarized electrode.

bulk, surface and adsorbed respectively. k_1 and k_2 are the reaction rate coefficients for the respective reduction processes. The current generated by this process is the sum of the number of electrons used in the reduction of O_2 to H_2O_2 and the reduction of H_2O_2 to H_2O, as given by the equation,

$$i = 2 F A k_1 C_{O_2}^S + 2 F A k_2 C_{H_2O_2}^S \qquad (1)$$

where i = electrode current, F = Faraday's constant, A = electrode surface area, $C_{O_2}^S$ and $C_{H_2O_2}^S$ are the surface concentrations of O_2 and H_2O_2 respectively.

   To generate a working model from this equation one must consider the reaction balance in the steady state for these two molecular species. The O_2 balance is between the rate of diffusion from the bulk media to the electrode surface and the rate of reduction to H_2O_2:

O_2 Balance: $$4D_{O_2} R (C_{O_2}^b - C_{O_2}^s) = A k_1 C_{O_2}^s \qquad (2)$$

The H_2O_2 balance is between the rate of production of H_2O_2 and its rate of reduction to H_2O plus its rate of diffusion into the bulk media.

H_2O_2 Balance: $$A k_1 C_{O_2}^S = A k_2 C_{H_2O_2}^S + 4 D_{H_2O_2} R C_{H_2O_2}^S \qquad (3)$$

D_{O_2} and $D_{H_2O_2}$ are the diffusivities of O_2 and H_2O_2 respectively. Solving for the surface concentrations of O_2 and H_2O_2, $C_{O_2}^S$ and $C_{H_2O_2}^S$, and substituting into the current equation yields the current expressed by the following equation:

$$i = 8 F D_{O_2} R \left[\frac{C_{O_2}^b}{1 + \dfrac{4 R D_{O_2}}{A k_1}} + \frac{C_{O_2}^b - C_{O_2}^s}{1 + \dfrac{4 R D_{H_2O_2}}{A k_2}} \right] \qquad (4)$$

For O_2 diffusion limited conditions, $4 R D_{O_2}/A k_1 \ll 1$ by definition and $C_{O_2}^{S} = 0$, thus simplifying the current description to:

$$i = 8 F D_{O_2} R C_{O_2}^{b} \left[1 + \cfrac{1}{1 + \cfrac{4 R D_{H_2O_2}}{A k_2}} \right]$$ (5)

This is the working equation to which the remainder of this paper is directed. Note that i is proportional to the bulk concentration of oxygen which is the basis for this method, and that the factor $4 R D_{H_2O_2}/A k_2$ is a ratio corresponding to the H_2O_2 diffusion pathway divided by the H_2O_2 reduction pathway.

There are three aspects of equation (5) of particular interest. First, if the quantity $4RD_{H_2O_2}/Ak_2 \ll 1$, that is, if the dominant pathway for H_2O_2 is reduction to H_2O, the bracketed factor

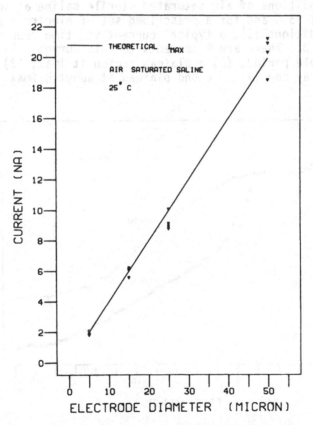

Fig. 2. Theoretical plot of Imax vs. electrode diameter
compared to experimental data.

becomes 2 and i becomes

$$i = Imax = 16 \ F \ D_{O_2} \ R \ C_{O_2}^b \qquad (6)$$

For bare disc platinum electrodes in air saturated saline at 25°C, values for Imax vs electrode diameter are shown in Fig. 2. Any current above the value shown for a given electrode diameter must be due to some reaction other than O_2 reduction. Most of the data to follow will relate to 15μm diameter electrodes which have an Imax = 6 na.

The second point of interest in equation (5) is that when $4RD_{H_2O_2}/Ak_2 \gg 1$, that is, the dominant pathway for H_2O_2 is diffusion into the bulk media, the bracketed factor reduces to 1, and i becomes ½ Imax. The third aspect of interest is that in a constant environment, the only possible variable with time in equation (5) is k_2.

Under conditions of air saturated sterile saline at constant temperature of 25°C and for a prescribed set of electrode pre-treatment conditions (3), a typical current vs. time response is shown in Fig. 3. There are 4 segments to this curve: (1) An initial unstable period, (2) a plateau region at Imax, (3) a region of current decay and (4) a second plateau at about ½ Imax. Since

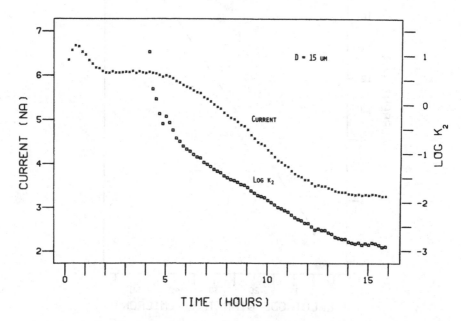

Fig. 3.   Typical CURRENT response for a pretreated 15μm diameter electrode and a plot of LOG k_2 associated with the decay region of the CURRENT curve.

the two plateaus were at these levels, it was considered a good possibility that there was a degradation in the H_2O_2 reduction step. If this is true, one can obtain knowledge of k_2 from the decay region.

An exponential decay with time was assumed for k_2, as shown in equation 7:

$$k_2 = C_1 \, EXP \, (- C_2 t) \qquad (7)$$

C_1 and C_2 are constants of the system and t is time. When k_2 was evaluated in the decay region and plotted on a semi-Log Scale (see Fig. 3), a linear relationship was obtained, verifying the hypothesis. The constants C_1 and C_2 can be evaluated from the Log k_2 vs t plot. C_1 is the intercept with the ordinate and C_2 is the slope of the line. From a number of plots of Log k_2 vs t, using the responses of 15 μm diameter electrodes, C_1 and C_2 values were obtained. These values were C_1 = 15 cm/sec and C_2 = 0.75 hr^{-1} (Fig. 4). Using these values of C_1 and C_2, theoretical curves were generated and compared to experimental data for 5 μm and 50 μm diameter electrodes. These comparisons are shown in Figs. 5A and B respectively. While the theoretical fit for the 50 μm diameter electrode data is reasonably good, the data of Fig. 5A are quite scattered, probably due to variations in electrode diameter, and

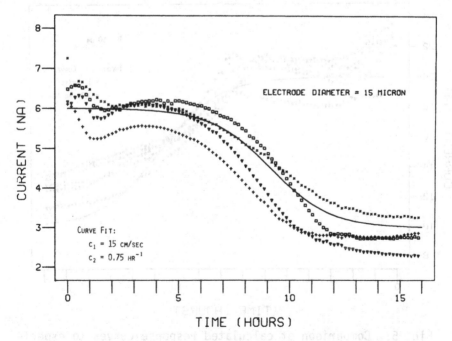

Fig. 4.   Comparison of experimental responses to theoretical
          curve fit obtained with averaged C_1 and C_2 values.

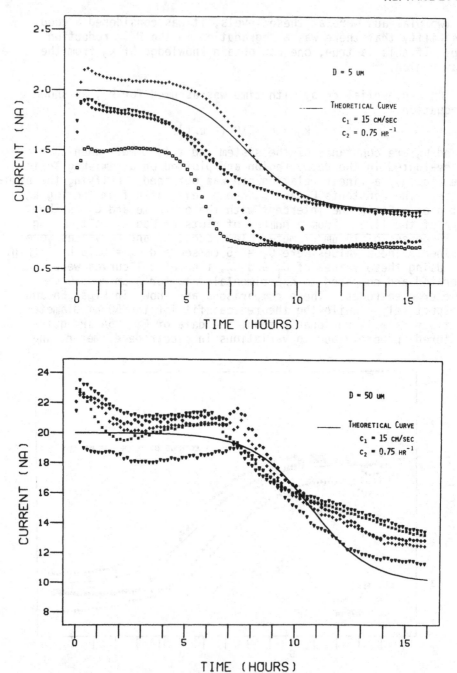

Fig. 5.   Comparison of calculated response curves to experi-
          mental curves for A. 5µm and B. 50µm diameter
          electrodes.

hence a good model fit was not obtainable.

It is concluded that the model presented is a good working model from which further understanding of the operating of oxygen reduction at noble metal microelectrode surfaces should be forthcoming. The most salient feature of the model is that it assesses the importance of the H_2O_2 reduction step and the importance of the competing H_2O_2 diffusion into the bulk media.

REFERENCES

1. Silver, I.A. (1967) Polarography and Its Biological Applications. Phys. Med. Biol. 12:285-299.

2. Forbes, M. and Lynn, S. (1975) Oxygen Reduction at an Anodically Activated Platinum Rotating Disk Electrode. AICHE Jour. 21:763-769.

3. Barr, R.E., Tang, R.E. and Hahn, A.W. (1977) Variations on the Response Characteristics of Oxygen Electrodes. In 'Oxygen Transport to Tissue III' ed. by I.A. Silver, Plenum Publ. Corp., New York.

VARIATIONS ON THE RESPONSE CHARACTERISTICS OF OXYGEN ELECTRODES

R. E. Barr, T. E. Tang and A. W. Hahn

John M. Dalton Research Center, University of Missouri
Research Park, Columbia, Missouri. 65201

A multiple pathway process for the reduction of oxygen at a platinum electrode was described by Forbes and Lynn (1). Using their descriptive process, Tang, et al. (2) developed a mathematical model, eq. 1, which appeared to satisfactorily explain the electrode current vs. time response obtained.

$$i = 8 F D_{O_2} R c_{O_2}^b \left[1 + \frac{1}{1 + \frac{4 R D_{H_2O_2}}{A k_2}} \right] \qquad (1)$$

However, only after a prescribed electrode pretreatment protocol had been followed, could the equation be applied to the electrode response for an extended period of many hours. It is the purpose of this paper to describe this protocol and responses one obtains when varying pretreatment protocol and experimental conditions.

Electrode Pretreatment Protocol. The principle conditions of pretreatment that yielded electrode current responses described in the previous paper (2) were as follows. Disc shaped electrodes were first polished and then were cathodically polarized at 700 mv with respect to a SCE in sterile saline at 25°C for periods exceeding 15 hours. They were then ultrasonically cleaned in distilled H_2O and anodized at two volts with respect to a SCE for five minutes in 1.0 N H_2SO_4. Following this they were ultrasonically cleaned in distilled H_2O, alcohol and again in distilled H_2O, five minutes each. The test cathodic runs were then conducted.

Table 1 is a list of factors that are known to influence electrode current characteristics. Some of these factors are obvious

17

TABLE 1. PARAMETERS CONTROLLING ELECTRODE RESPONSE CHARACTERISTICS.

Cathodization Voltage	Anodization Solution
Electrode Diameter	Saline
Preconditioning	H_2SO_4
Anodization	Other
Cathodization	Membrane Coating
Electrode History	Operating Time(s)
Fresh Surface	Electrode Shape
Used Surface	Periodic Anodization

and well known; a few are not well recognized. Some of these factors will be addressed in this paper.

<u>Cathodization Voltage</u>. The quantity k_2 is a positive exponen-
tial function of the applied cathodic voltage (3). For a larger
cathodic potential difference between the reference electrode
(Standard Calomel Half Cell (SCE)) and the recording electrode, the
effect of the k_2 dependency on voltage is seen as a delay in current decay from Imax (2) and a slower current decay to the ½ Imax
plateau. An example is shown in Figure 1. A response curve for
an applied potential of 700 mv is compared to the current responses
for three 15µm diameter electrodes polarized at 850 mv.

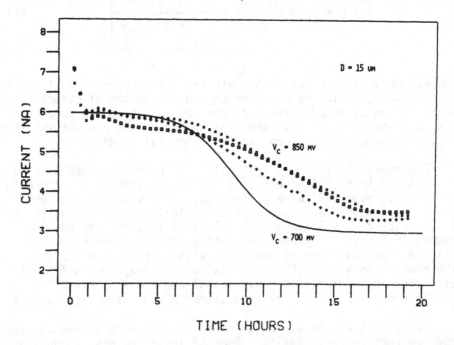

Fig. 1. Comparison between electrode responses for V_c = 700 mv
and V_c = 850 mv. The 700 mv curve is an averaged
composite of 4 electrode responses.

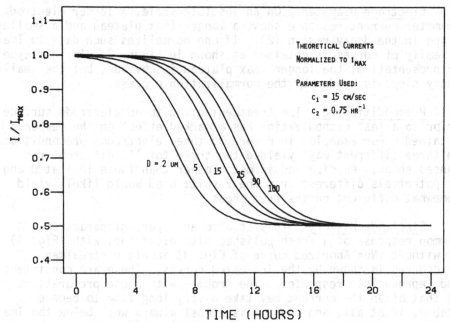

Fig. 2. Plots of current responses normalized to Imax for
         electrodes with diameters of 2,5,15,25,50 and 100μm.

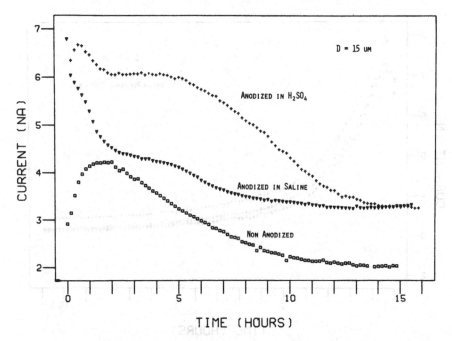

Fig. 3. Current responses for three electrodes pretreated in
         three different ways as described in the text.

Electrode Diameter. On an absolute scale, a larger electrode
diameter current response shows a longer Imax plateau and a smaller
slope in the decay region (2). If one normalizes such data to Imax,
a family of curves is obtained as shown in Figure 2. In this type
of presentation, the longer Imax plateau is obvious, but the smaller
decay slope is hidden by the normalization process.

Preconditioning. The treatment given to an electrode surface
prior to a test cathodization has a marked effect on the response
obtained. For example, in Figure 3, three electrodes preconditioned
in three different ways yielded the three totally different responses shown. Anodization in media other than those indicated and
at potentials different from the 2 volts used would likely yield
somewhat different curves from these.

Electrode History. This is also an important parameter. A
common response of a fresh polished disc electrode, with (Fig. 4)
or without (Non Anodized curve of Fig. 3) anodic pretreatment
procedures is shown by the indicated curves. These are consistent
and reproducible responses. The problem with these preparations
is that often the current may take a very long time to become
stable, if at all, and then it is almost always well below the Imax
level. A used surface may give an entirely different response, as
shown in Figure 5. These data were obtained using the same elec-

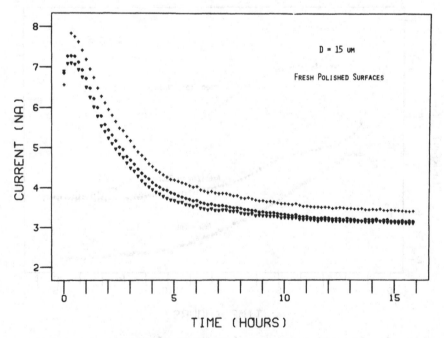

Fig. 4. Current responses of three freshly polished, anodized
electrodes.

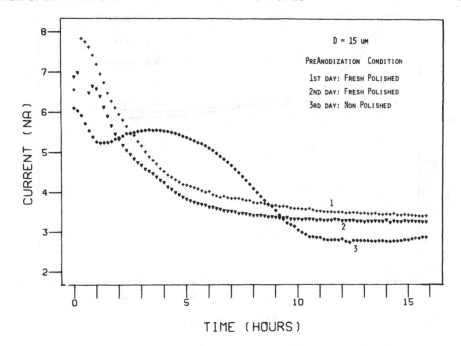

Fig. 5. Current responses for one electrode for three consecutive runs before which the electrode was 1) fresh
polished, 2) fresh polished and 3) not fresh polished,
respectively, and then anodized in H_2SO_4.

trode which was freshly polished before the first two runs and was
not polished for the third run. Before each cathodic current response shown, the anodization and cleaning process described above
was followed. It is clear that freshly polished surfaces and
used surfaces yield totally different responses.

Anodization Solution. It is apparent from Fig. 3 that a
significant difference in current response is obtained when
different types of solutions are used for electrode anodization.
Although we have only used 0.15 M NaCl (Saline) and 1.0 N H_2SO_4, it
is our suspicion that the presence of chloride ions may be the
most significant factor associated with the differences observed.

Membrane Coating. A membrane coating that has a smaller O_2
and H_2O_2 diffusivity will increase the length of time an electrode
operates at its Imax plateau. The reduced O_2 diffusivity will
decrease the Imax value, while the reduced H_2O_2 diffusivity reduces the competing H_2O_2 diffusion into the bulk media. Also the
surface is protected against molecules that may slowly change surface conditions. An example is shown in Figure 6. All three of
these electrodes operated at Imax for almost two days. That the

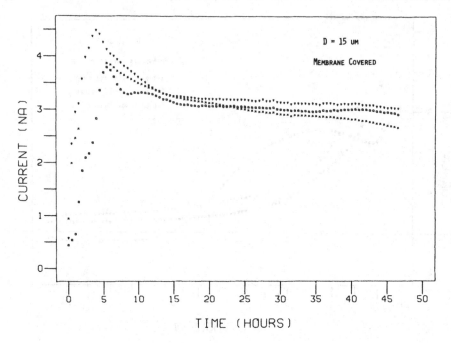

Fig. 6. Current responses for three pretreated electrodes
covered by a dialysis membrane.

current levels shown were indeed Imax values for the membrane
covered electrodes was demonstrated by the fact that, after re-
moving the membranes while the electrodes were polarized, the resulting bare tipped electrode currents were at theoretical Imax
levels.

To summarize: The works presented in this and the previous
paper (2) have produced an operational model for describing the
oxygen reduction process in common medical grade sterile saline
media at a platinum disc shaped electrode with a fairly specific
surface conditioning. This paper has illustrated some of the
variations possible in electrode current responses. An important
feature of these data is that they are highly consistent and
repeatable and can be discussed in terms of the model.

However, the question still remains: What is the aging process?
Is it due to a decrease of active sites for the electrochemical reduction process, brought about by the reduction process itself, or
is it a process caused by other species in the media? To answer
these questions, it may be necessary to employ some of the sophisticated techniques such as angle-resolved photoelectron spectroscopy
(4) and extended x-ray absorption fine structure (5), available today
for the study of atomic and molecular arrangements on solid surfaces.

REFERENCES

1. Forbes, M. and Lynn, S. (1975) Oxygen Reduction at an Anod-
    ically Activated Platinum Rotating Disk Electrode.   AICHE
    Jour. 21:763-769.

2. Tang, T.E., Barr, R.E., Murphy, V.G. and Hahn, A.W. (1977)
    A Working Equation for Oxygen Sensing Disk Electrodes.   In
    "Oxygen Transport to Tissue III. Ed. by I.A. Silver, Plenum
    Publ. Corp., New York.

3. Delahay, P. (1954) New Instrumental Methods in Electro-
    chemistry.   Interscience Publ., New York, p. 34.

4. Robinson, A.L. (1977) Surface Science (I): A Way to Tell
    Where the Atoms Are.   Science 196:1306-1308.

5. Robinson, A.L. (1977) Surface Science (II): An X-Ray
    Probe for Adsorbed Molecules.   Science 197:34-36.

DIRECTLY HEATED TRANSCUTANEOUS OXYGEN SENSOR

H. P. Kimmich, J. G. Spaan and F. Kreuzer

Department of Physiology, Medical School

University of Nijmegen, The Netherlands

Transcutaneous measurement of blood gases is gaining increasing interest in patient monitoring, mainly due to its non-invasiveness. In spite of many practical successes (Huch and Huch, 1975, Eberhard et al., 1975), especially in monitoring of newborns, this technique is not without disadvantages. Some of these problems are of little importance in patient monitoring such as the deviation at high PO_2 obtained during oxygen therapy due to venous admixture. Other problems such as the necessity of heating the sensor to 43 or 44 °C, as well as the variability of the ratio $tcPO_2/P_aO_2$ from patient to patient and in a single subject from hypoxia to hyperoxia (Goeckenjan and Strasser, 1977) and with changing blood flow, restrict the applicability of the method.

The heating problem is generally circumvented by applying two or more electrodes and by operating them intermittently or by changing the position of a single electrode from time to time. By directly heating the cathode, the heated area can be well limited and the construction can be simplified such that incorporation of several electrode systems (cathode and anode) in a single electrode is possible. In addition such an arrangement allows utilization of the fact that hyperemization remains for a certain time after discontinuation of heating the skin, allowing continuous measurement of $tcPO_2$ at body temperature.

In the literature the variability of the ratio $tcPO_2/P_aO_2$ is generally attributed to different degrees of hyperemization, or referred to as not yet fully understood. Based on a theoretical model it can, however, be shown that such changes are to be expected due to the oxygen transport from the hyperemized tissue to the electrode, even under conditions of ideal hyperemization.

MODEL OF OXYGEN TRANSPORT FROM THE CAPILLARIES TO THE SKIN SURFACE AND SENSOR

In the practical situation of tcPO$_2$ measurement (figure 1, left side), oxygen is transferred from the dermis (layer 5) through four layers to the cathode area of the polarographic cell. In layer 5 hyperemization is assumed to be ideal and thus the mean capillary PO$_2$ to be equal to the arterial PO$_2$. Since, however, the temperature is higher than 37 °C, P$_c$,O$_2$ is higher than normal P$_a$O$_2$ at 37 °C, due to the right shift of the dissociation curve. In layers 1 to 4 the PO$_2$ gradually drops from P$_c$, to zero. The drop is governed by pure diffusion in the electrolyte and membrane of the electrode (layers 1 and 2) and the cuticle (stratum corneum) of the epidermis (layer 3), but significantly for the measurement by both diffusion and oxygen consumption of the cells in layer 4.

If the resistance to diffusion in layers 1 and 2 is large as compared to that of layers 3 and 4, i.e. if the electrode is consuming little oxygen, then it may be written:

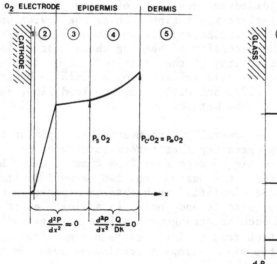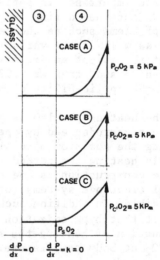

Fig. 1: (left) Model of oxygen transport from the arterialized capillaries of the dermis (5) to the cathode of the polarographic cell. For explanation see text. 1 = electrolyte of the electrode, 2 = membrane of the electrode, 3 = epidermis, dead tissue (cuticle), 4 = epidermis, living tissue.

(right) Model of the situation without heating. Oxygen consumption of the cells in layer 4 can thus be assessed.

$$tcPO_2 \approx P_sO_2 = P_aO_2 + \Delta P_aO_2(Tl) - P_QO_2$$

where: P_sO_2 = skin PO_2 = PO_2 at the border of layers 3 and 4

P_aO_2 = arterial PO_2 at body temperature of 37 °C!

$\Delta P_aO_2(Tl)$ = temperature correction term for $Tl \neq 37$ °C

P_QO_2 = PO_2 drop across layer 4 due to cell metabolism

Tl = temperature of the mean capillary blood

The ratio $TR = \dfrac{tcPO_2}{P_aO_2} = 1 + \dfrac{\Delta P_aO_2 - P_QO_2}{P_aO_2}$

will be 1 if $\Delta P_aO_2(Tl) = P_QO_2$. It should, however, be noted that both terms are temperature dependent and additionally that ΔP_aO_2 (Tl) is a function of P_aO_2 itself. Thus a change in temperature in layers 4 and 5 (due to changing blood flow in the dermis) as well as changing P_aO_2 alter the ratio TR. In addition a change in the temperature Tl in layer 5 alters the heat flux from cathode to layer 5. Thus the temperature in layers 1 and 2 changes, altering the calibration of the polarographic cell. Therefore transcutaneous assessment of absolute P_aO_2 requires measurement at constant temperature, which is easy only for Tl = 37 °C. Then ΔP_aO_2 (37 °C) is zero and thus TR < 1. With a constant temperature Tl P_QO_2 can be expected to remain constant too.

P_QO_2 may be estimated from the model of the skin (figure 1, right side) and some practical measurements. We assume the epidermis to be covered by an ideal electrode which behaves like a glass plate. $P_c'O_2$ is equal to venous PO_2 without heating namely 5 kPa. At the border of the glass plate and layer 3 the flux dP/dx is zero, thus the PO_2 curve is horizontal. At the border of layers 3 and 4 the flux must be the same on both sides and zero since there is no flux in layer 3. We may now distinguish three cases as shown in figure 1. If the PO_2 at the border of layer 3 is larger than zero, which practically is always the case, we have situation C. Physiologically, situations A and B are unlikely. The values at the skin surface are in the order of 0.5 to 1 kPa, leaving 4 to 4.5 kPa for P_QO_2.

We may now calculate TR for different situations. If at normoxia (P_aO_2 = 13 kPa) a TR of 0.7 is found, then a TR of approximately 0.5 and 0.85 may be expected for hypoxia (7.7 kPa) and hyperoxia (26 kPa) respectively, ignoring the venous admixture at hyperoxia.

THE POLAROGRAPHIC CELL

<u>Single electrode configuration.</u> The design of the cell is based on
the principle of a circular cathode arrangement. The advantages of
such an electrode were described earlier (Kimmich and Kreuzer, 1969).

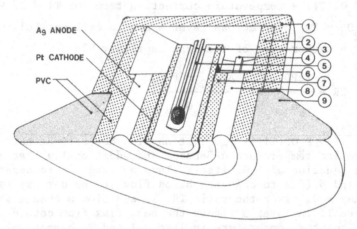

Fig. 2: Oxygen electrode for transcutaneous PO_2 measurements. 1, 2,
   7, 9 PVC insolation, 3 heat conduction cone (Ag), 4 anode
   connection, 5 thermistor, 6 Pt cathode and heating source,
   8 Ag anode, 9 ring, holding membrane.

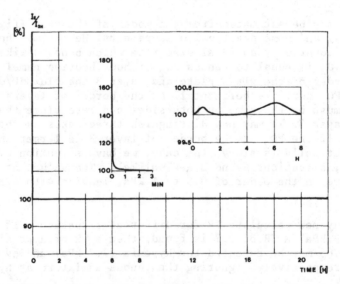

Fig. 3: Stability of the transcutaneous PO_2 electrode over 22 hours.
   Insets show the first few minutes after polarization and
   variations between 99.5 and 100.5 % during the first 8 hours.

The heat necessary for hyperemization is produced by passing a
current from one edge of the cathode (a 3 μm thick Pt foil) to the
other (pos. 6, fig. 2) and led to the skin surface by the heat conduction cone (pos. 3, fig. 2). Such an arrangement has a well-defined heating zone and a small temperature difference between thermistor (pos. 5, fig. 2) and skin surface. The characteristics of the
electrode are comparable to those described (Kimmich and Kreuzer,
1969). The stability is shown in figure 3. When compared with electrodes described by Huch and Huch, 1975, and by Eberhard et al.,
1975 our electrode shows identical reaction to breathing different
O_2 concentrations in normal subjects.

   Triple electrode arrangement. Three cathode/anode arrangements
have been combined in a single electrode (figure 4) for continuous
measurement at 37 ^{o}C. The switching cycle is shown in figure 5. If
an initial heating period of 15 minutes precedes the measurements,
then repeatable hyperemization of 10 minutes is obtained with subsequent heating periods of 1 minute. The heating (at approximately
43.5 ^{o}C), measurement (at 37 ^{o}C) and recovery (at 31 ^{o}C) of the
three electrodes are shifted in phase by 120° so that the PO_2 may
be measured continuously at 37 ^{o}C.

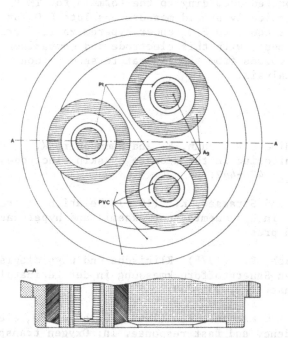

Fig. 4: Oxygen electrode for transcutaneous PO_2 measurement. Three
        cathode/anode systems similar to that of figure 2 are
        incorporated. For details see text.

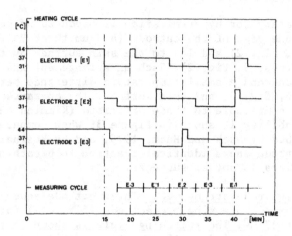

Fig. 5: Heating and measuring cycle of the triple electrode
        arrangement of figure 4.

CONCLUSIONS

When calibrated according to the formula for TR the oxygen
electrode theoretically should measure absolute P_aO_2 at 37 °C as
long as $P_{c'}O_2$ is equal to P_aO_2 under hyperemization. Preliminary
in-vivo measurements with this electrode and comparison of TR at
different P_aO_2 values from the literature seem to confirm the validity of this analysis.

References

Eberhard, P., Mindt, W., Jann, F. and Hammacher, K. (1975) Continuous pO_2 monitoring in the neonate by skin electrodes. Med. &
Biol. Engng., 13, 436-442.

Goeckenjan, G. and Strasser, K. (1977) Relation of transcutaneous
to arterial pO_2 in hypoxaemia, normoxaemia and hyperoxaemia. Bio-
telemetry 4 (in press).

Huch, A. and Huch, R. (1975) Klinische und physiologische Aspekte
der transcutanen Sauerstoffdruckmessung in der Perinatalmedizin. Z.
Geburtsh. Perinat. 179, 235-249.

Kimmich, H. P. and Kreuzer, F. (1969) Catheter PO_2 electrode with
low flow dependency and fast response. In: Oxygen transport to
Tissue. Ed.: F. Kreuzer. In: Progr. Resp. Res. Ed.: H. Herzog,
S. Karger, Basel, Switzerland, 3, 100-110.

A SELF-CALIBRATING, CONTINUOUS IN VIVO PO_2 AND PCO_2 MONITOR

J. S. Clark, W. D. Wallace, F. L. Farr,
and M. J. Criddle

Primary Children's Medical Center
320 12th Avenue
Salt Lake City, Utah 84103

Several in vivo blood gas monitoring systems have been developed which provide continuous monitoring of (1) PO_2 (systems which use miniature Clark-type electrodes), (2) PCO_2 (system of General Electric which uses a miniature and modified Severinghaus-type electrode), and (3) PO_2 and PCO_2 together using an in vivo gas collecting probe which feeds a mass spectrometer. While these systems are based on different principles, one feature common to all is the necessity for periodic calibration which requires collecting blood for analysis by a standard blood gas analyser. This paper describes a system for continuous monitoring of PO_2 and PCO_2 in body fluids which provides automatic calibration without removal of body fluids.

DESCRIPTION OF METHOD

The method utilized is shown in Figure 1. An in vivo probe contains a liquid which comes to equilibrium with body fluid gases. The probe consists of a gas permeable, liquid filled fiber and a smaller gas impermeable tube for transporting the liquid to gas sensors outside the body. Thus, the probe performs a function similar to that of the mass spectrometer probe in that gases from body fluids diffuse across a membrane for transport to gas sensors outside the body. However, unlike the mass spectrometer system, this probe acts as a tonometer in that the concentrations of gases within the probe liquid are a result of equilibration instead of the diffusion characteristics of the diffusion membrane and the body fluids.

Calibration is achieved by reversing the liquid flow in the

31

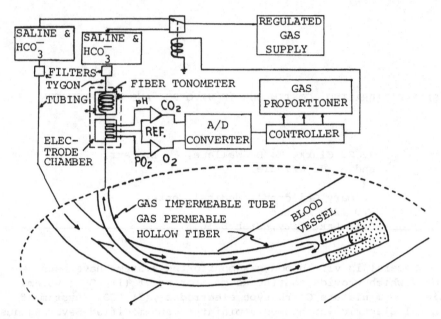

Figure 1: Self-Calibrating, in vivo system for monitoring PO_2
         and PCO_2

system so that the liquid which enters the sensor cuvette now
comes from the tonometer side.   Known gases for the tonometer are
provided by an electronically-controlled gas proportioning system.
High accuracy which is somewhat independent of electrode quality
is provided by adjusting the gas proportioner output until electrode output nulls are obtained with respect to probe values.   Of
course the equilibration in both the probe and the tonometer must
either be isothermal or mathematical corrections must be made
based on gas solubilities in the liquid and the temperature difference between probe and tonometer.

    The use of an 0.9% saline-bicarbonate solution as the liquid
in the system greatly simplifies the designs of the sensors and
the cuvette.   It allows the use of a bare pH sensor for detecting
CO_2 and permits a common reference for both sensors, the O_2 cathode
being of simple polarographic type.

                          GAS PROPORTIONER

    The accuracy of the system is determined by the accuracy of
the gas proportioner (refer to Figure 2).   The function of this

device is to produce a desired mixture of O_2, CO_2 and N_2 by controlling the 'open-times' on the three solenoid valves. The valves are operated under computer control and are programmed in sequence to give gas of desired composition. High accuracy is achieved through the following features.

1. An orifice common to all gases,
2. Temporal serial flow of each gas through the orifice,
3. Isobaric conditions for all gases at the input of the common orifice,
4. Choked flow conditions through all orifices shown in Figure 2.

To assure equal pressures all three gases are in common communication with a reservoir chamber. Initially flow of each gas is adjusted by its pressure regulator so that the flow through its orifice exceeds flow in the common orifice when its solenoid valve is open. This assures a sufficient flow of each gas toward the reservoir, preventing contamination of gases at the solenoid valve inputs. The push button valves and flow meter are provided for convenience in establishing these flows. The reference pressure in the reservoir chamber is determined by the net flow of the gases into the chamber and through the outlet orifice

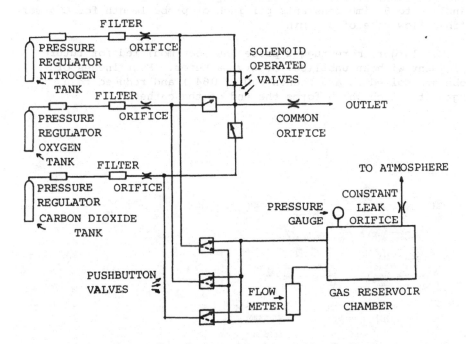

Figure 2: Gas proportioner block diagram

which provides a constant leak to atmosphere.

The accuracy of the gas proportioner is determined by the frequency response of the solenoid valves (LEE), which have an operation time variation of approximately 1 msec. The gas proportioner thus requires a duty period of 2 seconds to provide the 1 part in 1000 accuracy planned for this project.

PROBE DESIGN AND LIMITATIONS

The probe construction is shown in Figure 3. The probe under present study uses a .025"O.D., .012"I.D. Silastic gas permeable membrane and an inner 33 gauge stainless steel (.008" O.D., .004"I.D.) gas impermeable tube. The equilibrium time constants for the liquid-filled probe are 5 seconds for CO_2 and 1.5 seconds for O_2, which translates to one time constant per inch of probe length for CO_2 at a fiber fluid flow of 10 λ/min. This probe, while very rugged, is too large for radial artery placement in infants. The smallest probe we have made consists of a .010" O.D., .008"I.D. gas permeable fiber (G.E.'s MEM 213) with a 36 gauge stainless steel inner tube (.004"O.D., .002"I.D.), which is too delicate for practical clinical application. This probe has a time constant of 1.5 seconds for CO_2, 0.75 seconds for O_2 which translate to 6 time constants per inch of probe length for CO_2 for a fiber flow rate of 3 λ/min.

The larger, more rugged probe has been modified for future employment with an unbilical artery catheter. Four inches of probe are coiled to a 5 French O.D. (.064") and reduced to a length of 1 inch which forms the end of the catheter.

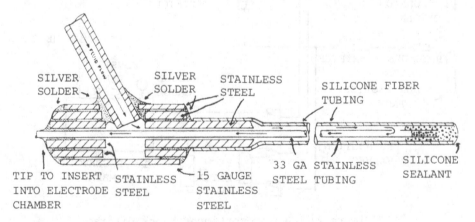

Figure 3: Diagram showing actual construction of gas probe

CALIBRATION PROTOCOL

The calibration cycle consists of an initial two point calibration for both O_2 and CO_2 sensors followed by   frequent single point calibrations as close as possible to the patient's actual values.   During monitor mode (electrodes measuring fiber fluid from the probe) the patient's blood gas values are continuously being measured and calculated based on the most recent calibration data.   Also during this time, the tonometer gas is continuously following the calculated patient values, which minimizes the subsequent calibration time.   Calibrations occur at regular intervals when the electrode outputs indicate that the patient is in a stable condition.   During such periods the system provides its theoretical (steady state) accuracy.   During rapid changes in patient status, however, calibrations are withheld to allow the system to follow the transient changes and the accuracy then depends on the size of the transient, electrode linearity, and the stability of the sensors since the last two point calibration.

EXPERIMENTAL STUDIES

A mechanical model representative of a lung and aortic circulation was used to test the system.   Water was substituted for blood in these experiments which represents a 'worst case' representation for both frequency response and accuracy because of the much reduced solubility of O_2 and CO_2 in water as compared to blood.   The entire system was maintained at room temperature.

Fig. 4 compares the response of the self-calibrating system (points) with that obtained from an electrode placed directly in the mechanical aorta induced by stepwise changes in the inspired gas applied to the 'lung'.   (The results are expressed as percentages of O_2 and CO_2).   The gas mixture was changed from 40 percent O_2 and 3 percent CO_2 to 20 percent O_2 and 7 percent CO_2 and then to 4 percent O_2 and 12 percent CO_2.   The voltages obtained from an O_2 electrode placed in the aorta at 40 percent and 4 percent O_2 were used as the calibration points for this electrode.   Intermediate O_2 percentages were calculated assuming linearity.   The fact that this electrode was non-linear is readily seen in the calculated O_2 values during administration of the 20 percent O_2.   This points out the need for calibrating at the patient's gas values when using such electrodes.   The CO_2 monitoring system also used a non-linear electrode.   Non-linearity (presumably due to an invalid slope from outdated two point calibration) adversely affected the values reported during the transition periods.   Once the patient stabilized, however, one point calibrations were done (they do not recompute slope) and subsequently reported values were correct.

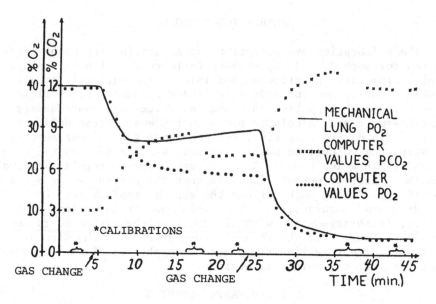

Fig. 4: Response of self-calibrating monitor to changes in the
PO_2 and PCO_2 of a simulated lung with water substituted for blood.
See text for details.

DISCUSSION

The results presented indicate that the system described above
can monitor blood gas values with precision and accuracy much
greater than standard blood gas analysers, assuming that gross
fibrin accumulation from blood does not occur.   Such an
occurrence seems unlikely in view of some preliminary in vivo
experiments with dogs and the generally good clinical experience
of others using Silastic in long term contact with blood.

The method could also have application in tissue gas monitoring
(using the smaller probe) where fluids are quite stagnant.   This
would require a control algorithm which in steady state takes no
appreciable gas from the system such as very frequent and equal
monitoring and calibration cycles.

THIN RING PO_2 ELECTRODE USING GOLD PASTE AND ITS APPLICATION TO THE STUDY OF THE EFFECTS OF VENOUS OCCLUSION ON SKIN PO_2

T. Koyama, S. Makinoda, T. Sasajima,
M. Ishikawa and Y. Kakiuchi
Research Institute of Applied Electronics
Hokkaido University
060 Sapporo, Japan

Elevation of venous pressure produces a rapid increase of capillary pressure to a level above the pressure in the veins (Landis and Pappenheimer, 1963). When capillary pressure is raised capillaries which were previously closed may open, resulting in an increase of oxygen transport to peripheral tissue. To examine this possibility we constructed a rapidly responding PO_2 electrode using gold paste.

A thin glass tube (OD 1.8 mm) is painted with diluted gold paste and heated for 60 minutes at a temperature of 400 °C. This tube is then inserted into another glass tube whose tip is closed. Air is removed from the tubes with a vacuum pump. The tube is

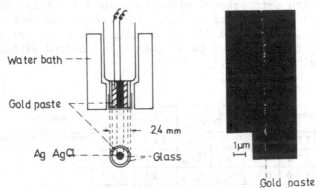

Fig. 1. Schematic illustration of the gold paste electrode covered with a teflon membrane and oil immersion microscopic photograph of a part of the gold paste electrode surface.

37

heated while the vacuum pump is running, which causes the outer tube
to melt and shrink ont·· the inner glass tube and insulate the gold
paste.   The tip of this tube, having an insulated circular gold
film in it, is cut and polished gently on an artificial leather with
cerium oxide powder, so that a smooth thin ring of gold film is
exposed on the surface.   Then a silver wire coated with silver
chloride is inserted into the glass tube and mounted in a suitable
position at the cut end by means of a resin.   This Ag-AgCl wire
serves as the reference electrode against the gold film, which is
charged at -0.7 v.

A photograph of a portion of the electrode surface pictured
through an oil immersion microscope is shown in Fig. 1.   Although
the whole electrode surface is circular, the photograph shows an
irregularly interrupted straight band.   This electrode has the
following properties: 1. a relatively high sensitivity (10^{-11}A/Torr),
2. slight dependence of oxygen current (5%) on fluid movements
tested by the current difference in bubbled and unbubbled saline
solution.   3. 90% response of 2 seconds to sudden change in PO_2
as roughly estimated by blowing a gas of different PO_2 on the
electrode when it is covered with 3μm teflon membrane.   4. A clear
plateau of oxygen reduction current over the range of applied
voltage -0.3 to -0.8 v.

The electrode covered with a 3μm teflon membrane was placed on
the left foot immersed in a water bath heated at 46°C.   Venous
occlusion was made by an inflation of a cuff placed around the leg
of subjects sitting on a bed while their legs were stretched
horizontally.   Venous occlusion tests were also made in the supine
position.   Two subjects whose skin PO_2 during sitting position was
nearly 0 mmHg during a control condition without any cuff inflation
were treated with α-tocopherol nicotinate (α-T.N., Eizai Pharmaceut-
ical Co. Tokyo) in a dose of 600 mg/day.   After two weeks treatment
their skin PO_2 increased to 22 and 25 mmHg.   Three other subjects
whose skin PO_2 ranged from 5 to 53 mmHg were studied without any
pharmacological treatments.

Subj	Mark	Age	Height; cm	B.W. ; kg	Blood Press. ♂ mmHg ↦o		PO_2 ; mmHg ♂	↦o	Remarks
T K	O	4 3	1 7 7	5 8	$^{154}/_{111}$	$^{137}/_{84}$	2 5.0	1 9.7	after taking α-T.N. 600mg/day for 14 days
Yo K	◑	4 3	1 7 0	7 0	$^{148}/_{115}$	$^{118}/_{88}$	1 6.7	1 0.0	do
T S	◐	3 0	1 6 0	6 0	$^{147}/_{106}$	$^{134}/_{80}$	9.3	8.2	
Yu K	◕	3 0	1 7 0	5 7	$^{176}/_{96}$	$^{144}/_{76}$	5 3.0	3 7.9	
S M	◖	2 6	1 7 6	6 5	$^{165}/_{120}$	$^{130}/_{102}$	5.3	4.8	

Table 1. Physical characteristics of the subjects studied.   Blood
pressure was measured on the underleg and skin PO_2 on the back of
the foot.

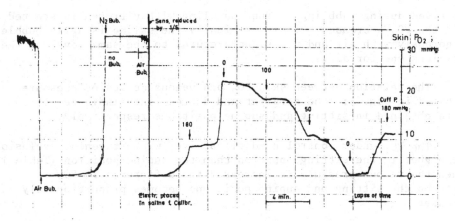

Fig. 2. An example of skin PO$_2$ recordings (read from right to left) and oxygen current obtained in the calibration vessel.

An example of actual measurements is shown in Fig. 2, where the subject is sitting. The skin PO$_2$ is first 10 mmHg. Then the cuff pressure is increased to 180 mmHg. The PO$_2$ starts to decrease with 10 seconds lag time and attains 0 mmHg in 2 minutes. On releasing the cuff pressure the PO$_2$ recovers to 10 mmHg. An increase in cuff pressure to 50 and 100 mmHg causes a step wise increase in PO$_2$. When the cuff pressure is decreased to 0 mmHg at the arrow with the marking 0, the PO$_2$ decreases quickly to 8 mmHg. Again the cuff pressure of 180 mmHg causes a decrease in PO$_2$ to 0 mmHg. Then the sensitivity of the pen recorder is decreased by 1/5 and the electrode is removed from the back of the foot and placed in the calibration vessel containing saline. The PO$_2$ signal fluctuates slightly for the first 1 minute, when the saline in in the vessel is bubbled with air. The bubbling is stopped for 2.5 minutes and the signal remains at the same level as

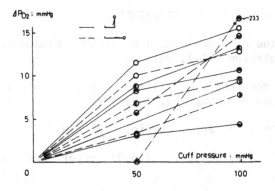

Fig. 3. Relation between skin PO$_2$ increase and cuff pressure.

observed during bubbling. Then bubbling with nitrogen is started and the PO_2 decreases quickly. Finally the saline is again bubbled vigorously with air and the signal returns to the same level as the previous one for air.

The relation between skin PO_2 and venous occlusion pressure is plotted in Fig. 3: the straight and dotted lines indicate the data obtained in sitting and supine positions respectively.

The PO_2 under control conditions, i.e. without venous occlusion, is higher in the sitting position than the supine position (Table 1). When the venous pressure is increased the difference in PO_2 between the sitting and supine positions becomes proportionately greater.

The increase in tissue PO_2 may be induced by two causes; the increase in the capillary diameter and opening of resting capillary. A model analysis using Krogh's tissue cylinder reveals that the increase in capillary diameter is insufficient to explain the PO_2 increase observed in this study. The opening of the resting capillary seems a more likely explanation.

The circular PO_2 electrodes have been described by several authors, using sputtered platinum (Saito and Mochizuki, 1965; Saito, 1967) and gold foil (Kimmich and Kreuzer, 1969). Gold paste also can be utilized as one of the materials for the circular electrode.

SUMMARY

A thin ring PO_2 electrode using gold paste is described and utilized for a study of the effects of venous occlusion on skin PO_2 of the foot. Venous occlusion causes an increase in skin PO_2 probably because it raises the capillary pressure and opens the resting capillaries.

REFERENCES

Landis, E.M. and Pappenhaimer, J.R. (1963) Handbook of Physiology. Sect. 2, Circulation Vol 2, 961.

Saito, Y. and Mochizuki, M. (1965) Digest of 6th Int. Conf. on Med. Electr. and Biol.Engning, Tokyo, 600.

Saito, Y. (1967) J. Appl. Physiol. 23, 979.

Kimmich, H.P. and Kreuzer, F. (1969) Progr. Resp. Res. 3, 100.

HOW TO QUANTIFY SKELETAL MUSCLE CAPILLARITY

James T. Loats, A.H. Sillau and Natalio Banchero

Dept.Physiology, School of Medicine, Univ. Colorado
Denver, Colorado 80262 U.S.A.

INTRODUCTION

The capillarity in skeletal muscle is not adequately defined
by either capillary density or by capillary to fiber ratio. Capillary density gives no clue as to the evenness of the distribution
of the capillaries in muscle cross sections but the reciprocal of
capillary density provides an estimate of the area of tissue cross
section served by the average capillary, a value used by Krogh and
other investigators (Tenney, 1974). The capillary to fiber ratio
renders no information on the area of tissue served by each capillary. Further, capillary density and C/F give no indication of the
maximal diffusion path length, important in assessing the capacity
of muscle for oxygenation. For these reasons, we have been interested in finding a better method of obtaining data that could be
used to estimate diffusion distances. This paper describes capillarity in skeletal muscle using several methods of quantification
that, we believe, provide a better understanding of the transport
of oxygen within the muscle.

METHODS

The solei muscles of guinea pigs, cats and rabbits were studied.
Because the fiber population in this muscle is quite homogenous
this selection minimized the influence of composition on capillarity.
The animals were sacrificed with an overdose of Na pentobarbital
and muscle samples were surgically removed. To minimize shrinkage
the samples were then quickly frozen in isopentane cooled (ca - 130°
C) with liquid nitrogen. After sectioning in a cryostat at 16 μm
the tissue slices were processed by the ATPase technique after pre-
incubation in an acid medium (pH 3.8 to 4.0). The reproducibility

and reliability of this technique, used to visualize capillaries, had been ascertained previously (Sillau and Banchero, 1977a). Photomicrographs were then made of the sections and projected on a screen at known magnification.

For some of the measurements the photomicrographs were projected on a system of circles. This "system" consisted of sets of four concentric circles (radii 1, 1.5, 2 and 2.5 cm) centered on each of the points in a square array (5.1 cm apart) as shown in figure 1. The usual point counting method for estimating areas (Elias, 1971) thus becomes a circle counting method. For each point in the array the largest circle around it, which contained no capillary, was recorded. In this way we were able to determine the percentage of muscle tissue in the cross section which was beyond or within a certain distance from the nearest capillary.

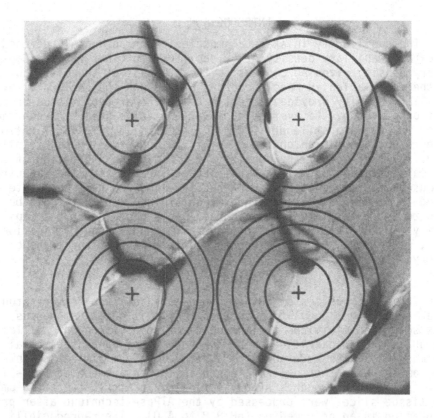

Figure 1. - Photomicrograph of soleus muscle with 4 sets of concentric circles.

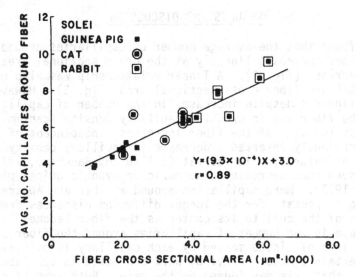

Figure 2.   Relationship between the number of capillaries around the fiber and fiber cross sectional area in the solei of 3 animal species.

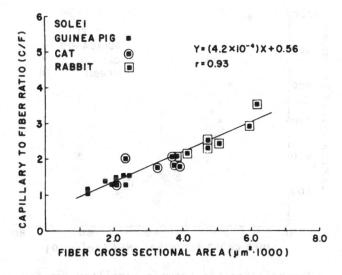

Figure 3.   Changes in capillary to fiber ratio with fiber cross sectional area.

RESULTS AND DISCUSSION

We found that the average number of capillaries around the muscle fiber increases linearly as the cross sectional area of the fibers increase (Fig. 2). A linear relationship was also observed between C/F and fiber cross sectional area (Fig. 3). However, as seen in figure 4 despite increases in the number of capillaries around the fiber and in C/F, the capillary density (cap/mm^2) decreases as the size of the fiber increases, independent of species. We had previously observed a decrease in capillary density as a function of maturation in the rat (Sillau and Banchero, 1977) but had not seen that decrease in normoxic or hypoxic guinea pigs (Sillau, 1977). More capillaries around a fiber are apparently needed to compensate for the longer diffusion distances from the periphery of the cell to its center as the fiber becomes larger. An increase in the number of capillaries around the fiber suggests that the area of tissue served by each capillary is maintained within certain limits. Previous work conducted in our laboratory indicates that this may indeed be the case. Both area of cross section and volume of skeletal muscle tissue perfused by a capillary tend to be kept below a certain value despite increases in the girth of the fibers (Sillau, 1977). The maximal area, or volume, of tissue served by a capillary varies in different muscles in relation to their particular fiber composition, being less in muscles with a high proportion of oxidative fibers than in muscles with a small population of these fibers.

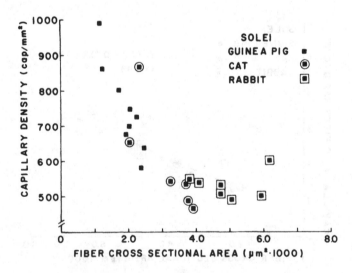

Figure 4. - The relationship between capillary density and fiber cross sectional area in the solei of 3 animal species.

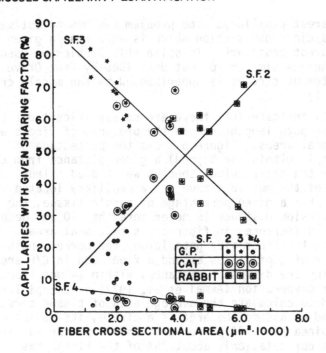

Figure 5. - Percent variation in capillary sharing factors in
relation to fiber cross sectional area.

The capillary sharing factor, i.e. the number of fibers the
capillary touches, was recorded for each capillary in the photomicrograph and then averaged. Plyley and Groom (1975) have made use
of these sharing factors in analyzing muscle fiber geometry. Figure
5 illustrates that in muscles in which fibers are of small cross
sectional area the majority of the capillaries are shared by 3 fibers
(s.f. = 3) whereas capillaries seldom occur between only two fibers
(s.f. = 2). Because more capillaries appear around fibers as they
increase their girth, the percentage of capillaries with a sharing
factor equal to 2 increases, while the percentage of capillaries
with a sharing factor of 3 decreases. No differences in the percentage of capillaries with a sharing factor of 4 or more were
observed.

It seems reasonable to expect that the diffusion distances in
muscles with large fibers would be greater than in those with fibers
of small cross sections. Not only is capillary density smaller in
muscles with large fiber cross sectional area (Fig. 4) but the large
fibers might have "pushed" the capillaries apart creating lacunae
in the capillary arrangement; i.e. portions of tissue unusually far

from the nearest capillary. The problem was how to estimate the amount of muscle cross section which is more than a given distance from the nearest capillary. To solve this problem we used a stereo-logical technique similar to that described by Cruz-Orive (1976) in which a system of circles is superimposed on the muscle cross sections (Fig. 1).

Our data indicate that there are no significant differences in the diffusion path lengths due to the presence of fibers with large cross sectional areas. Figure 6 shows the percentage of muscle tissue which is within (or beyond) a given distance from the nearest capillary in the three animal species we studied. Thus, for example, nearly 100% of the muscle tissue has a capillary located less than 50 µm away. For a given percentage of muscle tissue, the differences in diffusion distance is never more than 10 µm, despite very considerable differences in fiber cross sectional areas. This suggests that as the fiber size gets larger the corresponding increases in the number of capillaries around a fiber and in C/F are effective in maintaining the diffusion distances within values known to be adequate for oxygenation (Akmal et al, 1977). If capillary density is used to calculate the average area of tissue served by one capillary and we assume the area is a circle, its radius would be 21 µm for guinea pigs, 24 µm for cats and 25 µm for rabbits. Yet, according to our data, only about 75% of the tissue has a capillary within 25 µm. This indicates that estimating the radius of the

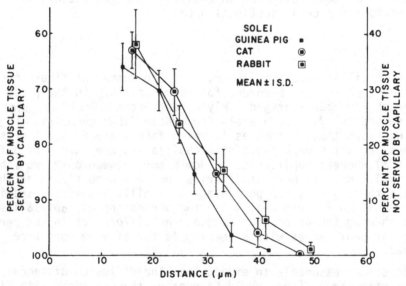

Figure 6. Actual distances through which O_2 molecules must diffuse from the capillary into the muscle. For example, in all three species approximately 75% of the muscle is within 25 µm from the nearest capillary and no muscle tissue is farther than 50 µm.

average tissue cylinder on the basis of capillary density does not
accurately represent the maximal diffusion distance. In fact,
figure 6 shows that the maximal diffusion distance may be twice
that long.

      In an effort to quantify the "pattern" of the capillary arrange-
ment, apart from variations in capillary density, the measurements
made for figure 6 were in fact originally done after each sample
was adjusted (via changes in magnification) so that the capillary
density was constant. The average area per capillary in each cross
section corresponded to the area of a circle with radius $r = 1.5$
(Fig. 7). These adjustments in magnification varied only by a
factor of 2, so that considerable variation in the fiber sizes was
present even after the adjustments were made.

      Figure 7 shows the percentage of the number of circles which
contain no capillaries plotted against the radii of these circles.
The capillary density for all these counts was kept constant. This
figure demonstrates that aside from possible variations caused by
the difference in capillary densities, one is no more likely to see
large gaps or lacunae in the capillary arrangment in the muscle of

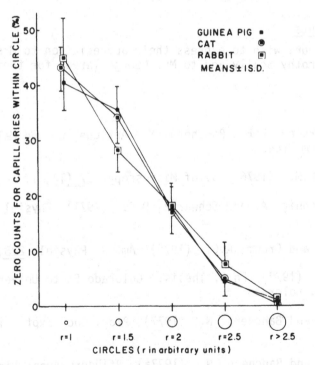

Figure 7. The number of circles containing no capillaries diminishes
progressively as the circles become larger. These measurements were
made after adjusting for constant capillary density.

rabbits than in that of cats or guinea pigs. This is in contrast to what could have been conjectured; namely, that the fibers with large cross sections might have "pushed" the capillaries apart creating lacunae.

CONCLUSIONS

Important changes in the capillarity of skeletal muscle occur as a function of fiber cross sectional area. These relationships appear not to be affected by species variability.

It is possible, with the aid of a system of concentric circles, to estimate the percentage of muscle tissue served or not served by a capillary located within a given distance. It has been shown that sixfold increases in the cross sectional area of the fibers in the solei of three different animal species appear to be compensated for by corresponding increases in the C/F and the average number of capillaries around the fiber. Moreover, in spite of decreases in the capillary density as fiber size increases, no muscle tissue is located farther than 50 μm from a capillary, a distance that is within limits that assure adequate oxygenation.

This work was supported by a grant from the USPHS, NHLI HL 18145.

Acknowledgments

The authors wish to express their appreciation to Mrs. Lynn Aquin and Dorothy Scally and to Mr. George Tarver for their assistance.

REFERENCES

Akmal, K., Bruley, D.F., Banchero, N., Artigue, R. and Maloney, W. (1977) Plenum Press.

Cruz-Orive, L.M.   (1976) J. of Microscopy 107 (1), 1.

Elias, H., Hennig, A. and Schwartz, D.E.   (1971) Physiol. Rev. 51, 1958.

Plyley, M.J. and Groom, A.C.   (1975) Am. J. Physiol. 228, 1376.

Sillau, A.H.   (1977) Ph.D. Thesis. Colorado State University, Fort Collins, Colorado.

Sillau, A.H. and Banchero, N.   (1977) Proc. Soc. Expt. Biol. Med. 154, 461.

Sillau, A.H. and Banchero, N.   (1977a) Pflügers Arch. (in press).

Tenney, S.M.   (1974) Respir. Physiol. 20, 283.

STAINING OF PO$_2$ MEASURING POINTS DEMONSTRATED FOR THE RAT BRAIN CORTEX

H. Metzger, S. Heuber, A. Steinacker, J. Strüber

Dept. of Physiology, Med. School Hannover,

Hannover, Fed. Rep. of Germany

INTRODUCTION

The local PO$_2$ distribution in the brain cortex is dependent upon the capillary arrangement and local blood flow,
as well as the cellular distribution and rate of oxygen
consumption within the tissue. As each part of the cortex is characterized by a specific cellular and capillary pattern, many authors have predicted that the local
PO$_2$ will vary accordingly (Thews, 1960; Metzger, 1976;
among others). Because of technical complications, however, differences in the PO$_2$ of the various cortical layers have not yet been investigated systematically. If
PO$_2$ microelectrodes are placed according to stereotaxic
coordinates large errors are to be expected. The
results already published use very different criteria,
such as race, sex and age as well as the histological
technique used for the preparation of the tissue. In order to overcome these difficulties it is necessary to
be able to localize the PO$_2$ microelelectrode tip by
combining polarographic and histological techniques. The
advantage of the experimental procedure described here
is the possibility of correlating local PO$_2$ values with
the specific brain layer where the PO$_2$ measurements had
been made as well as obtaining capillary data from the
same area of tissue.

METHODS AND RESULTS

Construction of a Combined Microelectrode

A double micropipette was used, one pipette for the PO_2 microelectrode constructed according to the procedure described earlier (Metzger, 1973), the other one filled with dye (Alcian Blue 8 GX) for injection into the tissue. Both pipettes were connected through a droplet of sealing-wax (tip-tip distance 2-5 μm). After the experiment the PO_2 microelectrode was retained while the closed dye pipette was discarded.

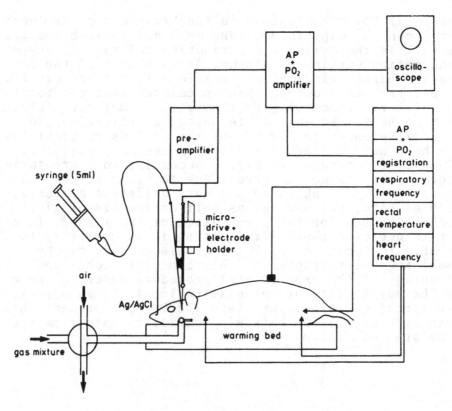

Fig. 1: Experimental set-up used for local PO_2 measurements and dye application.

Application of the Dye

In principal iontophoretic as well as hydrostatic application of the dye is possible.   As the FET input of the
PO_2 measuring device is sensitive to electrical charges
and leakage currents, the hydrostatic method is the better one.   The pH of Alcian Blue is 5.2 - 5.9 and vasodilatation is originated at the moment of injection giving
rise to an increase in local PO_2 which can be used as an
indication for the correct injection of the dye.

Experimental Procedure and Physiological Measurements

White rats (type Wistar, 180-250 g b. w., male) were anaesthetized with Urethane (750 mg/kg b. w.) injected intraperitoneally.   The animals were held in stereotaxic
equipment and were able to breath spontaneously through
a T-shaped cannula inserted into the tracheostoma.   The
combined microelectrode was inserted through a small
window of 4x7 mm drilled into the skull cap.   The microelectrodes were located in the visual cortex within a
distance of 1 - 1.5 mm from the brain surface.   Local
PO_2 values and extracellular action potentials were registered (experimental set-up see Fig. 1).   In order to
test the responsiveness of the animal and the measuring
system, short pulses of inspiratory hypercapnia (15% CO_2,
20.8% O_2, rest N_2) were applied.   An increase of the
local PO_2 was observed as described elsewhere (Metzger
et al, 1971).

PO_2 measurement lasted 30 minutes, at the end of which
Alcian Blue was injected causing a PO_2 increase.   After
the dye application Pancuroniumbromide was given to
relax the animal which was then artificially ventilated
so that the perfusion cannula could be inserted into the
left ventricle and the aorta.   The perfusion was performed with 50% Rheomacrodex with Liquimin (38°C) which
was followed by a 1% $AgNO_3$ solution in 50% Rheomacrodex
(4°C) as well as by a 10% p-formaldehyde solution (4°C)
for fixation.

Histological Technique

15µm sections were cut from the brain and examined under
the microscope.   If dye spots were seen, 5µm sections
were cut and stained with Cresylviolet for identification of the cortex layer.   The sites where measurements had been carried out were located within the neo-

and the archicortex and in two cases at the border between them. In Fig. 2 typical PO$_2$ values are seen with
higher mean PO$_2$ values within the neo- and lower within
the archicortex.

Television Image Analysis

Capillary data were obtained by means of a computer controlled image analysis. The results (see table) showed
that capillary volume and surface are larger in the neo-
than in the archicortex while the capillary distances
are smaller.

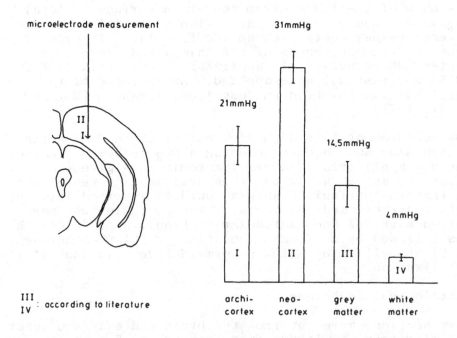

PO$_2$ distribution within different areas of the brain

Fig. 2: Graphical representation of the results. Left:
        location of the microelectrode; A 14 according
        to Craigie. Right: comparison of the local PO$_2$
        values.

TABLE: Results of the combined method of PO_2 measurements and staining by means of Alcian Blue. Capillary data are from the stained tissue area where local PO_2 has been measured.

V_r = relative capillary volume; L/V = capillary length per tissue volume; F/V = relative capillary surface per tissue volume; d = capillary distance.

No.	V_r (%)	L/V (mm/mm³)	F/V (mm²/mm³)	d (μm)	PO_2 (mmHg)	brain area
1	1.8	1162	15.3	50	29	neocortex
2	1.6	1083	14.2	55	27	neocortex
3	1.9	803	13.9	59	39	neocortex
4	1.0	871	10.9	56	32	neocortex
5	0.9	871	9.4	57	23	archicortex
6	0.6	735	8.5	65	12	archicortex
7	0.9	1112	11.1	51	28	archicortex
8	0.5	460	4.8	77	18	archicortex
9	1.5	922	13.4	55	22	archicortex
10	1.3	1073	12.7	55	27	border of white m.
11	1.6	991	13.6	55	23	border of white m.

DISCUSSION

The specific capillary and cellular arrangement of the different cortical layers described in the histological literature led to the following hypotheses:

a) The mean PO$_2$ level of the different brain layers is specific for each area.
b) A decreasing tendency of the mean PO$_2$ is to be expected when moving from the surface into the deep cortex, corresponding to the course and number of the cortical arteries supplying each region.

Many results published in the literature support these hypotheses: a mean surface PO$_2$ of 42 mmHg (Gleichmann et al, 1962) and decreasing PO$_2$ values from the pia to grey and white matter have been described (Metzger, 1971). Furthermore, a continuous PO$_2$ decrease from the pia into the deep cortical structures of the optical cortex have been reported for the cat (Nair et al, 1975) as well as for the rat (Metzger et al, 1977). Our results described above give further evidence for this hypothesis: the ontogenetically elder archicortex has a lower mean PO$_2$ than the younger neocortex. The same relationship is reflected in the capillary data which show greater capillary density in the neo- than in the archicortex.

Furthermore, it is assumed that the white matter has a very low PO$_2$ level. This has long been predicted on the basis of capillary data as well as theoretical considerations (Thews, 196o). Nevertheless, for final conclusions combined PO$_2$ measurements and histological investigations by means of the method described above are necessary.

SUMMARY

A combined physiological and histological technique was developed in order to determine the exact position of the tip of a microelectrode used for PO$_2$ measurements within the rat brain cortex.Using this method it was possible both to identify the tissue layer where PO$_2$ measurements had been performed as well as obtain information about the blood capillaries within the surrounding tissue. After the PO$_2$ had been measured small quantities of dye (Alcian Blue 8 GX) were injected through a micropipette attached to the PO$_2$ microelectrode (tip-tip distance 2-5 µm). Subsequently the tissue was fixed by perfusion, 5 µm sections were cut and stained with Cresylviolet. The points where measurements had been made could be seen under a light microscope as green coloured spots of about

100 μm in diameter. The capillary pattern could be demonstrated by silver nitrate perfusion. Information about the capillaries, such as length, distance and the gas exchange surface were obtained via computer analysis of a television image. This method was used to analyse the O_2 supply of the optical cortex of the rat. Correlation of the local PO_2 distribution with the capillary data revealed differences between the archi- and the neocortex of the rat brain.

REFERENCES

Gleichmann, U., Ingvar, D.H., Lübbers, D.W., Siesjö, B. and Thews, G. (1962) Acta Physiol. Scand. 55, 127.

Metzger, H. (1971) Habilitationsschrift, Mainz.

Metzger, H., Erdmann, W. and Thews, G. (1971) J. Appl. Physiol. 31, 751.

Metzger, H. (1973) In "Oxygen Supply" p. 164 (eds. Kessler, M., Clark, L.C., Lübbers, D.W., Silver, I.A. and Strauss, J.). Urban & Schwarzenberg, München.

Metzger, H. (1976) Mathem. Biosci. 30, 31.

Metzger, H., Heuber, S., Steinacker, A. and Strüber, J. (1977) XXVII Intern. Congress of Physiol. Sci. Paris.

Nair, P., Whalen, W.J. and Buerk, D. (1975) Microvasc. Res. 9, 158.

Thews, G. (1960) Pflügers Arch. ges. Physiol. 271, 227.

DISCUSSION OF PAPERS IN SESSION I

CHAIRMEN: DR. W. WHALEN and DR. M. KESSLER

PAPER BY : DR. ACKER et al

Dr. Metzger: a. Did you compare bitumen with epoxides?
               b. Is an insulation of 10^{12} Ω enough?

The principle of using a voltage clamp for the polarising voltage
was published by Kunke, Erdmann and Metzger. J. Appl. Physiol. in
1952.

Dr. Acker: a. Epoxides could be used but bitumen and glass
                  provide a very good contact.
            b. It is difficult to be sure if 10^{12} Ω is enough
                  but the impedance of bitumen may be better than
                  10^{12} Ω in any case.

PAPER BY: DR. KIMMICH et al

A number of points were raised on this paper among which were
those of Dr. Goeckenjan who commented that in patients under
intensive care they had seen an increase of $\dfrac{t_c PO_2}{PaO_2}$ ratio in the

first four to six hours of measurement. After that time the
$\dfrac{t_c PO_2}{PaO_2}$ dropped slowly. He wondered whether the method of

Dr. Kimmich gave the same results, whether any measurements had
been made in shock and whether there might possibly be burns at
the site of electrode application.

Dr. Lübbers was concerned that the transcutaneous PO_2 measurement might not give the values of arterial PO_2, if the authors did not ensure that their electrode was not dependent on blood flow. He quoted the theoretical analysis of t_cPCO_2 measurements by Huch, Lübbers and Huch in "Oxygen measurements in Biology and Medicine" (Eds. PAYNE and HILL, Butterworths, London and Boston 1975). These authors pointed out that in all measurements of transcutaneous PO_2 perfusion efficiency (defined as t_cPO_2 x 100 / P_aO = E) must be constantly determined. If the value decreased below 90 to 100% then the transcutaneous PO_2 measurement was no longer a reflection of the arterial PO_2. Dr. Puffer pointed out that temperature variation might have an effect on the response of the sensor.

PAPERS BY: DR. BARR et al

Dr. Metzger: Did you use any material other than platinum?
          We used gold which has a remakably small aging characteristic within the first twenty hours (less than 5 to 10%. See Metzger in Oxygen Supply, 1973, Urban and Schwarzenberg). I would not recommend the use of platinum myself.

Dr. Barr: We did not try any other materials.

Dr. Goldstick: You have presented an interesting new theory. However, we have never observed the kinds of plateaus you have shown in current with time. Other than the plateaus, do you have any other evidence that the diffusion of H_2O_2 plays an important role in oxygen electrodes as your theory proposes?

Dr. Barr: No, we have not obtained an alternate method to test for H_2O_2 diffusion into the bulk media. However, Forbes and Lynn (1975), using a ring-disc system, demonstrated a significant release of H_2O_2 from the electrode surface for their system. We also do not obtain the type of responses shown here when operating electrodes in the more common manner of only cathodic polarization without any specific pretreatment. Without anodic pretreatment, the electrode surface is not in an activated state. Hence, a current level corresponding to the four electron reduction process, i.e., Imax, is not obtained. Therefore, it is not possible to observe the Imax plateau.

Dr. Storey: When you put a teflon or some similar membrane over the tip, this would insure that the hydrogen peroxide would not diffuse away. The first thought that comes to mind is that it may be possible to put some catalase media between the electrode and the membrane to catalyze H_2O_2. Of course, the problem of electrode poisoning may interfere with such a test.

Dr. Barr: Thank you. It is certainly an idea to which one should give consideration. However, the catalytic action of catalase is to oxidize H_2O_2 to O_2. Thus, one could produce a complicated merry-go-round effect for which I am not sure what the electrode response would be. I will give further thought to this type of experiment.

Dr. Storey: We have found that one of the causes for drift is in the Ag/AgCl electrode. Thus, we routinely clean these reference electrodes in ammonia before using them. Do you know what process may be occurring at the Ag electrode?

Dr. Barr: Since this work was performed in an in vitro system in which size was of little concern, we used a standard calomel half cell as our reference. Therefore, our system was not influenced by potential changes in a Ag/AgCl reference electrode. I have had no other experience with the long term drift of Ag/AgCl electrodes, so I am sorry that I cannot give you a useful comment.

Dr. Kessler: I, too, would be interested to know if you have directly measured the liberated H_2O_2, or what evidence do you have that it is released?

Dr. Barr: We have not yet performed any experiments to directly measure H_2O_2. It would indeed be an important step in further validating our model.

Optical Methods

FIRST CRYOPHOTOMETRIC MEASUREMENTS OF THE HbO_2-SATURATION IN THE CAT CAROTID BODY

H. Acker, D.W. Lübbers, R. Heinrich and W.A. Grunewald*
Technical Assistance H. Grisar
Max-Planck-Institut für Systemphysiologie
46 Dortmund, West Germany
*Universität Regensburg

The cryophotometric method developed by Grunewald and Lübbers (1976) to define oxygen saturation of haemoglobin in blood vessels is suitable for determination of oxygen distribution within tissues. We therefore applied this method to the Glomus caroticum of the cat in order to verify the PO_2 distribution found by Acker et al (1971) in the carotid body tissue. Experiments were done on spontaneously breathing cats, anaesthetized with sodium pentobarbital (40 - 60 mg/kg). After preparation of the right carotid body and with controlled blood pressure, expiratory CO_2, tidal volume and arterial blood gases, the glomus caroticum was quickly frozen by Freon gas cooled in liquid nitrogen. The first figure shows such an experiment. Before the carotid body was removed the animal was ventilated with 5% O_2 in N_2. The tidal volume increased and consequently the expiratory CO_2 decreased. Blood pressure also decreased slightly. After examination of the blood gases the right carotid body region was quick-frozen as described above and excised. The whole procedure is quick and local and the animal does not show any reaction in blood pressure or respiration. This suggests that we are able to fix an actual physiologic state of the carotid body without disturbing the whole animal. The carotid body region, i.e. a small part of the common carotid artery, carotid sinus and external carotid artery, is now cut into slices of 11μm at a temperature of -80°C. Histological identification of single slices is used to delineate the carotid body from the surrounding tissues. This is the only method which can be used reliably to determine where typical carotid body tissue begins. For the cryophotometric measurement of the HbO_2 saturation a slice is brought into a measuring chamber (Grunewald and Lübbers 1976) and a photograph is taken to show the points of measurement.

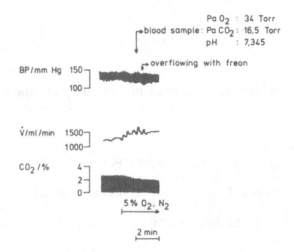

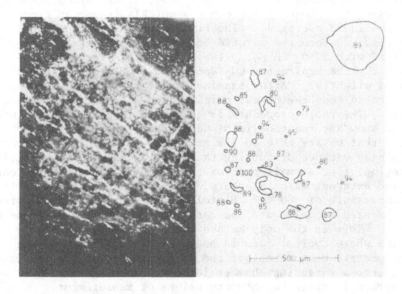

Fig. 1. Physiological condition under which the cat carotid body is quickly frozen in freon, cooled in liquid nitrogen, and excised from the animal.   From top to bottom: blood pressure (BP/mmHg), ventilation ($\dot{V}$/ml/min) and CO_2 content of the respiration air (CO_2/%). The time (2 min) is indicated as a bar.

Fig. 2. Left side: original photograph of a cryo-slice of the cat carotid body.   Right side: survey of vessels, in which red cells were found, and the measured HbO_2-saturation values.

Fig. 2 shows a Glomus caroticum taken out after being quickly
deep-frozen while the animal was breathing air.   Single vessels
filled with red cells can be seen but there are no details of the
specific carotid body tissue.   The HbO$_2$ values measured in
arteries, arterioles, venules and veins are marked in the photograph;   the high saturation values are striking.   Red cells were
rarely found in capillaries.   In one case we were able to obtain
8 cryo-cuts from one carotid body and to measure the HbO$_2$
saturation.   In Fig. 3, four of these 8 cryo-cuts are drawn
sequentially.   The vessels in which measurements were made and their
HbO$_2$ values are shown in this figure.   In the first and in the
eighth slice only high values were found whereas in the centre, i.e.
in the fourth slice, low HbO$_2$ values were also seen.   All HbO$_2$
values (n = 167) from this carotid body were recorded in a
frequency distribution curve.   More than half of all saturation
values were between 80 and 100%.   This frequency distribution can
be shifted by ventilation with 5% O$_2$ in N$_2$.   Fig. 4 demonstrates

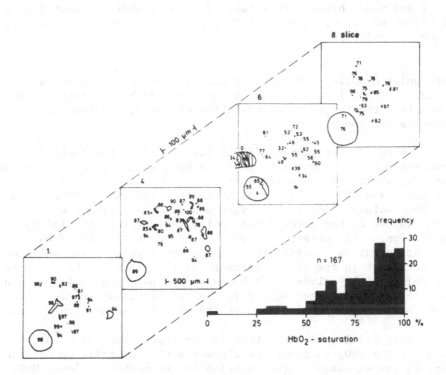

Fig. 3. Four out of eight cryo-slices of cat carotid body.   Vessels
in which red cells were found and the corresponding HbO$_2$ values are
drawn.   Insert: HbO$_2$-saturation values are shown by a distribution
curve.

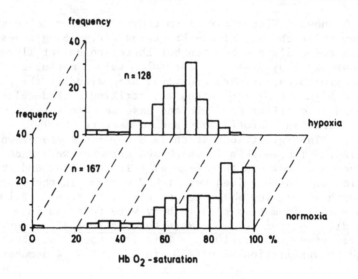

Fig. 4. HbO$_2$-saturation values under normoxia (n = 126, 1 carotid body) and under hypoxia (n = 128), 2 carotid bodies) plotted as a distribution curve. (x-axis = HbO$_2$ saturation, y-axis = absolute number of values).

that under hypoxia (n = 128, two carotid bodies) the peak value is at 45%. Also, low saturation values can now be observed. For comparison the frequency distribution of the HbO$_2$ values under normoxia are shown.

Grunewald and Lübbers (1976) found that in the rabbit myocardium under normoxia most of the HbO$_2$ values were between 20% and 40%, while under hypoxia most of the HbO$_2$ values were found between 0 and 10%. Thus it seems that in the rabbit myocardium the HbO$_2$ values reflect the oxygen supply of the tissue whereas the HbO$_2$ values of the carotid body mainly mirror the arterial O$_2$ saturation. The observation of a large number of high HbO$_2$ saturation values suggests that a high proportion of red cells do not take part in the oxygen exchange of the tissue. Furthermore the shift of the values under hypoxia does not necessarily mean a deterioration of oxygen supply (as in the rabbit myocardium) but that this change is a function of the arterial saturation values.

These results may mean that in our experiments we mainly measured the HbO$_2$ in shunt vessels where the red cells do not take part in gas exchange. The increase in the number of lower HbO$_2$ values under hypoxia may indicate that under this condition the red cells take part in the gas exchange within the specific tissue. This is in accordance with measurements of Acker and Lübbers (1976) who found an increase of plasma flow through the specific carotid body tissue under normoxia whereas under hypoxia more red cells flowed into the specific carotid body tissue. The discrepancy between the tissue PO$_2$ values found by Acker et al (1971) in the carotid body and the HbO$_2$ values observed in the present study under normoxia can be explained in the same way. With PO$_2$ micro-electrodes measurements are confined mainly to the specific carotid body tissue, i.e. to the capillary regions, whereas with the cryophotometric method we probably measure HbO$_2$ in shunt vessels. Low HbO$_2$ values found occasionally under normoxia may, however, justify the suggestion that low tissue PO$_2$ values can occur under these conditions.

In conclusion we can say that by using cryophotometry, and by scrutinizing the histological sections, HbO$_2$ saturations can be measured in vessels of the carotid body. The distribution curve found for HbO$_2$ values in normoxia and hypoxia suggest that measurements were mainly carried out in shunt vessels which do not take part in the gas exchange. Single low HbO$_2$ values indicate that low tissue PO$_2$ values can occur in the glomus caroticum.

REFERENCES

Acker, H., Lübbers, D.W. and Purves, M.J. (1971) Pflügers Arch. 329, 136-155.

Acker, H. and Lübbers, D.W. (1976) Pflügers Arch. 366, 241-246.

Grunewald, W.A. and Lübbers, D.W. (1976) In 'Oxygen Transport to Tissue II' (eds. J. Grote, D. Reneau and G. Thews) p. 55, Plenum Press, New York.

MULTIPLE WAVELENGTH REFLECTANCE OXIMETRY IN PERIPHERAL TISSUES

Peter W. Cheung, Setsou Takatani and Edward A. Ernst*

Department of Biomedical Engineering and
*Department of Anesthesiology, School of Medicine
Case Western Reserve University
Cleveland, Ohio 44106

INTRODUCTION

One of the principal functions of the circulatory system is to deliver oxygen from the lungs to tissues by the red cells. Therefore, an important measure of the effectiveness of the cardio-vascular and pulmonary system is the ratio of oxyhemoglobin (HbO_2) concentration to the total hemoglobin concentration in blood which is called the hemoglobin oxygen saturation (OS).

Since the introduction of transmission and reflection oximetry in whole blood, there have been continued interests in the application of these optical techniques to measure hemoglobin OS of microvasculature in tissues. The accurate measurement of hemo-globin OS in tissues is important especially in studies concerning oxygen transport and delivery to tissue because both the hemoglobin-bound oxygen and the dissolved oxygen in plasma and tissue fluids are governed by the oxyhemoglobin dissociation curve. For example, it is well known that the shape of the oxyhemoglobin dissociation curve depends upon such factors as pH, pCO_2, temperature and 2,3-DPG level in the red blood cell, among others. Therefore, for a complete description of oxygen microvasculatures in tissue as well as the local oxygen tension (pO_2) have to be known. A direct and accurate method for hemoglobin OS measurement in tissue under in vivo situations will be valuable for studies of oxygen transport to tissues. This paper describes our initial efforts in applying multiple wavelengths reflectance measurement in peripheral tissue towards the development of a solid state tissue reflectance oximeter.

INSTRUMENTATION

An electronic instrumentation system has been developed in this laboratory to obtain real time optical reflectance data from tissue. Figure 1 shows a block diagram of this tissue reflectance oximetry system.

The optical transducer in the tissue reflectance oximeter is custom fabricated with five light-emitting diode (LED) chips with peak emission wavelengths at 635, 665, 795, 900 and 940 nm, respectively. These five wavelengths are chosen arbitrarily based upon the commercial availability of LEDs. However, they do cover the red and near infrared wavelengths which are most useful for transmission and reflection oximetry in whole blood because of the low absorption by Hb and HbO_2 in these region. The LED chips are obtained from different semiconductor manufacturers and their sizes are approximately .5 X .5 mm. The reflected light from tissue is detected by two low noise PIN photodiode chips (2 X 2 mm) obtained from EG & G Inc., (Salem, Mass.). These two PIN photodiode chips are·placed at two different distances from the LED chips and are called the 'near' and 'far' channel depending upon their separation distance from the LED chips. Two Bi-FET operational amplifier chips (National Semiconductor LF 157) are connected adjacent to the

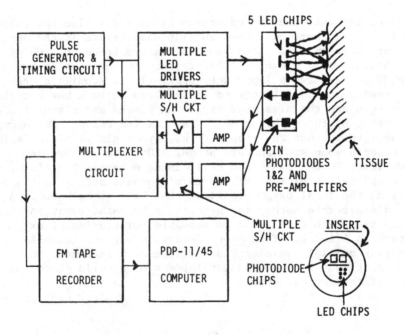

Figure 1. Block diagram of tissue reflectance oximeter.

PIN photodiodes as current-to-voltage preamplifiers to avoid noise pick up as well as to minimize stray capacitances. The outer diameter of the entire optical transducer is approximately 2 cm.

The reflectance oximeter operates by generating a set of 10 μs pulses at 1 K Hz to trigger the LED driver circuits to pulse the five discrete LEDs sequentially. The reflected light from tissue at each wavelength is measured at two discrete distances by the two PIN photodiodes. The output of the 'near' and 'far' channel amplifiers for each wavelength are sampled and held, filtered, and can be displayed on a front panel digital meter and recorded by a FM tape recorder. A total of 10 reflectance signals representing five different wavelengths and two separation distances from the LED chips can thus be recorded for off-line computer analysis using a PDP 11/45 computer.

EXPERIMENTAL

The optical reflectance data was obtained from the inner gut lining using an isolated gut preparation in dogs. Figure 2 shows the general experimental set up for the isolated gut experiments.

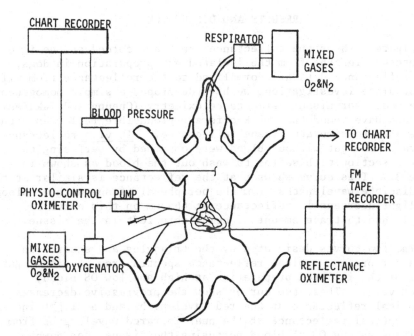

Figure 2.   Block diagram showing set up for _in vivo_ experiments.

Experimentally, the arterial supply and venous drainage of a small section of the dog's gut were tied off surgically. A major artery and vein from this isolated section were connected to an external pump and a small disc-oxygenator. The isolated gut section was then perfused extracorporeally with blood obtained from the same animal. Differences in arterial and venous hemoglobin OS were minimized by externally cooling the isolated gut section with cold saline to reduce the tissue's metabolism. A small incision was made on the gut wall and the optical reflectance transducer was inserted to record the tissue reflectance from the inner gut lining. Care was taken to avoid applying excessive pressure on the gut wall by the optical transducer. The OS of blood used to perfuse this isolated gut preparation were varied by controlling the % of oxygen going into the disc-oxygenator. Discrete blood samples were drawn at both the arterial inflow and venous outflow of the isolated gut section. These samples were analysed for their OS values and hemoglobin concentration using an Instrumentation Laboratory Oximeter (IL 182). These measurements provide absolute values of OS of blood perfusing the isolated gut section for correlation with the recorded tissue reflectance data. In addition, values of OS from the arterial inflow and the venous outflow of the isolated gut section were monitored closely to ensure that no significant difference in OS exists between them and that the entire isolated section is perfused with blood of the same OS value.

RESULTS AND DISCUSSION

Figure 3 shows the reflectance spectra recorded at the five discrete wavelengths from the isolated gut preparation in dogs. These reflectance data are normalized to the reflectance from milk. In a separate investigation, we have developed a simple homogeneous tissue model for tissue-reflectance oximetry (Cheung and Takatani, 1976) and have found that milk offers reproducible reflectance that can be used to simulate tissue reflectance. In vivo reflectance spectra of the gut without blood were obtained by perfusing the isolated section with saline to wash out the blood as shown in Figure 3. This curve shows that the reflectance is similar at the five discrete wavelengths from the peripheral tissue without blood. The slight decrease in reflectance at 665 nm on this curve is probably due to trace amount of hemoglobin left in the tissue.

The two curves designated by the triangles and squares in Figure 3 represent typical reflectance spectra from the inner gut lining of the isolated preparation at high and low OS blood, respectively. These two curves show the progressive decreases in the optical reflectance at the red wavelengths and a slight increase in the optical reflectance at the near infrared wavelengths from the tissue as the OS of blood perfusing the tissue goes down.

This result is in good agreement with the absorption characteristics of Hb and HbO_2 (Figure 3) which shows an increase in the optical absorption as the OS decreases. The reflectance spectra from the tissue yield the same reflectance for different OS at 795 nm which is close to the isobestic wavelength of 805 nm for Hb and HbO_2.

     In another series of experiments, the optical reflectance spectra from an intact gut section were recorded and compared with the arterial OS measured continuously with the Physio-Control in vivo Fiberoptic Oximeter (Redmond, Wash.). Figure 4 shows the arterial blood pressure, arterial OS and the red (665 nm) and infrared (940nm) reflectance recorded by the optical transducers from the intact gut. At point A in Figure 4, the dog was ventilated with low % of oxygen and the arterial OS droped rapidly as measured by the in vivo Fiber-optic Oximeter. The tissue reflectance obtained from the intact gut also shows a corresponding decrease in red reflectance (665 nm) with little change in the infrared reflectance (940 nm). At point B in Figure 4, the dog was given room air and the arterial OS and the tissue reflectance at the red wavelengths fully recover.

     From both the intact and isolated gut preparation experiments, our results show that the tissue reflectance at the red wavelength region is sensitive to changes in hemoglobin OS of microvasculatures in tissues. The infrared reflectance shows little change with tissue

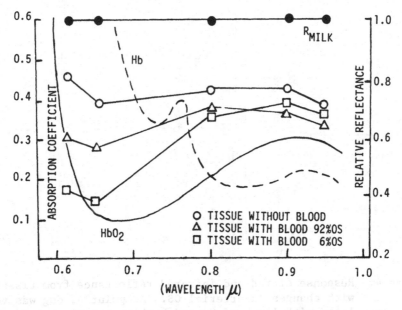

Figure 3. Absorption and reflection spectra of Hb, HbO_2 and tissue.

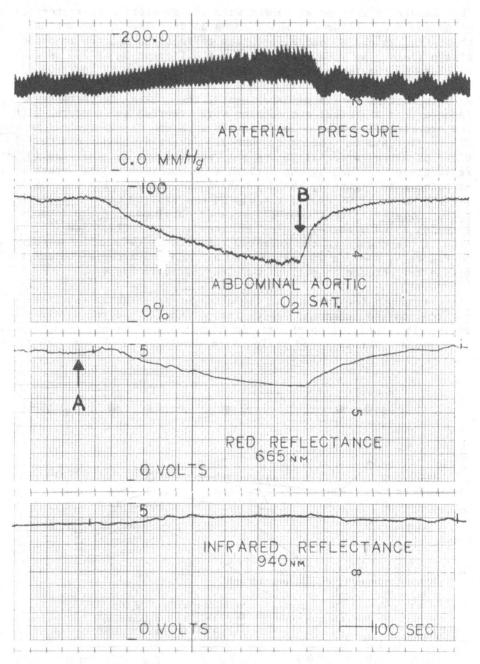

Figure 4.   Response of red and infrared reflectance from tissue
            with changes in arterial OS. At point A, dog was venti-
            lated with low % of O_2 and back to normal at point B.

OS and thus can best be used as reference to eliminate factors such as flow, non-homogeneity of tissue, varying red cell shapes flowing through microcapillaries, and variation in blood volume in the tissue as seen by the incident light sources.

Cohen and Wadsworth (1972) has constructed a skin reflectance oximeter using the red and infrared wavelengths. They have shown changes of the red reflectance from the forehead while the subject is holding his breath. However, their instrument cannot yield quantitative result due to the sensitivity to variation in skin pigmentation since only two wavelengths were used. Pittman and Duling (1975) measuring the optical transmittance at three wavelengths have avoided the effect of multiple scattering of red cells as well as the coloration of the vessel wall and other artifacts and obtained good quantitative measurement of OS on microvessels in the hamster cheek pouch. Lübbers(1973) had also described an empirical method of transforming the reflection spectrum from tissue into the absorption spectrum of Hb and HbO_2 by what he called the "Queranalyse" method which shows promise of quantitative estimation of OS from tissue using reflectance measurement at multiple wavelengths.

Our results show that optical reflectance measurement from tissue at multiple wavelengths in the red and near infrared region can yield good qualitative agreement with hemoglobin OS. We have further established an in vivo model using an isolated gut preparation for absolute calibration of OS in peripheral tissue. The measurement of hemoglobin OS in tissue is an important parameter for the study of oxygen transport to tissue. However, absolute measurement of hemoglobin OS in tissues awaits future progress and understanding in the theory describing the exact nature of optical propagation in tissues and its exact relationships with blood in the microvasculature.

REFERENCES

Cohen, A. and Wadsworth, N (1972) Med. and Biol Engr. 10, 385.
Cheung, P.W. and Takatani, S. (1976) Proc. of 29th ACEMB, 29 29.
Lübbers, D.W. (1973). In "Oxygen Transport to Tissue" p.45 (eds. Bicher, H.I. and Bruley, D) Plenum Press, New York.
Pittman, R.N. and Duling, B.R. (1975) J. of App/ Physiol. 38, 321.

ACKNOWLEDGEMENT

This work is supported by a grant from the National Institutes of Health, No. HL18710-01A1. The authors also wish to acknowledge Monsanto and Texas Instrument for supplying the LED chips and Physio-Control Corp. for the use of their in vivo Fiberoptic Oximeter. The help from Mr. Ralph Wiley in providing the illustrations is also appreciated.

MYOGLOBIN SATURATION AND CALCULATED PO_2 IN SINGLE CELLS OF RESTING GRACILIS MUSCLES

Thomas E. J. Gayeski and Carl R. Honig

University of Rochester School of Medicine & Dentistry
Department of Physiology
Rochester, New York 14642 USA

INTRODUCTION

Use of myoglobin (Mb) as an indicator of intracellular PO_2 has been dormant for half a century, chiefly because of difficulty in differentiating Mb from hemoglobin (Hb) when both are illuminated. We recently devised a microspectrophotometer with which light can be collected exclusively from either Hb or Mb. Spatial resolution is 2-5 μ. Since freezing arrests chemical reaction, saturation measurements on a large cell population can be interpreted as though all the measurements had been made simultaneously. In this way the purely spatial uniformity of O_2 delivery can be evaluated. Measurements can be made at several loci within one cell, at various loci in a cell cluster, or in cells selected at random from grossly different regions of the muscle. The method offers the further advantage that the contribution of local capillary recruitment to O_2 delivery can be evaluated.

METHODS

Dogs, 20-25 Kg body wt., were anesthetized with pentobarbital, 30 mg/Kg. Both gracilis muscles were isolated, taking care to preserve all 3 sets of vessels and the obturator nerve. The muscle surface was covered with Saran[R] and maintained at 37°C. Venous blood could be returned to the heart or diverted to a tared flask for flow and O_2 measurements. $\dot{V}O_2$ (O_2 consumption) was measured by use of the Fick principle. Immediately thereafter the Saran[R] covering was removed, and a 5 cm cube of copper, cooled to -196°C, was applied to the muscle at 0.09 Kg/cm[2] by use of an air-driven piston. In a representative experiment loci 600 μ from the surface reached 0°C in 470 msec, and -43°C in 1 sec. If $\dot{V}O_2$ is 2.5 μl/g·min,

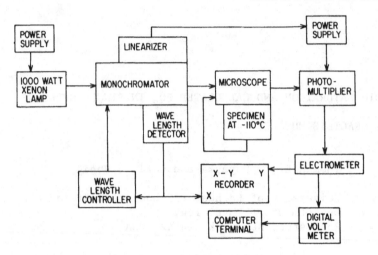

Fig. 1. Block diagram of microspectrophotometer.

Q_{10} is 2, and [Mb] is 0.5 mM, $\dot{V}O_2$ during cooling changes saturation by 10^{-5} per cent. The amount of O_2 physically dissolved is so small that the increase in O_2 affinity of myoglobin during cooling introduces a similarly trivial error. Though loci up to 2 mm deep are probably suitable in the resting state, measurements were made between 200 and 600 μ from the surface.

The muscle was transferred to liquid N_2 while still in contact with the copper block, and stored at -196°C. No change in the frequency distribution of saturation could be detected in muscles stored for 9 mo. The microscope cold stage consisted of a brass heat sink containing liquid N_2, to the base of which a brass column was attached. A well in this column was filled with 95% ethyl alcohol, regulated at -110°C ± 3°. At this temperature no change in the spectrum of fully desaturated Mb was observed over a 3 hr. period. The sample was positioned in the well so that a freshly cut muscle surface was just above the alcohol surface. Cells were observed in cross-section.

The specimen was viewed by reflected light with a Leitz orthoplan microscope and metallurgical head. Polarizers (extinction ∿ 1:5000) attenuated reflection from the film of viscid alcohol which coated the specimen. The alcohol prevented frost formation. A 1000 W Xenon lamp and monochromator (300 nm blaze) provided quasi-monochromatic light at wave lengths set ± 0.1 nm by a control circuit and stepping motor. A block diagram of the system is shown in Fig. 1.

Mb isobestic points at -110°C were located at 547, 568 and 588 nm. These values were, respectively, 4, 4 and 3 nm less than for Mb in solution (Gayeski and Honig, submitted). Isobestic points for Hb were shifted by the same amount. Mb saturation was computed with a 3 wave-length method for a non-isobestic point at 560 and another at 578 nm. The values were averaged. Since 560 is an extinction trough and 578 an extinction maximum for saturated Mb, errors attributable to light scattered from ice crystals tend to cancel. The measurement error was ± 5%.

To operate the system, the base line (maximum light intensity) was set for the 588 nm isobestic point, and the ammeter adjusted to give a signal of convenient magnitude on a digital voltmeter. The spectrum from 540-588 nm was also displayed on an x-y recorder. Data were accepted only if the absorption at 588 nm at the beginning and end of the scan differed by < 3%. Voltmeter readings were entered into a Dec 10 computer, together with cell diameter, coordinates of cell location, and number of capillaries/cell. Printouts include: 1) Various cell descriptors, table of isobestic and non-isobestic ratios, % saturation, and PO$_2$, 2) a graphic showing cells in cross-section, with locations of capillaries, locations of measurement sites and saturations at each site, 3) frequency histograms, non-parametric one way analysis of variance, multiple linear regression.

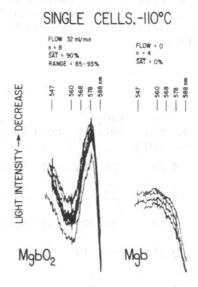

Fig. 2. Representative spectra from a well-oxygenated muscle (left) and anoxic muscle (right).

RESULTS

Representative recordings are shown in Fig. 2. The oxygenated spectra come from a muscle in which acute denervation had increased blood flow 8 fold. Spectra from 8 consecutive, randomly selected, widely separated cells 300-500 μ from the surface are shown. The maximum difference in location of the 578 nm peak was < .1 nm. Saturations ranged from 85-93%. Fig. 2B shows cells from a muscle stimulated at 4/sec for 5 min after clamping arterial inflow. Mb was fully desaturated in all cells sampled.

Results are summarized in Table 1. $\dot{V}O_2$ was independent of flow between 1.9 and 32 ml/min (2.4-40.3 ml/100 g·min, assuming 75g muscles). This confirms earlier work (Honig et al, 1971, Whalen et al, 1976), and is in accord with the fact that no $\dot{V}O_2$ could be detected in 2 cyanide-treated muscles (error in $\dot{V}O_2$ ∿ ± 5%). Muscles 2 and 4 were from the same dog. In the former reflex vaso-constriction was induced by hemorrhage; in the latter vasoconstrictor tone was abolished by denervation. Despite the 14-fold difference in flow mean Mb saturations were almost identical. In muscles 2, 3 and 4 (flow low, normal and high respectively) mean Mb saturation was > 85%, and no cells with Mb < 70% saturated were encountered. Blood flow was lowest in muscle #1, and its mean Mb saturation was lower than in the others (P < .001). Nevertheless, only 3 of 34 randomly selected cells contained Mb < 70% saturated. In each of the 4 muscles statistically significant differences in mean saturation were found in grossly different regions. This could reflect the regional heterogeneity of flow characteristic of skeletal muscle (Sparks and Mohrman, 1977). However, the differences were small, and the salient characteristic of the data is the uniformly high level of Mb saturation.

Muscle #	*Flow ml/min per 100 g	*$\dot{V}O_2$ ml/min per 100 g	PvO_2 mmHg	n	SATURATION Mean %	Range	P Value, ΔSat=0	PO_2 Mean mmHg	Range mmHg
1	2.40	0.26	28	34	77	95-29	<.001	29	3-79
2	2.75	0.33	22	16	86	96-71	.07	48	17-88
3	9.75	0.23	81	22	91	98-83	.07	65	30-92
+4	40.30	0.25	62	19	88	96-79		52	25-91

Table 1. Data summary; muscles 2 and 4 from the same dog. + = acutely denervated. * Assumes 75 g muscles.

PO$_2$ was calculated from saturation using a P$_{50}$ of 6.3. This value was determined in vitro for canine skeletal myoglobin at 37°C. Small errors in saturation on the plateau of the oxy-myoglobin dissociation curve lead to large errors in calculated PO$_2$. Since the error of the saturation measurement is ± 5%, several PO$_2$ values greater than PaO$_2$ were obtained in each muscle. These were set equal to PaO$_2$ in constructing the frequency histograms shown in Fig. 3. The open bars denote all 91 cells from muscles 1-4. The superimposed hatched bars represent the 34 cells in muscle #1, in which blood flow was lowest. All values < 20 mm Hg except one are from that particular muscle. The lowest value was 3 mm Hg. In all muscles the distributions appeared to be bimodal, for reasons which remain to be determined.

The number of erythrocyte-containing capillaries around a particular fiber varied from 0-9. (Capillaries are shared by two or more cells.) The linear regression of capillaries per fiber on Mb saturation was computed for all cells in the 4 muscles. The regression coefficient was not significantly different from 0 and the coefficient of determination was < .01, suggesting that satura-tion is maintained > 70% in part by local capillary recruitment.

In small animals, muscle $\dot{V}O_2$ increases with flow (Honig et al, 1971, Whalen et al, 1973). To determine whether anoxic regions exist in such muscles, Mb saturation was measured in one cat gracilis. The Mb concentration (and ratio of signal to noise) were much lower than in dog. Nevertheless, at many sites saturation (and hence PO$_2$) were indistinguishable from 0, while at other sites Mb was partly saturated.

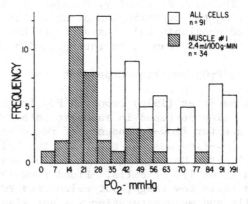

Fig. 3. PO$_2$ frequency histograms for all randomly selected cells from all muscles (open bars) and (superimposed hatched bars) from 1 flow-restricted muscle.

DISCUSSION

Facilitated Diffusion

Our principal finding is that Mb is highly saturated at almost all locations in resting dog gracilis, even if blood flow is severely limited by vasoconstriction. Consequently, in this muscle, and probably in large animals generally, Mb does not facilitate O_2 diffusion at rest. On the other hand, facilitated diffusion could play a significant role in resting muscles of small animals such as cat in which Mb appears to be substantially desaturated and $\dot{V}O_2$ is transport-limited.

Other Estimates of Mb Saturation

Coburn and Mayers (1971) calculated mean Mb saturation in dog from the distribution of CO. His mean value of 65% is less than the value observed by us, even for flow-limited muscles. Apart from many assumptions, Coburn's calculation requires mean HbO_2, PO_2 and PCO in capillary blood. These quantities cannot be determined accurately from samples of venous blood because of the enormous regional heterogeneity of muscle blood flow (Sparks and Mohrman, 1977).

Our preliminary data for cat gracilis are at variance with Millikan's claim (1937) that Mb is fully saturated in cat soleus. The explanation does not lie in the difference between soleus (red) and gracilis (mixed muscle), for the frequency distribution of PO_2 in cat soleus (Whalen et al, 1973) is also inconsistent with Millikan's result. Millikan did not control temperature, (a major determinant of the Mb dissociation curve) and this partly explains the discrepancy. The main difficulty, however, is that Millikan's method for evaluating the contribution of Hb to his signal is valid for fully saturated myoglobin only (Gayeski and Honig, submitted). His in vivo data therefore cannot be interpreted quantitatively.

P_TO_2 and Flow-Dependent $\dot{V}O_2$

Whalen and associates (1976) reported PO_2 frequency histograms in dog gracilis muscles perfused in an organ bath. They found lower values and greater flow-dependence of PO_2 than did we. For example, in their low-flow muscles about 1/2 the values were < 20 mm Hg and 1/4 < the Mb P_{50}. Even when flow was increased PO_2 was < 20 mm Hg in about 1/3 of cells. Blood flow in our muscle #2 falls well within their low range, but calculated PO_2 was < 20 mmHg in only 6% of cells and mean saturation was not significantly different from that in a high-flow muscle. Flow in muscle #1 was 1/3 less than the average for flow-limited muscles studied by Whalen et al, but mean PO_2 in muscle #1 was greater than that

reported for their high-flow muscles. A plausible reason for the
foregoing differences is that their muscles should have shortened
passively by about 20% when removed from the animal. The resulting
deformation of microvessels could produce small regions of low flow
and/or low capillary density. It is also possible that some of the
capillaries serving the cells they sampled were damaged or occluded
by the O$_2$ electrode.

Despite the quantitative discrepancies noted above, the main
conclusion of Whalen and co-workers is the same as ours, i.e. at
rest P$_T$O$_2$ does not limit $\dot{V}$O$_2$ in dog gracilis over the entire
physiological range of blood flow. Consequently, chemical pathways
for O$_2$ other than the classical respiratory chain probably do not
exist in the skeletal-muscle cells of large animals.

In cat and other small animals muscle $\dot{V}$O$_2$ is strongly dependent on flow (Honig et al, 1971, Whalen et al, 1973). Since PO$_2$
frequency histograms in cats are often similar to those in dogs it
is thought that lack of O$_2$ cannot account for the flow dependence
(Whalen et al, 1973, 1976). In view of the marked variability of
P$_T$O$_2$ among individual cats our preliminary data may not be representative. However, in the particular muscle we examined the
amount of potentially anoxic tissue was sufficient to account, at
least in part, for flow-dependent $\dot{V}$O$_2$. Though non-classical respiration in skeletal-muscle cells of small animals cannot be
excluded, it need not be assumed on the basis of present data.

Control of O$_2$ Delivery

The principal function of Mb in resting muscle appears to be
that of a short-term O$_2$ store. To perform this function Mb must
remain almost fully saturated despite large fluctuations in total
flow. Our data indicates that arterioles and pre-capillary
sphincters regulate P$_T$O$_2$ to that end. The mechanism of the regulation is built into vascular smooth muscle, for wall tension in
microvessels dissected free of skeletal-muscle cells varies with
PO$_2$ (Coburn, 1977). Since the set-point of the regulation is about
1000-fold higher than the PO$_2$ required for coupled oxidation by
isolated cardiac mitochondria (Chance et al, 1973) the O$_2$ sensor
could involve a variant of cytochrome a, a$_3$ of very low O$_2$ affinity
(Jöbsis, 1977). Alternatively, the sensor could depend on a process
which can be influenced by O$_2$ but is independent of the respiratory
chain. The latter need not actually consume O$_2$, and seems the more
likely possibility in view of Coburn's data (1977) on the O$_2$-depen-
dence of tension development by cyanide-treated vascular smooth
muscle.

REFERENCES

Chance, B., Oshino, N., Sugano, T. and Mayevsky, A. (1973)
Adv. Exper. Med. Biol. 37A, 277.

Coburn, R.F. and Mayers, L.B. (1971) Am. J. Physiol. 220, 66.

Coburn, R.F. (1977) Adv. Exper. Med. Biol. 78, 101.

Gayeski, T.E.J. and Honig, C.R. Resp. Physiol., Submitted.

Honig, C.R., Frierson, J.L. and Nelson, C.N. (1971) Am. J.
Physiol. 220, 357.

Jöbsis, F.F. (1977) Adv. Exper. Med. Biol. 78, 3.

Millikan, G.A. (1937) Proc. Roy. Soc. B 123, 218.

Sparks, H.V. and Mohrman, D.E. (1977) Microvasc. Research 13, 181.

Whalen, W.J., Buerk, D. and Thuning, C.A. (1973) Am. J. Physiol.
224, 763.

Whalen, W.J., Buerk, D., Thuning, C., Kanoy, Jr., B.E. and
Duran, W.N. (1976) Adv. Exper. Med. Biol. 75, 639.

ACKNOWLEDGEMENT

We thank Mr. James L. Frierson for technical assistance. This
research was supported by grants HLB 03290 and AM 01004 from the
U.S. Public Health Service.

THE MYOGLOBIN PROBED OPTICAL STUDIES

OF MYOCARDIAL ENERGY METABOLISM

M. Tamura*, N. Oshino** and B. Chance

Johnson Research Foundation, School of Medicine
University of Pennsylvania, Philadelphia, U.S.A.
*The Institute of Scientific and Industrial Research
Osaka University, Osaka, Japan
**Nihon Sherring, K.K., Osaka, Japan

INTRODUCTION

The oxygen supply to the heart is one of the fundamental parameters of the heart function, since cardiac contraction is supported by ATP produced by combustion of substrates, mainly at the mitochondrial level. Cardiac muscle contains myoglobin in cytosol and cytochromes in mitochondria, both of which participate in the respiratory mechanisms of the heart. The present paper describes an optical approach to myocardial energy metabolism with the intention of detecting the absorption changes of myoglobin during a single contraction-relaxation cycle.

The simultaneous measurements of oxygenation-deoxygenation of myoglobin and of the redox-changes of cytochrome aa_3 in the steady state provided a basis for the suggestion of a possible oxygen gradient between the cytosolic and mitochondrial spaces.

EXPERIMENTAL PROCEDURE

Haemoglobin-free perfused rat heart was obtained by the slightly modified method of Langendorf which included cannulation of the aorta and connection to a constant work load of 80 cm H_2O. The perfusate was Krebs-Ringer bicarbonate buffer containing 2.5mM Ca and 10 mM glucose. Absorption changes of myoglobin were measured by the triple beam method ('compensate') obtained by the slight modification of time-sharing dual wavelength spectrophoto-

This research was supported by USPHS Grants GM-12202 and HL-18708.

meter (Chance and Graham 1971).   A thin, flexible light guide of
0.8 mm diameter was inserted through the heart wall into the left
ventricle, and the light transmitted through the left ventricle
was guided into the phototube in the detection system (Tamura et al).

RESULTS

Oxygen gradient between cytosolic and mitochondrial spaces

Fig. 1A shows the steady state titration of myoglobin and
cytochrome aa_3 with oxygen in perfused heart.   After anaerobiosis
was achieved, the oxygen concentration in the inflowing perfusate
was increased in a stepwise fashion (arrow).   The signals of both
myoglobin and cytochrome aa_3 responded to each change in the oxygen
concentration, and reached new steady states.   When the fractional
saturation of myoglobin was plotted against the fractional oxidation
of cytochrome aa_3 (Fig. 1-8), it was found that two events were
apparently identical, resulting in a straight line.   When similar
titration experiments were performed in the reconstituted system
(i.e. 8:1 mixture of purified myoglobin and mitochondria), the
titration curve was not a straight line, but a 50% saturation of
myoglobin was accompanied by an oxidation level of more than 80%
of cytochrome aa_3.   This deviation from the straight line is
expected from the more than 10 fold difference in the oxygen affinity

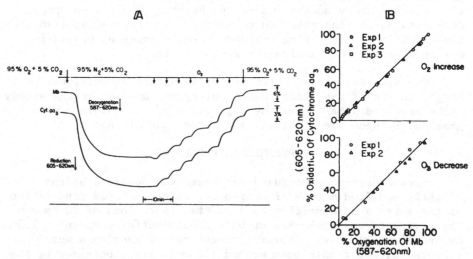

Fig. 1. Steady state titrations of myoglobin and cytochrome aa_3
with oxygen in the perfused rat heart.   The changes in the degree
of oxygen saturation of myoglobin (Mb) and in the redox state of
cytochrome aa_3 were measured spectrophotometrically at 587-620 nm
and 605-620 nm with a time constant of 10 s in the recording shown
in (A). The relative absorbance changes of cytochrome aa_3 were
plotted against those of myoglobin, as shown in (B).

between myoglobin and cytochrome aa_3 (Oshino et al, 1974). Thus, the straight line of Fig. 1B suggests that there is a sharp oxygen gradient between the cytosolic and mitochondrial spaces in the cardiac tissue.

Fluctuation of Intracellular Oxygen Concentration Associated with Contraction Relaxation Cycle

Fig. 2 shows the phase-relationships between the oxygenation-deoxygenation of myoglobin and left ventricular pressure (LVP) together with electrocardiogram (ECG) in the normal aerobic steady state. It is seen that the increase in LVP follows the ECG pulse in 10 msec, and 10 msec later the increased oxygenation is registered. Myoglobin is in the oxygenated state during systolic and diastolic periods and is then deoxygenated in the resting state. The oxygenation process during the contraction is found to be very rapid and has a half-time of few milliseconds. Under these aerobic conditions, approximately 10% of the total myoglobin undergoes the periodic oxygenation-deoxygenation cycle associated with the heart beat. This shows that the intracellular oxygen concentration changes periodically between 10^{-5}M and 10^{-4}M.

Respiration Rate During Single Cycle of Contraction

Fig. 3 shows the myoglobin absorption change during the contraction-relaxation cycle, where perfusion was performed with 50% oxygen saturated and substrate-free media. The heart was obtained from a rat kept without food for 16 hours. Under this condition the level of creatinephosphate in the cardiac tissue was lower than that observed in hearts obtained from fed animals perfused with 10mM glucose (Safer and Williamson, 1972; Tamura et

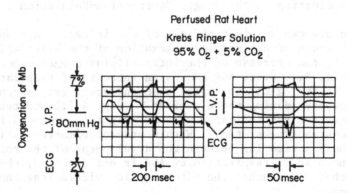

Fig. 2. Oxygenation-deoxygenation of myoglobin in relation to changes in LVP and ECG during a single contraction-relaxation cycle in perfused rat heart. Myoglobin absorption changes were measured by the triple beam (581 - $\frac{515 + 587}{2}$) nm. Aerobic state.

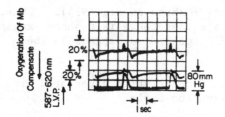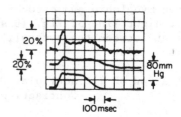

Fig. 3. Oxygenation-deoxygenation of myoglobin in the prolonged substrate free perfusion. The rat heart was perfused for more than 1 hour without any added substrate. Hypoxic condition with 50% oxygen saturated perfusate. Myoglobin absorption changes were measured as compensated $(581 - \frac{515 + 587}{2})$ nm and dual wavelength (587-620) nm.

al 1977). Both absorption signals (the compensated and the 587-620 nm) represent the oxygenation-deoxygenation of myoglobin and confirm the optical measurement using different wavelength pairs.

In contrast to the normal aerobic perfusion of Fig. 2, the deoxygenation occurs during the contraction and when the contraction reaches maximum, oxygenation starts (as shown by the sharp spike of the absorption change near the maximum of contraction). At the end of the diastole, myoglobin is again deoxygenated to a small but distinct extent and then reoxygenated during the resting state.

DISCUSSION

ADP-fluctuation in the Single Contraction-Relaxation Cycle

There are two distinct periods of the increase in respiration during one cycle of contraction-relaxation of the heart which are reflected by the decrease of the intracellular oxygen concentration shown in Fig. 3. Since ADP causes an increase of respiration (State 3) it is logical to expect that intracellular concentration of ADP increases during these periods. Fig. 4 illustrates the above suggestion and indicates when ADP might be released from the muscular contracting system. Within present time-resolution (few milliseconds) a time-lag between the development of the contraction and the increase of respiration by ADP is not detected, which suggests that ADP reaches the mitochondrion within less than 1 millisecond.

The increase of the respiration which appeared at the end of diastole seems rather puzzling. If it is due to increase in ADP, a possible interpretation is that ADP is being released from the

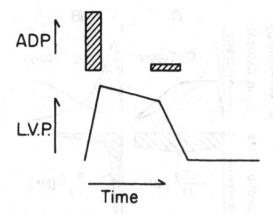

Fig. 4. A schematic presentation of the phase-relationship between
the increase of respiration or ADP and LVP.   The data was obtained
from the Fig. 3.

sarcoplasmic reticulum at the time of the reabsorption of calcium
ion.   Another possibility is that it is due to the change of
intracellular pH, which originates from the hydrolysis of ATP.
Further experiments are required to resolve this question.

Oxygen Supply from Circulating Systems

Prolonged substrate-free perfusion (Fig. 3) leads to a
decrease in the level of creatinephosphate in the cardiac tissue,
although the level of ATP remains constant (Williamson et al, 1972).
It is possible that the creatinephosphate-creatine system performs
a buffer function against the fluctuation of ATP-ADP, arising from
the contraction-relaxation cycle.   Thus, the results of Fig. 3
may arise from the absence of an effective creatine-creatine
phosphate buffer system, and reflect directly the behaviour of
ADP and ATP in cardiac tissue..   The increase of the oxygenation
level during systolic and diastolic periods observed in normal
aerobic steady state (Fig. 2) can be explained by the creatinephosphate dependent modulation of the respiration, which is shown in
Fig. 5.

In Fig. 5A (normal aerobic perfusion) we assume that oxygen is
supplied in a pulse-like fashion from the circulation into tissue
during contraction, (dotted line of the top column).   Under this
condition, the respiration rate is maintained constant through the
1 cycle of contraction by the creatinephosphate-creatine system
(middle column).   The oxygen supply overcomes the respiration

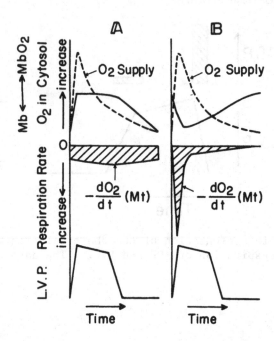

Fig.5. A tentative model describing the oxygen supply from
circulating system to the cardiac tissue and the respiration during
a single cycle of contraction-relaxation.   A. A normal aerobic
condition, where creatinephosphate-creatine system prevents the
fluctuation in ADP levels and leads to constant respiration rate
through the whole cycle.   B. Absence of the creatinephosphate-
creatine system (c.f. Fig. 3) where the 'burst' of respiration is
found during the contraction.   In the middle column, respiration
rate, the areas of (A) and (B) are the same and correspond to the
same amounts of oxygen utilized during one cycle of contraction.
Dotted line on the top column represents the pulse-like oxygen
supply from capillary into tissue.   The oxygen concentration
(solid line) is the difference between the oxygen supply (dotted
line) and respiration (middle column).

during the systolic and diastolic period.   This causes the
increase of the intracellular oxygen concentration as monitored by
the myoglobin absorption change (solid line of top column).   During
the resting state, the respiration overcomes the oxygen supply,
causing the decrease of the intracellular oxygen concentration.

In Fig. 5B (the absence of creatinephosphate-creatine system), the respiration increases during the contraction (cf Fig. 3 and 4), which overcomes the oxygen supply from the circulation, resulting in the decrease of the intracellular oxygen concentration during this period. However, the mechanism of oxygen supply from the circulation into the heart tissue is at present unknown. Thus, the tentative schemes of Figures 4 and 5 should be considered only as working hypotheses and the solution of the problem must await future work.

ACKNOWLEDGEMENT

One of the authors (M.T.) is greatly indebted to Professor Yuji Tonomura at Osaka University for his critical discussions on the behaviour of ADP and ATP during the muscular contraction.

REFERENCES

Chance, B. and Graham, N. (1971) Rev. Sci. Inst. 42, 941.

Oshino, N., Sugano, T., Oshino, R. and Chance, B. (1974) Biochem. Biophys. Acta. 368, 298.

Safer, B. and Williamson, J.R. (1973) J. Biol. Chem. 248, 2570.

Tamura, M., Oshino, N., Chance, B. and Silver, I. Biochem. J. (in press)

THE INTRACELLULAR HETEROGENEITY OF OXYGEN CONCENTRATIONS AS MEASURED BY ULTRAVIOLET TELEVISION MICROSCOPY OF PBA FLUORESCENCE QUENCHING BY OXYGEN

I. S. Longmuir, J. A. Knopp, Tei-Pei Lee, D. Benson and A. Tang

Department of Biochemistry, North Carolina State University, Raleigh, NC, U.S.A.

If oxygen moves through the cell along special channels (Longmuir, 1977) and the mean solubility coefficient for oxygen in liver cells is rather low as Zander (1976) has shown, then there should be considerable intracellular heterogeneity of oxygen concentration even in a non-respiring cell with uniform P_{O_2} throughout. Since the polarographic electrode measures P_{O_2} (Longmuir and Allen, 1960), this heterogeneity cannot be detected by this method. However, the fluorescence of pyrenebutyric acid (PBA) is quenched in proportion to the concentration of oxygen in a volume of a few hundred Augstrom's radius around each photofluor molecule (Longmuir and Knopp, 1976). Thus, this method, with a theoretical geometric resolution of 0.2 µm appears to have this capability.

The relationship between fluorescence intensity is given by the Stern Volmer equation:

$$\frac{Fo}{F} = 1 + K \alpha P_{O_2}$$

where Fo is the fluorescence intensity in the absence of oxygen; F in the presence of oxygen (P_{O_2}) in Torr, α is the local solubility coefficient, and K is a quenching constant.

METHOD

Individual liver cells stained with PBA suspended in a
substrate-free medium, so that they do not respire, were placed as
a thin film in a hanging drop chamber. The chamber was illuminated
with light of 334 nm from a Xenon arc lamp through a Ploem illumination microscope and a 54X objective and the emitted light measured
on a SIT TV camera after passing a 420 nm interference filter.
The signals from the camera were digitized and stored. The chamber
was ventilated at seven different values of oxygen tension from
0-700 Torr. Two thousand five hundred areas of about 0.3 μm^2 of a
cell were separately examined and the value of αK at each point
calculated from the best fitting value of a regression line of the
Stern Volmer plot on the seven data points from each area.

RESULTS

Figure 1 shows the distribution of Fo across a liver cell
about 30 μ in diameter. Figure 2 shows F across the same cell.
Although the picture is qualitatively similar to the first, the
levels of fluorescence intensity are diminished. Figure 3 shows

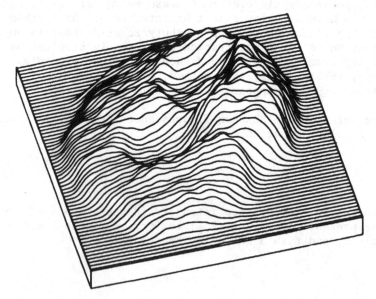

Fig. 1. Contour diagram of fluorescence intensity of an
anoxic non-respiring hepatocyte; lines scanned at 0.3 μ intervals;
upward deflection is a measure of intensity.

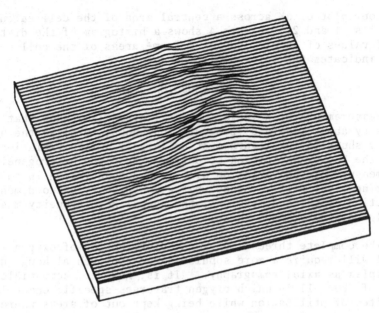

Fig. 2. The same cell in the presence of oxygen showing reduction in intensity.

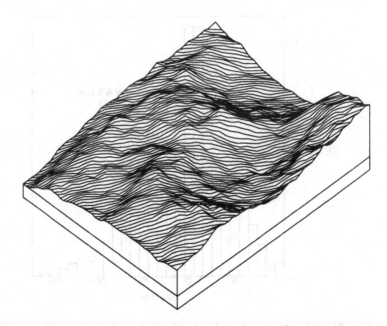

Fig. 3. Contour diagram of αK across part of the cell calculated from Figs. 1 and 2.

a contour plot of αK across a central area of the cell calculated
from Figs. 1 and 2.   Figure 4 shows a histogram of the distribution of values of αK of 2,500 of 0.3 μm² areas of the cell.   The
arrow indicates the value of αK for water.

DISCUSSION

Measurements of K in various cell organelles show that it
varies by about two-fold (Longmuir and Knopp, 1976) so the heterogeneity shown in the figure must be largely due to variations in α.
Since the PO_2 by definition is uniform, then the heterogeneity must
be a measure of the variation of oxygen concentration in this non-
respiring liver cell.   Since what we observe is a two dimensional
projection of three dimensions, the actual heterogeneity must
clearly be greater than shown.

The complete three dimensional distribution of oxygen within
a cell will require a more sophisticated approach although nothing
as complex as axial tomography.   It is, however, compatible with a
model of the cell in which oxygen traverses specific channels to
the sites of utilization while being kept out of areas where it
may damage certain enzymes (Longmuir, 1977).

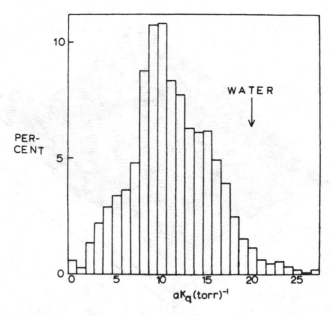

Fig. 4.   Distribution of values of αK in Fig. 3.   The arrow
indicates the value for water.

ACKNOWLEDGMENT

This paper is a contribution from the Department of Biochemistry, School of Agriculture and Life Sciences and School of Physical and Mathematical Sciences, and is supported in part by NIH Grant No. HL 16828.   Paper No. 5333 of the North Carolina Agricultural Experiment Station, Raleigh, North Carolina 27607.

REFERENCES

Longmuir, I.S. (1977) Search for alternative cellular oxygen carriers.   In 'Oxygen and Physiological Function' (Jöbsis, F.F. ed.), Professional Information Library, Dallas.

Longmuir, I.S. and Allen, F. (1960) J. Polarographic Soc. 8, 63.

Longmuir, I.S. and Knopp, J.A. (1976) J. Appl. Physiol. 41, 798.

Zander, R. (1976) Proc. Second OTT.

APPLICATION OF THE OPTODE TO MEASUREMENTS OF SURFACE Po_2

AND Pco_2 OF THE ISOLATED GUINEA-PIG HEART

N. Opitz, H. Weigelt, T. Barankay, D.W. Lübbers

Max-Planck-Institut für Systemphysiologie

4600 Dortmund, Rheinlanddamm 201, GFR

We described in previous papers that the so-called optode
(LÜBBERS and OPITZ, 1975 and 1976) was especially well suited for
the quantitative determination of Po_2 and Pco_2. For the measurement of Po_2, the flourescence quenching of the indicator pyrene
butyric acid by oxygen (VAUGHAN and WEBER, 1970; KNOPP and
LONGMUIR, 1972) and for Pco_2, the change of the fluorescence
indicator β-methylumbelliferone with pH was used (OPITZ and
LÜBBERS, 1975). In summary, the characteristical details of this
optode-device are:

1.   A few microns thick indicator layer is separated from the
medium to be measured by a gas-permeable membrane which prevents
possible toxic influences and spectral distortions by interactions
of the indicator molecules with molecules of the substance.
2. The indicator film is tightly held between a quartz window
(on the excitation side) and the membrane so that no changes in the
indicator concentration can occur.
3. The optode is located in front of the biological object so that
the filter effect of the tissue is avoided.

Finally, as a result of the optode design, we can use solutes of
high solubility suitable for the indicators so that tissue fluorescence is negligibly small or can even be reduced completely by
blackening one membrane face or by sputtering a reflecting layer
onto its surface. Using such an optode, we tested its applicability
to the Guinea-pig heart by measuring the surface oxygen and carbon-
dioxide tension.

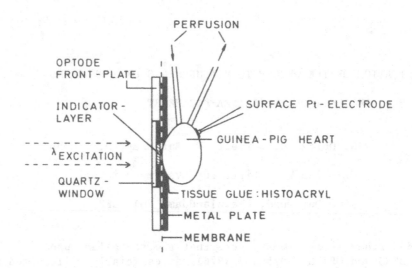

Fig. 1 Schematic view of the optode-device, as coupled
        onto the Guinea-pig heart

Owing to the specific construction of the optode (Fig. 1), the
animal's heart had to be brought in close contact to the teflon
membrane of the optode. Hermetical adaptation could be achieved by
using the tissue glue Histoacryl$^{(R)}$. The measuring field of the
indicator layer in the optode was about 6 mm in diameter. For the
Po_2-optode , we use 10^{-9} M solutions of pyrene butyric acid in
dimethylformamide and stabilize the fluid indicator film by adding
agarose to this solution till saturation. This procedure brings
about high-viscous indicator mixtures, which enable measurements of
a high degree of stability for hours. For the Pco_2-optode, saturated solutions of β-methylumbelliferone in solute mixtures of 10^{-3} M
$NaHCO_3$ (9 parts) and dimethylformamide (1 part) were used, which
also were stabilized by addition of agarose. Using a 6 μm teflon
membrane, the response time for the Po_2-optode amounted to 2 - 3
sec (90% of the final value), for the Pco_2-optode 3 - 4 sec (90%)
(Fig. 2). The measurements were performed with the "corrected
spectra measuring spectrofluorometer" (BOLDT and LÜBBERS, 1971).
Since the fluorescing indicator in this apparatus is firmly
fixed,   the investigations were performed with the isolated heart.

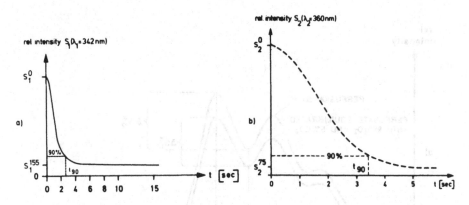

Fig. 2 a) Response time of the Po_2-optode
          b) Response time of the Pco_2-optode
          (6 μm teflon membrane were used in both cases)

The Guinea-pig (average weight 465 g ± 49.4 g) was anesthetized with
Nembutal[R] (initial dose 40 mg/kg). The heart was exposed during
artificial ventilation and the coronary vessels were perfused via
the aorta according to O. Langendorff's method (LANGENDORFF, 1895)
so that the heart beat   spontaneously. Examination of the tissue
fluorescence of the Guinea-pig heart showed that no interferences were
recognizable in the corrected excitation spectra of either fluorescence indicators. Fig. 3a shows fluorescence excitation spectra at
two different Po_2 values recorded on the surface of the Guinea-pig
heart. The change of the relative intensity is due to the oxygen
quenching of the fluorescence of pyrene butyric acid. To eliminate
additive interfering disturbances (e.g. straylight), which may
originate from the manipulations necessary to couple the heart to
the optode, the spectra were evaluated at two nearby wavelengths,
λ_1=342 nm and λ_2=333 nm, between which a high signal difference of
the corresponding signals, S_1 and S_2, existed. In a calibration
curve (Fig. 4a), the difference of the fluorescence intensities of
the corresponding signals, $\Delta S_{12}{}^x = S_1{}^x(\lambda_1) - S_2{}^x(\lambda_2)$, was reciprocally
plotted versus Po_2, where $\Delta S_{12}{}^0$ is the signal difference at a Po_2
of 0 Torr. This way we obtained a corrected calibration curve which
was well reproducible. The wavelengths used for evaluation must be
sufficiently close to each other so that the relative intensities
of the additive interfering disturbance are only slightly different.

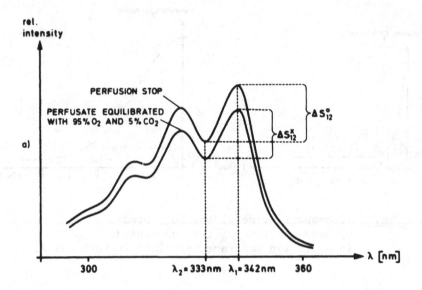

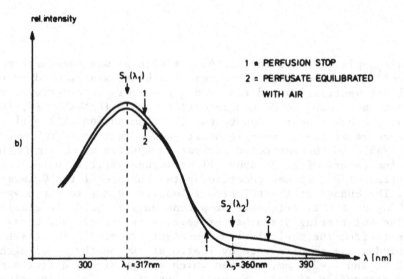

Fig. 3. a) Corrected excitation spectra of pyrene butyric acid
(λ_{em}=395 nm).

b) Corrected excitation spectra of β-methylumbelliferone (λ_{em}=445 nm).

(Both spectra were recorded from the system consisting
of optode and Guinea-pig heart)

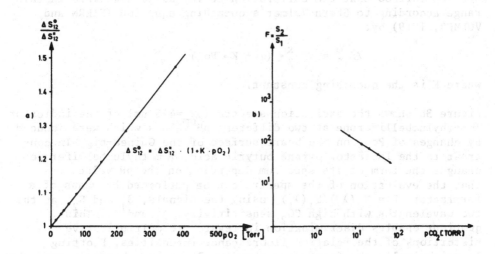

Fig. 4 a) Calibration curve of the P_{O_2}-optode

   b) Calibration curve of the P_{CO_2}-optode

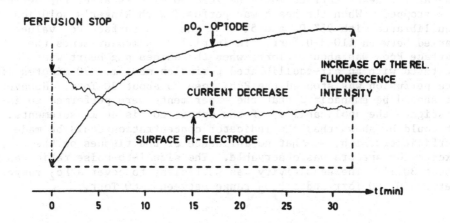

Fig. 5 Decrease of surface P_{O_2} of the Guinea-pig heart
measured simultaneously with an optode and a platinum
electrode.

Fig. 4a shows a good linearity of the Po_2-optode in the range of 0 - 400 Torr so that the calibration curve can be described in this range according to Stern-Volmer's quenching equation (STERN and VOLMER, 1919) by:

$$\Delta S_{12}^{o} = \Delta S_{12}^{x} \cdot (1 + K \cdot Po_2)$$

where K is the quenching constant.

Figure 3b shows the excitation spectra (λ_{em}=445 nm) of the indicator β-methylumbelliferone at two different pH values which were induced by changes of Pco_2 on the heart surface of the Guinea-pig. In contrast to the indicator pyrene butyric acid, β-methylumbelliferone changes the form of its spectrum depending on the pH value so that the evaluation of the spectra can be performed by means of a formfactor, $F = S_2(\lambda_2)/S_1(\lambda_1)$, using the signals, S_1 and S_2, at the two wavelengths with high CO_2 sensititivity, λ_1 and λ_2. This quotient enables discrimination in regards to multiplicative distortions of the relative fluorescence intensities. Plotting logarithmically the formfactor F versus Pco_2, one obtains a straight line of the calibration curve in the physiologically relevant Pco_2 range from 1 - 80 Torr (Fig. 4b).

With the aid of a Po_2 surface platinum electrode that was placed on the left ventricle of the heart, the Po_2 measured continuously by the fluorescence technique was checked polarographically. Both methods showed that Po_2 changes occurred in the same direction and nearly the same time course on the heart surface (Fig. 5).

For the quantitative evaluation of the Po_2 it was assumed that the Po_2 at the heart surface would be zero 30 minutes after the perfusion was stopped. When the heart was perfused with Ringer's solution equilibrated with 95% O_2 and 5% CO_2, the mean surface Po_2 values varied between 110-370 Torr. In initial Pco_2 measurements the surface Pco_2 was about 7 Torr, when the Guinea pig heart was perfused with an air-equilibrated perfusion medium. 30 minutes after the perfusion was stopped the Pco_2 rose to about 30 Torr. However, it should be emphacized that the experiments were performed to investigate the applicability of the optode to tissue measurements. It could be shown that the indicator concentration could be made sufficiently high, so that no influence of the tissues on the excitation spectra was observable. The signal-to-noise ratio was about 300:1. The sensitivity was sufficient to cover a Po_2 range between 0-400 Torr and a Pco_2 range between 1-80 Torr.

References

Boldt, M. (1971) Dissertation Marburg/Lahn

Knopp, J. A. and Longmuir, I. S. (1972) Biochim. Biophys. Acta, 279, 393

Langendorff, O. (1895) Pflüg. Arch. 61, 6, 291-332

Lübbers, D. W. and Opitz, N. (1975) Z. Naturforsch. 30c, 532

Lübbers, D. W. and Opitz, N. (1976) In "Oxygen Transport to Tissue - II" (eds. Thews, G., Grote, J., Reneau, D. D.) Plenum Publ. Corp. New York

Opitz, N. and Lübbers, D. W. (1975) Pflüg. Arch. 355, Suppl. 1975, p. R120

Stern, O. and Volmer, M. (1919) Physikal. Z. 20, 183

Vaughan, W. M. and Weber, G. (1970) Biochem. 9, 464

A NEW METHOD FOR MEASURING THE OXYGEN CONTENT IN MICRO-LITER SAMPLES OF GASES AND LIQUIDS: THE OXYGEN CUVETTE

R. Zander, W. Lang, and H. U. Wolf[+]

Inst. of Physiology, Mainz University, and

Dept. of Pharmacology[+],Ulm University, F.R.G.

Gas analytical processes for the determination of oxygen content or concentration are based partly on physical principles (e.g. mass spectrometry, gas chromatography, paramagnetic methods) and partly on chemical methods (e.g. gasometric, titrimetric, electrochemical or photometric methods).

In 1976, Wolf et al. described an experimental arrangement for a simple and precise photometric determination of oxygen with very high sensitivity. This method was modified to the so-called oxygen cuvette (ZANDER et al., 1977).

Principle

The principle of this method is the colour reaction between oxygen and an alkaline catechol solution containing Fe^{2+} ions. The sample to be analyzed is brought into contact with this reaction solution in a closed cuvette and the resulting increase in absorbance is measured in a photometer at a wavelength of 490 nm. The absorbance of the cuvette is proportional to the oxygen content within the cuvette.

Production

The oxygen cuvette is prepared inside an oxygen free glove box by filling 2.5 ml of the reaction solution into a cylindrical glass cuvette (light path about 9 mm). The cuvette is filled up with pure nitrogen and closed by an airtight membrane with a screw cap.

Measurement procedures

The gaseous or liquid sample of which the oxygen content is to be measured is injected by a precision syringe through the membrane into the cuvette. If a liquid sample is injected a correction factor in relation to dilution must be considered (e.g. in the case of 10 μl a value of 0.4 %). If the sample, e.g. in the case of blood, is coloured, the measured absorbance difference must be compared with a blank value. The blank value is calculated from a cuvette which is filled with the same quantity of liquid but without the reagents used for the oxygen test. In the case of blood, the blank value of absorbance, which is proportional to the Hb concentration, has to be subtracted from the measured value. Measurement of absorbance can be carried out between 30 seconds and some hours after injection of the sample.

Calibration

The cuvette is calibrated by injection of 10 μl of a 5 mM potassium iodate solution with a precision syringe. Physically dissolved oxygen in this solution is eliminated by equilibration with pure nitrogen for a short time. The solution yields 1.5 moles of oxygen per mole of iodate, i.e. 1.681 μl of oxygen corresponds to 10 μl of the standard solution.

KIO_3 for use in calibration has the advantage of being commercially available as a primary standard with a high degree of purity and of being fairly stable in aqueous solution (the absorbance is corrected by 0.4 % for dilution).

Using 46 cuvettes of the same production series, the injection of 10 μl of this standard solution three times into each cuvette results in an increase of absorbance of 0.283 per 1 μl of oxygen (STPD) (n = 138).

This calibration factor is a very constant one for cuvettes of different production series.

Linearity between absorbance and oxygen content

30 cuvettes were tested in relation to the question of linearity between oxygen content and absorbance. To this end, 10 μl of air were injected many times into the cuvettes. The results are shown in Fig. 1. Obviously, the proportionality between oxygen content (corrected to STPD conditions) and absorbance holds up to an absorbance of about 1.5; above this value a slight decrease of 3 % at an absorbance of 2.0 has been found.

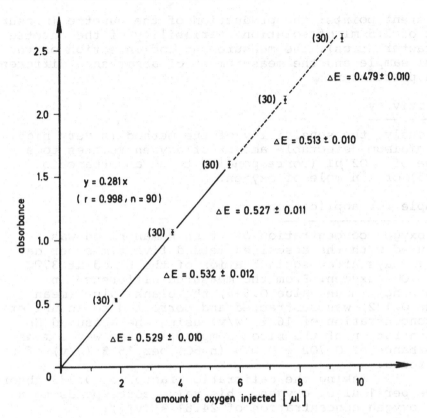

Fig. 1: Absorbance as a function of the amount of oxygen
(μl, STPD) injected five times into each of 30
cuvettes.

Accuracy

In Fig. 1, the accuracy of the described method is
also demonstrated. The mean value of 90 measurements of
oxygen content in air (corrected to STPD conditions) is
0.281 absorbance per 1 μl of oxygen. In comparison with
the calibration value of 0.283 absorbance per 1 μl of
oxygen, an accuracy of 1 % is attained.

Reproducibility

The reproducibility of the measurement of oxygen
content or concentration by the oxygen cuvette is ± 2 %
of the measured value. This has also been tested by
injection of 10 μl of air into 30 cuvettes as can be
seen in Fig. 1. This reproducibility includes many

different points: the production of the cuvette (measurement of 2.5 ml of solution, variability of the cuvette
characteristics), the measurement and injection of the
10 µl sample and the measurement of absorbance difference
in a photometer.

Sensitivity

Obviously, the sensitivity of the method is very high.
The minimum detectable amount of oxygen relates to a
value of 0.02 µl (corresponding to an absorbance of
0.005) or 1 n mole of oxygen.

Example for application

The oxygen concentration of fresh human blood was
measured with the described method five times per day
for 10 days after equilibration of the blood at 37°C
with 100% oxygen. From the measured difference in
absorbance (mean value 0.648) the blank value (mean
value 0.122) was subtracted and corrected to an uniform
Hb concentration of 16 % (w/v) using the measured Hb
concentration of the blood sample. In this way a mean
absorbance of 0.702 $\pm$ 0.019 (n=50) per 16 % (w/v) of Hb
was found.

Taking the calibration factor of 0.283 absorbance per 1 µl of oxygen, this value corresponds to a
mean oxygen concentration of 24.81 % (v/v).

The true oxygen concentration for fresh human
blood with an Hb concentration of 16 % (w/v) should be
24.36 % (v/v) at an oxygen partial pressure of 700 mmHg,
taking into account a Hüfner factor of 1.36 ml oxygen
per 1 g of Hb and an oxygen solubility for fresh human
blood of 0.0282 ml/ml atm (ZANDER et al., unpublished
data).

The difference between the expected and the
measured value amounts to 1.8 %.

Conclusions

For scientific research as well as for clinical
medicine the advantages of the described method are
obvious:

1) The determination of oxygen content in a microliter
    sample is possible within one minute with high
    accuracy (1-2%) and reproducibility (2%).

2) The measurement is extremely simple to carry out:
injection by a precision syringe, shaking, reading
of the absorbance.
3) The oxygen determination is possible in both gases
and liquids.
4) When measuring the oxygen content of a liquid sample,
extraction or elution of the gas from the liquid
phase can be dispensed with.
5) Due to the presence of an alkaline medium in the
cuvette, all cells and membranes undergo lysis and,
therefore, measurement of oxygen can be carried out
also in those biological liquids in which the oxygen
concentration would be greatly altered by respiration
of the material.
6) A sample of only 10 - 100 µl is necessary, e.g. in
the case of blood (10 µl) the sample can be taken
from the ear lobe or the scalp in infants.
7) Measurement of the oxygen concentration can be
carried out in a mobile unit if a portable,
battery-operated photometer is used, e.g. the
diagnosis of oxygen concentration of human blood
can be carried out on the spot, in emergency and
accident cases (medical ambulances) in diving, air
travel and space travel medicine (submarines,
aircraft) and in sports and industrial medicine.

References
WOLF,H.U., ZANDER,R., LANG,W.: An automated continuous
determination of oxygen with high sensitivity.
Anal. Biochem. 74, 585-591 (1976)

ZANDER,R., LANG,W., WOLF,H.U.: Oxygen cuvette: a simple
approach to the oxygen concentration
measurement in blood.
Pflügers Arch. 368, R 16 (1977)

FACTORS INFLUENCING THE CORRECTION FACTOR USED TO ELIMINATE THE APPARENT NADH FLUORESCENCE CHANGES CAUSED BY ALTERATIONS IN CEREBROCORTICAL BLOOD CONTENT

E. Dóra and A.G.B. Kovách

Experimental Research Department
Semmelweis Medical University
Budapest, Hungary

The so-called blood flow artifact is a serious challenge to the interpretation of in vivo NADH fluorometry (Chance et al., 1962; Harbig et al., 1976; Jöbsis et al., 1971). The apparent NADH fluorescence changes induced by alterations in blood content can be avoided by the method of Harbig et al. (1976), which is based on the artificial dilution of the cerebrocortical blood. As yet the analysis of the different factors which might influence the value of the correction factor (k) has not been done systematically and the purpose of the present study was to summarize our experimental results in this respect.

METHODS

The experiments were performed on 30 cats anaesthetized with 60 mg/kg α-D glucochloralose, immobilized by 2-4 mg/kg gallamine-thiethyl-iodide and artificially respired. For the NADH fluorescence and reflectance measurements a micro-fluoro-reflectometer was used. The correction factor was determined by injection of 0.1 - 0.3 ml oxygen-saturated saline into the lingual artery. The 'k' changes were investigated in the following conditions: at different illumination angles, during haemorrhagic shock and graded arterial hypotension before and during electrical stimulation of the cerebral cortex. The parameters of the stimulation were 10 V, 0.5 msec and 15 Hz. Haemorrhagic shock was induced by bleeding the animals via the femoral artery into a buffer-reservoir system. As 30-35 mmHg MABP was reached this arterial blood pressure level was maintained until 50-70% of the shed blood returned spontaneously into the animals. After this the shed blood remaining in the reservoir was reinfused. In case of graded arterial hypotention

the arterial blood pressure was decreased from the control level in
a stepwise fashion to 80, 60 and 40 mmHg.   Each arterial blood
pressure step was maintained for 25-30 min.   After the hypotensive
periods the shed blood was reinfused into the animals.

RESULTS

In the first series of experiments the cerebral cortex was
illuminated through an Ultropak of 6.5 with illumination angles of
90° and 54° respectively.   The cortex was stimulated at both.
angles and the correction factor was determined before and during
stimulation.

Electrical stimulation of the cortex caused an increase in
fluorescence of equal extent at both angles but the stimulation-

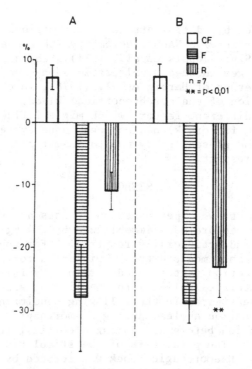

Fig. 1. Effect of electrical stimulation of the cerebral cortex on
the cortical corrected NADH fluorescence (CF %), NADH
fluorescence (F %) and reflectance (R %) with the 6.5
Ultropak at an illumination angle of 90° (1A) and of 54°
(1B).   The vertical lines closed at both ends on the
columns represent the ± SEM.   The number of the
experiments marked by n, the degree of the significance
by asterisks.

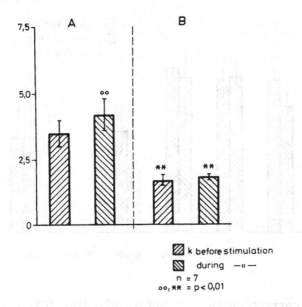

Fig. 2. The correction factors for the same experiments as in
        Fig. 1 before and during cortical electrical stimulation at
        90° and 54° illumination angles.   The degree of significant
        changes between the correction factors determined before
        and during stimulation is marked by o.   The degree of
        significant changes between the correction factors
        determined at an illumination angle of 90° (2A) and of 54°
        (2B) is marked by asterisks.

induced reflectance decrease was significantly greater at 54° than
of 90° (Fig. 1).

     One can see in Fig. 2 that the correction factor decreased
significantly when the illumination angle was decreased from 90°
(Fig. 2A) to 54° (Fig. 2B).   Furthermore electrical stimulation
of the cortex significantly increased the value of 'k' as compared
to the value before stimulation (Fig. 2A).

     In the second series of experiments the cortex was illuminated
perpendicularly with an Ultropak of 11.   The correction factor
which was determined in the control period before electrical
stimulation of the cortex (Fig. 3) was much smaller than when the
cortex was excited with a 6.5 Ultropak (Fig. 2A).   From the results
listed above it is concluded that the value of the correction factor
is greatly influenced by the extent of the cerebrocortical mirror
reflectance.   If more mirror reflectance is measured 'k' is greater
as compared to its value when less mirror reflectance is measured.

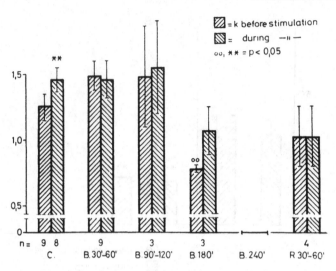

Fig. 3. The correction factors before bleeding (C), during bleeding
       (B) and after reinfusion (R).   In these experiments the
       cerebral cortex was illuminated through an Ultropak 11
       with an illumination angle of 90°.   The degree of the
       significant changes between the correction factors
       determined before and during stimulation is marked by
       asterisks.   The degree of the significant changes in the
       correction factors as compared to the control (C) values
       is marked by o.

    Another important factor which might influence the value of
the correction factor is the integrity of the cerebrocortical
capillary network.

    Kovách et al (1976) showed that haemorrhagic shock leads to a
gradual decrease and finally to the cessation of the cerebrocortical blood flow.   It can be seen in Fig. 3 that when serious
flow disturbances begin the value of the correction factor
decreases significantly (B.180') as compared to its value before
bleeding.

    In the third series of experiments the cortex was excited
through the 6.5 Ultropak with an illumination angle of 54°.   The
graded decrease of arterial blood pressure shifted the cerebrocortical NAD-NADH redox state towards reduction (Kovách et al.,

this volume).   Electrical stimulation of the cortex in the control
period resulted in an increase in corrected NADH fluorescence
which was replaced by a decrease in corrected NADH fluorescence
during arterial hypotension (Fig. 4).   Fig. 5 shows the values of
'k' before and during stimulation in the control period, at 80, 60,
40 mm Hg MABP and after reinfusion.   It can be seen that the value
of the correction factor is greatly influenced by the direction of
the NAD-NADH redox change.   The arterial hypotension which shifted
the cortical NAD-NADH redox state towards reduction resulted in a
significant increase in the value of 'k'.   Electrical stimulation
of the cortex in arterial hypotension which caused oxidation of
NADH decreased the value of the correction factor, as compared to
its value before stimulation.

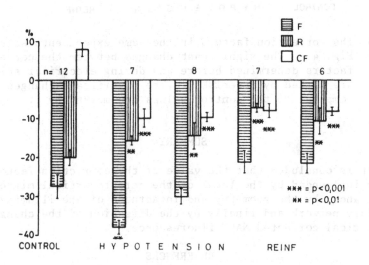

Fig. 4. Effect of cortical electrical stimulation on the corrected
        NADH fluorescence (CF %), NADH fluorescence (F %) and
        reflectance (R %) in the control period, at 80, 60, and
        40 mm Hg MABP levels and after reinfusion (REINF.).   In
        these experiments the cortex was illuminated through an
        ultrapak 6, 5 at an illumination angle of 54°.   The degree
        of the significant changes as compared to the control
        values is marked by asterisks.

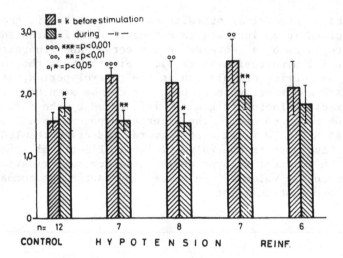

Fig. 5. The correction factors in the same experiments as shown in
Fig. 4.   The significant changes between the correction
factors determined before and during electrical stimulation
are marked by asterisks.   The significant changes as
compared to the control values are marked by o.

SUMMARY

It is concluded that the value of the correction factor is
vastly influenced by the level of the cerebrocortical mirror
reflectance, by the geometry and intactness of the illuminated
capillary network and finally by the direction of the changes in
the cortical corrected NADH fluorescence.

REFERENCES

Chance, B., Cohen, P., Jöbsis, F., Schoener, B. (1962)   Science
137, 499.

Harbig, K., Chance, B., Kovách, A.G.B., Reivich, M.   (1976)
J. Appl. Physiol. 41, 480.

Jöbsis, F.F., O'Connor, M., Vitale, A., Vreman, H.   (1971)
J. Neurophysiol. 34, 735.

Kovách, A.G.B., Dóra, E., Gyulai, L., Eke, A.   (1976)   Fed. Proc.
35, 526.

Kovách, A.G.B., Dóra, E., Hamar, J., Eke, A., Szabó, L.   (1977)
This volume.

ORGAN ABSORBANCE AND FLUORESCENCE SPECTROPHOTOMETRY AND ITS APPLICATION TO OXYGEN-DEPENDENT PARAMETERS

Helmut Sies and Helmut Schwab

Institut für Physiologische Chemie, Physikalische Bio-

chemie und Zellbiologie der Universität München, Germany

The application of absorbance--in contrast to reflectance--spectrophotometry to solid tissues such as the intact isolated perfused rat liver(Brauser, 1968) has opened possibilities of the detection of O_2-dependent enzyme intermediates and cytochromes in the spectral region now extending from the near-infrared to the ultraviolet. Thus, by directing light of appropriate wavelengths to a lobe of perfused liver and measuring light transmitted through the tissue, considerable information has been accumulated in recent years by application of organ absorbance spectrophotometry(see below).

While the early investigations in our group have been carried out with a modified Rapidspektroskop of Niesel et al(1964) that previously had been successfully applied to the perfused organ for reflectance photometry of cytochromes in the alpha-band region(Schnitger et al, 1965), the apparatus used in measurements on the perfused organ by Chance's group at the Johnson Research Foundation in Philadelphia was a modified time-sharing organ fluorometer(Theorell et al, 1972; Chance et al, 1975).

We have designed and constructed an organ spectrophotometer and fluorometer that combines advantages of such photometers. The apparatus has been successfully applied with the perfused liver and with suspensions of isolated hepatocytes since a few years(Sies et al, 1974; Sies & Großkopf, 1975). Due to its usefulness in applications related to the topic of this conference on oxygen transport to tissue(see Sies, this volume), we find it appropriate to briefly describe the apparatus. A general scheme of its arrangement in conjunction with the perfusion system is given in Fig.1.

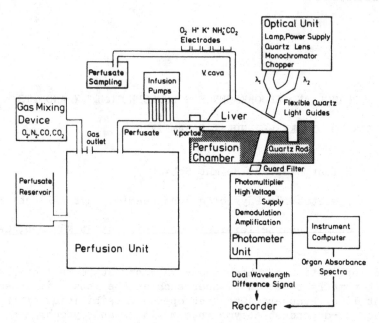

Fig.1. Schematic representation of organ spectrophotometer setup
in conjunction with the system of perfused liver.

DESIGN OF ORGAN SPECTROPHOTOMETER

Optical Unit

Illumination is provided by two interchangeable light sources.
For measurement from 340-750 nm the source is a 100 W tungsten lamp,
whereas from 200-400 nm a 150 W xenon lamp is used. The lamps are
placed in an air-cooled lamp housing and provide light of sufficient
intensity and stability. The light passes through a Farrand grating
monochromator. The monochromator exit is either one slit or a pair
of neighboring slits to provide either one beam or two beams of selectable wavelength difference, the difference being 10, 15, 20, 30,
40 or 50 nm; the slit width can be 1, 3 or 5 nm. The wavelength
may be scanned by driving the monochromator grating with a step mo-
tor(0.25 nm/step) with scan speeds selectable in the range between
0.05 and 16 nm/sec.

The two light beams of different wavelength are collected by
two arms of a branched flexible light guide after passing through a
chopper disc. The common light path is formed by a solid quartz rod
of 8 mm diameter. A small heating coil at the end of the rod brings
its temperature slightly above the $37^{\circ}C$ of the perfused organ in order to avoid moisture condensation. The rod is positioned to direct

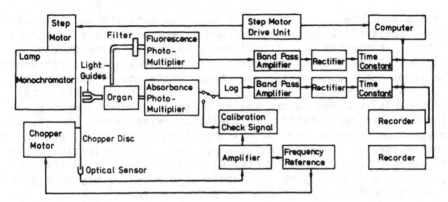

Fig.2. Block diagram of organ spectrophotometer and fluorometer.

the light through the liver lobe(Fig.1), and the transmitted light
is collected by another quartz rod from beneath the liver and directed to an end-on photomultiplier after passing through appropriate
guard filters. The photomultipliers are EMI 9592B in the visible
spectral region, and EMI 9601B in the ultraviolet.

Photometer Unit

The electronics is designed to allow for either dual-wavelength
reading or spectral scanning.

Dual-wavelength mode. A double slit is used at the monochromator exit. According to the chopper frequency of 120 Hz, the anode
current of the photomultiplier tube represents adjacent rectangular
pulses corresponding to the alternating light intensities I_1 and I_2
of the two wavelengths 1 and 2. Since the signal is fed into a log
amplifier(Fig.2), the peak-to-peak amplitude of the resulting square
wave is equal to $\log I_1 - \log I_2 = \log(I_1/I_2) = \Delta A$, i.e. the absorbance difference between the two wavelengths. The signal is further
processed by a narrow-band amplifier for elimination of hum and
noise(suppression of line frequency harmonics better than 30 dB) and
rectification before serving as an output for a strip chart recorder.
A damping network allows for time constants of 0.3, 1 or 5 sec.
Because of the narrow bandwidth of the amplifier(10 Hz between 3 dB
points), the chopper frequency is stabilized by feedback control.
From the feedback system, a reference signal is derived which serves
for ready checking of the calibration of the apparatus.

Spectral scanning mode. A single slit is employed at the monochromator exit, so that illumination of the object now alternates
between light energy at the selected wavelength and zero energy.

The log amplifier is placed after the time constant block in this mode. Spectral sweeps are performed by means of a step motor so that the photometer output delivers a signal of absorbance as a function of wavelength, containing the spectral characteristics of the lamp, the monochromator and other components of the optical system. In the presence of the organ in the light path, the total spectrum is recorded in the memory of an instrument computer and stored(12 bit resolution). Following an experimental change, another spectrum representing the new condition is recorded, and the difference spectrum between this new spectrum and the initial(reference) spectrum is obtained by digital subtraction. The difference spectrum may be viewed on the screen of a scope or may be plotted by an xy-recorder. An example is given in Fig.3.

Light attenuation in the liver lobe is of the order of 10^2 to 10^6 in the red and ultraviolet, respectively. Nevertheless, the apparatus described here provides a signal of sufficiently low noise even in the ultraviolet region(Sies et al, 1974) so that single slow scans proved adequate. Thus, in routine use with the perfused organ, sweep speed is 1-2 nm/sec and spectra are usually scanned twice to ensure steady state conditions. This is adequate, since the transition time of the organ is of the order of 10 sec.

Organ spectrofluorometer. As the relative fluorescence yield of compounds provides information e.g. on their state of binding, recording of fluorescence intensity emitted from the surface of the organ at the site of the incident light is a useful addition. As indicated in Fig.2, a flexible light guide is used to feed fluorescence intensity to a second photometer unit after passing appropriate cut-off filters, allowing for the simultaneous recording of fluorescence and absorbance, either in the dual-wavelength mode or the spectral scanning mode.

Since its introduction in a single-wavelength setup by Chance & Jöbsis(1959), the surface fluorescence of pyridine nucleotides has been monitored from a variety of organs. Studies on the enhancement of pyridine nucleotide fluorescence in liver have been performed (Bücher et al, 1972; Sies et al, 1974), and striking differences became evident in metabolic transitions involving the mitochondrial and cytosolic compartments. In other words, transitions comprising similar changes of reduced pyridine nucleotides in terms of nmol/g tissue may be represented by largely different changes in fluorescence intensity.

PERFORMANCE OF ORGAN SPECTROPHOTOMETER

Due to the special requirements of photometry of solid tissue, the main objectives in designing the instrument were low noise (to

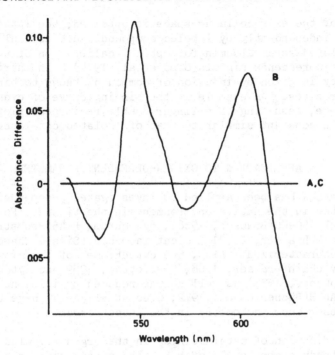

Fig.3. Liver absorbance difference spectrum 2 min after addition of
0.8 mM NaCN to perfusate(B).   Control spectra before and after are
shown as (A) and (C).   Signal corresponds to approx. 20x10⁶ cells.

detect small experimental changes in the presence of high basal absorbance)and high stability(to allow for prolonged experimental periods) in a compact and readily accessible setup.   Actual noise is
approx. 0.001 A when light attenuation cause by the organ is 4-5 A.
Stability was achieved by a stable mechanical design and by using a
common channel(time-sharing) in dual-wavelength monitoring.   Drift
is of the order of 0.001 A/hr; sporadically, spontaneous spikes due
to arc instabilities were encountered with the xenon lamp. In spectral scanning in the presence of the organ, drift is higher than
without an object, particularly in the blue or ultraviolet.   This is
due to slight shifts in the position of the organ on the perfusion
table.   Such baseline drift is observed as parallel(not inclined)
lines in the difference spectrum in the absence of any metabolic changes; usually, this drift also is negligible.

Calibration.   A check of the calibration of the instrument is
performed as mentioned above.   A special problem in measurement with
the organ, however, is the calibration of a measured change in terms
of optical pathlength, or ultimately of nmol/g tissue.   A solution to
this problem is given by the use of absorbent(and for fluorescence
yields, also fluorescent)compounds known to be non-penetrant, so that

a measure of the extracellular space is obtained; the latter may be determined independently by labeled compounds such as inulin. We have used dansylated serum albumin for optical calibration of the absorbance and fluorescence signals(Sies et al, 1974). An intrinsic check of linearity is given by infusion of compounds known to bind to intracellular sites. An example is the binding curve of cyanide to catalase heme, resulting in a linear double reciprocal plot and a dissociation constant similar to that of isolated catalase(Sies et al, 1973).

APPLICATION TO OXYGEN-DEPENDENT PARAMETERS

The method has been applied to investigate O_2-dependent enzyme intermediates in the native environment in the tissue. For example, cytochrome P-450-CO(Brauser, 1968), cytochrome P-450-substrate complexes(Sies & Brauser, 1970) and catalase-H_2O_2(Sies & Chance, 1970) have been characterized. Also, the cytochromes of the mitochondrial respiratory chain(Brauser, 1968; Sies et al, 1969)and cytochrome b_5 (Sies & Großkopf, 1975) as well as the reduced pyridine nucleotides NADH and NADPH(Bücher et al, 1972; Sies et al, 1974) have been measured by absorbance photometry in the intact organ.

Identification of catalase-H_2O_2 in the organ revealed the existence of steady state levels of H_2O_2, and steady state analysis allowed a calculation of the rate of H_2O_2 formation(Oshino et al,1973) even in the intact anaesthetized animal(Oshino et al, 1975a). Further, the method allowed a comparison of kinetic properties of catalase in situ with those in vitro, over an approx. 1000-fold concentration difference(Sies et al, 1973). More recently, the properties under different degrees of oxygenation have been analyzed(Oshino et al, 1975b; Sies, 1977), and the use of such O_2-dependent parameters as O_2 concentration indicators in different subcellular compartments may provide new tools in the study of intracellular and intercellular O_2 concentration profiles(for further discussion, see Sies, this volume).

Acknowledgements

Thanks are extended to Th.Bücher and B.Brauser for discussions on optical problems, and to H.Strobel, H.Erk and K.Metzner for their excellent electronic and mechanic work. Supported by Deutsche Forschungsgemeinschaft, SFB 51, Grants D/8 and F/1.

REFERENCES

Brauser, B.(1968) Z.analyt.Chem.237,8

Bücher, Th, Brauser, B., Conze, A., Klein, F., Langguth, O. & Sies, H.(1972) Eur.J.Biochem. 27,301

Chance, B. & Jöbsis, F.F.(1959) Nature 184, 195

Chance, B., Legallais, V., Sorge, J. & Graham, N.(1975) Anal. Biochem. 66, 498

Niesel, W., Lübbers, D.W., Schneewolf, D., Richter, J. & Botticher, W.(1964) Rev.Sci.Instr. 35, 578

Oshino, N., Chance, B., Sies, H. & Bücher, Th.(1973) Arch.Biochem. Biophys. 154, 117

Oshino, N., Jamieson, D., Sugano, T. & Chance, B.(1975a) Biochem. J. 146, 67

Oshino, N., Jamieson, D. & Chance, B.(1975b)Biochem.J. 146, 53

Schnitger, H., Scholz, R., Bücher, Th. & Lübbers, D.W.(1965) Biochem.Z. 341,334

Sies, H.(1977) in 'Tissue Hypoxia and Ischemia' p.51(eds. Reivich, M., Coburn, R., Lahiri, S. & Chance, B.) Plenum Press, New York

Sies, H., Brauser, B., Bücher, Th.(1969)FEBS Lett. 5, 319

Sies, H. & Brauser, B.(1970) Eur.J.Biochem. 15, 531

Sies, H. & Chance, B.(1970) FEBS Lett. 11, 172

Sies, H., Bücher, Th., Oshino, N. & Chance, B.(1973) Arch.Biochem. Biophys. 146, 106

Sies, H., Häussinger, D. & Großkopf, M.(1974) Hoppe-Seyler's Z. physiol.Chem. 355, 305

Sies, H. & Großkopf, M.(1975) Eur.J.Biochem. 57, 513

Theorell, H., Chance, B., Yonetani, T. & Oshino, N.(1972) Arch. Biochem.Biophys. 151, 434

AN EXPERIMENTAL MODEL OF THE KROGH TISSUE CYLINDER:

TWO DIMENSIONAL QUANTITATION OF THE OXYGEN GRADIENT

Bjørn Quistorff,* Britton Chance, and Axel Hunding**

Johnson Research Foundation, University of Pennsylvania
*Department of Biochemistry A, Panum Institute
**Institute of Chemistry, Faculty of Medicine, University
of Copenhagen

We have observed very steep regional redox ratio transitions
In Vivo in various tissues (1,2,3,4). The most obvious example
beeing the transition across the borderline of an ischemic area as
first described by *Barlow and Chance* for an artificially produced
infarct in a rat heart (5). We believe that the steep redox state
transition may reflect similarly steep tissue oxygen gradients (6)
and in order to probe that we have devised a simple model in which
the ischemic borderzone in terms of oxygen gradient can be reproduced. The model is essentially a *Krogh Tissue Cylinder* (7) in macro scale, approximately 1:200, where the oxygen concentration
profile perpendicular to the capillary may be recorded photographically in two dimensions. The model allows for independent variation of capillary oxygen tension, tissue oxygen consumption rate and
facilitation of oxygen diffusion.

As oxygen indicator we have used Photobacterium Phosphoreum[x].
Suspended in a hyperosmotic medium these bacteria will emit a green
luminescence when oxygen is present as shown in Fig. 1 which is
taken from *Sugano, Oshino and Chance* (8). The figure gives the
relative luminescence intensity versus oxygen concentration in the
medium. Saturation is achieved at rather low oxygen concentrations,
approximately 1 μM which corresponds to 0.75 Torr. 10% luminescence intensity is reached at an oxygen concentration about two
orders of magnitude lower. Thus, the photobacteria is an excellent

[x] The bacteria was kindly provided by Dr. Y. Nakase.

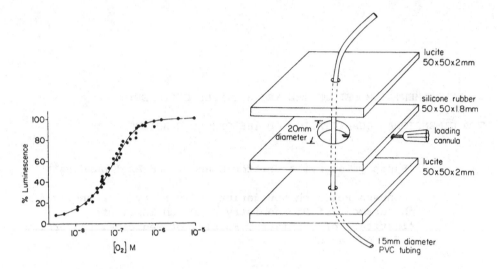

Fig. 1 (left). Relation between luminescence intensity of Photobacterium Phosphoreum and oxygen concentration. *Taken from T. Sugano, N. Oshino and B.Chance* (8).

Fig. 2 (right). Schematic diagram of the macro model of *The Krogh
tissue Cylinder* (1). See text for further details.

indicator of oxygen concentration in the region of Km for oxygen
for isolated mitochondria (8-10) Luminescence intensity which may
be recorded photographically is therefore a convenient measure of
respiratory activity in response to oxygen concentration.

Our model of the *Krogh Cylinder* is shown schematically in
Fig 2. Two plexiglas plates spaced by a silicone rubber membrane
in which a circular hole has been punched out from the chamber.
An axially located PVC tube runs through the chamber. The suspension of the Photobacteria containing 4% gelatine is introduced
into the chamber via the syringe needles and allowed to form a gel.
When the gel is stable, which it becomes after 10-15 min in the
refrigerator, the PVC tube may be pulled out leaving a perfect
channel in the gel. This channel constitutes the capillary of the
macro *Krogh Cylinder* through which oxygen is supplied as a gas.
Mitochondria and suitable substrates as well as myoglobin may be
added to the gelatine suspension prior to injection into the chamber in order to vary oxygen consumption rate or facilitate oxygen

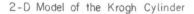

2-D Model of the Krogh Cylinder

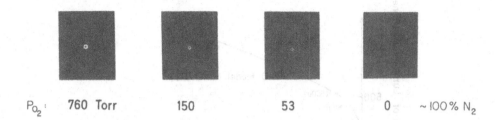

P_{O_2}:   760 Torr   150   53   0   ~100% N_2

Fig. 3. Photographic recording of luminescence intensity of Photobacterium Phosphoreum in the chamber shown in Fig. 2. Bacteria (4
mg wet weight/ml) was suspended in hyperosmotic medium (0.5 M NaCl,
0.1 M Na_2HPO_4, 10 mM glucose) with 4% gelatine. Polaroid film
(3000 Type 107) exposed for 2.5 min at f-stop 4.5. Image: object
ratio was 0.9:1.

diffusion in the gel respectively. Oxygen will diffuse from the
capillary into the gel and at steady state the bright luminescence
zone will indicate the area around the capillary with oxygen tension above approximately 0.5 Torr. The luminescence zone is recorded photographically through one of the plexiglass plates with the
optical axis of the camera aligned with the capillary.

     Steady state recordings of the luminescence zone at 4 diffe-
rent values of capillary oxygen tension are shown in Fig. 3. The
composition of the bacteria suspension is given in the figure legend. The oxygen/nitrogen gas mixtures were flushed through the capillary at a rate of 1 l/min, there was therefore no intra capillary oxygen gradient present. Oxygen consumption rate was calculated to 0.03 µmol/min x ml based on the time period elapsing from
an instantaneous oxygen/nitrogen transition in the capillary until
complete disappearance   of the luminescence. This estimate will
of course represent a maximum value because some oxygen will escape consumption in the gel by diffusing back into the capillary.
There are two interesting observations to be made from Fig 3 .
First, the borderzone transitions appear to be as sharp as the redox ratio changes we observe In Vivo, even with the much lower oxygen consumption rate of the model experiments. Second, a non-linear relationship exists between capillary oxygen tension and width
of the luminescence zone as also shown in Fig. 4.

     On this basis we decided to calculate the exact location and
steepness of the luminescence transition. The distance required

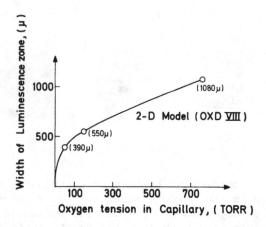

Fig. 4. Relation between width of luminescence zone and capillary oxygen tension. The width of the luminescence zone was recorded microdensitometrically with an accuracy of ±50 μ. Points of 50% intensity (≡ I_{50}) in the transition from luminescence to non-luminescence zone were taken as border lines in estimating the width.

for a decrease of luminescence intensity from 80% to 20% is taken as a measure of the steepness of the transition - in terms of isolated mitochondria that would be approximately the distance over which a 'full function/no function' transition would occur. The following equation describes oxygen diffusion for the circular geometry of our model:

$$\frac{\partial C}{\partial t} = D\left[\frac{\partial^2 C}{\partial r^2} + \frac{1}{r}\frac{\partial C}{\partial r}\right] - k_1 \frac{k_2 \, C^n}{k_3^n + C^n} \tag{I}$$

and at steady state

$$\frac{\partial^2 C}{\partial r^2} + \frac{1}{r}\frac{\partial C}{\partial r} = \frac{k_1 k_2}{D} \frac{C^n}{k_3^n + C^n} \equiv K \frac{C^n}{k_3^n + C^n} \tag{II}$$

D is diffusion constant for oxygen, k_1 is oxygen consumption rate, k_2 is the proportionality constant between oxygen consumption rate and luminescence intensity for a particular concentration of bacteria, k_3^n is K_m for oxygen for luminescence emission, n is the Hill coefficient, C is oxygen concentration and r the variable radius in the *Krogh Cylinder*. Values of 0.067 Torr and 1.5 may be obtained from Fig. 1 for k_3^n and n respectively.

For $C^n \gg k_3^n$ (II) has the following solution, as found by *Erlang*

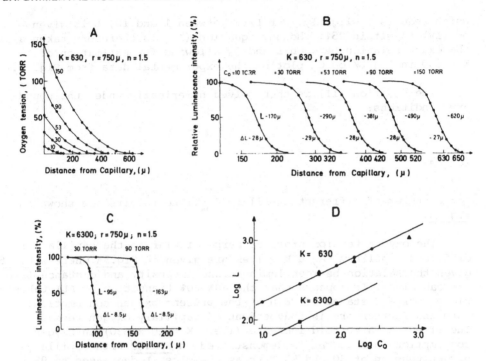

Fig. 5. A: Computer calculated oxygen tension profiles perpendicular to the capillary. B: Computer calculated luminescence intensity
profiles showing the transition zone at 5 different capillary P_{O_2}
at an oxygen consumption rate of 0.03 μmol/min x ml. C: Same as
B but calculated for a 10 times higher oxygen consumption rate at
capillary P_{O_2} of 30 and 90 Torr. D: The values for L and C_o plotted in a log/log diagram. ● is data from Fig. 5B, ■ from Fig.5C
and ▲ the experimentel data from Fig. 4. See text for further details.

$$C = C_0 - \alpha \ln \frac{r}{r_0} + \frac{K}{4} (r^2 - r_0^2) \qquad\qquad (III)$$

with r_o radius of the capillary. For C= 0, $\frac{dc}{dr}$ = 0 and r = R
radius of the *Krogh Cylinder*: $\alpha = \frac{K}{2} R^2$. With L defined as the
width of the luminescence zone, i.e., L ≡ $r - r_0$, (III) gives
for L << r_0

$$L \simeq \sqrt{\frac{2C_0}{K}} \qquad\qquad (IV)$$

For L >> r_0, (IV) is again obtained but with a correction factor which reduces L slightly. For L/r_0 between 1 and 10, L is given by (IV) to within 25%, though. Equation (IV) is therefore taken as the exact relation between L and C_0 allowing for estimation of K = 630 in log L/log C_o plot of the experimental data from Fig. 4.

The equation (II) is then solved numerically under the boundary conditions:

$$c = c_0, \quad r = r_0$$

$$\frac{dc}{dr} \rightarrow 0, \quad c \rightarrow 0$$

for a number of different capillary P_{O_2}. The results are shown in Fig. 5.

The oxygen tension profiles perpendicular to the capillary for different capillary P_{O_2} & K values are given in Fig.5A whereas Fig.5B gives the relation between luminescence intensity and distance from the capillary. It appears that the 80%-20% transition ($\equiv \Delta L$) takes place over a distance of 28 μ at the present oxygen consumption rate and furthermore is independent of capillary oxygen tension. The effect of a 10 fold increase (i.e., K = 10 x 630) in oxygen consumption on L and ΔL is demonstrated in Fig.5C with capillary oxygen tension of 30 and 90 Torr as examples. L decreases to 95 μ and 163 μ for 30 Torr and 90 Torr respectively, whereas ΔL decreases to 8.5 μ. In Fig. 5D the calculated L values of Fig. 5B and 5C are plotted together with the experimental data in a log/log plot of L versus C_0. In agreement with equation (IV) a slope close to 0.5 as well as a reasonable fit to the experimental data is obtained. A decrease in capillary diameter by two orders of magnitude to physiological dimensions (from the experimental 1500 μ to 8 μ) does not cause any change in the calculated ΔL. However, as may be predicted from equation (III), the width of the luminescence zone decreases, (from 163 μ to 106 μ, K = 6300, C_0 = 90 Torr). Finally, with physiological values for both oxygen consumption rate, 3 μmol/ min x ml, and capillary diameter, 8 μ, ΔL and L may be calculated to 2.7 μ and 33 μ respectively at a capillary oxygen tension of 90 Torr.

Even though the gelatine model is not directly comparable with the capillary unit In Vivo the present results indicate that anoxic zones may develop due to only a moderate decrease in arterial oxygen tension or to occlusion of single capillaries in a tissue with high oxygen consumption as for example brain where the average intercapillary distance is about 60 μ. Furthermore the results emphasize the point made by *Chance* (6) that the normoxic/anoxic transition in a tissue with high oxygen consumption can be expected to divide a single cell into a functional and a non-functional compartment.

References

1. Quistorff,B. and Chance,B. In 'Oxygen and Physiological Function' (F.F.Jöbsis ed.). Professional Information Library, Dallas.
   In Press.

2. Chance,B., Quistorff,B., Matschinsky,F., Mayevsky,A., Itsak,F.
   and Nakase,Y. This Meeting.

3. Quistorff,B. and Chance,B. Am. Physiol. Soc. Meet. Chicago 1977.
   Abstract 1358.

4. Quistorff,B., Barlow,C., and Chance,B. Biophys. Soc. Meet. New
   Orleans 1977. Abstract F-POS-P5.

5. Barlow,C. and Chance,B. Science, 193 p. 909 (1976).

6. Chance,B. Circulation Res. Suppl. I,38 p. 69 (1976).

7. Krogh,A. J. Physiol. 52 p. 409 (1918-1919).

8. Sugano,T., Oshino,N. and Chance,B. Biochem. Biophys. Acta 347
   p. 340 (1974).

9. Oshino,N., Sugano,T., Oshino,R. and Chance,B. Biochem. Biophys.
   Acta 368 p. 298 (1974).

10. Schindler, F. (1964). Oxygen Kinetics in the Cytochrome
    Oxidase-Oxygen Reaction PhD Dissertation. Univ. of Pennsylvania.

DISCUSSION OF PAPERS IN SESSION 2

CHAIRMEN DR. I. LONGMUIR and DR. D.W. LÜBBERS

PAPER BY: DR. LONGMUIR et al

Dr. Buerk: From your slides showing the CO_2 and the PO_2 profiles with distance based on quenching intensity, the apparent K_m appears to

be significantly higher than that indicated by PO_2 microelectrode profile measurements (Buerk and Longmuir, 1976 ISOTT Symposium) which give a K_m of 2.2 torr in liver (Buerk and Saidel, 1977 this Symposium) Can you comment on this difference?

Dr. Longmuir: I agree there is a discrepancy between the micro-electrode and the fluorescence measurements but there is some uncertainty in the PO_2 scale of this plot.

Dr. Chance: I presume that the sensitivity of the present instru-ment (as published in reference two) will be   7 mmHg = 10% change of fluorescence for the liver cell. A reference which is relevant to the   discussion describes the large variability in the penetration of BPA into single cells together with inhibition of glucose metabolism by the probe and should be taken note of in connection with the use of pyrene   butyric acid as a probe of oxygen distribution in single cells(see Kohen, E., Falmon, J.M., Kohen, C. and Bengtsson, G., (1974) Experimental cell research 89, 105-110).

PAPER BY: DRS; GAYESKI & HONIG

Dr. Meldon: With regard to your conclusion that there is no myoglobin-facilitated O_2 transport at rest, is the resolution of your technique sufficiently good to be capable of measuring the possibly very small areas of tissue that have a sufficiently low PO_2 to cause desaturation of myoglobin?

Note 1. Since the hyperbolic O_2-myoglobin dissociation curve is quite steep at low PO_2 it would be expected that most of the myoglobin would still be close to 100% saturated at these tensions.

    2. The location of importance is the <u>venous end</u> of tissue where PO_2 is lowest and the possibility of <u>facilitation</u> greatest.

<u>Dr. Honig</u>: Our technique is currently capable of measuring areas as small as 2 microns on each side so that areas of desaturation of this size can be detected. Of course, areas of desaturation smaller than this would be recorded as an average of the myoglobin saturation in the field.

We make our observations on cross-sections and cannot distinguish the location of our measurements along capillary length. With a sample of several hundred cells (not all reported here) we would have expected to have encountered some anoxic cells if capillary geometry influenced myoglobin saturation at rest.

PAPER BY: DR. TAMURA et al

<u>Dr. Kovách:</u> During the contraction phase of heart activity we know that there is a decrease in myocardial blood flow in the normal heart. May be in your isolated perfused hearts it was different. Did you measure phasic blood flow changes at the same time as the myoglobin oxygenation.

<u>Dr. Tamura</u>: I did not measure the blood flow (in this case perfusate flow) during one cycle of heart beat. I suppose it might be extremely difficult to measure the velocity of capillary flow (as apposed to venous outflow) with a few millisecond time resolution. I agree with you that our data conflicts with the well-known data of 'Contraction Ischaemia'. Here I would like to emphasise that present measurements demonstrate the extremely rapid increase of intracellular oxygen concentration during systole, though the mechanism is unknown. It must be noted that the decrease or cessation of coronary flow and decrease of intracellular oxygen concentration has to be differentiated especially from the kinetic viewpoint.

Model Systems

MULTI-CAPILLARY MODEL FOR OXYGEN TRANSPORT TO SKELETAL MUSCLE

Khan Akmal, Duane F. Bruley,* Natalio Banchero,**
Ronald Artigue, and Wiliam Maloney
Dept. Chemical Engineering, Tulane Univ., New Orleans,LA
70118, *Dept. Chemical Engineering, Rose-Hulman Inst. of
Technology, Terre Haute, IN 47803, and **Dept. Physi-
ology, Sch. Med. Denver, CO 80262   USA

Systems of nonlinear, unsteady-state, partial differential
equations have been developed to model oxygen transport in the
microcirculation of brain using the Krogh cylinder as the basic
anatomical unit (Reneau, Bruley and Knisely, 1967). The models
have been solved to predict trends in behavior but it has been
impossible to test them against accurate in-vivo quantitative data
from brain because of the experimental difficulties in determining
the exact position of PO_2 eletrodes in the capillary-neuron network. Because of this we have tried to find an animal model that
would reduce the histological complexity of the system and allow
us to test the validity of the mathematical models.

Recent work has shown that in some animals the cross sections
of skeletal muscle resemble hexagons with six capillaries around
them, that is, a capillary to fiber ratio of two. Important
changes in this arrangement occur as a result of maturation and
increases in body weight (Sillau and Banchero, 1977). The ATPase
reaction used for the visualization of capillaries has allowed
better understanding of some of the capillary-fiber arrangements
(Loats et al, 1977).

MODEL

This model is an extension of the Krogh cylinder modified in
order to accommodate a three dimensional arrangement of capillaries
around muscle fibers based on actual measurements of skeletal
muscle geometry.

The number of capillaries surrounding a skeletal muscle
fiber is proportional to the size of the cross sectional area of

the fiber (Loats et al, 1977). Six capillaries are arranged at the apices of the hexagon when the fiber has a cross sectional area of about 3000 μm^2 (Fig. 1). On internalizing such a capillary with no-flux boundaries through each of the hexagons, an equilateral triangle is obtained in the cross section which is completely supplied by the capillary. In a three dimensional view a 3-corner prism is inserted in the tissue. We have used this particular arrangement in modelling O_2 transport. This model requires concurrent flow and for this condition to be satisfied the capillaries, of identical length, are so arranged that all arterial ends are in the same plane. In addition, the blood flow through the capillaries is identical inasmuch as PO_2 is concerned.

Oxygen transport from the capillaries to the tissue and within the tissue is entirely due to diffusion. Since the convective term of blood flow is very large compared to the axial diffusion, and under normoxia axial gradients within the tissue are small, axial diffusion in the capillary and tissue is neglected. It is assumed that no other mechanism contributes to the transport of O_2. Fick's first law describes this diffusion transport.

To facilitate the mathematical solution, employing symmetrical considerations, triangular micro-units with the hypotenuse equal to 33 μm were used (Fig. 1). This dimension was selected because in several species it is half the distance between two diagonally opposite capillaries in a fiber that has a cross sectional area of about 3000 μm^2. Triangular micro-units lends the approach to treatment of shapes other than hexagons simply by a change of dimensions.

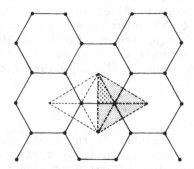

Figure 1. A hexagonal fiber area is completely supplied by the six capillaries at its apices, but only a 1/3 of each capillary faces a given hexagon. Each capillary participates in the supply of 3 adjacent fibers. The equilateral triangle (stippled area) is divided by bisectors into 6 triangular (30-60-90°) micro-units (coarse stippled area) with the hypotenuse equal to 33 μm.

A recently developed model (Artigue, personal communication) was used to determine the PO_2 conditions within the capillary. In order to use conventional mathematics, blood is lumped into two compartments-red blood cells (RBC) and plasma-both homogeneous within themselves, with mass transfer existing from the RBC to the plasma. The hemoglobin-bound oxygen dissociates according to the well known Hb-O_2 curve. The plasma PO_2 is used for the capillary boundary condition. Diffusion in more than one direction is described by partial differential equations. The tissue oxygen consumption is assumed to be constant, that is, independent of spatial position and PO_2 value.

The equations describing the model are:

CAPILLARY:

RBC
$$\frac{\partial P_{RBC}}{\partial t} + v\frac{\partial P_{RBC}}{\partial Z} = \frac{nA_c\,N_c\,(P_{RBC} - P_P)}{\alpha_{RBC}\,H + N_{Blood}\,\frac{\partial \Psi}{\partial P_{RBC}}}$$

PLASMA
$$\frac{\partial P_P}{\partial t} + v\frac{\partial P_P}{\partial Z} = \frac{nA_c\,N_c\,(P_{RBC} - P_P)}{\alpha_P\,(1-H)} - \frac{2J}{(1-H)\,R_1\alpha_P}$$

TISSUE:
$$\frac{\partial P}{\partial t} = D_t\frac{\partial^2 P}{\partial x^2} + \frac{\partial^2 P}{\partial y^2} - \frac{A}{S_t}$$

INTERFACE:
$$P_i\Big|_{Blood} = P_i\Big|_{Tissue}$$

$$D_b S_b\frac{\partial P}{\partial r}\bigg|_{\substack{r=R_1 \\ Blood}} = D_t S_t\frac{\partial P}{\partial r}\bigg|_{\substack{r=R_1 \\ Tissue}}$$

For an explanation of the symbols refer to the nomenclature.

The partial differential equations were reduced to difference equations and the Gauss-Seidel method with "successive over-relaxation" was used for the numerical solution. In order to employ these numerical methods the micro-unit is divided by a mesh in Cartesian coordinates to give representative grid points. The result is a simple mesh which affords an ease of programming due to its repeated geometrical pattern.

All points inside the capillary were given a value of zero at the beginning of the solution to the tissue equation. Since there is no-flux across the triangular boundary, the oxygen tension for grid points bounding it is equal. Mathematically the boundary conditions and the corresponding difference equations are given as:

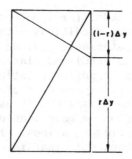

Figure 2. A line is drawn from each of the exterior points normal
to the boundary. The line is then extended until it intersects
one of the grid lines joining 2 of the interior points. $r\Delta y$
distance between intersection and lower grid point. $(1-r)\Delta y$ distance between intersection and upper grid point, where $0 < r < 1$.

(i) $P(x) = 0.0$ for $0 < x < R_1$

(ii) $\dfrac{\partial P}{\partial x} = 0.0;\ y = 1,\ J;\ x = R_2$

       $P(I - 1, J) = P(I + 1, J)$

(iii) $\dfrac{\partial P}{\partial y} = 0.0;\ x = 1,\ I;\ y = 0$

       $P(I, J + 1) = P(1, J - 1)$

(iv) $P(I, J) = (1 - r)\, P(I + 1, J - 1) + r\, P(I + 1, J).$

       $0 < r < 1$

The points lying on a line parallel to the irregular boundary are
approximated as shown in figure 2. The approximated value of the
dependent variable is then calculated as the weighted average of
the values at the two adjacent grid points. Since the grid points
do not lie on the capillary surface, the points immediately surrounding the capillary are given values calculated in terms of the
flux out of the capillary for a Krogh cylinder:

$$P(I, J) = P_{cap} + J \cdot \frac{\alpha}{\Delta x}$$

where, α is the distance between the capillary and the grid point
and Δx is the size of mesh in the x direction.

The steady state solution of the various equations was obtained on a CDC 6400 computer with an average processing time of
1500 sec. Normally reported values were used for the parameters

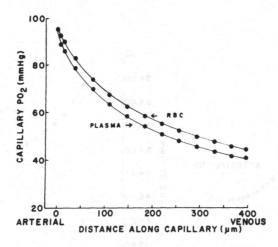

Figure 3. PO_2 profiles along capillary for the RBC and the plasma phases. Each set of 2 points at any given distance represent instantaneous values.

in the equations. The "over-relaxation" factor was calculated according to methods described in the mathematical literature.

RESULTS AND DISCUSSION

Diffusion being the limiting factor in the O_2 transport in the capillary, exponentially decreasing PO_2's for RBC and plasma phases are expected (Fig. 3). Profiles of PO_2 in resting muscle are shown for the shortest and longest distances (Figs. 4 and 5). Close to the capillary the PO_2 profiles are identical for both distances. However, the interaction of neighboring capillaries is more evident for the short distance reducing the pressure drop between the capillary and a given point in the muscle tissue. The Krogh-Erlang equation, when solved for the parameter values used in our study, indicated a pressure drop, at rest, of 0.75 mm Hg at the venous end whereas by our method it is only 0.48 mm Hg, nearly 36% less. In the case of exercising muscle, the corresponding decreases at the venous end were 7.5 mm Hg and 3.24 mm Hg respectively, a reduction of 57%. The PO_2 profile for exercising tissue at the venous end is illustrated in figure 6. It is evident that O_2 supply to any region in the tissue is enhanced by the presence of five capillaries in the neighborhood of any given capillary.

Figure 7 shows the PO_2 at the farthest points in the tissue parallel to the capillary. In resting muscle this line follows very closely the plasma PO_2 because the decrease in pressure within the tissue is small.

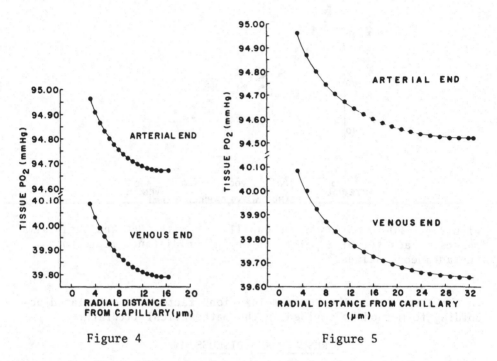

Figure 4   Figure 5

Figure 4.   PO$_2$ profiles in tissue at radial points away from capillary. Values for the shortest distance are shown.

Figure 5.   PO$_2$ profiles in tissue at radial points away from capillary. Values for the longest distance are shown.

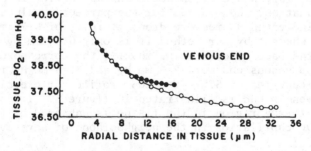

Figure 6.   PO$_2$ profiles for the longest and the shortest radial distances in exercising muscle.

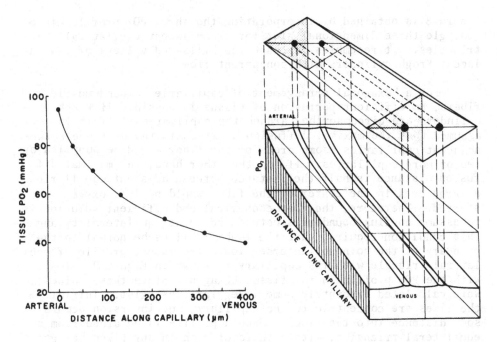

Figure 7.   PO$_2$ profiles in the tissue at farthermost points from capillary.

Figure 8.   Three dimensional view of PO$_2$ profiles along 2 adjacent capillaries and tissue prisms.

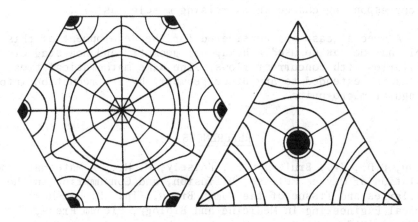

Figure 9.   Schematic representation of isobars around capillaries. Hexagonal arrangement on the left and triangular on the right.

Figure 8 is obtained by incorporating the three PO_2 profiles into a single three dimensional plot for two adjacent equilateral triangles. It resembles in shape the hills-and-valleys of two adjacent Krogh cylinders with concurrent flow.

For a hexagonal arrangement of capillaries around muscle fibers, no efficient perfusion of tissue is possible if Krogh cylinders are circumscribed around the capillaries. If it is assumed that the maximal diffusion distance is the distance between adjacent capillaries, some areas of the fiber would be supplied by two or more capillaries. If, on the other hand, the maximal diffusion distance is half the distance between adjacent capillaries a large area in the center of the fiber would be left oxygen starved. Therefore, the most economical and efficient solution is to assume no-flux boundaries between adjacent equilateral triangles. This condition requires that the isobaric lines be normal to the boundary at the point of intersection. The isobar profile of equilateral triangle with its capillary is shown in Figure 9, along with the PO_2 profile in the tissue hexagon. Since these values were calculated discretely some irregularities exist. Initially the lines are concentric to the capillary, but inversion occurs some distance into the fiber. Such a profile is obtained from six equilateral triangles, with a third of each in any given hexagon.

CONCLUSION

This multi-capillary model can be used to predict O_2 tensions in the tissue. The influence of surrounding capillaries on a given equilateral triangle of tissue results in an enhanced PO_2 at any point. For resting conditions the maximal pressure drop between proximal and distant points from the capillary was estimated to be about 36% lower than that obtained by the Krogh-Erlang equation. The corresponding change in exercising muscle was 57%.

A special case was considered for the development of this model inasmuch as we used a hexagonal geometry and non-staggered capillaries with concurrent flows. The same mathematical treatment can be extended to any other geometry by its reduction into triangular micro-units.

REFERENCES

Reneau, D.D., Jr.; Bruley, D.F.; Knisely, M. H.: A Mathematical Simulation of Oxygen Release, Diffusion, and Consumption in the Capillaries and Tissue of the Human Brain. In: D. Hershey: Chemical Engineering in Medicine and Biology, Plenum Press, New York, 1967.

Loats, J.T., Sillau, A.H. and Banchero, N. (1977) Plenum Press.

Sillau, A.H. and Banchero, N. (1977) Proc. Soc. Exp. Biol. Med. 154, 461.

Sillau, A.H. and Banchero, N. (1977a) Pflugers Archiv. (in press).

ACKNOWLEDGMENTS

This work was supported by grants from the USPHS, NIH: 5R01 NS 12009 and NHLI HL 19145.

The authors wish to express their appreciation to Mrs. Lynn Aquin, Mrs. Ruthanne Bastian and Mr. George Tarver for their assistance.

NOMENCLATURE

P_0	=	95.0 mm Hg	Arterial PO_2
t	=	sec	Time
v	=	0.04 cm/sec.	Blood velocity
η	=	9.3×10^{-7} ml $O_2 \cdot$ cm/ml sec mm Hg	RBC mass transfer coeff
A_c	=	1.63×10^{-6} cm^2	Wet surface area of RBC
N_c	=	5.4×10^9 cells/ml	Number density of RBC
αRBC	=	$S_b = 3.42 \times 10^{-5}$ ml O_2/ml·mm Hg	Solubility coeff RBC
αp	=	$S_b = 3.42 \times 10^{-5}$ ml O_2/ml·mm Hg	Solubility coeff plasma
H	=	0.45 ml·RBC/ml blood	Hematocrit
NBlood	=	0.204 ml O_2/ml	Oxygen capacity of blood
ψ	=	Dimensionless	Percent conc. of O_2
J	=	ml O_2/cm^2 sec	Flux out of capillary
R_1	=	3×10^{-4} cm	Radius of capillary
R_2	=	4×10^{-3} cm	Radius of Krogh cylinder
Db	=	1.7×10^{-5} cm^2/sec	Diffusivity in blood
Dt	=	1.7×10^{-5} cm^2/sec	Diffusivity in tissue
St	=	3.2×10^{-5} ml O_2/ml mm Hg	Solubility coeff tissue
A (rest)	=	4×10^{-5} ml O_2/ml sec	Tissue consumption
A (exercised)	=	4×10^{-4} ml O_2/ml sec	Tissue consumption
L_{CAP}	=	4×10^{-2} cm	Length of capillary

DYNAMIC HYPOXIC HYPOXEMIA IN BRAIN TISSUE: EXPERIMENTAL AND THEORETICAL METHODOLOGIES

William J. Dorson, Jr. and Beuford A. Bogue

Department of Chemical and Bioengineering, Arizona
State University, Tempe, Arizona 85281, U.S.A. and
HOSPAL Medical Corporation, 391 Chipeta Way-Research
Park, Salt Lake City, Utah 84108, U.S.A.

An experimental system was assembled to study feline cerebral cortex cellular and extracellular pO_2 response to rapid changes in carotid artery oxygen levels. The system has been described in prior articles in this series and elsewhere (Bogue and Dorson, 1973; Dorson and Bogue, 1973; Dorson and Bogue, 1976; Bogue, 1974). Changes in carotid artery oxygen level could be accomplished either by varying the ventilatory gas composition or by a carotid-jugular computer controlled exchange method. The latter technique involved cannulation of both internal carotid arteries and jugular veins. All other perfusion routes were supressed by compression. Relatively open flow was allowed in both directions with exchange between venous and arterial blood on an equal volume flow basis. This system resulted in the most rapid possible input change while maintaining close to normal physiological function. Many different types of changes were investigated, and this report will concentrate on oscillatory inputs caused by both the ventilation gas and blood exchange methods. No difference in response was noted up to the upper frequency limit of the ventilation method of 0.1 Hz while the exchange method was capable of 1.0 Hz oscillations.

Microelectrodes were used to measure arterial pO_2, intracellular pO_2 (and action potentials), and venous pO_2. Other continuous measurements included EKG, temperature, arterial blood pressure, and total carotid brain blood flow. Serial arterial and venous samples were drawn for pH, pCO_2, pO_2 (calibration check), Hb, hematocrit, and O_2 content. The serial measurements were used to calculate the total brain metabolic O_2 consumption which, on a per 100 gm basis, determined the physiological condition of the preparation at that time.

The theoretical model contained three capillary blood compartments (in series) with mass transfer to two parallel interstitial
fluid compartments. Two cellular compartments were then placed in
series with the extracellular compartments. To simulate the experimental arrangement both a time delay and mixing compartment
separated the appropriate capillary compartment from either the
arterial or venous measurement site. A four step kinetic metabolic
model was included into each of the two intracellular compartments.
Theoretical calculations could be compared to the experimental data
in several ways (see Dorson and Bogue, 1973; Dorson and Bogue, 1976
for more details). For any arterial oxygen waveform a direct comparison of predicted and experimental tissue or venous pO_2 with
time was possible. For oscillatory waveforms the entire test period
could be signal averaged to produce tissue (or venous) to arterial
pO_2 amplitude ratios for comparison purposes. The third method was
to produce auto- and cross-correlations between any two recorded
or predicted signals. This technique again averaged the response
over the entire test period and eliminated any unrelated noise.

The problem with these experiments, in addition to the instrumental complexity, is that total brain perfusion values are combined
with single cell measurements. The brain is both inhomogeneous and
subject to selective recruitment in response to changing perfusion
conditions. The tissue probe location variable could be easily
accounted for through the pO_2 absolute value with the transfer
coefficients. This straightforward approach is also consistent
with multiple probe observations in the brain cortex during extended
hypoxia induced by ventilatory gas composition changes (Leniger-
Follert et al, 1976). However, significant variations in local
blood flow rate changes were also noted in the referenced work.

The lack of exact correspondence between local and total brain
blood flow is an obstacle to the application of theoretical predictions herein. For temporal comparisons this situation could be
partially overcome by obtaining a large number of similar experiments and using a global average response. A less satisfactory
approach for oscillatory waveforms would be to assume that the
average local tissue response over an extended test period would be
directly related to the total brain input and response changes.

RESULTS

The major goal of the exchange system was to achieve extremely
rapid carotid artery pO_2 waveforms. This is also a significant
difference between these results and prior investigations. Exchange
system step changes were analogous to a square wave arterial pO_2
input while ventilation gas changes were analogous to a slow ramp
function.

The most important determinant of the type of response was the animal's physiological condition (Dorson and Bogue, 1976). This is summarized in the table with the definitions G (Good Condition), DS (Depressed Signs), RPC (Reversible Pathological Condition), and IPC (Irreversible Pathological Condition). Contained in the table are some representative values for the measured metabolism ranges (which defined the condition), the normalized brain blood flow rate, the transfer coefficients determined both from steady-state measurements just prior to the test period (K_{ss}) and from the mean oscil= lating values during the test (K_m), and ratios of arterial pressure to brain blood flow determined prior to (R_{ss}) and during the test (R_m). Some characteristic responses emerge. First, cats in good condition exhibit highly efficient transfer which opposes rapid hypoxic exposure. The first line of defense is hyperemia which occurs quickly, in the order of the arterial-capillary transit time. Arterial blood pressure either changes little or actually decreases in these cats. In prior studies it was shown that the kinetics of cellular metabolism also provides protection against rapid hypoxic changes in that tissue O_2 is conserved over short time periods.

In contrast to the tight control of cellular pO_2 exhibited by cats in good condition, as their physiological condition deteriorates blood pressure starts responding ahead of blood flow rate, and tissue/venous pO_2's start to mimic the input signal. In the DS and RPC conditions the cellular pO_2 has been frequently observed to either oppose the change (elevated cyclic pO_2) or follow the change directly. This difference in response is attributed to the local to total relative blood flow phenomena along with depressed cellular metabolism. By the time a cat is in IPC there is neither blood pressure nor flow response and both tissue and venous pO_2's passively follow any input signal.

An unusually low cortical tissue pO_2 region was found for a cat defined to be in good condition. The exchange system oscillations were initiated and the resultant response is shown in Figure 1. A sharp tissue pO_2 decline slightly preceded the total brain blood flow response. However, localized protective mechanisms (presumably recruitment) rapidly drove the tissue pO_2 to

AVERAGE RESPONSES TO DYNAMIC HYPOXIC OSCILLATIONS
GRADED BY PHYSIOLOGICAL CONDITION

Condition(#)	M_c (ml O_2/100gm-min)	Q/W (ml/min-gm)	K'_{ss}/K'_m (cm^3/sec)	R_{ss}/R_m (mmHg-min/ml)
G (2)	≥ 6.0	1.38	30.5/35.5	2.4/1.9
DS (4)	4.0-5.9	0.78	13.2/16.0	3.9/3.9
RPC (6)	2.0-3.9	0.57	9.0/16.2	3.9/4.5
IPC (2)	≤ 1.9	0.35	1.0/ 1.0	4.5/4.4

elevated values during and following the hypoxic test period. After the experiment, tissue pO_2 returned to a low value. Note also the negative arterial pressure response in this experiment.

Transfer coefficients were evaluated in two ways. With the assumption that $K_1' = K_2' = K_{ss}$ or K_m a set of steady state (ss) or mean (m) oscillating data values could be used to calculate K_{ss} or K_m respectively. Alternately, when oscillating data was used in conjunction with the compartment model, optimum values of K_1' and K_2' could be derived. The latter procedure required extensive computation time. K_1' represents the transfer from 1/3 of the capillary volume into adjacent extracellular fluid. K_2' represents transfer from 1/2 the extracellular fluid into 1/2 the intracellular fluid. The following list compares the different values during two experiments where the coefficients are all reported in cm^3/sec. The

Condition	K_{ss}'	K_m'	K_1'	K_2'
G	60	70	54.4	75.1
RPC	18	20	21.1	10.1

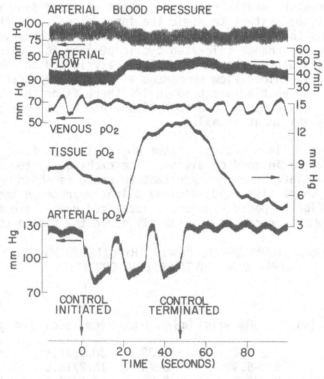

Figure 1. Observed Response to 0.06 Hz Control Induced Oscillations ($pCO_2 \sim 40$ mmHg, Test 74-1147, Good Condition).

optimum values are seen to bracket K'_{ss} and K'_m. Again, cats in good
condition exhibit highly efficient transfer. Also, the K'_2 and K'_1
magnitudes might be indicative of both cellular active transfer and
well perfused tissue. For the cat in RPC capillary oxygen still
equilibrates with extracellular fluid (though slightly less efficient, see Dorson and Bogue, 1976) but the intracellular transport
is highly inefficient.

The calculated dynamic responses expressed as amplitude ratios
were not affected by the transfer coefficients until high frequencies (>0.1 Hz) were reached. Conversely, the level of metabolism
only affects the low frequency response. Both arterial flow and
pO_2 have large effects at all frequencies. Although entire test
periods could be signal averaged, direct comparisons of predicted
and actual responses were difficult due to changing conditions and
limitations of this theoretical method. Figure 2 and 3 show observed and calculated responses which demonstrate the type of general agreement, in this case due to flow rate, which resulted. One
problem which was encountered involved the time period for averaging
data. In order to maintain the cat in good condition only short,
low trauma experiments could be used. For many of these tests not
enough time was available to eliminate high frequency noise by signal averaging. Thus, it was common (7 of 10 experiments) to have
an equal or higher observed amplitude ratio at high frequencies
than the low frequency ratios when the cat was in good condition.

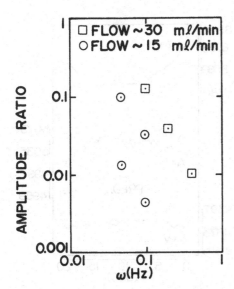

Figure 2. Observed Tissue/
Arterial pO_2 Amplitude Ratio
(pCO_2 ~ 30mmHg, Test 76, Good
Condition).

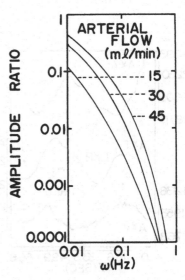

Figure 3. Predicted Tissue/
Arterial pO_2 Amplitude Ratio for
M_c =3.4, $K'_1 \equiv K'_2$=30, W=25, Arterial
pO_2=75.

The response shown on Figure 2 was one of the exceptions. The possibility exists that there is a high frequency metabolic transfer effect. For cats in deteriorating condition longer experiments were used, including pseudo-random noise, and all observed responses consistently fell off similar to the calculated responses shown on Figure 3.

The final method of comparison involved cross-correlations which also averaged the response over the entire test period and was less subject to noise since major interrelations would dominate. Figures 4 (RPC) and 5(G) contain the data auto- and cross-correlations of arterial pO_2 (AxA), tissue and arterial pO_2 (AxT), and venous and arterial $\bar{p}O_2$ (AxV) (these correspond to Figures 5 and 4, respectively, from Dorson and Bogue, 1976). The predictions were calculated from the compartment model and the offset is caused by the error limit used to restrict the extensive computation time. The results support the prior conclusions that the response of a cat in good condition opposes the dynamic hypoxic change, neither venous pO_2 nor blood pressure had an oscillating component related to the arterial pO_2, and the theoretical compartment model contains all the major control quantities (effect, not cause). The opposition to hypoxic oscillatory changes would be ascribed primarily to the flow response since it was used in the prediction, and the local intracellular pO_2 was directly related to the overall brain blood flow changes. Figure 4 demonstrates a loss of control (blood pres-

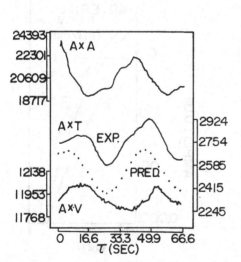

Figure 4. Observed pO_2 Correlations with Predicted AxT ($pCO_2 \sim 40mmHg$, Test 68-775, RPC) in $mmHg^2$.

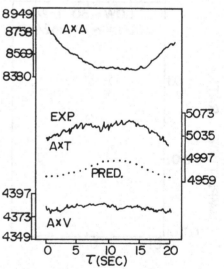

Figure 5. Observed pO_2 Correlations with Predicted AxT ($pCO_2 \sim 40mmHg$, Test 68-237, Good Condition) in $mmHg^2$.

sure also had a strong oscillatory component with arterial pO_2) but the local tissue pO_2 was still directly related to the total brain blood flow response.

Although microcirculation responses to ventilatory gas O_2 step changes have been observed to be highly variable, the total impact of the selective recruitment process seems to be to relate local cortical tissue response to the arterial flow response when consistent variations are observed. The inconsistent tissue pO_2 responses observed, such as shown on Figure 1, would also be as-cribed to the recruitment process, but stimulated by local protective mechanisms. In prior theoretical comparisons on a time basis it was established that the cellular metabolic kinetics were important in predicting rapid tissue pO_2 responses. However, constant metabolism was used for the prediction of average responses over the entire test period herein. The correspondence between theory and data seems to justify this assumption, at least at the frequencies investigated so far.

Acknowledgement: This work was supported in part by the Faculty Grant-In-Aid program, Arizona State University.

NOMENCLATURE

K_1^i Capillary to extracellular fluid transfer coefficient (cm^3/sec)
K_2^i Extracellular to intracellular transfer coefficient (cm^3/sec)
M_c Normalized cellular O_2 metabolism (ml O_2/100 gm-min)
Q Total brain blood flow rate (ml/min)
W Brain weight (gm)

REFERENCES

Bogue, B.A. and Dorson, Jr., W.J. (1973) In 'Oxygen Transport to Tissue: Pharmacology, Mathematical Studies, and Neonatology' p.903 (eds. Bruley, D.F. and Bicher, H.I.). Plenum Publishing Corp., New York.

Bogue, B.A. (1974) Feline Brain Tissue pO_2 Response to Step and Oscillating Arterial pO_2 Changes. Ph.D. Thesis, Arizona State University.

Dorson, W.J. and Bogue, B.A. (1973) In 'Oxygen Transport to Tissue: Instrumentation, Methods, and Physiology' p.251 (eds. Bicher, H.I. and Bruley, D.F.). Plenum Publishing Corp., New York.

Dorson, Jr., W.J. and Bogue, B.A. (1976) In 'Oxygen Transport to Tissue-II' p. 343 (eds. Grote, J., Reneau, D., and Thews, G.). Plenum Publishing Corp., New York.

Leniger-Follert, E., Wrabetz, W., and Lübbers, D.W. (1976) In 'Oxygen Transport to Tissue-II' p.361 (eds. Grote, J., Reneau, D., and Thews, G.). Plenum Publishing Corp., New York.

MATHEMATICAL MODEL OF RESPIRATORY GAS EXCHANGE AT STATIONARY CONDITIONS

A. Grad and S. Svetina

Institute of Biophysics, Medical Faculty and
J.Stefan Institute, University of Ljubljana
Ljubljana, Yugoslavia

Exchange of respiratory gases in an organism is a corporate process in which the ventilatory, circulatory and metabolic functions are involved (Wasserman et al, 1967). The properties of the respiratory gases exchange system are determined by a number of regulatory mechanisms and the oxygen and carbon dioxide carrying properties of the blood. The system is multivariant with many inputs and outputs therefore the mathematical models can be considered as an important tool in understanding its behaviour. In this communication a simple mathematical model is introduced for studying the respiratory gases exchange at stationary conditions, in which the ventilation is regulated by the arterial values of carbon dioxide and oxygen, and the blood flow is assumed to depend on the metabolic needs of the tissue. The input parameters are external pressures of oxygen and carbon dioxide, oxygen consumption rate in tissue and respiratory quotient. The outputs are arterial and venous concentrations of oxygen and carbon dioxide, arterial and venous pH, ventilation and blood flow.

Constituent parts of the model are based upon the following properties of the system. The steady state behaviour of the ventilatory part of the respiratory gases exchange system is treated as proposed by Milhorn and Brown (1971). The controlling equation relating ventilation to the alveolar partial pressures of carbon dioxide and oxygen obtained by Lloyd and Cunningham

(1963) is used. From the given values of the partial
pressures of oxygen and carbon dioxide, oxygen consumption rate and respiratory quotient, the alveolar
partial pressures of oxygen and carbon dioxide are
determined.

It is assumed that arterial blood is in equilibrium with the alveolar gas. The amounts of oxygen and
carbon dioxide in arterial and venous blood are determined by employing a simple model of blood chemistry,
in which blood is considered as an one-compartment
system, and the binding of oxygen and carbon dioxide
as well as their mutually dependent binding to blood
are taken into account. The arterial pH is obtained
from the arterial concentrations of oxygen and carbon
dioxide and the values of oxygen concentration (0.122
mM/l), carbon dioxide concentration (1.28 mM/l) and
pH (7.4) at the reference state.

Arterial values are used then as the input of a
subsystem describing the exchange processes in tissue.
The outputs of this subsystem are venous oxygen, venous
carbon dioxide, venous pH, and relative value of the
blood flow. The essential property of the proposed
model is that it includes the local blood flow regulation according to the metabolic needs of the tissue
(Guyton et al, 1973). Although the detailed mechanisms
involved in the regulation of blood flow have not yet
been elucidated, several models for the tissue blood
flow regulation have been proposed by introducing the
concept of the critical level of tissue oxygen concentration. The comparison between the controlling mechanisms employed in these studies is presented in Fig.1.

The characteristic property of the model used here
(Fig.1C) is the inclusion of the structural features of
the microvascular system. It is well established that
there is a correlation between the constriction of the
blood vessels in the precapillary region and the metabolic needs of the tissue (Wiedeman et al, 1976) and
that the flow through the capillaries is of pulsative
nature (Johnson and Wauland, 1967). Additional evidence
of such behaviour is a reduced number of open capillaries when oxygen is supplied to the tissue also from
the suffusing solution (Prewitt and Johnson, 1976).

The model behaviour is tested with regard to its
behaviour at elevated oxygen consumption rate ($\dot{O}_2$). To
obtain a reasonable dependence of the blood flow on $\dot{O}_2$

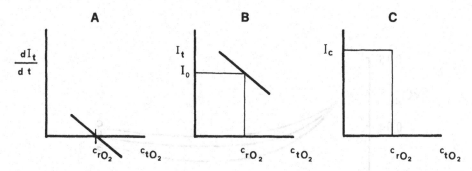

Fig. 1. Examples of the control equations which have been employed in the models of the local blood flow regulation.

A. Model of Duvelleroy et al. (1973): changes in coronary blood flow (dI_t/dt) are proportional to the negative value of the difference between the tissue oxygen level (c_{tO_2}) and its regulative value (c_{rO_2}).

B. Model of Mitchell et al. (1972): tissue blood flow (I_t) is proportional to the negative value of the difference between c_{tO_2} and c_{rO_2}.

C. Model of Smolej and Svetina (1975): capillary blood flow (I_c) is zero if $c_{tO_2} > c_{rO_2}$ and has a constant value if $c_{tO_2} < c_{rO_2}$. Tissue blood flow in this model is proportional to the I_c and the number of open capillaries. The relative number of open capillaries as a function of the oxygen consumption rate is determined in the model by calculating the time during which a capillary is closed.

it was necessary to assume that $\dot{O}_2$ influences the critical oxygen level. A possible meaning of this assumption is that the precapillary vessels are influenced also by an effector the amount of which is under steady state conditions proportional to $\dot{O}_2$. The following function for the dependence of the control tissue level of oxygen is used:

$$c_{rO_2} = \frac{K + 1}{K + q}\, c_{rO_2}(o)$$

q is the ratio between the $\dot{O}_2$ and the oxygen consumption rate at the reference state. K is an adjustable constant

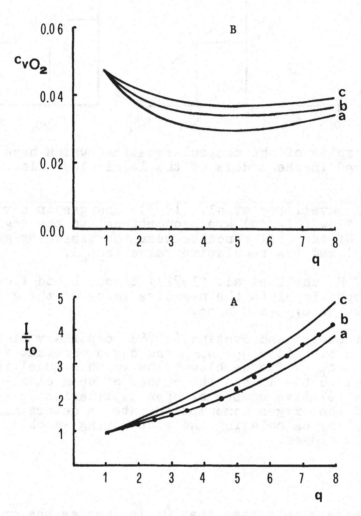

Fig. 2. A. Relative blood flow (I/I_0) as a function of relative oxygen consumption rate (q). Dotted curve are experimental data.

B. Venous oxygen concentration $(c_{vO_2}$, in mM/l) as a function of relative oxygen consumption rate (q).

Calculated curves are given for three values of the parameter K: 1(a), 2(b), 3(c).

and $c_{rO2}(o)$ is chosen in such a way (Smolej and Svetina, unpublished) that at $q = 1$ (reference state) it has a value with which the model predicts the reference value of the venous oxygen concentration.

In Fig. 2 the relative blood flow (I/I_0) and venous oxygen concentration (c_{vO2}) are presented as a function of relative oxygen consumption rate for different values of the parameter K and compared with the experimental data for blood flow. It can be seen that by a proper choice of the adjustable parameter K the measured data are described quite satisfactorily. The calculated venous properties of blood are also in a good correlation with the experimentally obtained levelling of the c_{vO2} curve at higher oxygen demand (Fig.2B) and with a more pronounced decrease in pH of the venous blood as compared with the decrease in pH of the arterial blood (Doll et al, 1968). Changes of external oxygen pressure, external carbon dioxide pressure and the value of the respiratory quotient give the responses of the model which are qualitatively in accord with general behaviour of real systems. However, some predictions of the model are not a priori obvious. For instance: blood flow is slightly lower at higher values of respiratory quotient provided all other properties of the system are unchanged. The relative blood flow is also decreasing by increasing the external carbon dioxide partial pressure.

The model introduced is based on a large number of simplifications so that in the present form it can not be used to fully simulate the real systems. The results presented here indicate that tissue oxygen level as well as tissue oxygen consumption control the blood flow so that there should be at least two substances involved in this process. The inclusion of the ventilatory gases exchange process is important in studying the mechanism of the tissue oxygen release as it brings about changes in arterial blood properties which accompany the changes in tissue parameters.

REFERENCES

Doll, E., Keul, J. and Maiwald, C. (1968) Amer.J. Physiol. 215, 23.

Duvelleroy, M.A., Mehmel, H. and Laver, M.B. (1973) J. Appl. Physiol. 35, 480.

Guyton, A.C., Jones, C.E. and Coleman, T.G. (1973)
Circulatory Physiology: Cardiac Output and its Regula-
tion. W.B. Saunders Company, Philadelphia, London and
Toronto, Ch. 19.

Johnson, P.C. and Wayland, H. (1967) Amer. J. Physiol.
212, 1405.

Lloyd, B.B. and Cunningham, D.J.C. (1963) A quantitative approach to the regulation of human respiration.
In 'The Regulation of Human Respiration' (eds. Cunningham, D.J.C. and Lloyd, B.B.). F.A. Davis Co.,
Philadelphia.

Milhorn, H.T., Jr. and Brown, D.R. (1971) Comput.
Biomed. Res. 3, 604.

Mitchell, J.W., Stolwijk, J.A.J. and Nadel, E.R. (1972)
Biophys. J. 12, 1452.

Prewitt, R.L. and Johnson, P.C. (1976) Microvas.
Res. 12, 59.

Smolej, V. and Svetina, S. (1975) Biosystems 7, 209.

Wasserman, K., Van Kessel, A.L. and Burton, G.G. (1967)
J. Appl. Physiol. 22, 71.

Wiedeman, M.P., Tuma, R.F. and Mayrovitz, H.N. (1976)
Microvas. Res. 12, 71.

CALCULATION OF THE FACILITATION OF O_2 OR CO TRANSPORT BY HB OR MB

BY MEANS OF A NEW METHOD FOR SOLVING THE CARRIER-DIFFUSION PROBLEM

L. Hoofd and F. Kreuzer

Department of Physiology, University of Nijmegen

Geert Grooteplein Noord 21a, Nijmegen, The Netherlands

A new analytical approximation is used for calculating facilitated diffusion in flat layers. It is applied to oxygen or carbon monoxide diffusion through flat layers containing myoglobin or hemoglobin, where it can be applied to all situations. Calculations for the total gas flux are in good agreement with data from the literature. New calculations for the facilitated diffusion of CO show non-equilibrium facilitation over a wide range of layer thicknesses and CO pressures.

THEORY

The facilitation of substrate diffusion by a carrier diffusing simultaneously leads to mathematical problems which cannot be solved exactly. Even in such a simple case as diffusion of oxygen through a flat layer containing myoglobin the differential equations describing the system contain nonlinear terms which cannot be neglected. If the carrier (myoglobin) is denoted by C and the transported substrate (oxygen or carbon monoxide) by S, these substances reversibly react to form a carrier-substrate complex CS:

$$S + C \underset{k}{\overset{k'}{\rightleftharpoons}} CS \tag{1}$$

Considering simultaneous diffusion of these species in steady state leads to the following set of differential equations:

$$D_S \frac{d^2[S]}{dx^2} = D_C \frac{d^2[C]}{dx^2} = -D_{CS} \frac{d^2[CS]}{dx^2} = k'[C][S] - k[CS] \tag{2}$$

163

where the concentration of each species X is denoted by $[X]$ and its diffusion coefficient by D_X.

An approximate analytical solution is developed by splitting the term for the substrate concentration into a carrier- and a position-dependent part:

$$[S] = e([C]) + f(x) \tag{3}$$

Now the position-dependent part $f(x)$ is solved for the conditions near the boundaries, $x=0$ and $x=L$, where

$$\frac{d[C]}{dx} = \frac{d[CS]}{dx} = 0 \qquad \text{for} \quad x=0,L \tag{4}$$

since the carrier cannot leave the layer. This also means that all $[C]$-dependent terms may be regarded as constants and, without going into detail now, we get the solutions:

$$e([C]) = \frac{k[CS]}{k'[C]} \tag{5}$$

$$f(x) = -\frac{J_S\lambda}{D_S} \frac{\sinh\{(\tfrac{1}{2}L-x)/\lambda\}}{\cosh(\tfrac{1}{2}L/\lambda)} \tag{6}$$

$$\frac{1}{\lambda^2} = \frac{k'[C]}{D_S} + \frac{k}{D_{CS}} + \frac{k[CS]}{D_C[C]} \tag{7}$$

J_S is the total substrate (O_2 or CO) flux. Note that the term $e([C])$ implies chemical equilibrium and that its 'correction' $f(x)$ disappears in the middle part of thick layers ($x(L-x)>>\lambda^2$). The validity of this approximation for a prediction of substrate diffusion (Hoofd and Kreuzer, in preparation) facilitated by Mb or Hb may be seen from the following.

COMPARISON WITH DATA FROM THE LITERATURE

In practical situations the remaining boundary conditions are imposed by the given substrate concentrations at either side of the layer (or by a combination with flux). Experimentally this is done by maintaining constant gas pressures outside the layer; the total substrate flux will be driven by the concentration differences in both free and bound substrate:

$$J_S L = D_S([S]_{x=L}-[S]_{x=0}) + D_{CS}([CS]_{x=L}-[CS]_{x=0}) \tag{8}$$

Now for each situation a unique solution for the set of equations (3),(5)-(8) exists, which can be found by a trial and error procedure.

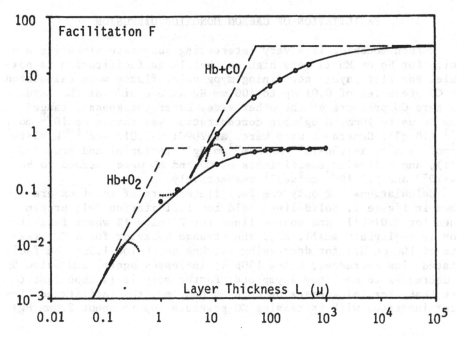

Fig. 1. Facilitation of O_2 and CO by Hb (solid lines). Dotted lines: analytical approximations of Smith et al. (1973). Circles: numerical calculations of Kutchai et al. (1970). Broken lines are asymptotes.

A comparison was made with calculations found in the literature concerning facilitation of CO or O_2 by Hb or Mb (where Hb is thought to react as a monomer according to equation (1)). A typical example is shown in figure 1. Here the facilitation F – the bound substrate flux divided by the free substrate flux – is shown for a large range of layer thicknesses. The present theory can be proven to neatly approximate the asymptotes for both thick and thin layers (broken lines), as may be seen from the course of the solid lines in figure 1. Separate approximations for thick and thin layers applied by Smith et al.(1973) gave results indicated by the dotted lines; these lines coincide with our calculations in the range of their applicability. Kutchai et al.(1970) used a numerical technique; their results are represented by the open circles. The deviations in facilitation for L=1µ and 2µ lead to a difference of about 1% for the total flux; these were the largest differences encountered.

Equations (5)-(7) are solutions for the boundary layers only but they can also be applied to calculate profiles of [S],[C] and [CS] through the whole layer. Predictions for [S] turned out to be very accurate whereas the profile for [C] was too low sometimes.

FACILITATION OF CARBON MONOXIDE DIFFUSION

Carbon monoxide is a very interesting substrate since its affinity for Hb or Mb is very high so that large facilitation is possible. For flat layers containing myoglobin, fluxes were calculated
for CO pressures of 0.01 up to 100 mm Hg at one side of the layer
and zero CO pressure at the other side. Layer thicknesses ranged
from 1μ up to 10cm. Myoglobin concentration was chosen as 10^{-5} mol.
cm^{-3} (18 g%). Constants used were, at 20°C: k=0.017 sec^{-1}, k'=5×10^8
$cm^3 mol^{-1} sec^{-1}$, α=1.36×10^{-9} mol cm^{-3}mm Hg^{-1} (Antonini and Brunori,
1971), and diffusion coefficients of CO and Mb were assumed to be
1.4×10^{-5} and 5.3×10^{-7} $cm^2 sec^{-1}$ respectively.

Calculations for only the facilitated part of the flux are
shown in figure 2. Solid lines hold for facilitation F>1, broken
lines for 0.01<F<1, and dotted lines for F below 1% where facilitation is negligibly small. Note the strange behavior for a CO pressure of 100 mm Hg: for decreasing thicknesses below 1.5mm the facilitated flux decreases, below 150μ it increases again, and below 5μ
it decreases to meet the asymptote. Furthermore it is important to
note that, for thicknesses between 5μ and 1mm, the facilitated flux
first increases with increasing CO pressure (up to about 2.5mm Hg)

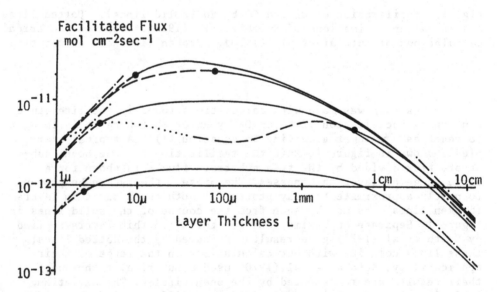

Fig. 2. Facilitated CO flux through layers containing 18 g% Mb at
20°C. See text for constants used. Lines calculated for CO pressures of (from top to bottom) 1, 10, 0.1, 100, and 0.01 mm Hg against
0 mm Hg. In each line a heavy dot indicates where the pure diffusion
flux equals the facilitated flux (F=1); below this value the line is
dashed, or dotted where F<1%. ——·—— asymptotes for small and for
large thicknesses.

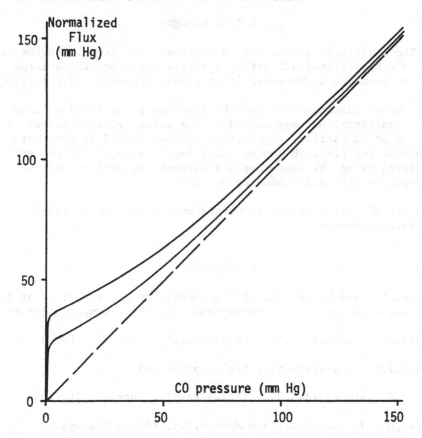

Fig. 3. Normalized total CO flux (JL/Dα) through a layer containing
Mb (upper line) or Hb (lower line); situation of Murray and Wyman
(1971). ──── ──── identity line (no facilitation). At 100 mm Hg the
facilitation still amounts to 6% for Mb and 3% for Hb.

and then decreases again, the same though more pronounced effect as
found for Mb + O_2 (Kreuzer and Hoofd,1972). Also note that even for
L=10cm the facilitation has not yet reached its equilibrium value
in spite of the fact that the Damköhler number kL^2/D_{CO} here is as
large as 1.2×10^5 ! (Goddard et al.,1974)
    The decrease in facilitated flux with increasing pressure is
also demonstrated in figure 3 where a 'normalized flux' (JL/Dα) is
shown for a layer thickness of 220μ according to the situation of
Murray and Wyman (1971). They predicted no facilitation, but figure 3 shows a facilitation of 6% by Mb and of 3% by Hb at a CO pressure as high as 100mm Hg. With low CO pressures the facilitated flux
is much larger than the flux of free CO diffusion (broken line).

CONCLUDING REMARKS

The analytical approximation sketched here is well suited to calculate facilitated diffusion in single cases or over a large range of parameters. Moreover it is straightforward and relatively simple.

Another advantage is that the reaction rates k and k' need not be constants, but may depend on the actual concentrations of free and bound carrier, since these are considered as constants in solving for f(x). This means that facilitation by Hb can be calculated using the same approach without the need of assuming a one-step reaction for binding O_2 or CO.

Part of this work was supported by a grant from Stiftung Volkswagenwerk.

REFERENCES

Antonini,E., and Brunori,M. (1971) Hemoglobin and Myoglobin in their Reactions with Ligands. North-Holland Publishing Company, Amsterdam.

Goddard,J.D., Schultz,J.S., and Suchdeo,S.R. (1974) AIChE J. 20, 625

Hoofd,L.J.C., and Kreuzer,F. (in preparation)

Kreuzer,F., and Hoofd,L.J.C. (1972) Respir. Physiol. 15, 104

Kutchai,H., Jacquez,J.A., and Mather,F.J. (1970) Biophys. J. 10, 38

Murray,J.D., and Wyman,J. (1971) J. Biol. Chem. 246, 5903

Smith,K.A., Meldon,J.H., and Colton,C.K. (1973) AIChE J. 19, 102

THE EFFECT OF DEOXYGENATION RATE OF THE ERYTHROCYTE ON OXYGEN

TRANSPORT TO THE CARDIAC MUSCLE

Masaji Mochizuki and Tomoko Kagawa

Department of Physiology
Yamagata University School of Medicine
990-23 Yamagata, Japan

Up to the present time O_2 delivery to the cardiac muscle has been studied theoretically by many authors (1, 2, 11, 12) using a Krogh's cylinder model. However, relatively little attention has been paid to the influence of deoxygenation of red blood cells (RBC) on the O_2 delivery. Mochizuki (8) measured the O_2 dissociation rate of oxygenated hemoglobin and RBC by using a rapid flow method, and found that the deoxygenation rate of RBC was proportional to the Po_2 difference between RBC and surrounding medium, suggesting that the diffusion inside RBC and across the cell membrane was a rate limiting factor. The rate factor, Fc', which is given by dividing the O_2 quantity taken up by 1 ml RBC by the Po_2 difference between RBC and surrounding medium, was 0.02 - 0.03 $sec^{-1} \cdot mmHg^{-1}$. Recently, Tazawa et al (10) reported that the deoxygenation rate of RBC in the chorioallantoic capillary of chick embryos ranged from 0.008 to 0.009 $sec^{-1} \cdot mmHg^{-1}$. In contrast to our observations, Lawson and Forster (5) previously described that the Po_2 difference between RBC and plasma in tissue was negligibly small, when the rate factor measured by them in a RBC suspension mixed with hydrosulfite (4) was used. Their Fc' value was 6 to 7 times as great as the author's and about 20 times greater than Tazawa's value. In addition, they assumed in their calculation that hemoglobin was distributed homogeneously within the capillary lumen. The diffusion rate in RBC depends in general on RBC shape (9). Therefore it is unreliable to calculate the Po_2 difference without taking into consideration the structure or the boundary conditions of RBC. Thus, we studied again the Po_2 difference by using a RBC model and our previous data on the deoxygenation rate of RBC.

1) Relationship between the Deoxygenation Rate of RBC and Diffusivity across the Barrier Surrounding It

   Because RBCs deform when flowing through the capillary (7),
we calculated the deoxygenation rate by using two, (disc and
cylinder) models (Fig. 1). The diffusivity across the diffusion
barrier was expressed by a unique coefficient ζ, which will be referred to as the transfer coefficient. First, we solved the differential equation (11) analytically, assuming the slope of the O_2
dissociation curve of RBC to be constant. Then, using a computer
we derived a numerical solution by using a standard O_2 dissociation
curve for Pco_2 of 40 mmHg in order to evaluated the effect of the
non-linearity on the reaction rate. One of the most important
parameters is the diffusion coefficient within RBC. According to
Longmuir and Roughton (6), Klug et al (3) and Grote and Thews (2)
the O_2 diffusion coefficient ranged from 0.8×10^{-5} to 0.47×10^{-5}
$cm^2 \cdot sec^{-1}$ at 37°C. In order to make the calculated So_2 curve in
the deoxygenation process well fit to the experimental, however, it
was necessary to assume a restrictive barrier around RBC, even if
the lowest coefficient obtained by Klug et al was used. Thus,
their value, 0.47×10^{-5} $cm^2 \cdot sec^{-1}$ was used throughout this study.

   Space averages of So_2 obtained from the numerical solution in
the disc model are depicted against the reaction time in Fig. 2,
where Po_2 outside RBC was abruptly reduced from 100 to 0 mm Hg and
the ζ value was varied from 0.1×10^{-5} to 0.35×10^{-5} $cm \cdot sec^{-1} \cdot mm$
Hg^{-1}. The deoxygenation rate within RBC varied from one section
to another, the rate at the boundary layer being the highest. The
average So_2 curves tended to show simple exponential functions of
time and the half-time ranged from 90 to 270 msec. In the analytical solution the Fc' value initially decreased and attained a
steady state value within 0.2 sec. However, in the numerical solution of the differential equation in which the non-linear term of
the O_2 dissociation curve was involved the initial decrease in Fc'

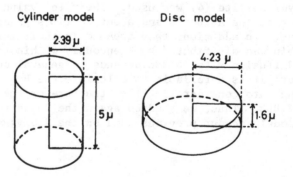

Fig. 1. Red cell models used for the calculation.

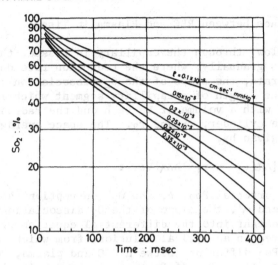

Fig. 2.   Changes in S_{O_2} calculated when P_{O_2} in outer medium was
abruptly reduced, at varying ζ value.

was enlarged and prolonged. In Table 1 are tabulated the Fc' values obtained from the analytical solution at the steady state and
those obtained from the numerical solution at 0.2 sec. Since the
latter values were evaluated at the transition stage, they were
greater than the former, whereas a good agreement was seen in a
higher ζ range. The Fc' values obtained in the disc model was 60
to 100 % greater than those in the cylinder model.

Table 1.   The rate factor of deoxygenation, Fc' in the disc and
the cylinder models obtained from both analytical and
numerical solutions at varying ζ values.

ζ	Fc' ($sec^{-1} \cdot mmHg^{-1}$)			
x 10^{-5}	Disc		Cylinder	
	Analytical	Numerical	Analytical	Numerical
0.10	0.0131	0.0172	0.0082	0.0115
0.15	0.0176	0.0217	0.0104	0.0143
0.20	0.0214	0.0250	0.0120	0.0165
0.25	0.0246	0.0273	0.0132	0.0175
0.30	0.0273	0.0300	0.0141	0.0184
0.35	0.0296	0.0313	0.0147	0.0186

2) Po_2 Difference between RBC and Plasma in Tissue

When RBC flow through the capillary in tissue, the PO_2 in plasma decreases gradually, where the reduction rate depends on the O_2 consumption rate, the slope of the O_2 dissociation curve and the η value. Let the length of a capillary segment which is occupied by a single RBC with a volume of Ve be h and the radiuses of the capillary and tissue cylinder, r_1 and r_2. The space average of Po_2 in RBC, $\overline{Pc}$ may be given by,

$$\overline{Pc} = Pa - [A\pi(r_2{}^2 - r_1{}^2)h/\alpha'Ve]\cdot t \tag{1}$$

where Pa is the arterial Po_2, A, the O_2 consumption rate per 1 ml tissue (sec^{-1}) and α', the slope of the O_2 dissociation curve. Putting α' = constant into the differential equation of diffusion in RBC, we derived an analytical solution, from which we further calculated the Po_2 difference between RBC and plasma, $\overline{Pc} - P_p$, so as to satisfy Eq. (1). The difference was proportional to the O_2 consumption rate, but was independent of the slope of the O_2 dissociation curve (Fig. 3). The values of the parameters used in Fig. 3 were as follows : $r_1 = 3 \mu$, $r_2 = 14 \mu$, h = 7.1 μ and Ve = 90 μ^3. The time course of $\overline{Pc}$ and P_p obtained from numerical solution agreed well with the values calculated from the analytical solution.

3)   Change in PO_2 in the Heart Muscle

Since the slope of the O_2 dissociation curve of myoglobin is hyperbolic, the diffusion equation in the muscle also becomes non-

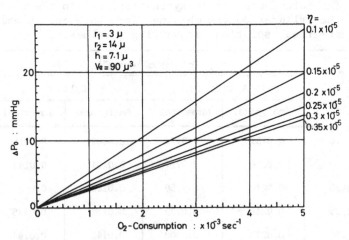

Fig. 3. Po_2 difference between RBC and plasma plotted against O_2 consumption rate at varying η value.

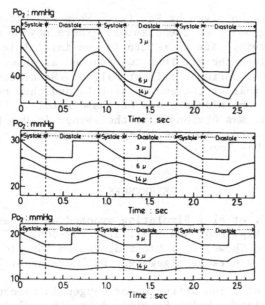

Fig. 4.   Cardiac change of tissue Po_2 at three radial distances of
3, 6 and 14 μ. The decrease in plasma Po_2 was caused by
a stop of blood flow in the systole. O_2 consumption was
kept at 1.94×10^{-3} sec^{-1}.

linear. In the derivation of an analytical solution, however, we
assumed the slope to be constant and evaluated the effect of myoglobin on the Po_2 change. The solution was given by a linear combination of the first 4 _eigen_ functions. The relation between the
time constant of those functions and the Po_2 value was obtained by
using the parameter values described by Grote and Thews (2) for the
heart muscle. The time constant of the first _eigen_ function was
the longest and was about 0.1 sec at Po_2 = 40 mm Hg, increasing to
1 sec at 7 mmHg. It seemed to become about 10 sec at the lowest
Po_2.

When the O_2 consumption rate increases, the Po_2 difference between RBC and plasma as well as the Po_2 gradient in the tissue increases, and the Po_2 level in the tissue decreases. When the blood
flow is reduced, the tissue Po_2 decreases according to a drop of
Po_2 in RBC. Whatever the cause of Po_2 change in the tissue may be,
it is markedly buffered by the O_2 dissociation from both hemoglobin
and myoglobin. An example of the Po_2 distribution is illustrated
in Fig. 4 : The curves were obtained at three radial distances of
3, 6 and 14 μ. The Po_2 pattern at 3 μ or the capillary boundary
was calculated by assuming that the blood flow stops at the systole
and begins to flow at the diastole. When the blood flow stops during the systole, the change in plasma Po_2 at a certain site along

the capillary may be given by Eq. (1). When the blood flow is re-
sumed at the beginning of the diastole, there may be a delay for
Po_2 at the observing site to return to the initial level until
fresh blood arrives there. Thus, we assumed as shown in Fig. 4
that the Po_2 level during the first half of the diastolic phase
was the same as that at the end of systole and then returned to the
initial level at the middle phase of the diastole. From the curves
for 6 and 14 μ it was obvious that the change in Po_2 became smaller
as the Po_2 decreased. A phase delay even appeared at the distal
site with a low Po_2 level.

REFERENCES

1. Bruley, D. F. et al : Simulating myocardium oxygen dynamics,
Advances in Exp. Med. and Biol. <u>37B</u>, 859–866, 1973.
2. Grote, J. and Thews, G. : Die Bedingungen für die Sauerstoffversorgung des Herzmuskelgewebes. Pflügers Arch. <u>276</u>, 142–165,
1962.
3. Klug, A. et al : The diffusion of oxygen in concentrated hemoglobin solutions. Helv. Physiol. Acta, <u>14</u>, 121–128, 1956.
4. Lawson, W. H. Jr. et al : Effect of temperature on deoxygenation rate of human red cells. J. Appl. Physiol. <u>20</u>, 912–917,
1965.
5. Lawson, W. H. Jr. and Forster, R. E. : Oxygen tension gradient
in peripheral capillary blood. J. Appl. Physiol. <u>22</u>, 970–973,
1967.
6. Longmuir, I. S. and Roughton, F. J. W. : The diffusion coefficients of carbon monoxide and nitrogen in hemoglobin solutions.
J. Physiol. <u>118</u>, 264–275, 1952.
7. Miyamoto, Y. and Moll, W. : Measurements of dimensions and
pathway of red cells in rapidly frozen lung in situ. Resp.
Physiol. <u>12</u>, 141–156, 1971.
8. Mochizuki, M. : On the velocity of oxygen dissociation of
human hemoglobin and red cell. Jap. J. Physiol. <u>16</u>, 649–657,
1966.
9. Mochizuki, M. : Graphical analysis of oxygenation and CO-com-
bination rates of the red blood cells in the lung. Hirokawa
Publ. Co. Tokyo, 1975.
10. Tazawa, H. et al : Oxygenation and deoxygenation factors of
chorioallantoic capillary blood. J. Appl. Physiol. <u>40</u>, 399–
403, 1976.
11. Thews, G. : Ueber die mathematische Behandlung physiologischer
Diffusionsprozesse in zylinderförmigen Objekten. Acta Bio-
theoretica. <u>10</u>, 105–138, 1953.
12. Thews, G. : Die Sauerstoffdrucke im Herzmuskelgewebe. Pflügers
Arch. <u>176</u>, 166–181, 1962.

GAS TRANSFER THROUGH THE SKIN: A TWO-LAYER MODEL RELATING

TRANSCUTANEOUS FLUX TO ARTERIAL TENSION

John A. Quinn

Department of Chemical and Biochemical Engineering
and Institute for Environmental Medicine
University of Pennsylvania
Philadelphia, Pennsylvania, U.S.A.

Recent developments in clinical application of transcutaneous blood-gas sensors show promise for continuous, noninvasive monitoring of arterial oxygen and carbon dioxide tensions (Huch et al., 1975). In practice, a probe placed in contact with the skin is used to measure the flux of gas between the skin and the gas space within the probe. The probe or skin electrode is calibrated to relate measured gas flux to arterial tension. Since the flux through the skin depends on many variables an accurate correlation between measured flux and blood-gas tension requires a basic understanding of the overall skin permeation process.

To identify the variables which control gas transfer through the skin a simplified, two-layer model for skin permeation has been derived. The model incorporates gross anatomical and circulation details while introducing a minimum of physicochemical and blood-flow parameters. The resulting linear equation shows the skin flux related to five quantities: (1) the arterial tension relative to that at the surface of the skin, (2) the permeability of the epidermis, (3) the specific rate of skin metabolism, (4) the effective permeability of the vascularized dermis, and (5) the thickness of the skin.

Preliminary animal studies on transcutaneous gas exchange have been carried out at the Institute for Environmental Medicine. In these experiments transfer rates were measured for six different inert gases permeating through the skin of anesthetized pigs (Col-

lins, 1976). These data interpreted in light of the present model
provide insight into the relative roles of perfusion and diffusion
in gas transfer through the skin.

In this paper we describe our two-layer model for skin transfer.
Limiting forms of the flux equation are examined along with a discussion of possible methods for parameter evaluation. Finally, sample data from our on-going animal studies of the simultaneous transfer of several inert gases are presented.

MASS TRANSFER

Our model for the skin is that of "a bilayer membrane laminate,
the outer layer of which (the epidermis) is about 100 μm thick and
unvascularized, while the inner layer (the dermis) is several hun-
dreds of microns in thickness and interlaced with capillaries."
(Michaels et al., 1975). A single, open capillary is the basis for
our steady-state mass balance on the permeating gas which enters
with (or leaves) the blood flowing through the capillary and eventually exits (or enters) through the outermost skin layer. We assume
negligible gas exchange between the dermis and underlying subcutaneous tissue. Assume that the dissolved gas tension, or partial
pressure, P_b, is a function only of distance along the capillary, z,
and that outside the immediate vicinity of the capillary the gas
tension ($\overline{P}_d$) is uniform throughout the dermis. For capillary flow
rate, Q(cm^3/sec) and radius, R, a differential mass balance at
any point along the capillary yields:

$$-QH_b \frac{dP_b}{dz} = k_d(2\pi R) \ H_d(P_b - \overline{P}_d) \tag{1}$$

where k_d is a mass transfer coefficient governing exchange between
capillary and dermis, and H_b and H_d are Henry's law constants relating dissolved gas concentrations to partial pressures. Integrating Equation (1) over the length, L, of the capillary loop where
gas tension changes from $P_b(0)=P_a$ (entering, arterial value) to
$P_b(L)=P_v$ (leaving, venous tension) gives:

$$\frac{P_a - P_v}{P_a - \overline{P}_d} = 1 - e^{-\beta} \quad \text{and} \quad \beta = \frac{D_d}{\delta^2 \gamma q} \tag{2}$$

The following substitutions having been made: γ, the blood/dermis
distribution coefficient is equal to H_b/H_d; $k_d=D_d/\delta$, a film-type
mass transfer coefficient with D_d the diffusion coefficient in the
dermis and δ, the characteristic thickness of the dermis diffusion
barrier; an appropriate value for δ is V/2πRL, where V is the volume
of skin irrigated by one open capillary (obtained by dividing the

total skin volume by the total number of open capillaries -- a strongly temperature-dependent quantity) and δ is, therefore, the ratio of tissue volume to capillary surface area; q is Q/V, the specific blood flow, expressed as cm^3 of blood/cm^3 of skin/sec. (Scheuplein and Blank, 1971)

Events in the dermis are linked to the transcutaneous flux and to skin metabolism through an overall mass balance on V. Assume that the skin volume V has an outer surface area, A, and the trans- cutaneous flux across A is N (cm^3 of gas/cm^2 of skin/sec). The rate of metabolism of the skin is introduced as a zero-order reaction, i.e. independent of oxygen tension (Roughton, 1952) - this assump- tion would require modification at low O_2 tensions, a modification which can be introduced without undue complication. The specific rate of metabolism is m (cm^3 of O_2/cm^3 of skin/sec) for O_2 consump- tion, or -m for CO_2 production. The overall balance is then

$$QH_b(P_a-P_v) = AN + Vm \tag{3}$$

and N is represented as a film-type expression

$$N = k_e H_e(\overline{P}_d-P_o) = K(\overline{P}_d-P_o) \tag{4}$$

where k_e is the mass transfer coefficient for the epidermis, H_e is a Henry's law constant, and $K=k_e H_e$ is the permeability of the epi- dermis. P_o represents the environmental partial pressure of the permeating gas, i.e. the pressure at the outer surface of the skin.

Combining Equations (2), (3), and (4), and solving for N gives

$$N = \frac{KW}{K+W}[(P_a-P_o)-\frac{\tau m}{W}] \quad \text{and} \quad W = \tau q H_b(1-e^{-\beta}) \tag{5}$$

where W is the effective permeability of the dermis; and τ, the skin thickness, equals V/A. Equation (5) is the working equation which links measured transcutaneous flux, N, to arterial tension, P_a. Note that it assumes steady conditions (extension to the transient case is straightforward) and film-type mass transfer resistances.

LIMITING FORMS

Special cases which provide insight into evaluation of the various parameters in Equation (5) are the following. If skin flux is zero, then arterial supply just balances skin metabolism and

$$(P_a-P_o)\Big|_{N=0} = \frac{\tau m}{W} \tag{6}$$

By measuring N as a function of (P_a-P_o) with all else held constant, $\tau m/W$ could be obtained from the intercept of a plot of N vs. (P_a-P_o). For $K \gg W$, i.e. dermal resistance controlling,

$$N\Big|_{K \gg W} = W(P_a-P_o)-\tau m \tag{7}$$

and the converse case of the epidermis constituting the major resistance, $K \ll W$,

$$N\Big|_{K \ll W} = K(P_a-P_o) - \frac{K\tau m}{W} \tag{8}$$

Limiting cases indicating predominance of "diffusion" or "perfusion" in the dermis are associated with values of β, hence W:

Perfusion limited (β large)

$$W\Big|_{\beta \to \infty} = \tau q H_b \tag{9}$$

Diffusion limited (β small)

$$W\Big|_{\beta \to o} = \tau q H_b \beta \tag{10}$$

For inert gases, m=o

$$N\Big|_{m=o} = \frac{KW}{K+W}(P_a-P_o) \tag{11}$$

In addition, there are several other limiting forms corresponding to combinations of these cases. For example, the limits for inert gas transfer corresponding to the relative dominance of dermal and epidermal resistances can be obtained from Equations (7) and (8).

$$N\Big|_{m=o,K \gg W} = W(P_a-P_o) \tag{12}$$

$$N\Big|_{m=o,K \ll W} = K(P_a-P_o) \tag{13}$$

Equation (12) is the perfusion-limited case, i.e. flux is governed by conditions in vascularized dermis, and (13) corresponds to diffusion through the epidermis being the controlling factor.

TABLE 1. COMPARISON OF IN VIVO MEASUREMENTS OF TRANSCUTANEOUS INERT GAS EXCHANGE

Gas	Ambient Temperature(°C)	Refr.	$N/(P_a-P_o)$ (cm³/hr/M²/atm.)	Comments
Helium	26-28°	(1)	41	Efflux, forearm and hand (human)
"	"	(2)	54	Influx from He environment, whole body (human)
"	"	(3)	97	Efflux, forearm and hand (human)
"	"	(*)	46	Efflux, lower abdomen (pig)
"	37-38°	(1)	57	Efflux, forearm and hand (human)
"	"	(*)	60	Efflux, lower abdomen (pig)
"	40-41°	(1)	65	Efflux, forearm and hand (human)
"	"	(*)	65	Efflux, lower abdomen (pig)
Ethylene	26-28°	(4)	23	P_a unknown, est. 0.75 atm., efflux, forearm and hand (human)
"	"	(*)	41	Efflux, lower abdomen (pig)
Nitrous Oxide	26-28°	(4)	332	Efflux, forearm and hand (human)
"	"	(5)	306	Efflux, forearm and hand (human)
"	"	(*)	269	Efflux, lower abdomen (pig)

(1) Klocke et al., 1963.
(2) Behnke and Willmon, 1941.
(3) Adamczyk et al., 1966.
(4) Orcutt and Waters, 1933.
(5) Stoelting and Eger, 1969.
(*) Collins (this laboratory), 1976.

PARAMETER ESTIMATION

To apply Equation (5) to the calibration of skin probes, values
are required for the parameters K, W, τ and m. In principle, the
permeability of the epidermal layer, K, can be determined from in
vitro measurements using excised skin; Cullen and Eger (1972) have
reported such measurements. Alternatively, K can be estimated from
in vivo measurements with inert gases whose flux is limited by epidermal transfer, Equation (13). Correspondingly, W can be obtained
directly from measurements with a perfusion-limited inert gas; our
animal studies (Collins et al., 1977) indicate that helium may approximate this requirement. W can also be calculated from known
values of τ, q, H_b and β -- each of which can be determined separately. The skin thickness, τ, can be measured. The metabolic
ratio can be found by doing Warburg experiments on excised, minced
skin (Adams, 1949).

ANIMAL STUDIES WITH INERT GASES

In preliminary studies using piglets (Collins et al., 1977),
efflux rates for several inert gases were measured over a range of
skin temperatures (34 to 41°C) on the lower abdominal (midline) region. A collection cup sealed to the skin and covering a surface
area of about 40 cm^2 was used to collect samples of gas which per-
meated through the skin. Mixtures of inert gas were breathed to
permit comparison between the gases under identical physiological
conditions, thus eliminating in part the expected interanimal variation. Table 1 shows a comparison of our data for helium, ethylene,
and nitrous oxide with representative data on humans taken from the
limited literature on transcutaneous exchange. The experimental results are shown as a normalized flux -- efflux or influx -- calculated as the ratio of the measured skin flux (in units of cm^3 gas/M^2
skin/hr) to the partial pressure driving force, (P_a-P_o), (in atm.)
where P_a is taken to be approximately equal to the partial pressure
of the inspired gas. The overall agreement is reasonable indicating that the pig is an appropriate experimental animal. At this
time we have insufficient data on the parameters of Equation (5) to
make a detailed comparison of our analytical model. Studies are
currently underway to obtain the necessary measurements on these
animals.

Acknowledgement. This work was supported in part by the Institute for Environmental Medicine, University of Pennsylvania Medical
Center. The animal experiments were performed by Dr. J.M. Collins
as part of his Ph.D. dissertation (University of Pennsylvania, 1976).
This study stems from a continuing collaborative investigation of
physiological gas exchange carried out jointly with Professors D.J.
Graves and C.J. Lambertsen.

REFERENCES

Adamczyk, B., Boerboom, A.J., and Kistemaker, J. (1966) J. Appl. Physiol. 21, 1903.

Adams, P.D. (1949) Amer. Perfumer Ess. Oil Rev., 134.

Behnke, A.R. and Willmon, T.L. (1941) Amer. J. Physiol. 131, 627.

Collins, J.M., Lambertsen, C.J., and Quinn, J.A. (1976) Physiologist 19, 155.

Collins, J.M. (1976) Inert gas transfer in the body: Experimental Study and perfusion/diffusion modeling of transcutaneous and gas cavity exchange rates, Ph.D. Dissertation, University of Pennsylvania.

Collins, J.M., Lambertsen, C.J., and Quinn, J.A. (1977) Transcutaneous gas exchange: simultaneous measurement of multiple inert gases. (submitted for publication.)

Cullen, B.F. and Eger, E.I. (1972) Anesthesiology 36, 168.

Huch, R., Lubbers, D.W., and Huch, A. (1975) The transcutaneous measurement of oxygen and carbon dioxide tensions for the determination of arterial blood-gas values with control of local perfusion and peripheral perfusion pressure. Theoretical analysis and practical application. In "Oxygen Measurements in Biology and Medicine" p.121 (eds. Payne, J.P. and Hill, D.W.) Butterworths, London and Boston.

Klocke, R.A., Gurtner, G.H., and Farhi, L.E. (1963) J. Appl. Physiol. 18, 311.

Michaels, A.S., Chandrasekaran, S.K., and Shaw, J.E. (1975) A.I.Ch.E. Journal 21, 985.

Orcutt, F.S. and Waters, R.M. (1933) Anesthesia and Analgesia 12, 45.

Roughton, F.J.W. (1952) Proc. Roy. Soc. 140B, 203.

Scheuplein, R.J. and Blank, I.H. (1971) Physiol. Reviews 51, 702.

Stoelting, R.K. and Eger, E.E. (1969) Anesthesiology 30, 278.

ELECTRICAL POTENTIALS DURING CARBON DIOXIDE TRANSPORT IN HEMOGLOBIN SOLUTIONS

J. De Koning, P. Stroeve, and J.H. Meldon

Depts. of Physiol., Univ. of Nijmegen, Nijmegen

The Netherlands, and Univ. of Odense, Odense, Denmark

Transport of CO_2 in aqueous solutions is enhanced by the diffusion of HCO_3^- ions (Gros and Moll, 1971, 1974). This facilitated transport is dependent on the kinetics of CO_2 hydration (Enns, 1976; Otto and Quinn, 1971) and therefore on the concentration of carbonic anhydrase (CA). The role of charged proteins, if present in the solution, has remained unclear. It was suggested in the case of albumin that the protein serves mainly as a carrier of protons (Gros and Moll, 1974). However, since the macromolecules are nearly immobile, compared to the smaller bicarbonate ions, appreciable diffusion potentials can be generated by the imposition of a CO_2 gradient across a protein solution. These electrical potentials can significantly affect the facilitated CO_2 transport. An analysis which accounts for electrical potentials does in fact provide the explanation for what must be re-garded as a relatively low permeability of CO_2 in protein solutions (Meldon, 1975). We report here experimental results which demonstrate the induction of sizable diffusion potentials by the transport of CO_2 in hemoglobin solutions, and describe the influence of these po-tentials on CO_2 transport.

THEORY

The important reactions involved in CO_2 diffusion in a moderately alkaline layer of protein solution are:

$$CO_2 + H_2O \rightleftharpoons H_2CO_3 \rightleftharpoons HCO_3^- + H^+ \qquad\qquad I$$

$$Pr^{1-\nu} \rightleftharpoons Pr^{-\nu} + H^+ \qquad\qquad II$$

Reaction I is catalyzed by carbonic anhydrase, which is normally present in erythrocytes and certain tissues. Reaction II denotes the acid dissociation of macromolecule Pr with net negative charge $1-\nu$. At physiological pH, the formation of $CO_3^=$ can be neglected. The reactions are coupled during CO_2 transport. Therefore a CO_2 concentration gradient leads to concentration gradients of all other reactive species and their diffusion is described by the Nernst-Planck equation:

$$J_k = -D_k C_k \left(\frac{d}{dx} \ln C_k + z_k \frac{F}{RT} \frac{d}{dx} V \right) \tag{1}$$

Here J_k is the flux, D_k the diffusivity, C_k the molar concentration and z_k the charge of species k; F, R, and T are respectively the Faraday constant, ideal gas constant, and absolute temperature; x is the distance into the film from the high CO_2 partial pressure (pCO_2) boundary; dV/dx is the gradient of the electrical potential. In an electrically floating layer of protein solution exposed to gas phases of differing pCO_2, steady state fluxes J_i of inert species like Na^+, which are constrained to the film, must be zero everywhere. Therefore:

$$\frac{d}{dx} \ln C_i = -z_i \frac{F}{RT} \frac{d}{dx} V \tag{2}$$

which is readily integrated. An equation analogous to (2) describes the distribution of protein species, but since z_{Pr} varies with pH as well as CO_2 tension this equation is not readily integrated.

An expression for the local electric field may be derived by substitution of (1) into the zero-current relation ($\Sigma_k z_k J_k = 0$) and then applying electroneutrality ($\Sigma_k z_k C_k = 0$) and the corresponding differential ($\Sigma_k z_k \frac{d}{dx} C_k = 0$); with equation (2) for both inert species and proteins, retaining significant terms, we arrive at:

$$-\frac{d}{dx} V = -\frac{RT}{F} \left\{ \frac{1-\alpha}{C_{HCO_3^-} + \alpha(z_{Pr}^2 C_{Pr} + \Sigma z_i^2 C_i)} \right\} \frac{d}{dx} C_{HCO_3^-} \tag{3}$$

where $\alpha = D_{Pr}/D_{HCO_3^-} \approx 0.04$ (for numerical values see Fig. 1).

According to the equation of Linderstrøm-Lang (Cohn and Edsall, 1943) the relationship between average squared protein charge, $\overline{z_{Pr}^2}$, z_{Pr}, and buffercapacity, β_{Pr}, in the absence of CO_2 is:

$$\overline{z_{Pr}^2} = z_{Pr}^2 + \beta_{Pr}/2.3 .$$

Clearly the electrical field is a consequence of the bicarbonate-protein diffusivity difference. Taking K as an effective constant for the bracketed term in eq. (3), the potential drop across the film can be expressed as:

$$\Delta V = \frac{RT}{F} \, K \, \Delta C_{HCO_3^-} \qquad (4)$$

The expression for net CO$_2$ flux is:

$$J_{CO_2}^{net} = \frac{1}{L} \{ D_{CO_2} \Delta C_{CO_2} + D_{HCO_3^-} \, \Delta C_{HCO_3^-} \, (1 - K') \} \qquad (5)$$

L is film thickness and K' an effective constant for the product of C$_{HCO_3^-}$ and K. The last term on the righthand side of eq. (5) corresponds to the bicarbonate facilitated portion of net CO$_2$ transport.

The potential's consequences are twofold: 1) Inert anions accumulate at the high pCO$_2$ side, inert cations in the low pCO$_2$ region, and protein molecules behave according to the sign of z_{Pr}. The resulting boundary pH values ensure a smaller $\Delta C_{HCO_3^-}$ than in case of ΔV = zero. 2) The electrically driven HCO$_3^-$ flux opposes that stemming from its concentration gradient, i.e. $0 \le K' \le 1$. Both effects tend to decrease facilitation of the CO$_2$ flux.

EXPERIMENTAL

Two 25 cc gas chambers are separated by a horizontal layer of Hb solution (diameter 10 mm, thickness 0.5 - 1.7 mm). The liquid film is supported by a microporous polyethylene membrane, 29 μm thick, that has a negligible resistance to CO$_2$ diffusion. The gas compositions in the chambers are maintained by continuously sweeping humidified gases of known concentrations at 50 cc/min. Two micropipette electrodes (Ag/AgCl type) are vertically oriented by micrometers, one just in contact with the upper surface, the other with the lower surface of the protein solution. Potential differences across the film are measured directly by the electrodes, fed into a high-input impedance differential amplifier and recorded. Before an experimental run the same gas (pCO$_2$ = 2 mmHg in N$_2$) is flowing through both chambers, and any steady-state offset voltage ($\pm$ 1 mV) is compensated. Upon sudden change of the gas composition in the upper chamber to a higher pCO$_2$ an electrical potential ΔV_1 is gradually established. Returning to the original mixture causes the potential to decay to zero. If the composition in the lower chamber is switched to the CO$_2$-rich mixture, the measured diffusion potential, ΔV_2, is approximately equal to ΔV_1 (though opposite).

Hb solutions are prepared by hemolyzing fresh bovine red blood cells. After dialysis and concentration, the Hb solution is de-ionized and sodium bicarbonate is added as desired. All measurements were performed at room temperature (21 $\pm$ 0.5 $^{\circ}$C).

RESULTS AND DISCUSSION

Steady-state diffusion potentials measured in 4 mM Hb solutions are presented in Fig. 1 as a function of the concentration of added $NaHCO_3$. The imposed CO_2 gradient was 2 - 38 mm Hg in nitrogen. Experiments with active carbonic anhydrase (CA) are denoted by filled circles. Adding CA (1mg/ml) has no effect, which indicates that the enzyme normally present in Hb solutions as prepared is sufficient to ensure equilibrium of the CO_2 hydration reaction. Inhibition of CA with acetazolamide (1 mg/ml) reduces the signal to 60 % of the original value. Apparently the reaction is no longer at equilibrium and the potential is dependent on layer thickness (de Koning et al.,in prep.). Fig. 1 indicates satisfactory agreement between the observed fall in diffusion potential with increasing $NaHCO_3$ and theoretical results from an approximate analytical solution of the equations governing the reaction equilibrium case. The analysis suggests two reasons for the decline of ΔV: 1) Addition of sodium bicarbonate raises the solution pH which makes z_{Pr} more negative, and increases in equation (3) the term $z_{Pr}^2 C_{Pr}$. 2) Adding Na^+ produces an in-

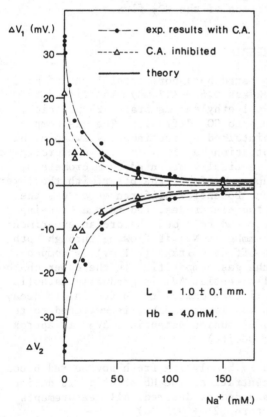

Figure 1

Steady-state diffusion potentials as a function of the concentration of sodium, added as $NaHCO_3$. ΔV_1 and ΔV_2 are the respective potentials with the high pCO_2 mixture above and below. ΔCO_2 = 2 - 38 mmHg . Numerical values used for calculation of the theoretical curve:

pK (reaction I) = 6.1

γ_{CO_2} = 4 x 10^{-5} M/mm Hg

D_{CO_2} = 8.5 x 10^{-6} cm^2/sec

$D_{HCO_3^-}$ = 4.9 x 10^{-6} cm^2/sec

(Gros and Moll, 1974)

D_{Hb} = 0.18 x 10^{-6} cm^2/sec

(Keller et al.,1971).

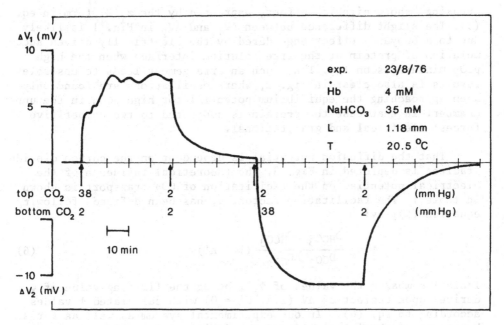

Figure 2. Record of an experiment with both an oscillatory and a steady diffusion potential. Oscillations do not occur when the layer density gradient in Hb is stable (ΔV_2).

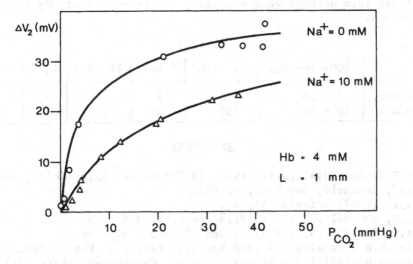

Figure 3. Steady-state diffusion potentials ΔV_2 at two different sodium concentrations as a function of pCO_2 in the lower chamber. In the upper chamber pCO_2 is maintained at 2 mmHg.

creasing "short-circuit" effect, expressed by the $z_i^2 C_i$ term in eq. (3). The slight difference between ΔV_1 and ΔV_2 in Fig. 1 is likely due to a buoyancy effect engendered by the electrically driven accumulation of protein at the free solution interface when the high pCO$_2$ mixture is on top. That such an arrangement leads to unstable results is also clear in Fig. 2, where oscillations are found only when approaching the equilibrium potential for high pCO$_2$ in the upper chamber. In that case the protein is subjected to two competitive forces: electrical and gravitational.

That the diffusion potential is dependent on the carbon dioxide gradient is depicted in Fig. 3. The theoretical influence of the electrical potential on the facilitation of CO$_2$ transport is shown in table 1. The facilitation factor, Φ, has been defined, following equation (5), by:

$$\Phi = \frac{D_{HCO_3^-} \, \Delta C_{HCO_3^-}}{D_{CO_2} \, \Delta C_{CO_2}} (1 - K') \tag{6}$$

Table 1 compares the values of Φ_0, being the limiting value of Φ derived upon neglect of ΔV (i.e. $K' = 0$) with calculated Φ values according to eq. (6). In our experimental system as well as for a hypothetical physiological case the facilitated portion of the CO$_2$ flux is profoundly reduced.

We therefore conclude that the ionic nature of the species participating in CO$_2$ transport as well as their relative mobilities must be taken into account when analyzing net transport of CO$_2$ in protein solutions.

Table 1

	ΔCO_2 (mm Hg)	Na$^+$ (mM)	V (mV)	Hb (mM)	Φ_0	Φ
this exp.	2 - 38	35	11	4	9	.6
physiol.	40 - 45	150	.2	5	3	.2

REFERENCES

Cohn,E.J. and Edsall,J.T. (1943) in "Proteins, Amino Acids, and Peptides", Reinhold, New York, p. 462.
Enns,T. (1967) Science 155, 44.
Gros,G. and Moll,W. (1971) Pflügers Arch. 324, 249.
Gros,G. and Moll,W. (1974) J. Gen. Physiol. 64, 356.
Keller,K.H., Canales,E.R.,and Yum,S.I. (1971) J. Phys. Chem. 75, 379.
Meldon,J.H. (1975) 5th Biophys. Congr., Copenhagen, abstr. 413.
Otto,N.C. and Quinn,J.A. (1971) Chem. Eng. Sci. 26, 949.

Supported in part by Stiftung Volkswagenwerk and FUNGO/Z.W.O.

INTERPRETATION OF OXYGEN DISAPPEARANCE RATES IN BRAIN CORTEX

FOLLOWING TOTAL ISCHAEMIA

D.D. Reneau and J.H. Halsey, Jr.*

Louisiana Tech University, Ruston, Louisiana 71270, USA.
*University of Alabama Medical Center, Birmingham,
Alabama 35294, USA.

INTRODUCTION

The purpose of this project was to attempt to obtain a more precise interpretation of the meaning of the rates of disappearance curves of PO_2 in brain cortex following complete ischaemia as measured with microelectrodes. The following three specific studies are discussed:

(1) Analysis of individual PO_2 disappearance as a function of time.

(2) Analysis of the rate of disappearance as a function of the initial tissue PO_2.

(3) Analysis of the rates of disappearance curves with respect to the possibility of prediction of local metabolic rates.

The method of analysis was by means of mathematical simulation. The change in tissue PO_2 with respect to time following cessation of capillary flow is a function of several factors including metabolic consumption, oxygen supply from oxyhaemoglobin trapped in the capillaries, and diffusivity parameters. These factors first were combined into a distributed parameter mathematical model for capillary source, radial diffusion, and tissue consumption; and the entire process of the disappearance rate was theoretically simulated.

EXPERIMENTAL

Using microelectrodes in the cerebral cortex of gerbils and rabbits, the time course of PO_2 changes following total ischaemia has been measured under a variety of conditions in numerous animals. Repetitive experiments in the same animal at the same locus can be obtained in the gerbil by means of bilateral carotid ligation. In rabbits only one curve per animal could be obtained since it was necessary to use cardiac arrest in order to achieve total ischaemia. For details see Halsey (1974) and Reneau et al (1976).

Figure 1 is a representative curve descriptive of the PO_2 time history following ischaemia. Note the straight line decrease of PO_2 during the first second of time which is followed by a tapered curvature that approaches zero torr assymptotically. In a prior communication, Reneau et al (1976) reported that the straight line portion of the curve was mathematically consistent with a constant metabolic rate and the curvature could be an indication of a changing metabolic rate. That analysis will be more fully explored in this paper. In some of the experiments when the initial tissue PO_2 is very high a curvature is noticed during the duration of the curve.

If the initial slope of the straight line segment of a series of curves similar to Figure 1 is measured (disappearance rate, mmHg/sec.) and plotted versus the initial PO_2, a curve is obtained similar to Figure 2 or Figure 3. The curve has the appearance of a straight line and the rate of disappearance of O_2 is directly proportional to the initial tissue PO_2. The curve is interesting

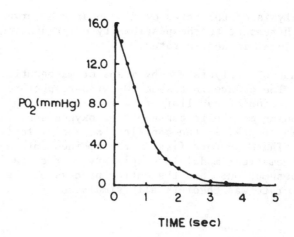

Fig. 1. The change in PO_2 in gerbil cortex with respect to time following bilateral carotid ligation.

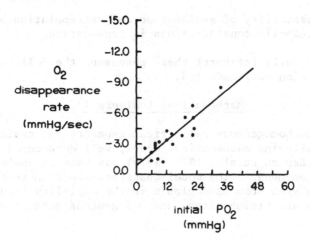

Fig. 2. Oxygen disappearance rate as a function of the initial
        tissue PO_2 in rabbit cortex.   Each point is taken from an
        animal killed by cardiac arrest.

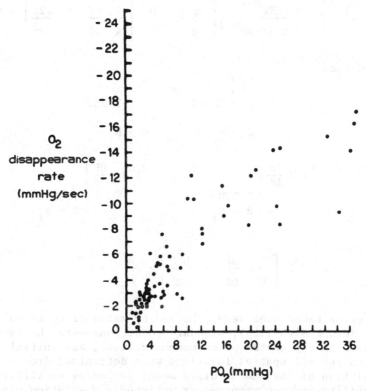

Fig. 3. Oxygen disappearance rate as a function of the initial
        tissue PO_2 in gerbil cortex. Every data point was measured
        in the same location with the same electrode and represent
        a variety of conditions.

since the possibility of explanation and extrapolation of interpretation to metabolic considerations is provocative.

To more fully interpret these phenomena the following mathematical simulation was conducted.

Mathematical Analysis I

Based on homogeneous cylindrical geometry and radial diffusion only, the following mathematical model, well documented in the literature (Reneau et al., 1970, 1976) was used to analyse the above presented phenomena. The model describes the transient non-linear release of oxygen from haemoglobin in the capillary, radial diffusion to all tissue sites, and homogeneous metabolic consumption.

Mathematical Model

Capillary:

$$V_x \left[1 + \frac{nNKP^{N-1}}{C_1(1+KP^N)^2} \right] \frac{\partial p}{\partial X} = D_1 \left[\frac{1}{R} \frac{\partial P}{\partial R} + \frac{\partial 2p}{\partial R^2} \right] \quad (1)$$

Interface:

$$\left. P_1 \right|_{\text{BLOOD}} = \left. P_1 \right|_{\text{TISSUE}} \quad (2)$$

$$R = R_1 \qquad R = R_1$$

$$\left. D_1 C_1 \frac{DP}{DR} \right|_{\substack{\text{BLOOD} \\ R = R_1}} = \left. D_2 C_2 \frac{DP}{DR} \right|_{\substack{\text{TISSUE} \\ R = R_1}} \quad (3)$$

Tissue:

$$D_2 \left[\frac{1}{R} \frac{DP}{DR} + \frac{D^2P}{DR^2} \right] - \frac{A}{C_2} = 0 \quad (4)$$

Solution techniques were achieved by means of numerical analysis (Crank-Nicholson), boundary conditions were the same as those given in the quoted prior communications, and initial conditions for all spatial locations were determined from steady state solution of the standardized model including capillary flow. Both stability and convergence was achieved and solution via the IBM 370 digital computer was rapid. Standard data as given for the human in the prior papers were used for the trend simulation.

SIMULATION RESULTS

Disappearance rates and metabolic prediction

Figure 4 represents the results of the theoretical analysis. By observing the lower curve note that the same results were obtained mathematically as were found experimentally, i.e. the oxygen disappearance rate is directly proportional to the initial tissue PO_2. The explanation for this occurrence is that the higher the PO_2 the less the quantity of O_2 released from haemoglobin per unit change in PO_2. At high tissue and blood PO_2 more O_2 is consumed from the oxygen physically dissolved in tissue fluid and less is supplied from trapped capillary haemoglobin than at low tissue PO_2. Hence at high tissue PO_2 the disappearance rate is greater. For an aid to understanding refer to the non-linear shape of the oxygen dissociation curve. These results are consistent with the constant metabolic rate.

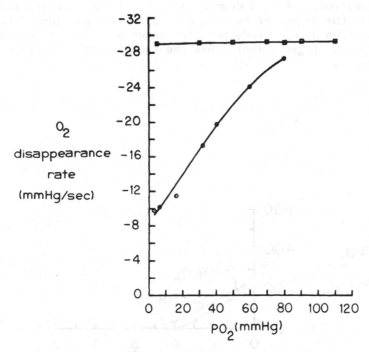

Fig. 4. Theoretically predicted oxygen disappearance rate curve as a function of initial tissue PO_2.

    ⊙ - PO_2 below haemoglobin saturation level.
    ▣ - PO_2 above haemoglobin saturation level or in the absence of haemoglobin.

The study predicts that the disappearance rate will have a
constant value at all tissue PO_2 values that are above the
haemoglobin saturation level or in the absence of haemoglobin.
This value is represented by the upper curve of Figure 4.
The disappearance rate under these conditions is exactly equal to
the metabolic rate divided by the tissue solubility.   As a result,
one should be able to determine the local metabolic rate directly
from the initial slope disappearance curve under hyperbaric oxygen
conditions or under conditions of perfusion without haemoglobin.

Individual PO_2 changes with time

The simulation also indicates that the straight line decrease of PO_2
initially found in Fig. 1 is consistent with a constant rate of
metabolism.   However at higher PO_2 values a curvature can be
expected during the course of the PO_2 change which reflects the
non-linear process for the release of oxygen from haemoglobin.
The more extensive curvature as PO_2 approaches zero torr can be a
function of a changing metabolic rate or the result of progressively
developing anoxic areas at radial regions beyond the electrode
measuring position.   Fig. 5 demonstrates the latter process and
suggests that the degree of curvature in the lower portion of Fig. 1
may be a function of electrode position between capillary supply and
developing anoxic regions (which has the same effect as a change in
metabolic rate).

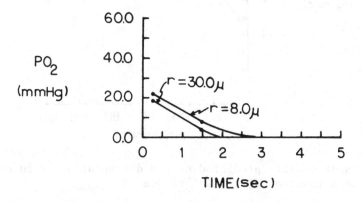

Fig. 5. PO_2 disappearance as a function of time at
different radial locations.

Diffusional Resistances

Following complete ischaemia, the steady state radial gradient between capillary and tissue changes to a new dynamic radial gradient within at least a few hundred milli seconds. This dynamic gradient is a function of the PO_2 level and is almost zero at very high PO_2 values since the source effect of haemoglobin is then absent; but the gradient increases as PO_2 decreases and reaches a maximum when tissue PO_2 is in equilibrium with capillary blood PO_2 above the S-shaped region at the lower end of the dissociation curve. If gradients were not substantial one would expect to find an increase in the disappearance rate at the very low end of Fig. 2. This has not been observed experimentally and offers possibilities for future conjecture concerning diffusional resistances in the microcirculation.

Mathematical Analysis II - Metabolic Prediction

In an attempt to extract information concerning metabolic rates from PO_2 disappearance rates at physiological tissue PO_2 values, a different approach was taken. If one assumes that spatial resolution can be sacrificed for this study, a lumped parameter model can be developed for the capillary and tissue and combined into the following simple differential equation:

$$\frac{dP}{dt} = \frac{A}{\alpha_T} \quad \emptyset \tag{5}$$

where,

$\dfrac{dP}{dt}$ = oxygen disappearance rate

$\dfrac{A}{\alpha T}$ = metabolic rate divided by tissue solubility

$\emptyset = \dfrac{1\,m}{1 + \dfrac{V_\beta N}{V_T \alpha_T \lambda}}$

$\dfrac{V_\beta}{V_T}$ = ratio at blood volume tissue volume

N = oxygen capacity of capillary blood

m = slope of O_2 dissociation curve at a particular condition

$\lambda = \dfrac{PO_2 \text{ of tissue}}{PO_2 \text{ of blood}}$

Note that $\emptyset$ is a dimensionless parameter related to the tissue vital capacity and is a direct measure of the degree of alteration of the rate of disappearance curve from the metabolic effect. The value of $\emptyset$ ranges from values approaching zero at low tissue PO_2 to a maximum of 1.0 for high PO_2 values that reflect haemoglobin saturation.

If for a given microregion $\emptyset$ is relatively independent of changes in metabolism at a given tissue PO_2, then equation (5) offers some interesting possibilities. To test the independence of $\emptyset$ from A/α_T at the same tissue PO_2, the distributed parameter model was used to generate rates of disappearance curves for a wide range of metabolic values and $\emptyset$ was calculated as a function of tissue PO_2 by the relationship,

$$\emptyset = \frac{(dP/dt)}{(A/\alpha_T)}$$

Results indicate that above a tissue PO_2 at 10 torr $\emptyset$ is approximately independent of changes in metabolism. The independence becomes more pronounced as tissue PO_2 increases.

Consequently if A/α_T is known for a given microregion under a given set of conditions, or is measured from disappearance curves under hyperbaric conditions as outlined earlier in this paper, then a $\emptyset$ versus tissue PO_2 curve can be constructed from disappearance curves and used to evaluate the metabolic pattern under a variety of conditions.

Figure 6 presents two experimentally measured rates of disappearance curves produced at the same locus in gerbil cortex under two different sets of conditions. The upper curve was measured under pure oxygen and the lower curve was measured under the suppressive influence of O_2-N_2O-diabutal. We have attempted to estimate the two metabolic rates from these curves in the following manner.

The distributed parameter model was used to simulate the rate of disappearance curve in normal gerbil cortex. A general metabolic rate was assumed and the O_2-dissociation curve was estimated by using the Schmidt-Nielsen weight equation for P_{50} (determined as 39.7 mmHg). The radial region of diffusion was taken to be that between the capillary of the mouse and rat brain or 24 microns. From the theoretical curves and the assumed A/α_T, a $\emptyset$ versus dP/dt curve could be generated. Using these values for $\emptyset$ and the experimental curves in Fig. 6, the metabolic rate in gerbil cortex for the two conditions was calculated as given below:

$A = 7.56$ cm$^3 O_2/100$ gm. tissue-minute (for 100% O_2)

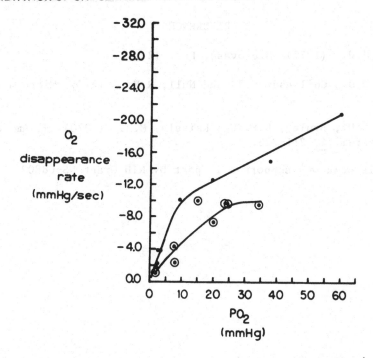

Fig. 6. O$_2$ disappearance rate as a function of tissue PO$_2$ in
gerbil cortex.

  • - 100% O$_2$.

  ⊙ - O$_2$-N$_2$O-Diabutal

and

$$A = 5.20 \text{ cm}^3 \text{ O}_2/100 \text{ gm. tissue-minute (for O}_2\text{-H}_2\text{O-diabutal)}$$

    At present the results are speculative and the methods outlined
in the above material must await further mathematical and
experimental development which is in progress. However theory and
experiment appear to be in good qualitative agreement.

REFERENCES

Halsey, J.H.   (1977) Microvasc. Res. 13.

Reneau, D.D., Guilbeau, E.J. and Null, R.E.   (1977)   Microvasc.
Res. 13.

Reneau, D.D., Bruley, D.F. and Knisely, M.H.   (1970)   J. Am. Assoc.
Med. Instrum. 4, 211-223.

This work was supported in part by NIH Grant NS-08802.

ANALYSIS OF OXYGEN TRANSPORT IN BULLFROGS

Hiroshi Tazawa and Masaji Mochizuki

Department of Physiology
Yamagata University School of Medicine
Yamagata 990-23, Japan

INTRODUCTION

The O_2 transport system in frogs is different from other higher vertebrates, because of the structure of their heart consisting of the two atria and one ventricle, and rather similar to the mammalian fetuses (Dawes et al., 1954) and avian embryos (Tazawa and Mochizuki, 1977). Both the arterialized blood from the lung and the venous blood from the systemic tissues become confluent in the univentricle, and the confluent flow goes on into the systemic and pulmocutaneous circulations simultaneously. The O_2 quantity in the systemic arterial blood was reported to be larger than in the pulmocutaneous artery, indicating a selective streaming in frog's heart (DeLong, 1962; Johansen and Ditadi, 1966; Emilio and Shelton, 1974). In the present report, we attempted to obtain the basic data on the O_2 transport in bullfrogs and present an analytical method for showing the O_2 distribution in the pulmocutaneous and systemic circulations.

BLOOD GAS PARAMETERS

Gas analyses were performed in blood drawn from the left atrium, the ventricle, the conus arteriosus and the sinus venosus of Rana catesbeiana (Table 1). There were no statistical differences in the blood gas parameters between the ventricle and the conus arteriosus. Because the bloods from these two sites were sampled through the direct puncture for a period of several heart beats, the samples were considered to be a 100 % mixture of the arterialized and venous bloods. The O_2 dissociation curve was determined with a microphotometric apparatus (Ono and Tazawa, 1975; Tazawa et al., 1967), and was expressed by the following equations:

Table 1.   Values of blood gas parameters in <u>Rana catesbeiana</u>.

	N	weight (g)	P_{O_2} (mm Hg)	P_{CO_2} (mm Hg)	pH	C_{O_2} (vol%)	O_2 cap. (vol%)	S_{O_2} (%)	Ht (%)
Left atrium	10	216 ±46	88.6 ±11.9	12.3 ±1.7	7.85 ±0.06	8.2 ±1.2	8.6 ±1.0	94.7 ±5.1	25.1 ±3.0
Ventricle + Conus arteriosus	12	232 ±35	55.9 ±10.5	15.9 ±3.2	7.76 ±0.07	6.0 ±1.1	9.4 ±1.2	63.9 ±10.5	27.6 ±3.3
Sinus venosus	12	241 ±43	43.5 ±6.1	18.1 ±5.1	7.72 ±0.08	4.3 ±1.2	9.6 ±2.0	44.9 ±10.8	27.9 ±5.6
Average	34	231 ±43					9.2 ±1.6		27.0 ±4.4

$$\log P_{O_2} = 3.694 - 0.266\ pH + 0.387\ \log S_{O_2}/(100-S_{O_2})$$

The P_{50} at pulmonary venous P_{CO_2} (12.3 mm Hg) was 40.4 mm Hg.   The O_2 uptake was 1.55±0.4 μl/min/g (N=10, the average body weight for 10 frogs was 269±51 g).   The values for O_2 affinity and O_2 uptake were almost comparable to the previously reported values (Lenfant and Johansen, 1967; Gottlieb and Jackson, 1976).

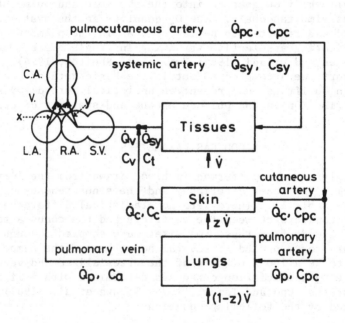

Fig. 1.   A simplified blood circulation model.

BLOOD CIRCULATION MODEL

Using the data obtained experimentally, the relationships between the rates of separation in the heart, blood flows and O_2
contents in the pulmocutaneous and systemic arteries were assessed on
the basis of a blood circulation model (Fig. 1). The model consists
of four compartments (the lungs, the skin, the systemic tissues and
the heart) and blood flow through them are as follows: Blood flow
entering into the pulmocutaneous artery is the sum of fractions of
pulmonary venous blood and of systemic venous blood. The other
fractions from the individual vessels proceed to the systemic artery.
Blood in the pulmocutaneous artery is divided into the pulmonary and
cutaneous circulations, and the venous return to the right atrium is
the sum of blood flows in the systemic and cutaneous circulations.
In addition to the distribution of blood flows, the O_2 uptake through
the lungs and skin is all consumed in the systemic tissues. The
equations relating to blood flow and O_2 quantity in individual compartments were derived as follows:

$$\dot{Q}_p = (1-z)\dot{V}/(C_a - C_{pc}) \tag{1}$$

$$\dot{Q}_c = z\dot{V}/(C_c - C_{pc}) \tag{2}$$

$$\dot{Q}_{sy} = \dot{V}/(C_{sy} - C_t) \tag{3}$$

$$\dot{Q}_{pc} = \dot{Q}_p + \dot{Q}_c \tag{4}$$

$$\dot{Q}_v = \dot{Q}_c + \dot{Q}_{sy} \tag{5}$$

$$(1-x)\dot{Q}_p + y\dot{Q}_v = \dot{Q}_{sy} \tag{6}$$

$$(1-x)\dot{Q}_p C_a + y\dot{Q}_v C_v = \dot{Q}_{sy} C_{sy} \tag{7}$$

$$\dot{Q}_v C_v = \dot{Q}_{sy} C_t + \dot{Q}_c C_c \tag{8}$$

where $\dot{Q}$, C and $\dot{V}$ stand for blood flow rate (ml/min), O_2 content (ml/
ml blood) and O_2 consumption in the tissues (ml/min), respectively.
x is a fraction of pulmonary venous blood ($\dot{Q}_p$), which proceeds to
the pulmocutaneous artery, and y, a fraction of venous return to the
right atrium ($\dot{Q}_v$), which proceeds to the systemic artery. z is a
fraction of O_2 uptake through the skin.

O_2 DISTRIBUTION THROUGH THE PULMOCUTANEOUS AND SYSTEMIC CIRCULATIONS

There are fifteen parameters in eight equations, in which we
know only C_a (8.2 vol %), C_v (4.3 vol %) and $\dot{V}$ (0.417 ml/min) and
the others are unknown. Thus, it was assumed that the blood passing
through the cutaneous capillaries was arterialized to the same level
as the pulmonary venous blood; i.e., both the O_2 contents are

identical ($C_c=C_a$). Furthermore, according to Gottlieb and Jackson (1976), the lungs of <u>Rana catesbeiana</u> were responsible for 80-90 % of total O_2 uptake. Then, we took z=0.1.

When the blood is completely separated in the ventricle; x=y=0, the pulmonary blood entirely enters into the systemic artery; $\dot{Q}_{sy}=\dot{Q}_p$ and $C_{sy}=C_a$=8.2 vol %. Similarly, $C_{pc}=C_v$=4.3 vol %. From Eqs. 1 and 2, $\dot{Q}_{sy}=\dot{Q}_p$=9.6 ml/min and $\dot{Q}_c$=1.1 ml/min.

When the arterialized and venous bloods ($\dot{Q}_p$ and $\dot{Q}_v$) are mixed completely in the heart, the C_{sy} and C_{pc} become equal to that of blood sampled from the ventricle; $C_{sy}=C_{pc}$=6 vol %. We obtained $\dot{Q}_p$=17.1 ml/min, $\dot{Q}_c$=1.9 ml/min and $\dot{Q}_{sy}$=20.2 ml/min.

When there is some selective streaming, the cardiac output changes within a range of 20 to 40 ml/min. We attempted to estimate the relationship between the blood flows and fractional separation of blood. From Eqs. 5-7, the separation ratios x and y are given by taking C_{sy} and C_{pc} as independent variables by

$$x = 1-\dot{Q}_{sy}(C_{sy}-C_v)/[\dot{Q}_p(C_a-C_v)] \tag{9}$$

and
$$y = \dot{Q}_{sy}(C_c-C_{sy})/[(\dot{Q}_{sy}-\dot{Q}_c)(C_a-C_v)] \tag{10}$$

where $\dot{Q}_{sy}$ is expressed by eliminating C_t, $\dot{Q}_v$ and $\dot{Q}_c$ from Eqs. 2,3,5 and 8 as follows;

$$\dot{Q}_{sy} = \dot{V}[1-z(C_a-C_v)/(C_a-C_{pc})]/(C_{sy}-C_v) \tag{11}$$

Substituting Eqs. 1 and 11 into Eq. 9, x is given by

$$x = 1+[z-(C_a-C_{pc})/(C_a-C_v)]/(1-z) \tag{12}$$

Since all the parameter values except C_{pc} in Eq. 12 are known, x can be given by a linear function of C_{pc}. On the other hand, $\dot{Q}_p$ and $\dot{Q}_c$ are evaluated by putting a certain value to C_{pc} in Eqs. 1 and 2. Thus, if C_{pc} is given, $\dot{Q}_p$, $\dot{Q}_c$ and x are all determined. The relations of $\dot{Q}_p$, $\dot{Q}_c$ and x to C_{pc} are illustrated in Cartesian nomogram shown in Fig. 2.

The separation ratio y is rewritten by substituting Eqs. 2 and 11 into Eq. 10 as follows;

$$y = [(C_a-C_{pc})-z(C_a-C_v)](C_a-C_{sy})/\{[(C_a-C_{pc})-z(C_a-C_{sy})](C_a-C_v)\} \tag{13}$$

The relationship between C_{pc}, C_{sy} and y is shown in Fig. 3. When C_{pc} and C_{sy} are given, $\dot{Q}_{sy}$ can also be estimated from Eq. 11, as shown in Fig. 4.

By substituting Eq. 11 into Eq. 3, C_t is obtained as

$$C_t = [(C_a-C_{pc})C_v-z(C_a-C_v)C_{sy}]/[(C_a-C_{pc})-z(C_a-C_v)] \tag{14}$$

Fig. 5 shows the relationship between C_t, C_{sy} and C_{pc}. The range of C_t value is rather small compared with C_{sy} and C_{pc}.

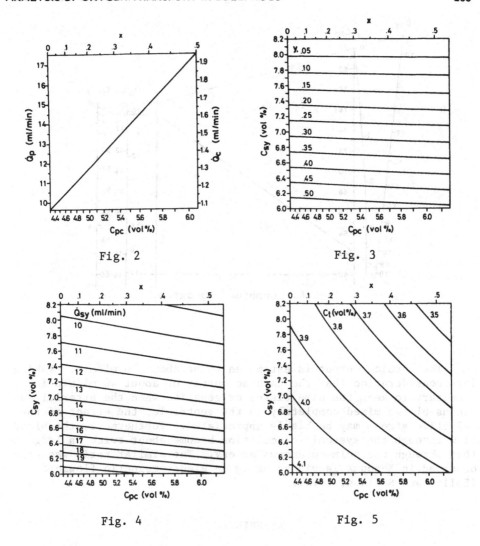

Fig. 2

Fig. 3

Fig. 4

Fig. 5

Figs. 2-4 indicate that C_{pc}, C_{sy} and flow rates in the model can be obtained for given values of x and y. Three figures are composed in one nomogram shown in Fig. 6, where a subsidiary line was used to connect the relation between Fig. 2 and Figs. 3 and 4. According to the data in <u>Rana catesbeiana</u> (DeLong, 1962), about 52 % of blood of the right atrium and 6 % of the left atrium proceed to the pulmocutaneous artery, and the remainder of blood, to the systemic circulations; i.e., x=0.06 and y=0.48. The solid line in the nomogram shows the blood flow rates and O_2 content in this case. The dotted line and broken line show the cases of complete separation and complete mixing of blood, respectively.

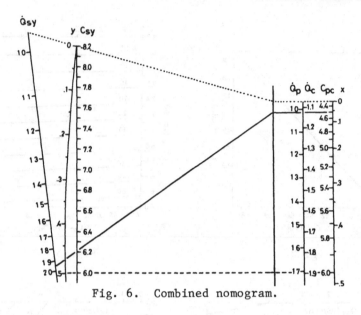

Fig. 6.　Combined nomogram.

The cardiac output is estimated to be about 30 ml/min. Taking into consideration that the cardiac output of about 40 ml/min is necessary to keep the same tissue oxygenation when the arterial and venous bloods mixed completely in the ventricle, the effect of the selective stream may be highly appreciated. Furthermore, the blood flow through the systemic circulation becomes about twice as large as that through the pulmocutaneous artery. The similar ratio was also observed in Xenopus laevis by using an electromagnetic flowmeter (Emilio and Shelton, 1972).

REFERENCES

Dawes, G. S., Mott, J. C. and Widdicombe, J. G. (1954). J. Physiol. 126, 563.

DeLong, K. T. (1962). Science 138, 693.

Emilio, M. G. and Shelton, G. (1972). J. Exp. Biol. 56, 67.

Emilio, M. G. and Shelton, G. (1974). J. Exp. Biol. 60, 567.

Gottlieb, G. and Jackson, D. C. (1976). Amer. J. Physiol. 230, 608.

Johansen, K. and Ditadi, S. S. F. (1966). Physiol. Zool. 39, 140.

Lenfant, C. and Johansen, K. (1967). Respir. Physiol. 2, 247.

Ono, T. and Tazawa, H. (1975). Jap. J. Physiol. 25, 93.

Tazawa, H., Ono, T. and Mochizuki, M. (1976). J. Appl. Physiol. 40, 393.

Tazawa, H. and Mochizuki, M. (1977). Respir. Physiol. (in press).

DISTRIBUTION OF INTRACAPILLARY O$_2$-SUPPLY AND TISSUE PO$_2$ IN CANINE LEFT VENTRICLE DURING NORMOXIA - AN ANALYSIS OF KRYOPHOTOMETRICALLY MEASURED HbO$_2$ SATURATION WITH A DIFFUSION MODEL

W.A. Grunewald and W. Sowa

Institute of Physiology, University of Regensburg

P.O. Box 397, D-8400 Regensburg, W. Germany

Recent studies concerning the O$_2$-supply of the myocardium do not yet show a uniform picture. According to PO$_2$ measurements of Schuchhardt (1971) and Whalen et al (1973) with microelectrodes in the canine and cat heart, the O$_2$ supply of the myocardial fibre at normoxia as well as at hypoxia seems to be kept at an essential minimum. Measurements of the myoglobin-bound oxygen (Coburn et al, 1973) show a mean PO$_2$ value of 6 mmHg in the canine myocardial fibre in normoxia. Under hypoxic conditions, this PO$_2$ value can decrease to around 1 mmHg. In contrast to these experimental findings, theoretical calculations (Thews 1962; Grote and Thews 1962) for the human myocardium predict more favourable conditions in the O$_2$ supply.

Thus we reconsidered the question of the intramyocardial O$_2$ supply and differentiated it as follows:

1. How is the i.c. O$_2$ content in the myocardium distributed under normoxia?
2. Does the i.c. O$_2$ content and its distribution change with increasing hypoxia?
3. Can transmural differences in the i.c. O$_2$ content be ascertained?
4. What consequences for the tissue PO$_2$ in myocardium can be inferred from the distribution of the i.c. O$_2$ content?

The kryomicrophotometric method (Grunewald and Lubbers, 1976) of the i.c. HbsO$_2$ measurement was used for answering questions 1 to 3. The distribution of the tissue PO$_2$, referred to in question 4, is calculated by means of a diffusion model which is based on so-called microcirculatory units (Grunewald and Sowa, 1977) and on experimental data.

In cooperation with Bassenge and co-workers tissue samples of the left ventricle of the beating heart were removed from anaesthetized (Neurolept-Barbiturat-N) and thoractomized dogs. The removal was timed immediately after the opening of the pericardium and carried out with specially cooled tongs. The transmural samples had a diameter of 2-3mm and were kryofixed in situ in sufficiently short a time. At the same time as the myocardial tissue samples were removed, a blood sample from the A. femoralis and from the sinus coronarius was taken for analysis of the O_2 content.

At approximately -60°C the tissue samples were cut into 12-16 μm thick slices on a microtome, and the subendocardial separated from the subepicardial ones. The Hb-absorption was measured in 10 blood vessels (diameter 2-15 μm) in each of these tissue slices at -100°C in a microscopkryostat by using the microscopphotometer UMSP 1 (Fa. Zeiss, Oberkochen). The i.c. HbsO$_2$ was calculated

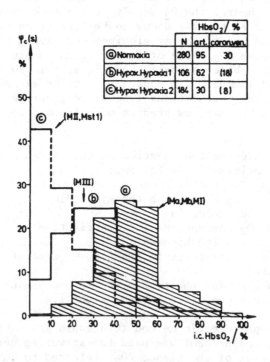

Fig. 1. Frequency distribution ψ_c(s) of the i.c. HbsO$_2$ of the total left ventricle of the canine myocardium, (a) at normoxia, (b) and (c) in hypoxia. The encircled parameters give the number of measurements N and the HbsO$_2$ in the A. femoralis as well as in the sinus coronarius.

from the measured i.c. Hb-absorption spectra by using multi component analysis (Bassenge et al, 1976). The frequency distribution of the endocardium and the epicardium respectively and of the total ventricle wall was calculated from the i.c. $HbsO_2$ values.

As shown in Fig. 1, approximately 300 i.c. $HbsO_2$ values measured over the total normoxic left ventricle wall are distributed with a frequency maximum between 40 and 50 sat.%. The arterial $HbsO_2$ averages 95 sat.%. the coronary venous $HbsO_2$ averages 30 sat. %. The lowest i.c. $HbsO_2$ values found ranged between 0 and 5 sat. %.

A reduction of the arterial O_2 content due to the breathing of hypoxic mixtures of O_2 and N_2O results, as further indicated in Fig. 1, in a shift of the frequency maxima of the i.c. saturation distributions towards lower $HbsO_2$ values. At an arterial HbO_2 saturation of 62 sat.%. (30 sat.%) and a coronary venous HbO_2 saturation of 18 sat.% (8 sat.%) the frequency maximum of the i.c. $HbsO_2$ values lies between 25 and 35 sat.% (0 and 10 sat.%).

Fig. 2 shows the dependence of i.c. $HbsO_2$ values with maximal frequency on the arterial $HbsO_2$ value of the blood of the A. femoralis. Starting from a value of 95 sat.% of the arterial

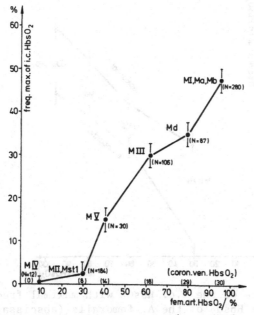

Fig. 2. Dependence of the frequency maximum of i.c. $HbsO_2$ of the total left ventricle of canine myocardium (ordinate) on the $HbsO_2$ of the A. femoralis (abscissa) during normoxia and increasing hypoxia.

blood at normoxia, the frequency maximum of the i.c. $HbsO_2$ systematically shifts to lower saturation values with increasing hypoxia.
The coronary venous $HbsO_2$ values, given in parenthesis above the
abscissa indicate that the frequency maximum of the i.c. $HbsO_2$
value always lies at or above the coronary venous value.   The
vertical lines crossing the dots of the curve indicate the size of
the most frequent class and not the standard deviation of the i.c.
$HbsO_2$.

    Differentiating between the frequency maxima of the i.c.
$HbsO_2$ values from the subendocardial area and the subepicardial
area results in transmural differences in the i.c. O_2 content as
shown in Fig. 3.   The differences are significant.   The figure
shows the subendocardial and the subepicardial frequency maxima of
the $HbsO_2$ value against the arterial $HbsO_2$ in increasing hypoxia.
The measured transmural difference of the O_2 content of the capillary blood indicates a higher O_2 extraction, i.e. an increased O_2
supply in the subendocardial area.   These findings are in accordance with blood flow measurements with the particle distribution
method (Bassenge et al, 1976).   The higher O_2 extraction and the
higher blood flow of the subendocardial area (Bassenge et al, 1976)

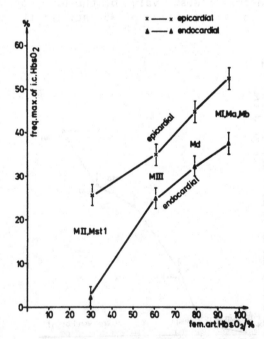

Fig. 3. Dependence of the i.c. $HbsO_2$ with maximal frequency
(ordinate) on the $HbsO_2$ of the A. femoralis (abscissa) during
normoxia and increasing hypoxia of the endocardial (lower curve)
and epicardial (upper curve) area of the left ventricle of the
canine myocardium.   The differences of the distribution of the
i.c. $HbsO_2$ in these areas are significant.

results from the fact that even in normoxia subendocardial O_2 consumption is higher than that of the subepicardial area.

The consequences for the tissue PO_2 resulting from these i.c. $HbsO_2$ measurements were considered in a capillary model by simulation of the microcirculation and O_2 diffusion. We assume that the capillary network consists of so-called microcirculatory units (MCUs). Such an MCU is shown in Fig. 4. Capillary distance d, capillary length 1, capillary radius r_c as well as the arterial inflows 'a' and venous outflows 'v' can be varied. Fig.5 shows MCUs with a varying arrangement of the capillary ends. The first four of these MCUs were chosen to be representative for the capillary network. We further assume (1) that the functional capillary distance in normoxia varies between 24.3 and 32.3 μm; (2) that the lowest capillary venous $HbsO_2$ equals the measured one of 2.5 sat.%; (3) that the mean value of all capillary venous $HbsO_2$ values is equal to the coronary venous $HbsO_2$ value of 30 sat. %; and (4) that the myocardial O_2 consumption lies between 10 and 12 ml/100g/min. By using an iteration process (Grunewald and Sowa, 1977) the i.c. $HbsO_2$ distribution can be calculated for each of the MCUs. From the i.c. $HbsO_2$ distributions of the respective MCUs the total distribution of the i.c. $HbsO_2$ is formed for the

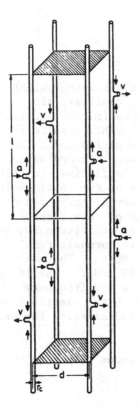

Fig. 4. Microcirculatory unit (MCU) for the simulation of the capillary network in the canine ventricle. d = capillary distance, 1 = capillary length, r_c = capillary radius, a = (arterial) capillary inflow, v = (venous) capillary outflow. The arrangement of the capillary ends can be chosen nearly at random along the length of the capillaries.

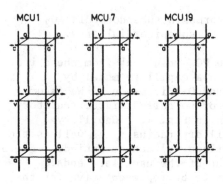

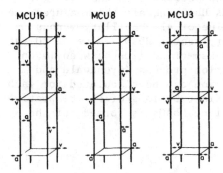

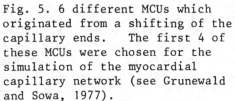

Fig. 5. 6 different MCUs which
originated from a shifting of the
capillary ends.   The first 4 of
these MCUs were chosen for the
simulation of the myocardial
capillary network (see Grunewald
and Sowa, 1977).

endocardial as well as the epicardial area by assigning weighting
factors to the respective MCUs with differing capillary distances
and differing O_2 content in order best to approximate the calculated total distribution to the measured one.   This results in an
O_2 consumption of 12 ml/100g/min for the endocardium and in an
O_2 supply of 10 ml/100g/min for the epicardium.   According to
these weighted parameters and the chosen MCUs a fictive, functional
capillary structure for the capillary network of the total canine
myocardium at normoxia results.   The frequency distribution of
the tissue PO_2 can be calculated for each MCU of this fictive
capillary network.   The total distribution of the tissue PO_2 in
the canine myocardium of the left ventricle in normoxia results
from the PO_2 distributions of the respective MCUs.   The maximum
of the total frequency distribution lies at 25 mmHg.   The lowest
PO_2 values lie between 1 and 5 mmHg and have a low frequency
(Fig. 6).   In the upper right corner of Fig. 6 the distribution
of the weights of the capillary distance is indicated.   The main
weighting is at 27 μm.

    In summary the measurements and calculations result in the
following:

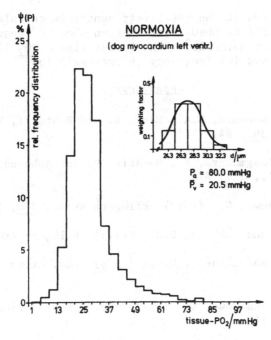

Fig. 6. Frequency distribution $\psi(P)$ of the myocardial tissue PO_2 in normoxia in the total left canine ventricle. This distribution results from the model calculation which is based on the measured i.c. $HbsO_2$ distribution $\psi_c(s)$ of the normoxic canine ventricle ventricle (see Fig. 1). The maximum lies at 25 mmHg. Tissue PO_2 values between 1 and 5 mmHg are rare. The relative weighting distribution of the capillary distance is indicated in the upper right corner. From the simulation, the main weighting for the functional intercapillary distance in the normoxic left canine ventricle is 27 μm.

(1) In normoxia, an i.c. $HbsO_2$ distribution with a maximum between 40 and 50 sat.% is seen in the left ventricle of the canine heart. The lowest i.c. $HbsO_2$ values lie between 0 and 5 sat.%.

(2) With increasing hypoxia the maximum of the i.c. $HbsO_2$ shifts to lower saturation values.

(3) A transmural difference in the O_2 content exists under normoxic as well as hypoxic conditions. The O_2 consumption of the endocardium of the left canine ventricle in normoxia is calculated to be 12 ml/100g/min and that of the epicardium 10ml/100g/min.

(4)   The tissue PO_2 of the total left ventricle calculated by using
the measured i.c. $HbsO_2$ distribution shows a frequency maximum
at 25 mmHg at normoxia.   The lowest tissue PO_2 lies between 1
and 5 mmHg and its frequency is extremely low.

REFERENCES

Bassenge, E., Grunewald, W.A., Manz, R. and Restorff, V.   (1976)
Pflügers Arch., 365, R4.

Coburn, R.F., Ploegmakers, F., Gondrie, P. and Abbound, R.   (1973)
Amer. J. Physiol., 224, 870.

Grote, J. and Thews, G.   (1962)   Pflügers Arch., 276, 142.

Grunewald, W.A. and Lübbers, D.W.   (1975)   Pflügers Arch., 353, 255.

Grunewald, W.A. and Lübbers, D.W.   (1976)   Adv. Exper. Med. Biol.
75, 55.

Grunewald, W.A. and Sowa, W.   (1977)   Rev. Physiol Biochem.
Pharmacol., 77, 149.

Lübbers, D.W. and Wodick, R.   (1969)   Appl. Optics. 8, 1055.

Schuchhardt, S.   (1971)   Pflügers Arch. ges. Physiol., 322, 83.

Thews, G.   (1962)   Pflügers Arch., 276, 166.

Whalen, W.J., Nair, P. and Buerk, D.   (1973)   In 'Oxygen Supply'
(eds. Kessler, M., Bruley, D.F., Clark, L.C., Lübbers, D.W.,
Silver, I.A. and Strauss, J.) p. 199-201, Urban and Schwarzenberg,
Munich.

ACKNOWLEDGEMENT

This work was supported by the Deutsche Forschungsgemeinschaft.

METABOLISM PREDICTION BASED ON MEASUREMENT OF PO_2 AND FLOW AT THE SAME LOCUS DURING SEIZURES AND BARBITURATE SUPPRESSION OF EEG

D.D. Reneau, *R.S. McFarland and *J.H. Halsey, Jr.
Louisiana Tech University, Ruston, Louisiana 71270, USA
*University of Alabama Medical Center,
Birmingham, Alabama 35294, USA

INTRODUCTION

The general purpose of this project was to determine the local state of oxygenation and metabolism in brain cortex during conditions of seizure and suppression.   The methods employed to achieve· these goals are outlined in the following list.

(1) Seizure or suppression was induced by drugs.

(2) Local PO_2 and local flow was simultaneously measured
     with the same microelectrode.

(3) The local metabolic changes associated with the measured
     parameters were predicted with the aid of a mathematical model.

Items (1) and (2) of the above list are discussed in a parent publication in this volume by McFarland et al, and the remainder of this paper will be specific to item (3).

MATHEMATICAL ANALYSIS

Based on the Krogh cylindrical geometry of the microcirculation a distributed parameter mathematical model was used for computation of quantitative changes in the oxygen consumption rate.   The model accounts for capillary blood flow, the non-linear release of oxygen from haemoglobin as blood flows through the capillary, the diffusion of oxygen throughout the tissue region, and homogeneous metabolic consumption at all tissue sites.   The model, which is presented below for steady-state (neglecting axial diffusion), has been in use for several years and details for this application are best found in Reneau et al (1969).

MATHEMATICAL MODEL

CAPILLARY:

$$\left[1 + \frac{NK_N P^{N-1}}{C_1(1+KP^N)^2} \right] \frac{\partial P}{\partial T} = D_1 \left[\frac{\partial^2 P}{\partial R^2} + \frac{1}{R} \frac{\partial P}{\partial R} \right] \tag{1}$$

INTERFACE:

$$P_I \Big|_{R=R_1} = P_I \Big|_{R=R_1} \tag{2}$$

$$D_1 C_1 \left. \frac{\partial P}{\partial R} \right|_{R=R_1} = D_2 C_2 \left. \frac{\partial P}{\partial R} \right|_{R=R_1} \tag{3}$$

TISSUE:

$$\frac{DP}{DT} = D_1 \left[\frac{D^2 P}{DR^2} + \frac{1}{R} \frac{DP}{DR} \right] - \frac{A}{C_2} \tag{4}$$

Boundary conditions applied to the model are listed below:

$$\text{BC1}: \quad \frac{\partial P}{\partial r} = 0 \qquad @ \ r = 0 \tag{5}$$

$$\text{BC2}: \quad \frac{\partial P}{\partial r} = 0 \qquad @ \ r = R_2 \tag{6}$$

$$\text{BC3}: \quad P = P_{arterial} \qquad @ \ X = 0, \quad 0 \leq r \leq R_1 \tag{7}$$

$$\text{BC4}: \quad P = P_i \qquad @ \ r = R_1, \quad 0 \leq X \leq L \tag{8}$$

Solution Technique. The capillary equation was solved by employing the Crank-Nicholson 6-point implicit numerical analysis method, using a special predictive method for the non-linearities, and combining the tissue effects through the interface equations. An analytical solution can be obtained for the tissue equation by applying the integrating factor method with the given boundary conditions. The tissue equation is identical to the Krogh-Erlan equation and is used for the aforementioned combination with the capillary equation solution by means of the interface equations.

Computation Rate. The system of equations for solution was programmed in fortran for the IBM 360 digital computer and each

solution required less than one minute of computational time.
Details for method rate, stability and convergence are found in
Reneau et al (1969).

Specific Procedure for Present Application.   Following standard-
isation of all circulatory, diffusional and metabolic parameters
for normal conditions, the model was used to determine changes in
metabolism during seizure and depression by using the experimentally measured values for micro flow and tissue PO_2.   Standardis-
ation was accomplished as outlined in the prior referenced publication, but the experimental data as given in McFarland et al (this
volume) was replotted versus an arbitrarily defined EEG index.
Fig. 1 is a plot of the experimental measurements as a function of
the EEG index.   Suppression is represented by an EEG index less
than 5, seizure is represented by an EEG index greater than 5; and
normalization of the model was accomplished by using data at an
EEG index of 5.

Fig. 1 is a graphical representation of the results obtained
from one animal (gerbil) and each of the 16 data points represent
separate measurements for a given EEG condition.   In standardizing
the model, normal respiratory conditions were present for arterial
blood and both the PO_2 and flow at an EEG of 5 were taken as
representative of normal conditions.   The calculation procedure for
all other points was as follows:

(1)   The PO_2 was taken as indicative of the value of lethal corner
      region in the Krogh cylinder and could be compared to the PO_2
      at an EEG of 5.

(2)   The change in flow could be expressed as a percent change from
      normal by comparing the actual flow change to the flow at an
      EEG of 5.

(3)   Since the arterial respiratory conditions were known, the local
      change in PO_2 from normal at the lethal corner region was known,
      and the percent change from normal in local flow was known, the
      parameters could be imposed in the normalized mathematical
      model and the change in metabolism could be calculated that
      would describe these experimentally measured values.   In this
      procedure a difference of approximately 19 mmHg between the
      PO_2 at the lethal corner and that of venous blood was calcul-
      ated for normal conditions.   This difference value was held
      constant in each calculation and agrees relatively well with
      values that could be predicted from PO_2 tissue histogram
      measurements in the literature.

                         RESULTS

After the local metabolism was determined for a specific set
of measurements, the degree of change from normality was expressed

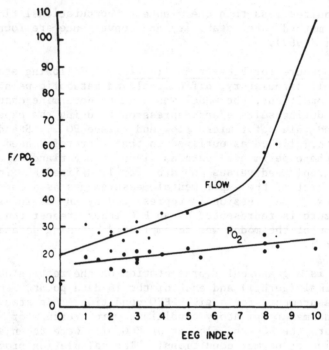

Fig. 1. Local flow (F) and local tissue PO_2 as a function of the EEG index. (F = cm^3 blood/100 gm. tissue-min; PO_2 = mmHg).

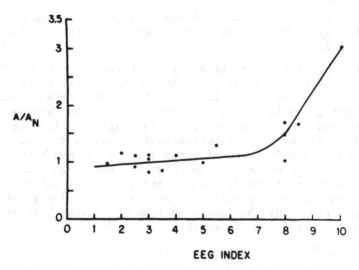

Fig. 2. The metabolic change is given as a function of the EEG index. (A = metabolic rate; A_N = normal metabolic rate at EEG=5).

as the ratio of predicted metabolic rate to the normal metabolic rate and then plotted as a function of the EEG.   Fig. 2 presents the results of the calculations for the experiment shown in Fig. 1.

An interesting relationship was obtained by calculating the oxygen supply rate ($cm^3 O_2$/sec) entering the capillary from arterial blood and presenting the change in supply rate as a function of the change in metabolic demand.   Fig. 3 illustrates this relationship and is representative of the experiments.   The straight line relationship is not a mathematical constrict even though both the abscissa and ordinate coordinates must always be (1,1).   In point of fact in one experiment where no change in metabolic rate was predicted, a correlation was not found between rate of supply and rate of demand.

DISCUSSION

Based on the experimental measurements represented by Fig. 1, neither tissue anoxia nor hypoxia was found during drug induced seizure or suppression.   A relatively small change in tissue PO_2 was measured and the trend indicated small increases during seizure. However, simultaneous measurements of local flow demonstrate that large increases occur during maximal stimulation.   The increase in tissue PO_2 suggests that the increase in flow is sufficient to not only satisfy the possible increase in metabolic demand, but also to overcompensate.

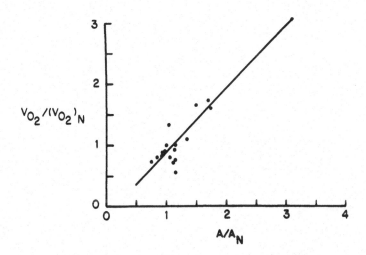

Fig. 3.   The change in oxygen supply rate is given as a function of the change in metabolic demand.
(VO_2 = O_2 supply rate; $(VO_2)_N$ = Normal O_2 supply rate)
(A   = metabolic rate; A_N = normal metabolic rate)

Based on theoretical predictions, represented by Fig. 2, the change in metabolic demand was found to increase as much as three times normal for conditions of high excitability and to decrease to approximately 70% of normal for cases of severe depression.   Figs 1 and 2 serve to demonstrate that the increased rate of delivery of oxygen was always greater than the increased metabolic demand for oxygen.   From Fig. 3 a straight line relationship was determined to exist between oxygen metabolic demand and oxygen supply rate from arterial blood.   These results are a strong indication of a highly precise control mechanism that operates in the presence of seizure or suppression.   The same trend was found in six of seven experiments performed on the cerebral cortex of gerbils.

REFERENCES

McFarland, R.S., Halsey, J.H. and Reneau, D.D.   (In this volume).

Reneau, D.D., Bruley, D.F. and Knisely, M.H.   (1970)   J. Am. Assoc. Med. Instrum. 4, 211-223.

ACKNOWLEDGEMENTS

This work was supported in part by NIH grant NS-08802.

A COMPUTER ANALYSIS OF GRADED ISCHEMIA IN BRAIN

Randal E. Null   Daniel D. Reneau

University of Virginia   Louisiana Tech University

Charlottesville, VA.   Ruston, LA.

Based on the Krogh tissue cylinder, a lumped parameter mathematical model was developed to describe multicomponent transport
and metabolic reaction processes in brain. Utilizing the mathematical model, computer solutions were obtained for a wide range of
patho-physiologic conditions. Varying degrees of ischemia were
imposed on arterial blood flow in order to examine the metabolic
state of brain tissue during reduced oxygen supply. The major
purpose of the study was to observe the effects created in tissue
at extremely low flow rates, including complete flow cessation.

Figure 1 illustrates the geometric model for a single capillary-
tissue cylinder. This particular formulation is simply a modification of the two compartment, blood-tissue model presented by
Krogh (1922). The structural modifications were introduced to
isolate the individual metabolic reaction cycles and include the
transport resistances of membrane separations between compartments.
Mass transfer between compartments was regulated by whole compartment
concentration differences, consumption and production rates, and
overall mass transfer coefficients. Formulation of overall mass
transfer coefficients was achieved by finite differencing the mass
flux equation to obtain the following relationship,

$$K = \frac{\pi r z D}{\Delta r},$$
(1)

where r = membrane radius
   z = compartment length
   Δr = midpoint to midpoint diffusion distance between adjacent
        radial compartments
and   D = component molecular diffusivity.

219

This procedure resulted in a typical mass balance of the form

$$\frac{dVC}{dt} = Q[C \text{ in} - C \text{ out}] + K[\Delta C] + R, \qquad (2)$$

where V = compartment volume,
     C = component concentration
     Q = volume flow rate,
    ΔC = concentration difference between adjacent radial
          compartments,
and   R = net reaction rate in the compartment.

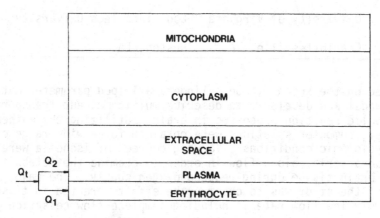

Fig. 1 Modified Krogh Tissue Cylinder

The three major metabolic reaction cycles of glycolysis,
Krebs cycle, and oxidative phosphorylation were chosen as the
kinetic basis of the model. Following the Embden-Meyerbof scheme
of glycolysis, a simplified version was developed through combinations of intermediate reactions into an overall reaction system.
A version of the reaction scheme presented by Chance, et al.
(1960) was the basis for the kinetic model representing Krebs cycle
and oxidative phosphorylation. A detailed description of the mathe-
mathical development and simplifying assumptions is presented by
Null (1976).

RESULTS

Beginning with a steady state concentration profile, step
changes of 0, 10, 25 and 50% of normal were imposed on the inlet
blood flow rates. The figures which are presented are all transient
profiles of extracellular component concentrations. Figure 3
shows the oxygen partial pressure profiles for the varying degrees
of ischemia. As an analysis of the tissue metabolic state, pH,

glucose, and lactic acid were observed.   Figures 4 through 6
illustrate these components' dynamic responses to reduced flow.

DISCUSSION

No significant variations in the tissue state were observed
until blood flow was reduced to 50% of normal.   However, as blood
flow was reduced below the 50% mark a progressive deterioration
in the chemical component balance was seen.   Figure 3 reveals the
rapid response of oxygen to ischemia.   Within ten seconds a new
oxygen steady state concentration was achieved.   The rapid response
time was partially attributed to the fact that a small volume
system was used and that the inlet alterations were imposed at the
capillary entrance.

Due to kinetic delays the transient responses of the additional
components were prolonged.   The acidic state of the tissue was
chosen as the detrimental indicator.   Figure 4 shows that at 25%
of normal flow and above, the pH levels rise.   This pH rise is
attributed to decreased carbon dioxide production.   However, at
the lower flow rates pH falls.   Several factors contribute to the
pH decline in severe ischemia.   Decreased carbon dioxide washout
is partially responsible for the fall, but the shift to anaerobic
metabolism and the subsequent lactate production becomes the
overriding process, forcing the pH down.   The most significant
effect seen in Figure 4 is the pH crossover in which the 10% of
normal flow rate results in a pH level below that for complete

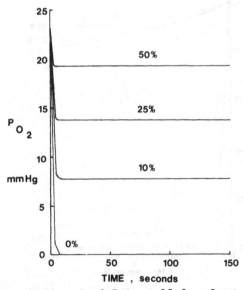

Fig. 2. Transient Response of Extracellular Oxygen to Reduced
Levels of Flow (Ischemia) Expressed as Percent of Normal.

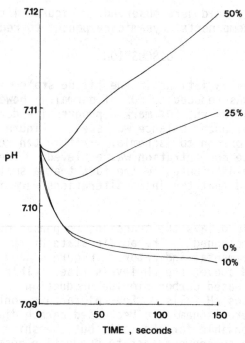

Fig. 3. Transient Response of Extracellular pH to Reduced Blood
Flow (Ischemia) Expressed as Percent of Normal.

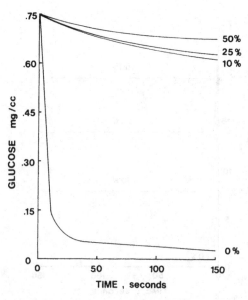

Fig. 4. Transient Response of Extracellular Glucose to Reduced
Blood Flow (Ischemia) Expressed as Percent of Normal.

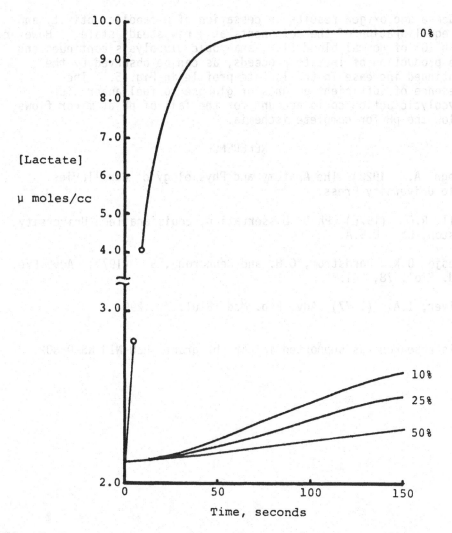

Fig. 5. Transient Response of Extracellular Lactate to Reduced Blood Flow (Ischemia) Expressed as Percent of Normal.

ischemia.   This pH crossover is of particular interest since experimental findings by Siesjo et al. (1976) and Silver (1977) have revealed a similar phenomenon.

A plausible explanation of the pH crossover is uncovered by examination of the glucose and lactate responses to ischemia, illustrated in Figures 4 and 5 respectively.   A rapid transient to a new steady state concentration is observed for all components during complete ischemia.   This response is due to the elimination of the metabolic supply components in zero flow.   The absence of

glucose and oxygen results in cessation of metabolic activity and
an equilibration of the components at a new steady state.   However,
with 10% of normal blood flow, anaerobic glycolysis continues and
the production of lactate proceeds, as can be observed by the
continued increase in the lactate profile in Fig. 5.   The
presence of sufficient amounts of glucose to fuel anaerobic
glycolytic action could account for the fall of pH at minor flows
below the pH for complete ischemia.

REFERENCES

Krogh, A.   (1922)   The Anatomy and Physiology of Capillaries.
Yale University Press.

Null, R.E.   (1976)   Ph.D. Dissertation, Louisiana Tech University,
Ruston, La., U.S.A.

Siesjo, B.K., Nordstrom, C.H. and Rehncrona, S.   (1977)   Adv. Exp.
Med. Biol. $\underline{78}$, 261.

Silver, I.A.   (1977)   Adv. Exp. Med. Biol. $\underline{78}$, 299.

This research was supported in part by grant   HEW-NIH-NS-08802.

A COMPARISON OF TWO NONCLASSICAL MODELS FOR OXYGEN CONSUMPTION IN BRAIN AND LIVER TISSUE

Donald G. Buerk[*] and Gerald M. Saidel[+]

*Department of Chemical Engineering
 Northwestern University
 Evanston, Illinois 60201   USA

+Department of Biomedical Engineering
 Case Western Reserve University
 Cleveland, Ohio 44106 USA

INTRODUCTION

Warburg-type experiments using tissue slices demonstrate non-classical chemical reaction kinetics [7]. Longmuir et al. [8] found that a Michaelis-Menten kinetic model more accurately. described experimental data from several different tissues. Brain tissue oxygen consumption was not significantly different from classical zero-order reaction kinetics, whereas liver tissue exhibited the most substantial deviation from the classical model. More recently, Buerk and Longmuir [2] have shown that oxygen consumption does not follow simple zero-order kinetics in either brain or liver tissue. The experimentally measured steady-state pO_2 profiles from this study have been compared with nonclassical models for oxygen consumption.

METHODS

Rat brain and liver tissue slices were bathed on one side by a flowing film of solution in a temperature regulated apparatus. The opposite surface rested on an oxygen impermeable glass base. For this experimental system, steady-state pO_2 profiles are established in a simple one-dimensional geometry. Recessed Whalen-type oxygen microelectrodes [10-11] were used to measure the pO_2 profiles. Data obtained in the tissue phase below 40 torr were

analyzed and normalized to compare with mathematical models for
oxygen consumption. The procedure requires much less time than
Warburg-type experiments. A more complete description of the
experimental method may be found elsewhere [2].

OXYGEN CONSUMPTION MODELS

The governing differential equation arising from consideration of the mass balance for oxygen in this experimental system is

$$Dk \frac{d^2 P}{dx^2} - Q(P) = 0 \quad , \qquad P_t < P < P_s, \quad x_t < x < x_s$$

The diffusivity-solubility product Dk is assumed to be constant.
The oxygen consumption rate $Q(P)$ may depend on the partial pressure
of oxygen P according to the chemical reaction kinetics assumed.

For a kinetic model assuming a change from zero- to first-
order kinetics at a critical partial pressure, the oxygen consumption rate in the zero order region is constant

$$Q(P) = Q_0 \quad , \qquad P > P_0$$

and varies linearly with partial pressure in the first-order
region below the critical value P_0

$$Q(P) = Q_1 P \quad , \qquad P < P_0$$

The zero- to first-order kinetic model has an analytical solution
[3], described in Appendix A. The model is characterized by
three independent parameters.

For a model assuming Michaelis-Menten kinetics, the oxygen
consumption rate follows a saturation form

$$Q(P) = \frac{Q_{max} P}{P + K_m}$$

where the rate falls to half-maximum at the partial pressure K_m.
The Michaelis-Menten kinetic model must be solved numerically
(see Appendix B). The model is also characterized by three
independent parameters.

The average oxygen consumption rate may be calculated for either model by integrating over the measured distance

$$Q_{avg} = \frac{1}{x_s - x_t} \int_{x_t}^{x_s} Q(P)dx$$

to compare with whole organ metabolic rates determined by other investigators.

RESULTS

The best parameter estimates for each model were obtained by minimizing the differences between the experimental data of Buerk and Longmuir [2] and model values. A Marquardt-type gradient method [1] was employed to obtain the minimum. The weighting function for the nonlinear least-squares was based on the experimental variance.

The corresponding pO_2 profiles for the optimum parameters of the zero- to first-order oxygen consumption model are shown for both tissues in Fig. 1. The critical value P_0, endpoint P_t, zero-order oxygen consumption rate Q_0 and average rate Q_{avg} tabulated in Table I were calculated from the optimum parameters obtained for each tissue.

The pO_2 profiles for the optimum parameters of the Michaelis-Menten oxygen consumption model are shown for both tissues in Fig. 2. The partial pressure K_m at half-maximum consumption, endpoint P_t, maximum Q_{max} and average Q_{avg} oxygen consumption rates tabulated in Table II were calculated from the optimum parameters obtained for each tissue. Thews' value for Dk [9] was used in all calculations. The lower endpoint values P_t predicted by the Michaelis-Menten model are more consistent with the expected resolution of sensitive oxygen microelectrodes. The average oxygen consumption rate Q_{avg} in brain tissue calculated for the Michaelis-Menten model is approximately 50% higher than the whole organ value determined by Eklof et al. [5]. The value calculated for Q_{avg} in liver tissue is also higher than values measured by Kessler [6].

For both tissues, the Michaelis-Menten oxygen consumption model provides a better fit of the experimentally observed pO_2 profiles than the zero- to first-order oxygen consumption model. For brain tissue the Michaelis-Menten model improves the fit slightly, reducing the χ^2 statistic by 6%. The improvement is more substantial for liver tissue, reducing the χ^2 statistic by 50% over the zero- to first-order model.

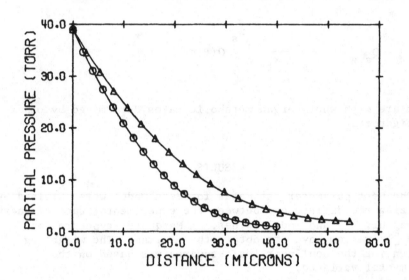

FIGURE 1:   ZERO- TO FIRST-ORDER OXYGEN CONSUMPTION MODEL
The pO_2 profiles shown (solid lines) are predicted from the
optimum parameters obtained by fitting the analytical solution
for the zero- to first-order consumption model to experimental
brain (circles) and liver (triangles) data.

TABLE I: OXYGEN PARTIAL PRESSURES, METABOLIC RATES AND MODEL FIT
FOR OPTIMUM PARAMETERS OF ZERO- TO FIRST-ORDER OXYGEN CONSUMPTION
MODEL

	BRAIN	LIVER
P_0 (torr)	4.01	7.06
P_t (torr)	1.02	2.04
$Q_0 \pm$ S.E.M. (μmoles O_2/min·cm^3)	7.81 ± 0.71	4.64 ± 0.53
$Q_{avg} \pm$ S.E.M. (μmoles O_2/min·cm^3)	6.60 ± 0.60	3.70 ± 0.43
χ^2 (d.f. = 16)	3.5×10^{-3}	1.0×10^{-2}

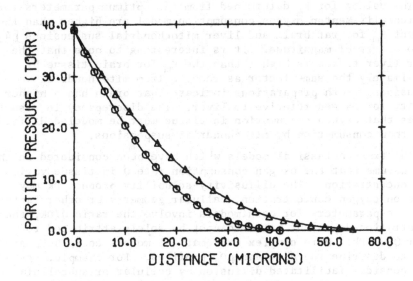

FIGURE 2: MICHAELIS-MENTEN OXYGEN CONSUMPTION MODEL
The pO_2 profiles shown (solid lines) are predicted from the optimum
parameters obtained by fitting the numerical solution for the
Michaelis-Menten oxygen consumption model to experimental brain
(circles) and liver (triangles) data.

TABLE II: OXYGEN PARTIAL PRESSURES, METABOLIC RATES AND MODEL FIT
FOR OPTIMUM PARAMETERS OF MICHAELIS-MENTEN OXYGEN CONSUMPTION MODEL

	BRAIN	LIVER
K_m(torr)	0.80	2.24
P_t(torr)	0.004	0.26
Q_{max} ± S.E.M. (μmoles O_2/min·cm^3)	8.66 ± 0.78	5.48 ± 0.63
Q_{avg} ± S.E.M. (μmoles O_2/min·cm^3)	6.77 ± 0.61	3.87 ± 0.45
χ^2 (d.f. = 16)	3.3×10^{-3}	5.2×10^{-3}

DISCUSSION

The values for K_m determined from the optimum parameters for the Michaelis-Menten oxygen consumption model are higher than the apparent K_m for rat brain and liver mitochondrial suspensions [4] by two orders of magnitude. It is interesting to note that the K_m for liver tissue is higher than the K_m for brain tissue by approximately the same factor as results from mitochondrial suspensions. Both preparations indicate that brain has a higher affinity for oxygen relative to liver. The discrepancy in results implies that oxygen consumption in tissue must be modeled differently than consumption by mitochondrial suspensions.

The two nonclassical models which have been considered in this paper assume that the oxygen consumption rate Q in tissue varies with concentration. The diffusivity-solubility product Dk may also depend on oxygen concentration, cellular geometry or other factors. Since the parameters for both models involve the ratio Q/Dk, the concentration-dependent nature cannot be solely attributed to either Q or Dk. More complex mathematical models could be postulated to describe the observed pO_2 profiles. For example, one might consider facilitated diffusion by cellular or subcellular oxygen carrier systems. The heterogeneous nature of biological tissues may also modify the mathematics, particularly if the intracellular permeability to oxygen is lower than in the extracellular phase. The sensitivity of other oxygen-requiring biochemical systems, such as aromatic amino hydroxylases [4], would also need to be considered for a more complete analysis of tissue oxygen consumption.

SUMMARY

Experimentally observed steady-state pO_2 profiles in tissue slices can be described by a Michaelis-Menten oxygen consumption model. Calculated values for K_m = 0.8 torr in brain tissue, and K_m = 2.2 torr in liver tissue are two orders of magnitude higher than K_m values determined from mitochondrial suspensions. Brain tissue has a higher metabolic rate and higher affinity for oxygen than liver tissue.

ACKNOWLEDGEMENTS

This study is supported in part by N.I.H. training grant GM 00894-15.

REFERENCES

1. Bevington, P.R., "Data Reduction and Error Analysis for the Physical Sciences", McGraw-Hill, pp. 204-246 (1969).
2. Buerk, D.G. and I.S. Longmuir, Microvas. Res., 13, 345-353 (1977).
3. Buerk, D.G. and G.M. Saidel, 29th A.C.E.M.B., p. 226 (1976).
4. Clark, J.B., W.J. Nicklas and H. Degn, J. Neurochem., 26, 409-411 (1976).
5. Eklof, B., N.A. Lassen, L. Nilsson, K. Norberg and B.J. Siesjo, Acta physiol. Scand., 88, 587-589 (1973).
6. Kessler, M., in "Oxygen Transport in Blood and Tissue", Georg Thieme Verlag - Stuttgart, pp. 245-251 (1968).
7. Longmuir, I.S. and S. Sun, Microvas. Res., 2, 287-293 (1970).
8. Longmuir, I.S., D.C. Martin, H. Gold and S. Sun, Microvas. Res., 3, 125-141 (1971).
9. Thews, G., Pflugers Arch. ges. Physiol., 271, 227-244 (1960).
10. Whalen, W.J., J. Riley and P. Nair, J.A.P., 23, 789-801 (1967).
11. Whalen, W.J., P. Nair and R.A. Ganfield, Microvas. Res., 5, 254-262 (1973).

APPENDIX A: Zero- to First-Order Model Solution

By introducing the dimensionless partial pressure and distance variables

$$P^* = \frac{P(x) - P_t}{P_s - P_t} \qquad\qquad x^* = \frac{x - x_t}{x_s - x_t}$$

the governing equations and boundary conditions lead to the following dimensionless analytical solutions (see ref. 3 for details).

In the zero-order region, $P_0^* < P^* < 1$, $x_0^* < x^* < 1$

$$P^*(x^*) = gx^{*2} + \left[\frac{1-h}{1-B} - g(1+B) \right] x^* + gB + \frac{h-B}{1-B}$$

In the first-order region, $0 < P^* < P_0^*$, $0 < x^* < x_0^*$

$$P^*(x^*) = \frac{2g}{A^2} \left[\frac{\sinh Ax^*}{\sinh AB} \right] + C \left[\frac{\sinh A(B-x^*)}{\sinh AB} - 1 \right]$$

The functions g and h are given by

$$g = A^2(h+C)/2,$$

$$h = \frac{1 + AC(1-B)[\text{csch } AB - \text{coth } AB - A(1-B)/2]}{1 + A(1-B)\text{coth } AB + A^2(1-B)^2/2}$$

where the three independent parameters that characterize the solution are

$$A = (x_s - x_t)\sqrt{\frac{Q_1}{Dk}}, \qquad B = \frac{x_0 - x_t}{x_s - x_t}, \qquad \text{and} \quad C = \frac{P_t}{P_s - P_t}$$

APPENDIX B: Michaelis-Menten Model Solution

Using the same dimensionless variables, the governing equation for Michaelis-Menten kinetics becomes

$$\frac{d^2 P^*}{dx^{*2}} - \frac{2A'(P^* + C')}{(P^* + B')} = 0$$

The numerical solution is obtained by solving a set of algebraic finite difference equations using Gaussian elimination. The solution is characterized by the three independent parameters

$$A' = \frac{Q_{max}(x_s - x_t)^2}{2Dk(P_s - P_t)}, \qquad B' = \frac{(K_m - P_t)}{(P_s - P_t)}, \qquad C' = \frac{P_t}{P_s - P_t}$$

MODELS FOR PULSED POLAROGRAPHIC ELECTRODES

Alfred C. Pinchak and Edward A. Ernst

Department of Anesthesiology, School of Medicine
Case Western Reserve University
Cleveland Metropolitan General Hospital, Ohio

Introduction

The proposed application of this work is to the measurement
of both tissue perfusion and tissue pO_2 with the same polarographic
probe. It is anticipated that membrane characteristics will markedly affect the overall flow sensitivity or insensitivity of a
particular probe when operated under pulsed conditions. Moreover
operation with very short pulse times requires consideration of
the rapid development of the "double layer" as the double layer
current can be significantly larger than the current due to the
polarographic reaction. The effect of the double layer formation
is specifically considered below along with the incorporation of
convective phenomena in the model.

One-Dimensional Flow Through Electrode

One of the models considered by us is a single sheet electrode
which freely permits the solution to flow through it. Because of
the particular flow geometry postulated here the governing equation
is simply:

$$\partial C/\partial t = D\partial^2 C/\partial x^2 - V\partial C/\partial x \qquad (1)$$

where V is the constant stream velocity directed toward the
electrode (V is assumed to be in the negative x direction in this
particular case). $C(x,t)$ is the concentration, D is the diffusion
coefficient, x is the distance perpendicular to the sheet
electrode and t is time.

Because this model probe is considered as having a membrane, the concentration of the reacting substance (oxygen) will not be zero at the surface of the probe (outer surface of the membrane). However, it will be assumed that the partial pressure of oxygen is zero at the inner surface of the membrane (Stuck et.al., 1971). The steady solution for equation (1) with an assumed linear gradient through the probe membrane is:

$$I_{pol} = I_o + \frac{F A_m D_m}{\Delta L} C_\infty \frac{V/(D_m/\Delta L)}{1 + (V/D_m/\Delta L)} \tag{2}$$

where F is the Faraday, D_m and A_m the membrane diffusion coefficient and electrode area respectively, and ΔL the thickness of the membrane. The term I_o has been added to equation (2) to indicate that there generally will be a finite diffusion current even under zero velocity conditions. Note that the diffusion coefficient of the stream does not appear explicitly in this particular equation. For the case of a vanishingly thin membrane, the complete solution to equation (1) can be obtained analytically (see e.g. Carslaw and Jaeger, 1959) in the following form:

$$C(x,t) = C_\infty - \tfrac{1}{2} C_\infty \exp (Vx/2D)\left[\exp(Vx/2D)\,\mathrm{erfc}\left[-x/(2\sqrt{Dt}) - \right.\right.$$
$$\left.\left. - (V/2)(\sqrt{t/D})\right] + \exp(-Vx/2D)\,\mathrm{erfc}\left[-x/2\sqrt{Dt} + (V/2)(\sqrt{t/D})\right]\right] \tag{3}$$

It may readily be shown that equation (3) provides the same steady-state concentration distribution as equation (2). Moreover, if the velocity (V) is set equal to zero, equation (3) provides a flux at the electrode surface which leads to the well-known Cottrell equation. If the complete transient solution to equation (1) is desired with a finite membrane thickness then the solution must be obtained numerically. (See below.)

One-Dimensional Model with Membrane and Developing Double Layer

The basis of this model is also equation (1); within the membrane the transport velocity (V) is neglected. At the electrode surface the reaction rate is initially charge-transfer limited. Our equivalent electronic circuit is similar to that of Saveant and Tessier (1977) with the (band pass limiting) series inductor eliminated. During the early stages of development of the double layer the polarographic voltage may be approximated by:

$$E_{pol} = E_{app} (1 - \exp(t/\tau)) \tag{4}$$

where E_{app} is the externally applied voltage and τ is the effective time constant for the development of the double layer. With the polarographic reaction considered irreversible the polarographic current may be written as (Delahay, 1954):

$$I_{pol} = n F A_m k C_e \ \exp \{(\alpha n F/RT)(E_{pol} - E_c^0)\} \tag{5}$$

where n is the number of electrons per mole of reactant reduced, k is the formal rate constant, C_e the O_2 concentration at the electrode surface, α the charge transfer coefficient, R the gas constant, T the absolute temperature and E_c^0 the equilibrium potential for the reaction. The electrode surface boundary condition then requires that the diffusional flux of O_2 to the surface match equation (5). This charge transfer limited reaction is considered in effect until the surface concentration at the electrode becomes zero at which time the boundary condition becomes $pO_2(0,t) = 0$. at the electrode surface.

A standard finite difference scheme is employed here to carry the diffusion process through the membrane and a similar method is also employed in the bulk region surrounding the membrane. At the interface between the membrane and the surrounding tissue or fluid, equality of transport fluxes is required.

Because of the presence of the double layer and the probe membrane there arise two naturally-occurring characteristic quantities: the characteristic time (τ) of formation of the double layer and the membrane thickness (ΔL) being the appropriate characteristic length. Currents are non-dimensionalized by the maximum, steady-state polarographic current. ($C = C_\infty$ at the membrane surface.)

$$I_{pol,max} = C_\infty D_m n F A_m /\Delta L \tag{6}$$

where C_∞ is the invariant concentration far from the probe. Another model parameter which must be specified is the ratio of peak double layer current and $I_{pol,max}$.

Results

A typical numerical solution for the pulsed membrane probe is shown in Fig. 1. Note that the true, time dependent, polarographic current exceeds $I_{pol,max}$. This is not unexpected when the double layer builds up very rapidly; a relatively high concentration of oxygen remains within the membrane and is available for the polarographic reaction. However, with larger values of τ the double layer grows more slowly and when diffusion-limited conditions are reached, the O_2 concentrations are sufficiently small near the electrode surface so that only relatively small polarographic currents are obtained. Recent observations in our laboratory with pulsed operation of two different probes (IBC electrode and a conventional Clark electrode) show a marked distinction in the transient pulse current. The IBC electrode has a single steady decay while the Clark electrode shows a "shoulder" as seen in Fig. 1.

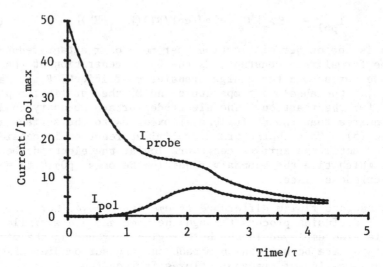

Fig. 1: Dimensionless current vs. time plot with τ the time constant of the double layer charging process and $I_{pol,max}$ the maximum, steady state, diffusion limited polarographic current.

However, as the maximum double layer current is relatively increased the "hump" due to the polarographic current will not be appreciated.

To eliminate the effect of the double layer, a sampling scheme has been developed involving current integration over a time interval equal to twice the "pulse on" time (Cheung and Ernst, 1976). The integration scheme effectively eliminates the effect of the double layer current as the integrated charge during double layer formation is canceled by a nearly equal charge integral during the dissolution of the double layer. Fig. 2 shows the results of operating a conventional IBC electrode with a relatively short pulse duration (5msec on and 8 sec off). Correlation of the data presented in Fig. 2 is reasonably good (r=0.995). With longer pulse durations, the probe demonstrates a marked velocity dependence.

Probe Operation in the Steady State

For the case of extremely long pulse duration, the current is expected to be given by a relation having the form of equation (2). It was of particular interest to compare the velocity dependence of equation (2) with actual probe data. Fig. 3 shows the comparison for an IBC type electrode. The free parameters in equation (2) were selected to give the best fit of the experimental data. However, this relatively good fit of the data would not be possible if the velocity dependence predicted by equation (2) were grossly in error.

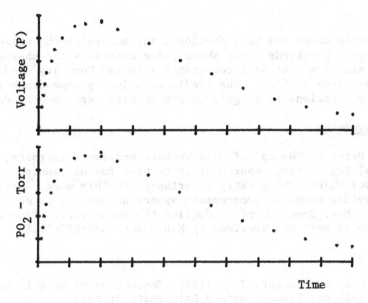

Fig. 2: Dual strip chart recording of pulsed polarographic electrode system (P) and Clark electrode (R). PO$_2$ range from 0-140 Torr.

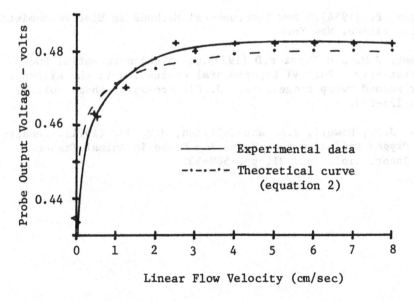

Fig. 3: Velocity dependence of IBC polarographic probe under
steady state operation.

Summary

A simple model has been developed for analyzing the pulsed polarographic electrode. For short pulse durations the charge transfer kinetics must be incorporated into the boundary condition at the electrode surface. The predicted velocity dependence for long pulse durations is in good agreement with experimental data.

Acknowledgements

Dr. Peter W. Cheung, of Case Western Reserve University, Biomedical Engineering Department is thanked for his assistance and counsel which have greatly contributed to this work. Ralph Wiley provided computer programming expertise and generated illustrations. Mrs. Donna Chorich compiled the manuscript. Financial assistance in part was provided by NIH Grant #GRS-642-9258.

References

Carslaw, H.S. and Jaeger, J.C. (1959) Conduction of Heat in Solids. Second Edition, Oxford, Oxford University Press.

Cheung, P.W. and Ernst, E.A. (1976). pO_2 Measurements with Flow-sensitive Polarographic Oxygen Probe: Flow Artifact or Information? Federation Proceedings Vol. 35, pg. 830.

Delahay, P. (1954). New Instrumental Methods in Electrochemistry. Interscience, New York.

Saveant, J.M. and Tessier,D (1977).Convolution Potential Sweep Voltammetry. Part VI Experimental evaluation in the kilovolt per second sweep range rate. J. Electroanal. Chem. Vol. 77 pp. 225-235.

Stuck, J.D., Howell, J.A. and Cullinan, H.T. Jr. (1971). Analysis of Oxygen Diffusion to a Measuring Probe in Animal Tissue. J. Theor. Biol. Vol. 31, pp. 509-532.

MATHEMATICAL SIMULATION OF OXYGEN AND CARBON DIOXIDE TRANSPORT

IN FETAL BRAIN

James M. Cameron   Daniel D. Reneau

TTU School of Medicine   Louisiana Tech University

Lubbock, Texas 79409   Ruston, Louisiana 71270

INTRODUCTION

Dynamic behavior of the fetal system during times of stress
is a topic of considerable interest. An understanding of the
physiological consequences of abnormal labor, cord occlusion, and
maternal death to the fetal system is critical. Also of interest
is the response of the fetal control systems during these stressful
situations. Quantitative analysis of fetal respiratory function
and cardiovascular dynamics using mathematical modeling can contribute to the understanding of these processes. The purpose of this
paper is to present a study of carbon dioxide and oxygen concentration in fetal brain tissue during times of stress using a mathematical model.

MATHEMATICAL DEVELOPMENT

A diagram of the fetal system is shown in Figure 1. Both the
fetal and maternal sides of the placenta are incorporated into the
fetal system. Also shown in Figure 1 are the divisions into which
the fetal system is divided in order to facilitate mathematical
development. On the diagram (Figure 1), the solid lines represent
flow exchange between compartments, and the arrows indicate the
direction of flow. The boxes represent organs, body divisions, or
major blood vessels. A dotted line within a box indicates that the
lump is represented by two compartments between which mass transfer can take place by diffusion but not by bulk flow.

A complete development of the mathematical model is given in
Cameron et al. (1977) and will not be repeated here. Relationships
of the variables are shown in the schematic of a typical organ
lump given in Figure 2. The organ division is shown with capillary and tissue sections. The inlet concentrations are those

239

leaving the preceeding lump. Diffusion of chemical components
between blood and tissue is governed by individual mass transfer
coefficients. Control signals act to change the local resistance
which governs flow characteristics. Outlet values of the compartment are assumed to be the same as the values within the compartment, that is, the compartment is assumed to be uniform.

Equations are derived for each of the model divisions. These
equations can be classified into five groups.

I.   Mass balances
      A.   Total
      B.   Oxygen
      C.   Hydrogen ions
      D.   Carbon dioxide

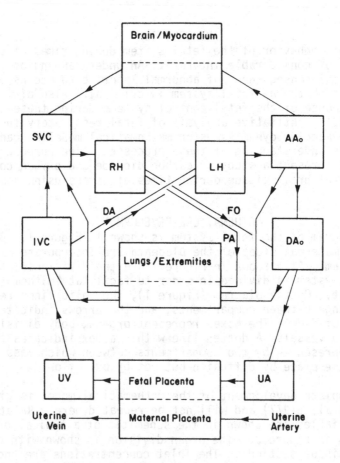

Fig. 1 A Lumped Representation of the Fetal System for Mathematical Modeling.

RESULTS

The response of fetal brain tissue carbon dioxide and oxygen partial pressure to (1) complete cord occlusion, (2) labor with cord compression, and (3) maternal death were determined using the mathematical model. Additionally, blood supply to the brain, brain tissue pH, fetal arterial pressure, and fetal heart rate are plotted. These results are shown in Figures 3, 4, and 5. In all the figures the dashed lines correspond to the simulation of total umbilical cord occlusion; lines of alternating dashes and dots represent the simulation of labor with cord occlusion; the solid lines are the results of the simulation of maternal death. In the labor study, a contraction was assumed to start at time 0, slowly build to a maximum at 0.7 of a minute and return to 0 at 1.5 minutes. A second contraction started at 2 minutes. Both maternal death and cord occlusion started at time 0.

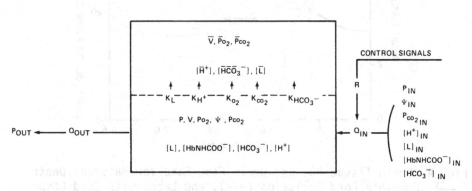

Fig. 2 An Organ Lump Demonstrating Relationship of Variables.

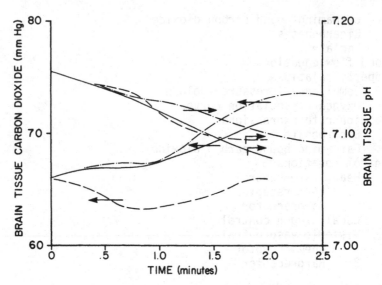

Fig. 3 Brain Tissue Carbon Dioxide Partial Pressure and pH Calculated for Maternal Death (———), Complete Cord Occlusion (---),
and Labor with Cord Compression (-·-).

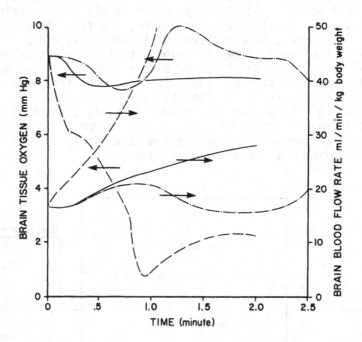

Fig. 4 Brain Tissue PO_2 and Brain Flow Rate for Maternal Death
(———), Complete Cord Occlusion (---), and Labor with Cord Compression (-·-).

Labor with cord compression was simulated by varying umbilical cord blood flow resistance proportional to the intrauterine pressure. Umbilical flow fell to about 30% of normal. This resulted in a proportionate increase in arterial pressure. Because of this, the timing of the contraction corresponds very closely to the arterial pressure plot shown in Figure 5. During compression, fetal control systems responded by producing a dip in the fetal heart rate. This is mainly a cardiovascular response to the arterial pressure variations. The brain oxygen concentration falls during the contraction due to the partial loss of oxygen supply to the fetus. The oxygen partial pressure curve shows an overshoot following reoxygenation of the blood following the contraction. This overshoot is a result of a controlled increase of blood flow to the brain.

Maternal death was simulated by stopping the maternal blood supply to the placenta at time 0. The response of the fetal cardiovascular system was an increase in arterial pressure. This resulted from vasoconstriction which was a controller response to

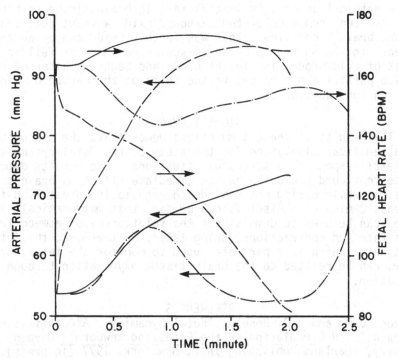

Fig. 5 Fetal Arterial Pressure and Heart Rate Calculated for Maternal Death (——), Complete Cord Occlusion (---), and Labor With Cord Compression (-·-).

lowered oxygen concentrations measured by chemoreceptors in the aorta. The chemoreceptor also caused the fetal heart rate to rise initially but later the fetal heart rate leveled out and began to drop as the fetal arterial pressure control systems began to take effect. It can be seen that the control systems have managed to protect the brain oxygen during the two minutes of the simulation as evidenced by the maintenance of near normal values following a small initial dip. This is accomplished by increased blood flow supply to the brain (Figure 3). Carbon dioxide partial pressure showed a gradual increase resulting from acid production in the extremeties which caused a shift in the carbon dioxide-hydrogen ion equilibrium curve.

Simulation of complete occlusion of the umbilical cord was done by stopping all umbilical blood flow. The immediate response was an increase in the arterial pressure due to the loss of a major flow channel. Instantly the fetal heart rate dropped due to the baroreceptor control system. Flow supply to the brain increased greatly both because of the increase in arterial pressure and lower blood flow resistance due to local oxygen control. It can be seen that constriction of the umbilical cord has an immediate effect on the brain oxygenation as opposed to a slower effect during maternal death. An initial fall in brain tissue carbon dioxide resulted from accelerated carbon dioxide washout due to an increased brain blood flow. This was further evidenced by an initial increase in the pH of the brain tissue. The pH later fell as a result of acid production in the brain and began to alter carbon dioxide partial pressure due to the shift of the carbon dioxide hydrogen ion equilibrium.

SIGNIFICANCE

The results of these simulations demonstrate the usefulness of mathematical simulation for the study of the fetal system and the fetal responses to stressful situations. The results demonstrate that cord occlusion has an immediate effect on brain oxygenation, while during maternal death, anoxia is forestalled for at least 2 minutes. Also, it can be seen that mathematical simulation can be used to demonstrate the relationships between fetal heart rate and contractions during labor. Furthermore, the fetal heart rate, which is a parameter used to monitor the fetus during labor, can be related to the brain tissue oxygenation through simulation.

REFERENCES

Cameron, J.M. and D.D. Reneau, "Fetal Dynamics: A Quantitative Approach," IN Circulation in the Fetus and Newborn: Oxygen Delivery, Garland Publishing Inc., New York, 1977 (in press).

This research was supported in part by grant #HEW-NIH-NS-08802.

SOME EFFECTS OF HIGH ALTITUDE AND POLYCYTHAEMIA ON OXYGEN DELIVERY

D.D. Reneau* and I.A. Silver

Department of Pathology, University of Bristol

Medical School, Bristol BS8 1TD, England

INTRODUCTION

The purpose of this project was to investigate by means of mathematical analysis some of the implications of polycythaemia at high altitude on tissue oxygenation with special emphasis on the human cerebral cortex.   Experimental data concerning arterial oxygen saturation, haematocrit, and corresponding blood viscosity was collected from the literature and used as input data for the predictive study.   Tissue oxygenation of brain cortex was evaluated for a variety of cases using a mathematical model and solution techniques for the mapping of oxygen deficient tissue zones as described in prior publications but specifically in Reneau et al (1970).   In addition, the effect of changes in specified variables was analysed in an effort to evaluate the effectiveness of possible protective mechanisms.   Specific effects investigated included a rightward shift in the oxygen dissociation curve as found in polycythaemic patients due to hypercapnia, increased capillary density and flow rate accommodation.

Mathematical Model

As stated the model used in this study is well documented in the literature, (Reneau et al 1970) and is essentially as described elsewhere in this volume, Reneau et al (1977).   The model is based on the idealized Krogh capillary tissue cylindrical geometry and describes the interactions between blood flow, diffusion, tissue O_2

* Permanent address : Louisiana Tech University, Ruston, Louisiana 71270, U.S.A.

consumption and oxygen release from haemoglobin.   For the present
study the model is restricted to steady state and is used to
investigate oxygen distribution in the axial and radial direction
for the entire cylindrical arrangement.

RESULTS

Increased haematocrit and variable capillary flow rate

An increase in haematocrit without a change in flow rate results
in increased oxygenation of tissue as would be expected.   Fig. 1
represents simulated PO_2 profiles along the length of a capillary
for conditions under which the haematocrit has increased from 45%
to 80%.   The parameters represent variable flow rates and each is
compared to the normal (second curve from the top).   Note that an

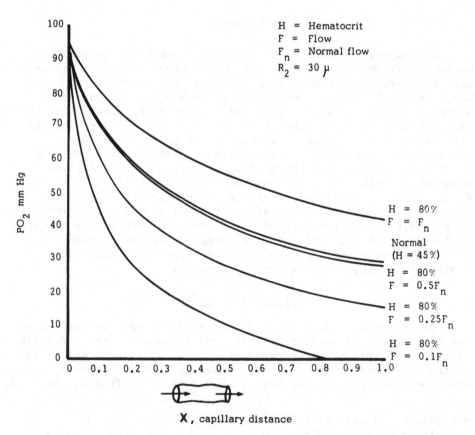

Fig. 1. A plot of capillary oxygen tension changes with respect to
      capillary length.   Parameters reflect changes in haematocrit
      and flow rate as listed, with all other factors normal.

increased haematocrit to 80% can be accompanied by a 50% reduction
in flow rate and still maintain an almost normal tissue oxygenation
profile.   However as flow is reduced to 25% of normal, hypoxia
develops and if flow rate is reduced to 10% of normal anoxia
develops in the capillary.

Figure 2 is a diagramatic representation of the region of
anoxic tissue that would be present if the haematocrit was 80% and
flow rate 10% of normal.   Almost 40% of the tissue would be anoxic
and much more hypoxic.

Figures 1 and 2 are calculations that demonstrate the trend
of development that would occur if haematocrit increased rather
quickly in man before any compensatory changes could occur.   One

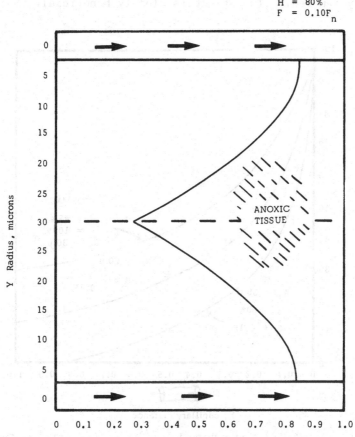

Fig. 2. A mapping of the quantity of anoxic tissue ($PO_2 < 0.5$ mmHg)
between capillaries when the haematocrit is 80% and flow
rate is reduced to 10% of normal.   All other factors are
maintained at normal levels.

possible compensating effect would be increased capillary density
(reduced intercapillary distances) Cassin et al. (1966) that would
reduce the radial diffusion zone and improve the blood supply for
oxygen.

Increased capillarity

Figure 3 demonstrates, theoretically, the effectiveness of
decreasing intercapillary distance during polycythaemia such that
the effective radial diffusion zone is reduced from 30μ to 20μ.
These particular curves were determined by holding capillary length
constant.   Thus the volume of tissue supplied per capillary as
well as the diffusion zone was reduced.   Note that although the
oxygenation picture is not returned to normal capillary anoxia is
avoided and the region of anoxic tissue given in Fig. 2 is
completely removed.   The effect is clearly beneficial.

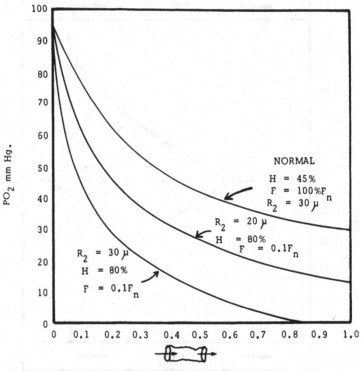

X, capillary distance

Fig. 3. A comparison of the PO_2 change in the capillary with
respect to length as the capillary density, flow rate, and
haematocrit change from the normal.   All other factors
maintained normal.

However the question arises as to the extent to which increased
capillarity can occur.   Using equations derived by Thews (1960)
for determining the effective radial region of supply in tissues
when the capillarity has been measured, one can assume radial
regions of supply and, in reverse, calculate capillarity.   The
results of these calculations are shown in Fig. 4.

The normal capillarity of brain tissue in man is represented
by a tissue radius of 30μ.   As this radius is reduced the necessary

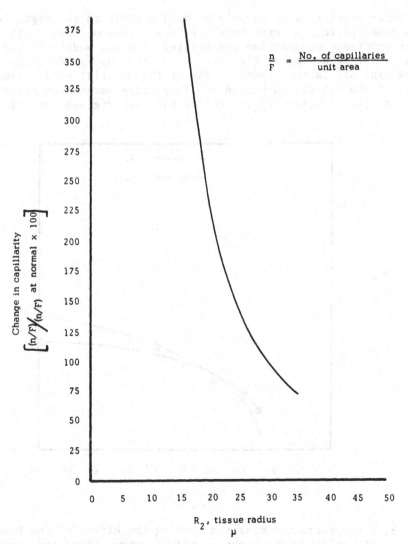

Fig. 4. Theoretically predicted change in capillary needed to
meet the indicated tissue diffusion zones, R_2.

capillary density begins an exponential increase.   For instance for
a capillarity yielding a radial diffusion zone of 25μ, 20μ and 10μ,
the capillarity would have to increase 1.44, 2.25 and 9.0 times
beyond normal, respectively.   Clearly a point of diminishing
returns is reached that probably rather quickly limits the degree
of useful compensation that can be achieved by reducing intercapillary distance.

Oxygen Dissociation Curve Shift

Under conditions of chronic hypoxia a shift to the right is
often observed for the oxyhaemoglobin dissociation curve.   The
effect on tissue oxygenation was studied with our model and the
findings are presented in Fig. 5.   This study was produced by
maintaining all factors constant except the arterial oxygen tension.
In Fig. 5 the calculated venous PO_2 is plotted versus the arterial
PO_2.   A plot of tissue PO_2 at the lethal corner gives the safe trend.

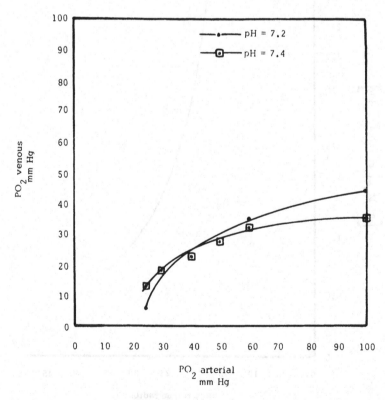

Fig. 5. A theoretical comparison showing the effect of the BOHR
        ODC shift to the right on tissue oxygenation, for conditions
        of progressively developing hypoxic-hypoxia.   ODC's taken
        from 'Blood and Other Body Fluids'.

TABLE I:

THEORETICAL PREDICTIONS OF BRAIN OXYGENATION AT 4,300 METERS
AND A COMPARISON OF POSSIBLE PROTECTIVE MECHANISMS

DATA			CALCULATED		VENOUS PO_2		ODC – SHIFT		CAPILLARIZATION		FLOW ACCOMMODATION FOR NORMAL P_T	
λa	Hematocrit	Viscosity	F_2/F_1	λv	P_v (pH=7.4)	P_v (pH=7.2)	P_{Tissue} (pH=7.4)	P_T (pH=7.2)	$R_2(P_T=O.O^+)$ pH=7.4	$P_2(P_T=O.O^+)$ pH=7.2	F/F_{PN} (pH=7.4)	F_{PN} (pH=7.2)
0.95	45	2.0	1.00	0.625	33	-	11.4	-	-	-	-	-
0.84	45	2.0	1.00	0.515	27	33.0	5.4	11.4	-	-	1.51	1.0
0.84	48	2.9	0.69	0.40	23	28.0	1.4	6.4	-	-	1.41	0.94
0.84	53	3.3	0.61	0.389	22.5	27.5	0.9	5.9	-	-	1.28	0.86
0.84	58	3.8	0.53	0.365	21.6	26.6	0.0	5.0	30 μ	-	1.17	0.78
0.84	65	4.5	0.44	0.33	20.0	25.0	-1.6	3.4	29.2	-	1.04	0.70
0.84	72	5.8	0.34	0.24	17.0	21.6	-4.6	0.0	27.7	30 μ	0.94	0.63
0.84	79	8.5	0.24	0.07	8.0	11.0	-13.6	-10.6	20.5	23 μ	0.86	0.57
0.84	86	10^+	0.20^-	0.00	0.0	0.0	-21.6	-21.6	impossible	impossible	0.79	0.53

Note that the rightward shift in the ODC is beneficial as long as the arterial PO_2 is sufficiently high. As the arterial PO_2 is reduced the beneficial effect of the right hand shift in the ODC is reduced until a crossover occurs, and the right hand shift in the ODC becomes a liability. In other words under certain conditions of low arterial PO_2, a left hand shift in the ODC is beneficial to tissue oxygenation and is seen in the truly adapted high altitude camelids such as the Llama (Monge and Whittembury 1972). The reason for this phenomena is that at low arterial PO_2 values the arterial saturation of blood is so much less for the right shifted ODC that tissue oxygenation is adversely affected. These studies are substantiated by the recent experiments of Bakker (1977) and predictions of Turek et al (1973).

Oxygenation at 4,300 meters

In an effort further to examine tissue oxygenation, Table 1 was prepared to investigate possible brain tissue oxygenation at 4,300 meters. The first three columns are data from the literature that was used in the mathematical model, and the first row of numbers represent normal conditions for comparison purposes. Saturation of arterial blood was taken as 0.84 at 4,300 meters and maintained constant for all calculations. F_2/F_1 represents predicted fractional changes in flow rates from normal and were determined by use of the Hagen-Poiseulle equation with the given viscosity data. Based on this data venous oxygen saturation, λv, venous PO_2, Pv and the PO_2 at the lethal corner, P_{tissue}, was calculated. Comparisons are given for (1) an ODC shift, (2) increased capillarization that would keep the lethal corner PO_2 slightly above zero torr, and (3) flow adjustment that would be necessary to maintain a normal oxygenation status. The negative values for P_{tissue} indicates the degree of anoxia present.

In this study the ODC has a beneficial effect until a haematocrit of 72 is attained. Increased capillarization is beneficial, probably, until a haematocrit 70-80 is reached. Flow accommodations appear to be of the greatest value but local measurements seem to be completely absent in the literature and no effective evaluation of the F_2/F_1 column or the last two columns in Table 1 is possible. In all cases it appears that as haematocrit rises above 80, adequate tissue oxygenation is impossible because of increased blood viscosity.

REFERENCES

Bakker, J.C. (1977) Thesis, University of Amsterdam.

Cassin, S., Gilbert, R.D. and Johnson, E.M. (1967) U.S.A.F. Report AD-633091 Contract AF41 (609)-2421.

Monge, C. and Whittembury, J. (1972) Naturwissenschaft.

Reneau, D.D., Bruley, D.F. and Knisely, M.H. (1970) J. Am. Ass. Med. Instrum. 4, 211.

Reneau, D.D., McFarland, R.S. and Halsey, J.H. (In this volume).

Thews, G. (1960) Pflügers Arch. ges. Physiol. 271, 197.

Turek, Z., Kreuger, F. and Hoofd, L.J.C. (1973) Pflügers Arch. ges. Physiol. 342, 185.

This work was supported in part by NIH Grants NS-08802 and NS-10939.

THE THEORETICAL EFFECT OF DPG UPON OXYGEN DIFFUSION

IN ERYTHROCYTES

Jerry H. Meldon

Physiology Department, Odense University

5000 Odense-C, Denmark

The physiological significance of intra-erythrocyte haemoglobin (Hb)-facilitated oxygen transport (HFOT) has been debated since the observation (Wittenberg 1959; Scholander 1960) that steady-state O_2 transfer across a thin layer of solution is accelerated by this heme-bearing protein. An authoritative review has been published by Kreuzer (1970).

If diffusion of oxyhaemoglobin contributes to the flux of O_2 within red cells en route from blood to tissue, then ΔPO_2^1 (the O_2 tension drop between red cell interior and capillary wall) must be correspondingly smaller than that dictated by diffusion of physically dissolved gas alone. A lower capillary flow rate would therefore be required to maintain adequate tissue PO_2.

Most theorists (Thews 1960; Lawson and Forster, 1967; Lightfoot 1974) estimate ΔPO_2^1 to be less than 5 mmHg; a low value compared with that between capillary and tissue (Kessler 1974). However, an alternative view in which ΔPO_2 is much higher, has recently been put forward by Hellums (1977) but will not be considered here.

This paper deals with a generally neglected aspect of HFOT; the effect of 2,3-diphosphoglycerate (DPG), one of the 3 primary physiological factors affecting O_2-Hb equilibrium. The effects of H^+ (Fox and Landahl, 1965; Bright 1967) and of CO_2 (Ulanowicz and Frazier, 1970) have already been considered.

DPG binds selectively to deoxy-Hb (Benesch et al, 1968); thus a decreasing Hb affinity for O_2 follows an increase in total DPG concentration, $[DPG]_T$. A PO_2 gradient induces, therefore, not

255

only a similarly directed gradient in fractional Hb saturation with O_2 (Y), but also an oppositely directed one in its saturation with DPG.   Since the mobility of the relatively small DPG molecule must well exceed that of the DPG-protein complex, the free DPG concentration profile must be rather flatter than that of its bound form. Consequently a PO_2 gradient must induce a directionally opposed $[DPG]_T$ gradient, and this promotes O_2 binding at higher PO_2 with release at lower values and therefore facilitation of O_2 transport. The following analysis suggests that $\Delta[DPG]_T$ may be responsible for up to 1/3 of HFOT at the venous end of skeletal muscle capillaries.

ANALYSIS

We invoke the simplified model (Keller and Friedlander, 1966) of a semi-infinite, planar layer of solution, of thickness L and exposed at its respective surfaces to constant PO_2^O and PO_2^L ($<PO_2^O$). O_2 conservation dictates the following steady-state relationship:

$$DO_2\alpha O_2 PO_2 + 4D_{Hb}[Hb]_T Y = -\phi_1 x + \phi_2 \tag{1}$$

where αO_2 is the O_2 solubility coefficient, $[Hb]_T$ is total Hb tetramer concentration (a constant), x is the distance from the high PO_2 boundary and Fick's law of diffusion has been applied to the analysis (i.e. electrical effects have been neglected). ϕ_2 is a constant determined by PO_2^O and Y^O.   With the surfaces permeable to O_2 only, ϕ_1 is the net O_2 flux.   From eq. 1 applied at x = 0 and x = L, it follows that:

$$\phi_1 = D_{O_2}\alpha O_2 (PO_2^O - PO_2^L)(1+F)/L \tag{2}$$

where F, the flux augmentation factor due to HFOT, is equal to $\{D_{Hb}[Hb]_T(Y^O - Y^L)\}/\{D_{O_2}\alpha O_2(PO_2^O - PO_2^L)\}$.

The problem then is to determine Y^O and Y^L, the boundary values of Hb saturation with O_2.   Even when we assume reaction equilibrium (which overestimates $Y^O - Y^L$ (Keller and Friedlander, 1966), although the extent is likely small at 37°C), such values cannot be read off an O_2-Hb dissociation curve (ODC) since the latter is always determined at essentially constant $[DPG]_T$.   Thus a model for O_2-Hb-DPG interaction is required, and we resort to that often invoked (e.g. Duhm 1975) to derive equilibrium constants for DPG binding to oxy- and deoxy-Hb from the variation of P_{50} (PO_2 at Y = 0.5) with DPG concentration, i.e.:

$$4A + B = A_4B \qquad K_1 = [A_4B]/(PO_2)^4[B]$$

$$P' + B = P'B \qquad K_2 = [P'B]/[P'][B]$$

$$P' + A_4B = P'A_4B \qquad K_3 = [P'A_4B]/[P'][A_4B]$$

where A=O_2, B=Hb and P'=DPG.   Denoting by P_{50}^o the P_{50} value for
DPG-free (i.e. "stripped"), Hb, then $K_1 = (P_{50}^o)$.

The shortcomings of the model with respect to molecular biology are considerable (Szabo and Karplus, 1976); to be more
rigorous one might admit DPG binding to $(O_2)_2$Hb and $(O_2)_3$Hb.   None-
theless, for standard in vivo conditions of $[Hb]_T$=5.3 mM, $[DPG]_T$=
5.0 mM, pH 7.2 and 37°C, the ODC may be approximated (Fig. 1) by
setting P_{50}^o at 16 mmHg (Duhm 1975) and assuming K_2 and K_3 are
respectively 4 and 4 x 10^{-2} $(mM)^{-1}$ (values comparable with those
obtained from P_{50}-[DPG] data (Duhm 1975) and direct binding measurements (Garby and De Verdier 1971; Berger et al, 1973) under ∿in
vivo conditions).

Finally, local and global conservation of DPG species
respectively require that:

$$D_{DPG} [P'] + D_{Hb}([P'B] + [P'A_4B]) = \text{constant} \qquad (3)$$

$$\int_o^' ([P'] + [P'B] + [P'A_4B]) \, d(x/L) = \overline{[DPG]}_T \qquad (4)$$

where $\overline{[DPG]}_T$ is overall $[DPG]_T$ and D_{Hb} has been assumed applicable
to all Hb species.   Eq. 2 implies the effective constancy of $[P']$
for large D_{DPG}/D_{Hb}.   Assuming D varies as $1/\sqrt{\text{molecular wt.}}$, then
D_{DPG}/D_{Hb} is ∿16.   Gel chromatography data (Berman et al, 1971)

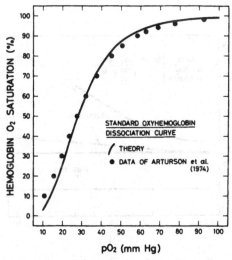

Fig. 1. Fit of standard dissociation curve (Arturson et al, 1974)
with assumed values for K_1, K_2 and K_3 (see text).

however suggest a lower ratio at physiological pH, and since PB +
$[P'A_4B]$ may be several times $[P']$ (see Fig. 2), it is important to
keep in mind that finite D_{DPG}/D_{Hb} yield lesser effects than those
described below.

The assumption that $[P']$ is constant (though unknown prior to
solution) makes analysis of eqs. 1, 2 and 4 constrained by the
reaction equilibria, a matter of algebra and integration which will
not be pursued here.   Results were calculated assuming physiolog-
ical $[Hb]_T$= 5.3 mM; K_1, K_2 and K_3 as above, α_{O2}=1.4 x 10^{-2} mM/mm
Hg (Roughton and Severinghaus, 1973) and D_{Hb}/D_{O2} = 0.01 (Kreuzer
1970) at 37°C.   No L value need be assigned for present purposes,
in as much as reaction equilibrium has been assumed.

RESULTS AND DISCUSSION

Fig. 2 depicts DPG concentration profiles for cases of maximal
and minimal effects of $\Delta[DPG]_T$ upon HFOT.   In fact, it is the case
with the far greater $\Delta[DPG]_T$ (i.e. the solid lines) which involves
<u>minimal</u> facilitation effects: the Y values at 0 and 100 mm Hg are
0 and ~1.0 irrespective of DPG concentration, which yields an F
value of 1.5 under all circumstances.   On the other hand, both Y
and Hb saturation with DPG are rather sensitive to PO_2 in the 20-25
mmHg range, with $[DPG]_T$=3 mM; and it is found that Y^0 and Y^L are
respectively 0.59 and 0.37 in the rigorously calculated case as
opposed to 0.55 and 0.40 when the difference between D_{DPG} and D_{Hb}
is neglected.   Thus F is calculated to be 6.6, which is nearly
50% greater than the value arrived at by traditional means.   This
indicates a potentially appreciable $\Delta[DPG]_T$ effect under conditions

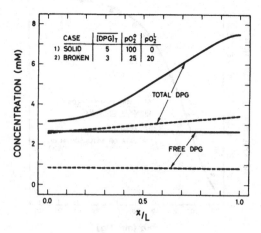

Fig. 2. Concentration profiles of free and total DPG in two
cases examined.

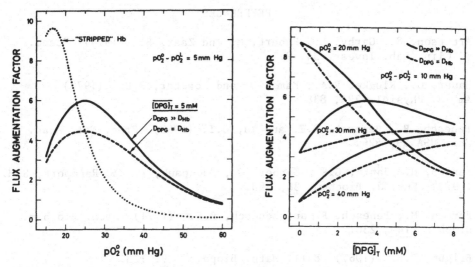

Fig. 3. Comparison of F values assuming $D_{DPG} \gg$ and $= D_{Hb}$, at varying levels of (a) PO_2 and (b) $[DPG]_T$.

found in the venous end of skeletal muscle microcirculation (Thompson et al, 1974). In addition, the large $[DPG]_T$ gradient in the 100 mmHg ΔPO_2 case, although insignificant in the present equilibrium framework, would be advantageous in cases of finite Hb-O_2 kinetics, since the degree of HFOT is then limited by Hb deoxygenation rates at the low PO_2 boundary (Meldon et al, 1973) and the latter are generally increased by DPG (Bauer et al, 1973).

Figures 3a and 3b illustrate, respectively, the dependence of F (for both D_{DPG} much greater than and equal to D_{Hb}) upon PO_2 level and overall DPG concentration, for cases of small PO_2 driving forces. The curves maximise where the relevant ODCs are steepest (i.e. where $Y^o-Y^L)/(PO_2^o-PO_2^L)$ is greatest); and the significance of DPG gradients is seen to behave somewhat similarly. For a normal $[DPG]_T$ value of 5 mM, its gradient is cause for a maximal increase in F of some 35%.

In conclusion, total DPG concentration gradients are potentially important in regard to Hb-facilitated O_2 diffusion under simulated physiological conditions. The maximum effect is estimated, using a highly simplified model of O_2-Hb-DPG interaction and physical conditions, to be an increase in the degree of facilitation of some 30-50% by comparison with traditional methods of analysis.

REFERENCES

Arturson, G., Garby, L., Robert, M. and Zaar, B.   (1974)   Scand.
J. Clin. Lab. Invest. 34, 9.

Bauer, C., Klocke, R.A., Kamp, D. and Forster, R.E.   (1973)
Am. J. Physiol. 224, 838.

Benesch, R., Benesch, R.E. and Yu, C.I. (1968)   Proc. Nat. Acad.
Sci. USA 59, 526.

Berger, H., Jänig, G.R., Gerber, G., Ruckpauk, K. and Rapoport, S.M.
(1973)   Eur. J. Biochem. 38, 553.

Berman, M., Benesch, R. and Benesch, R.E.   (1971)   Arch. Biochem.
Biophys. 145, 236.

Bright, P.B.   (1967)   Bull. Math. Biophys. 29, 123.

Duhm, J.   (1975)   In 'Erythrocyte Structure and Function' (ed.
Brewer, G.), A.R. Liss, New York.

Fox, M.A. and Landahl, H.D.   (1965)   Bull. Math. Biophys. 27, 183.

Garby, L. and De Verdier, C.H.   (1971)   Scand. J. Clin. Lab. Invest.
27, 345.

Hellums, J.D.   (1977)   Microvasc. Res. 13, 131.

Keller, K.H. and Friedlander, S.K.   (1966)   J. Gen. Physiol. 49,663.

Kessler, M.   (1974)   Microvasc. Res. 8, 283.

Kreuzer, F.   (1970)   Respir. Physiol. 9, 1.

Lawson, W.H. and Forster, R.E.   (1967)   J. Appl. Physiol. 22, 970.

Lightfoot, E.N.   (1974)   In 'Transport Phenomena in Living Systems
Wiley-Interscience, New York.

Meldon, J.H., Smith, K.A. and Colton, C.K.   (1973)   Adv. Exper. Med.
Biol. 37a,199.

Roughton, F.J.W. and Severinghaus, J.W.   (1973)   J. Appl. Physiol.
35, 861.

Scholander, P.F.   (1960)   Science 131, 585.

Szabo, A. and Karplus, M.   (1976)   Biochem. 15, 2869.

Thews, G. (1960) Pflügers Arch. <u>271</u>, 197.

Thomson, J.M., Dempsey, J.A., Chosy, L.W., Shahidi, N.T. and Reddan, W.G. (1974) J. Appl. Physiol. <u>37</u>, 658.

Ulanowicz, R.E. and Frazier, G.C. (1970) Math.Biosci. <u>7</u>, 11.

Wittenberg, J.B. (1959) Biol. Bull. <u>117</u>, 402.

DISCUSSION OF PAPERS IN SESSION 3

CHAIRMEN: DR. D. RENEAU and DR. D. BRULEY

PAPER BY: DR. AKMAL et al

Dr. Metzger: 1. Did you use hexagonal co-ordinates?
2. Was there convergence for over-relaxation?

Dr. Bruley: We did not do the entire hexagonal configuration cal-culation. Because of symmetry it was possible to use the 30-60-90 triangular prism described to determine PO_2 throughout the hexa-gon. Certainly it would be possible to treat the whole hexagon, but unnecessary.

2. We did not have any serious convergence problems using Grain-Siedel with the over-relaxation factor. The steady state solution was obtained on a CDC-640 computer with an average processing time of 1500 seconds.

Dr. Metzger: 1. Would it not be necessary to include a cellular compartment in the model because glucose diffusion through the cell membrane is much more time consuming than diffusion through the extra-cellular space?

2. Have you done calculations on hypoglycaemia?

Dr. Bruley: 1. The numerical solutions for the multi-component model are already very tedious. If we are to maintain the distri-bution parameter nature of the model it would be virtually impossi-ble to compartmentalise the tissue equations and still be able to solve the problem with conventional mathematical techniques. There may be a possibility of doing this with the probabalistic models which we are now looking at.

263

2. Not yet but we plan to.

Dr. Goldstick: It seems to me that the value of a simulation is
its ability to represent the average behaviour of the physiological
system and that one does not know if the simulation is accurate
unless one tests it against an experiment. If the simulation
behaves identically to the average behaviour of the physiological
system when both are subjected to the same stress then it is a
good simulation. That is the test of the simulation; not its
resemblance to the geometry of the physiological system.

Dr. Bruley: In general I would agree with this statement although
I feel that the closer you can come to reality with the model the
better off you are. Many physiological systems are so complex
that it will never be possible to simulate them exactly.

Dr. Chance: Would you be more likely to find appropriate geometric
models in the liver?

Dr. Bruley: It is my understanding that a hexagonal arrangement
of capillaries does exist in the liver so it is definitely one
possibility. However, it would probably be more difficult to perform in vivo polarographic experiments in liver plus, as a
theoretician you have to locate someone who is willing to do the
experimental work.

Unnamed questioner: I regret that the capillary circulation in
skeletal muscle is far more complex than has been believed in the
past.

1. Hexagonal geometry is but one of the several models consistent
with Dr. Banchero's data.

2. His data pertain only to the situation when all capillaries
are open. This never happens, even in maximal exercise in normal
muscle, for at least one third of the motor units remain at rest
under such conditions.

3. Functional capillary density follows no discernable pattern
whatever if erythrocyte-containing capillaries are mapped from
sectioned freeze-clamped muscles.

4. There is no fixed capillary length or transit time in muscle.
The former ranges from 150 to 300 µm and the latter from 50 m sec.
to 43 sec. This diversity must be taken into account. Since the
anatomy is so indeterminate and plays such a large role in the
calculations I suggest that skeletal muscle circulation is too
complex for the purpose that you have in mind.

Dr. Bruley: The points you have made are well understood.
However, the purpose of the study is to try and find tissue that
is less complicated than the brain in order to determine the validity of our non-linear, distributed parameter (PDE), time-depen-
dent system of equations representing oxygen and other component
transport in the micro-circulation. Our interest is in predicting
local values of oxygen tension, etc. and our main concern is to
attempt a verification of our numerical solutions in an in-vivo
preparation. Even though not exact I am sure that tests in
skeletal muscle would be easier to perform and provide a more
accurate comparison than those in brain tissue. We are not trying
to play-down or ignore the complexities of any physiological
system but merely to find the simplest model possible for testing
the equation.

Dr. Banchero has results showing the hexagonal pattern in some
samples of tissue. His technique for staining, etc. is an
improvement because it illustrates all of the capillaries around
the muscle fibre whether they are open or closed. For experiments
with micro-electrodes we would probably open all capillaries with
the proper drug to do the testing and use the method of Metzger
to locate the tip of the electrode relative to the capillary network (see his presentation in this symposium). Certainly I would
be happy if someone could suggest a better tissue to test the
equations on.

Dr. Fletcher: Have you compared a Krogh cylinder of comparable
size to your triangular model to see if the boundary complications
are worth the effort?

Dr. Bruley: First the boundary considerations of the triangular
model are no more complicated than those of the Krogh Cylinder
model, The computations are of about the same degree of difficulty.
Second, we did not compare the numerical solutions of the triangles
with the numerical solutions of the Krogh Cylinder, however we did
compare with the Krogh-Erlang analytical solution. It was found
that the influence of surrounding capillaries on a given equilateral triangle of tissue results in an enhanced PO_2 at any point.
For resting conditions the maximal pressure drop between proximal
and distal points from the capillary was estimated to be about 36%
lower than that obtained by the Krogh-Erlang equation. The
corresponding change in exercising muscle was 57%.

PAPER BY: DRS: GRAD & SVETINA

Dr. Metzger: What can be the physiological mechanism of your con-
sumption-controlled sphincter?

2. What values for A (consumption rate) do you use for what tissue?

Dr. Svetina: The model presented is based on the assumption that the blood flow through a capillary or group of capillaries can be described approximately by an on/off control of their opening. It is possible to calculate the input/output characteristics of a system exhibiting such behaviour without knowing the detailed mechanism of this process. To obtain reasonable results from the model we have to assume that there are two effectors operative. The amount of one being proportional to the oxygen tension and the amount of the other being proportional to the steady state of oxygen consumption. The results of the calculations are relative values of the blood flow with respect to a certain reference state of the system and can be used to describe different tissues exhibiting local blood flow regulation according to the metabolic needs.

PAPER BY: DRS. HOOFD and KREUZER

Dr. Chance: What are the conditions under which you would expect to find significant facilitated diffusion within a single cell. For example, by haemoglobin in a yeast cell or by P_{450} inside a hepatocyte?

1. See Oshino et al E.J.B. 35 23-33 (1973).

2. See Longmuir ISOX Symposium Discussion.

PAPER BY: DR. MOCHIZUKI

Dr. Chance: Do you compute a time constant for the response of myoglobin to increases of oxygen concentration that agrees with those observed experimentally by Tamura (in this book)?

Dr. Mochizuki: Yes, the PO_2 in the heart muscle may be evaluated from the solution for any change in O_2 consumption. When the O_2 consumption rate increases the PO_2 decreases as the O_2 is consumed. But the PO_2 increase, due to a reduction of O_2 consumption may not occur so rapidly, as stated by Dr. Tamura, since it obeys the time constant of the diffusion.

PAPER BY: DR. QUINN

Dr. Goeckenjan: In adults with normal circulation we found a decrease of $\frac{t_c PO_2}{PaO_2}$ ratio from hyperoxaemia (approx. 0.9-0.95) to

normoxaemia (approx. 0.8-0.85) and to hypoxaemia (PaO_2 approx. 45-50 mmHg, $\frac{t_c PO_2}{PaO_2}$ approx. 0.45-0.5). It would be interesting if the reason for this behaviour could be derived from your mathematical model.

PAPER BY: DRS. RENEAU & HALSEY

Dr. Fletcher: The " ϕ factor" you have described looks very much like the limiting coefficient I derived in my 1975 OTT Conference Paper in which it was predicted that the haemoglobin dissociation properties would be the limiting factor at lowered PO_2 s! I did not do any ischaemia studies but it seems clear that the conclusions would apply. The expression I refer to was, I believe,

$$\frac{1}{1 + C\,\frac{d\Psi}{dP}} \quad \to \quad 1 \text{ as } P \to \infty$$

Where c, is blood capacity and Ψ is the oxy-haemoglobin dissociation curve; P of course, is O_2 pressure. Are these factors and analyses referring to the same phenomena?

Dr. Reneau: The relation you describe appears to be similar to our Ψ factor with the exception of V_0, λ and α_T.

Dr. Goldstick: I wonder if its' possible that your observation that the initial slope depends upon the initial PO_2 may be an artifact created by the O_2 consumption of the electrode itself which leads to an apparent non-constant mitochondrial O_2 consumption near the electrode tip. If the diffusion field created by the electrode tip extends into the tissue then the PO_2 might be sufficiently reduced near its tip to give the nonlinearity you observe. Of course, the haemoglobin nonlinearity will also be present.

Dr. Reneau: We do not feel that the factors you describe are significant enough to affect the general conclusion of our results. (cf. the answer given by Friedli).

Dr. Friedli: In answer to the objection of Dr. Goldstick to Dr. Reneau's paper, I have observed the same decrease in the rate of PO_2 drop with initial PO_2 below 100 mmHg in response to increased O_2 consumption in isolated cervical ganglia containing some capillary haemoglobin. This was observed with a recessed PO_2 micro-electrode of <u>very small consumption</u> which sould have 90% of its PO_2 field within its recess. Consequently I do not feel that the observations were artifactual due to electrode consumption.

Cellular Respiration and O₂ Transport

ON THE MECHANISM OF REGULATION OF CELLULAR RESPIRATION. THE

DEPENDENCE OF RESPIRATION ON THE CYTOSOLIC [ATP],[ADP] AND [PI]

Maria Erecińska and David F. Wilson

Department of Biochemistry and Biophysics

University of Pennsylvania, Philadelphia, Pa. 19104

Mitochondrial oxidative phosphorylation consists of two types of reactions: electron transfer reactions and ATP-synthesizing reactions. Electron transfer from the reducing substrates to molecular oxygen occurs down the electrochemical potential gradient and is therefore accompanied by a negative free energy change. ATP synthesis is, on the other hand, an energy-requiring process which cannot occur spontaneously unless it is linked to another energy yielding reaction. In vivo in the cell, the obligatory coupling between the mitochondrial redox reactions and ATP synthesis provides the latter with the necessary "energetic push".

It has been demonstrated by the experiments of Chance and Hollunger (1961) and Klingenberg and Schollmeyer (1961) that the redox reactions between the NAD and cytochrome c couples can be reversed on addition of ATP. This indicated that, in principle, equilibrium could exist between the two redox couples and the adenine nucleotide system. If we ignore simple proton uptake, the equilibrium is depicted by equation (1).

$$\text{NADH} + 2\text{cyt } c^{3+} + 2\text{ADP} + 2\text{Pi} \rightleftharpoons \text{NAD}^+ + 2\text{cyt } c^{2+} + 2\text{ATP} \quad (1)$$

which allows us to define the equilibrium constant K, where

$$K = \frac{[\text{NAD}^+]}{[\text{NADH}]} \times \frac{[\text{cyt } c^{2+}]^2}{[\text{cyt } c^{3+}]^2} \times \frac{[\text{ATP}]^2}{[\text{ADP}]^2 [\text{Pi}]^2} \quad (2)$$

Since the possibility of establishing equilibrium does not necessarily mean that that equilibrium actually exists in the functioning system, systematic studies were undertaken both in isolated mitochondria (Erecińska et al, 1974) and in suspensions of cells

(Wilson et al, 1974 b, c; Wilson et al, 1977 b) to determine the
free energy relationships between the redox reactions and ATP
synthesis under various metabolic conditions. The results of
experiments on suspensions of isolated mitochondria respiring in
the presence of substrate and oxygen, and on suspensions of various
cells are summarized in Table I. It can be seen that the equilibrium relationship of equation 1 holds when the [NAD$^+$]/[NADH]
ratio of the mitochondrial matrix and the extramitochondrial
(cytoplasmic) concentrations of ATP, ADP, and Pi are employed.
It should be indicated that in equation 2, the [NAD$^+$]/[NADH] refers
to the ratio of the free nicotinamide-adenine dinucleotides as
calculated, for example, from the measured concentration of
acetoacetate and 3-OH-butyrate and the equilibrium constant for
the 3-OH-butyrate dehydrogenase reaction (Williamson et al, 1962;
1967). The [cytochrome c^{2+}]/[cytochrome c^{3+}] ratio can be determined spectrophotometrically, while the concentrations of ATP, ADP,
and Pi can be measured by standard analytical procedures.

The demonstration that the first two sites of oxidative
phosphorylation are at near equilibrium with the extramitochondrial
[ATP]/[ADP][Pi] allows us to describe the overall respiratory rate
by combining equation 2 and the rate expression for the oxidation
of reduced cytochrome c by molecular oxygen. Equation 2 states

Table I

Free-Energy Relationships Between the Oxidation-Reduction Reactions of the Respiratory Chain and ATP Synthesis (Experimental)

Type of Material	E_H Cytochrome c (volt)	E_H NAD (volt)	ΔE (volt)	ΔG_{OX-RED} (kcal/2e$^-$)	ΔG_{ATP} (kcal/2ATP)	$\Delta\Delta G$ (kcal)	Reference
Liver cells (no substrate)	0.272	-0.242	0.514	23.7	23.8	-0.1	Wilson et al (1974)
Liver cells (lactate + ethanol)	0.269	-0.260	0.529	24.4	24.2	0.2	"
Perfused liver (no substrate)	0.253	-0.263	0.516	23.8	23.6	1.2	"
Ascites tumor cells	0.260	-0.270	0.530	24.4	23.6	0.8	"
Cultured kidney cells	0.271	-0.252	0.523	24.1	24.2	-0.1	Wilson et al (1977)
Tetrahymena pyriformis cells	0.251	-0.236	0.487	22.5	22.4	0.1	Erecińska unpubl.
Pigeon heart mitochondria (succinate)	0.270	-0.343	0.613	28.4	29.8	-1.4	Erecińska et al (1974)

$$\Delta E = E_{HNAD} - E_{HCYT\ c}\ \ \text{where}\ E_H = E_M + \frac{2.3RT}{nF}\ \log \frac{[ox]}{[red]}\ ;\ \ \Delta G_{OX-RED} = -n\ F\Delta E;$$

$$\Delta G_{ATP} = \Delta G_0' + 1.36\ \log \frac{[ADP]\ [P_i]}{[ATP]}\ ;\ \ \ \Delta\Delta G = \Delta G_{OX-RED} - \Delta G_{ATP}$$

that the concentration of reduced cytochrome c and thus the respiratory rate itself must be dependent on the phosphorylation state
of the adenine nucleotide system. [The redox state of cytochrome c
is also dependent on the concentration of oxygen which enters
directly into the rate equation (see Wilson et al, 1977 a, and this
symposium)]. In agreement with this, it has been shown (Holian
et al, 1977) that in suspensions of tightly coupled mitochondria
isolated from various sources, the respiratory rate was dependent
on [ATP]/[ADP][Pi] and not on the [ATP]/[ADP] ratio.

In as much as mitochondrial oxidative phosphorylation is the
primary source of cellular [ATP] and the primary sink for cellular
[NADH], [ADP], and [Pi], it follows that the activities of other
metabolic pathways which utilize these co-factors may also be
dependent on [ATP]/[ADP][Pi] ratio and not on concentrations of
the individual reactants. This suggests that the [ATP]/[ADP][Pi]
might be an important regulatory factor of cellular homeostasis
and that the intracellular [Pi] contributes in equal measure to
the regulatory phenomena along with the concentrations of [ATP]
and [ADP].

To test this hypothesis we have chosen to investigate the
changes in intracellular [Pi] and their impact on cellular metabolism.

Table II

The Effect of Glycerol on Concentrations of Metabolites in Isolated Liver Cells

METABOLITE OR METABOLITE RATIO	CONTROL	2 MIN.	10 mM GLYCEROL 5 MIN.	15 MIN.
ATP[*]	2.02 ± 0.27	1.66 ± 0.33	1.29 ± 0.35	0.95 ± 0.42
ADP[*]	0.48 ± 0.15	0.76 ± 0.30	0.79 ± 0.27	0.75 ± 0.33
AMP[*]	0.45 ± 0.07	0.47 ± 0.07	0.42 ± 0.11	0.42 ± 0.06
Pi[*]	3.38 ± 0.04	1.39 ± 0.13	1.01 ± 0.03	0.80 ± 0.10
ATP/ADP	4.2 ± 1.5	2.60 ± 0.15	1.99 ± 0.14	1.57 ± 0.25
ATP/ADP x Pi (M^{-1})	1346 ± 329	1203 ± 165	1380 ± 204	1277 ± 381
ENERGY CHARGE	0.76 ± 0.01	0.68 ± 0.01	0.65 ± 0.04	0.58 ± 0.02
$\frac{\text{3-OH-BUTYRATE}}{\text{ACETOACETATE}}$	1.41 ± 0.4	1.40 ± 0.35	1.45 ± 0.52	1.62 ± 0.48
$\frac{\text{CYT } C_{OX}}{\text{CYT } C_{RED}}$	5.12 ± 2.0	4.74 ± 2.0	4.50 ± 2.0	4.46 ± 1.6
O_2 UPTAKE (µMOLE/MIN/G)	1.57 ± 0.4	1.64 ± 0.56	1.41 ± 0.47	1.20 ± 0.43

[*] VALUES EXPRESSED IN µMOLES/G WET WEIGHT. RESULTS FROM FOUR INDEPENDENT EXPERIMENTS ± S.D.

The experimental material used in the studies was either suspensions
of isolated liver cells incubated with metabolites which lower the
intracellular [Pi], or yeast (Candida utilis) grown in media
containing various concentrations of inorganic phosphate. As shown
in Table II, liver cells incubated in the presence of glycerol show
a rapid fall in inorganic phosphate and a decrease both in ATP and
in total adenine nucleotides concentration, in agreement with the
results of other authors on perfused liver (Raivio et al, 1969;
Woods et al, 1970). During the 15 minute incubation, the [ATP]/[ADP]
ratio decreased from 4.2 to 1.6, and the energy charge (defined as
([ATP] + [½ ADP])/([ATP] + [ADP] + [AMP]) declined from 0.76 to
0.58. However, the redox states of mitochondrial NAD couple and of
cytochrome c, the respiratory rate and the [ATP]/[ADP][Pi] all
remained essentially unaltered. The same, although more striking
effects were observed in the liver cells incubated with fructose
(Erecińska et al, 1977).

Marked changes in concentrations of intracellular phosphate was
found in the yeast, Candida utilis, grown in the presence of
different [Pi]. As shown in Table III, the concentration of
intracellular phosphate in cells grown in 50 mM Pi rose to 25.9
μmoles/g wet weight, while it was 11.6 μmoles/g wet weight in cells
grown in 5 mM Pi and 2.9 μmoles/g wet weight in cells grown in
1 mM Pi. The increase in the intracellular [Pi] was paralleled by
an increase in the level of ATP, which rose from 1.2 to 1.3 μmoles/g
wet weight in cells grown in either 5 mM or 1 mM Pi to about 4
μmoles/g wet weight in cells grown in medium containing 50 mM Pi.
The concentrations of ADP were the same irrespective of whether the
cells were grown in the high or in the low phosphate medium.

Table III

Concentrations of the Adenine Nucleotides and Pi in Candida utilis
Yeast Grown in the Media Containing Various Pi

THE RESPIRATORY SUBSTRATE WAS 25 mM ETHANOL. CONCENTRATIONS OF ATP, ADP, AND
PI ARE EXPRESSED IN μMOLES/G WET WEIGHT.

PI IN THE GROWTH MEDIUM	ATP	ADP	PI	ATP/ADP	ATP/ADP x PI	∆G$_{ATP}$ (KCAL)	TN E⁻/SEC/CYT c
50 mM	4.17±0.07	0.12±0.004	25.9±1.9	33.8±1.4	1322±151	11.84	52±5
5 mM	1.32±0.04	0.12±0.004	11.6±1.8	11.5±0.7	1109±141	11.74	50±3
1 mM	1.22±0.07	0.15±0.02	2.9±0.7	8.3±0.7	3140±602	12.36	35±0.3

Although the [ATP]/[ADP] ratios were significantly higher in cells grown in 50 mM Pi than in cells grown in 5 mM Pi, the [ATP]/[ADP][Pi] values were the same within experimental error, because the high [ATP]/[ADP] ratios in the former were compensated by the high intracellular Pi levels. The respiratory rates (turnover numbers for cytochrome c) were the same in cells grown in 50 mM and 5 mM Pi while they were slower in cells grown in 1 mM Pi, in agreement with the observed higher [ATP]/[ADP][Pi].

The experiments described above were designed to gain insight into the nature of the regulatory phenomena of cellular metabolism. Two fundamentally different regulatory parameters have been proposed: the energy charge, defined by Atkinson (1966, 1968) as ([ATP] + [½ADP])/([ATP] + [ADP] + [AMP]) and the phosphorylation state of the adenine nucleotide system (Wilson et al, 1974 a) (as defined by the ratio [ATP]/[ADP][Pi]). The first of these parameters, the energy charge, encompasses the diverse effects exhibited by individual adenine nucleotides within a single parameter with a theoretical range from 0 to 1. In order to perform the cellular regulatory function in vivo, the energy charge must be maintained close to or within the range of 0.85 - 0.90. On the other hand, the second parameter, [ATP]/[ADP][Pi], is directly related to the ∆G for ATP hydrolysis and incorporates, in addition to the effects exhibited by ATP and ADP, those induced by Pi. Thus, while the latter stresses the primary importance of intracellular [Pi], the former ascribes no role to the phosphate concentration, but involves AMP as a primary regulator. (In regulation by [ATP]/[ADP][Pi] the concentration of AMP enters only indirectly through the adenylate kinase reaction.) It should also be emphasized here that experimentally, the more sensitively the metabolic activities of the cell respond to variations in the regulatory parameter the less it will be seen to vary in vivo because the homeostatic mechanisms will tend to oppose any large changes under physiological conditions.

The independence of the value for the energy charge parameter from [Pi] means that the energy charge can perform its regulatory function solely by maintaining constant ratios in the adenine nucleotides pool and those need not be affected by changes in the concentration of inorganic phosphate. In contrast, in order to maintain the [ATP]/[ADP][Pi] constant, if the [ATP]/[ADP] varies, the [Pi] must change. The results described above showed that variations in intracellular [Pi] induced simultaneous readjustments in the [ATP]/[ADP] so that the [ATP]/[ADP][Pi] was maintained at a constant value. Since the respiratory rate remained unchanged under the same conditions, in spite of the large changes in the individual concentrations of ATP, ADP, and Pi as well as in the energy charge, the conclusion can be drawn that cellular respiration is regulated by the phosphorylation state of the adenine nucleotide

system and not by the energy charge. It should, however, be pointed
out here that although the $[ATP]/[ADP][Pi]$ is still the primary
regulator of cellular metabolism under conditions when the
intracellular $[Pi]$ does not vary and adenylate kinase is near
equilibrium, (see for example Beis and Newsholme, 1975), the
energy charge under these conditions will behave essentially the
same as does the $[ATP]/[ADP][Pi]$. Both parameters will tend to
be maintained constant under most physiological conditions.

It also follows from the above considerations that changes in
$[ATP]/[ADP][Pi]$ (and thus in cellular metabolic rates) can be
induced solely through variations in $[Pi]$. In tissues such as
brain and muscle where maintaining a nearly constant level of ATP
is required for metabolic reasons, the stimulation of respiration
can occur through hydrolysis of phosphocreatine to creatine and
phosphate since that would tend to decrease the $[ATP]/[ADP][Pi]$.
Moreover, in cells and tissues in which the intracellular $[Pi]$
is high, greater $[ATP]/[ADP]$ are to be found so that the
$[ATP]/[ADP][Pi]$ ratios seem to be maintained in various systems
in a relatively narrow range of values from $7 \times 10^2 M^{-1}$ to
$4 \times 10^3 M^{-1}$.

We have shown here that cellular respiration is dependent on
the $[ATP]/[ADP][Pi]$, with the other variables being the mitochondrial $[NAD^+]/[NADH]$ and the oxygen tension (Wilson et al, 1977 b
and Wilson et al, this symposium). It has been repeatedly reported
that the respiratory rates of cell suspensions remain almost
independent of O_2 concentrations to quite low O_2 values (Warburg
and Kubowitz, 1929; Longmuir, 1957). Because the cellular ATP
utilization per se is independent of O_2 concentration, this
deceptively small K_m value may arise from a continuously decreasing
$[ATP]/[ADP][Pi]$ and/or decreasing mitochondrial $[NAD^+]/[NADH]$
which can maintain the respiratory rate at a constant value despite
decreasing $[O_2]$. Our preliminary results (Wilson et al, 1977 b)
on suspensions of cultured kidney cells showed that as the extracellular O_2 concentration was lowered, a decrease in the respiratory rate was accompanied by a decrease in the $[ATP]/[ADP]$ and a
progressive reduction of cytochrome c. These observations are,
however, in contrast with the results obtained in other laboratories
on whole freeze-clamped brain which show that the levels of ATP,
ADP and phosphocreatine remain unaltered even in severe hypoxia,
after the electrical activity of the brain cortex ceased to exist
(see e.g. Duffy et al, 1972; Bachelard et al, 1974). It is obvious
that more experiments are needed under well-defined conditions to
resolve this question. It is also clear that the hypothesis
outlined in this meeting (see Wilson et al) and in the previous
publications (Wilson et al, 1974 a, b, c; 1977 a) has been very
fruitful in explaining cellular behavior under various metabolic
conditions, and useful in designing future experiments.

REFERENCES

Atkinson, D.E. (1966) Ann. Rev. Biochem. 35, 85-124.

Atkinson, D.E. (1968) Biochemistry 7, 4030-4034.

Bachelard, H.S., Lewis, L.D., Pontén, U., and Siesjo, B.K. (1974) J. Neurochem. 22, 395-401.

Beis, I., and Newsholme, E.A. (1975) Biochem. J. 152, 23-32.

Chance, B., and Hollunger, G. (1961) J. Biol. Chem. 236, 1577-1584.

Duffy, T.E., Nelson, S.R., and Lowry, O.H. (1972) J. Neurochem. 19, 959-977.

Erecińska, M., Veech, R.L. and Wilson, D.F. (1974) Archiv. Biochem. Biophys. 160, 412-421.

Erecińska, M., Stubbs, M., Miyata, Y., Ditre, C.M., and Wilson, D.F. (1977) Biochem. Biophys. Acta in press.

Holian, A., Wilson, D.F. and Owen, C.S. (1977) Archiv. Biochem. Biophys. 181, 164-171.

Klingenberg, M., and Schollmeyer, P. (1961) Biochem. Z. 235, 243-262.

Longmuir, I.S., (1957) Biochem. J. 65, 378-382.

Raivio, K.O., Kekomäki, M.P. and Mäenpää (1969) Biochem. Pharmacology 18, 2615-2624.

Warburg, O., and Kubowitz, F. (1929) Biochem. Z. 214, 5-18.

Williamson, D.H., Lund, P., and Krebs, H.A. (1967) Biochem. J. 103, 514-527.

Williamson, D.H., Mellanby, J. and Krebs, H.A. (1962) Biochem. J. 82, 90-96.

Wilson, D.F., Erecińska, M., and Dutton, P.L. (1974 a) Ann. Rev. Biophys. Bioeng. 3, 203-230.

Wilson, D.F., Owen, C.S. and Holian, A. (1977 a) Archiv. Biochem. Biophys. in press.

Wilson, D.F., Erecińska, M., Drown, C. and Silver, I.A. (1977 b) Amer. J. Physiol. in press.

Wilson, D.F., Stubbs, M., Oshino, N., and Erecińska, M. (1974 b) Biochem. 13, 5305-5311.

Wilson, D.F., Stubbs, M., Veech, R.L., Erecińska, M., and Krebs, H.A. (1974 c) Biochem. J. 140, 57-64.

Woods, H.F., Eggleston, L.V., Krebs, H.A. (1970) Biochem. J. 119, 501-510.

This research was supported by U.S.P.H.S. Grant GM21524. M.E. is an established investigator for the American Heart Association.

REGULATION OF MITOCHONDRIAL RESPIRATION IN INTACT TISSUES: A MATHEMATICAL MODEL

David F. Wilson, Charles S. Owen and Maria Erecińska

Department of Biochemistry and Biophysics

University of Pennsylvania, Philadelphia, Pa. 19104

INTRODUCTION

Adenosine triphosphate [ATP] synthesized by mitochondrial oxidative phosphorylation is utilized in most of the biosynthetic pathways of the cell as well as for maintenance of the intracellular ion balance and for specialized functions such as muscle contraction and nerve transmission. This central role in cellular metabolism requires that mitochondrial oxidative phosphorylation (respiration) be subject to precise regulation by the cell. Understanding of this regulatory mechanism both qualitatively and quantitatively is essential to our knowledge of cytosolic-mitochondrial interrelationships and of overall cellular metabolism.

Recent experimental and conceptual advances have been made on three levels which, taken together, have encouraged us to develop a quantitative model for the control of mitochondrial oxidative phosphorylation. First: in both intact cells and isolated mitochondria, phosphorylation sites 1 and 2 in the mitochondrial respiratory chain from NADH to cytochrome c were observed to be in near equilibrium with the extramitochondrial [ATP]/[ADP][Pi] ratio (Erecińska et al, 1974; Wilson et al, 1974 a, b). This implies that the mechanism for respiratory control originates in the third site (cytochrome c oxidase) and not at sites 1 or 2. Second: the rate of mitochondrial respiration was shown to be dependent on the extramitochondrial [ATP]/[ADP][Pi] for suspensions of mitochondria isolated from several tissues and the quantitative relationship was measured (Owen and Wilson, 1974; Holian et al, 1977). Third: major advances have occurred in understanding the mechanism of cytochrome c oxidase, including demonstration of a role for the "invisible copper" in the reduction of oxygen to water (Lindsay

279

and Wilson, 1974; Lindsay et al, 1975) and evidence for a stable
bound peroxide intermediate in the reaction (Lindsay and Wilson,
1974; Lindsay et al, 1975; Orii and King, 1972; Greenwood et al,
1974; Chance et al, 1975). An earlier model which attempted to
describe cellular respiration (Owen and Wilson, 1974) was only
partially successful due to the use of an incomplete expression
for the reaction of cytochrome c oxidase with oxygen.

Figure 1 is a schematic presentation of the model we have
chosen as most accurately representing our current knowledge of
the mechanism of cytochrome c oxidase. The complete derivation of
the rate expression is presented elsewhere (Wilson et al, 1977)
and will be only summarized here. Each operating cycle reduces
one mole of oxygen to produce two moles of H_2O and two moles of
ATP. Water and hydrogen ions are not explicitly shown since these
are implicit in the rate constants. The oxygen reactive site of
cytochrome c oxidase contains two redox components, cytochrome a_3
and the "invisible copper". Reduction of the "invisible copper"
(reaction 1) opens the reaction site to oxygen (Wilson et al, 1975,

Figure 1

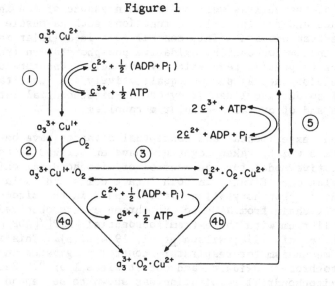

A schematic representation of the reaction of the cytochrome a_3-
"invisible copper" portion of cytochrome oxidase with cytochrome c
and oxygen. For simplicity, no intermediate compounds are indicated which couple the redox reactions to ATP synthesis. Similarly
intermediates in the electron transport pathway between cytochrome
c and the a_3-Cu complex have been omitted. In both cases the
omitted compounds are not considered to be important at rate
limiting stages in the respiration process (Wilson et al, 1977).

1976) which enters with a diffusion limited rate of 1×10^8 $M^{-1}sec^{-1}$ (Gibson and Greenwood, 1964; Chance et al, 1973). Once oxygen is in the site it binds to either the form $a_3^{3+}-Cu^{1+}$ or, following internal electron transfer, $a_3^{2+}-Cu^{2+}$(reaction 3). The addition of the second electron to the reaction site initiates a very rapid and strongly exergonic (George, 1965) reduction of the oxygen to bound peroxide (reaction 4). The cycle is completed in a fully reversible reaction which further reduces the bound peroxide to water and regenerates the oxidized form of cytochrome oxidase.

In the model, reactions 4a and 4b are always considered to be irreversible while reactions 1 and 2 are reversible only under conditions of limiting oxygen. Reactions 3 and 5 are considered to be at near equilibrium. Solution of the rate equations for steady state conditions gives the desired expression:

$$v = \frac{k_2 \, a_{3T}[O_2]}{1 + \alpha[O_2]} \tag{1}$$

where

$$\alpha = \frac{k_2}{k_1[c^{2+}]} \left\{ 1 + \frac{k_1(1 + K_3)}{k_{4b} + K_3 k_{4a}} + K_5^{-1} \frac{[ATP]}{[ADP][Pi]} \left[\frac{c^{3+}}{c^{2+}} \right]^2 \right\} \tag{2}$$

The rate constants are designated with lower case letters (k) and the equilibrium constants by capitol letters (K).

The equilibrium constant for reaction 3 (K_3) is expressed:

$$K_3 = Q \, 10^{(E_{ma3} - E_{mcu})}/0.059 \tag{3}$$

where Q is the relative affinity of O_2 for $a_3^{3+} - Cu^{1+}$ and $a_3^{2+} - Cu^{2+}$ and E_{ma_3} and E_{mcu} are the half reduction potentials of cytochrome a_3 and the "invisible copper" respectively. Experimentally the E_m value for cytochrome a_3 has been observed to be dependent on $[ATP]/[ADP][Pi]$ according to the equation

$$E_{ma3} = E_{ma3}^{*} - 0.059 \log \frac{0.16 \, M^{-1} + A}{1 \times 10^3 \, M^{-1} + A} \tag{4}$$

where E_{ma3} is the half reduction potential of cytochrome a_3 measured in the presence of 6 mM ATP (Wilson and Brocklehurst, 1973; Lindsay et al, 1975) and A is $[ATP]/[ADP][Pi]$. The E_m value of "invisible copper" is 0.34 V and is dependent on neither $[ATP]/[ADP][Pi]$ nor pH.

Application of the Model to Suspensions of Isolated Mitochondria

The reaction from cytochrome c to oxygen. The steady state

reduction of cytochrome c and the respiratory rate have been
measured for suspensions of pigeon heart mitochondria at defined
[ATP]/[ADP][Pi]. Progressive stepwise reduction of cytochrome c
was achieved by adding aliquots of N,N,N',N'-tetramethylpara-
phenylene diamine in the presence of 4 mM ascorbate. It can be
seen from Figure 2 that at low [ATP]/[ADP][Pi] the respiratory
rate was proportional to the reduced cytochrome c with a maximal
turnover number of approximately 70 sec^{-1} at 100% reduction. When

Figure 2

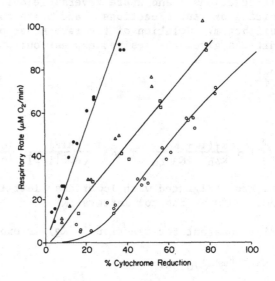

The dependence of the mitochondrial respiratory rate on the reduction of cytochrome c at pH 7.0. The experimental points represent
data obtained by suspending pigeon heart mitochondria at approximately 0.2 μM cytochrome a in a medium containing 0.2 M sucrose,
0.04 M morpholinopropane sulfonate, and 0.2 mM ethylene dinitrilo-
tetraacetate pH 7.0. Sodium ascorbate (5 mM), ATP, ADP, and Pi
were added to stimulate respiration. The respiratory rate and the
reduction of cytochrome c (550 nm minus 540 nm) were measured
simultaneously and the resulting data plotted in the figure. The
added concentrations of ATP, ADP, and Pi were 4 mM ATP (o); 5 mM
ATP, 1 mM ADP, and 1 mM Pi (□); 1 mM ATP, 1 mM ADP, and 1 mM Pi
(Δ); and 3 μg oligomycin plus 0.023 μM S-13 (●). Control measurements with 3 μg oligomycin plus 0.023 μM S-13 in addition to the
indicated ATP, ADP, and Pi were indistinguishable from those of
just oligomycin and S-13. The solid curves are the simulated
behavior of a suspension of mitochondria at a concentration of
0.4 μM cytochrome c (0.2 μM cytochrome a) and [ATP]/[ADP][Pi]
values of 10^{-1}M^{-1} (B) and 4 x 10^{5}M^{-1} (C).

3 mM ATP was added ($[ATP]/[ADP][Pi]$ assumed to be $2 \times 10^5 M^{-1}$)
the respiratory rate was inhibited at all levels of cytochrome c
reduction but the inhibition was greater when the cytochrome c
was more oxidized. The solid lines in Figure 2 are computed
according to equation 1. The equilibrium and rate constants which
yield the best fit of calculated curves to the data are given in
Table I. In the fitting procedure the turnover number of 100%
reduction of cytochrome c is determined by the value of Q (in K_3)
while the curvature at low $[c^{2+}]$ is determined by the value of K_5.

The [ATP], [ADP] and [Pi] dependence of the rate of mitochondrial oxidation of NAD linked substrates. The quantitative
dependence of the mitochondrial respiratory rate on [ATP], [ADP],
and [Pi] has been measured (Holian et al, 1977) and is presented
in Figure 3. The data points represent the respiratory rate of

Table I

The kinetic and equilibrium constants used in the model

Constant	Value	Constant	Value
k_1	$8.5 \times 10^7 M^{-1} sec^{-1}$	k_{4a}	$8.5 \times 10^7 M^{-1} sec^{-1}$
k_2	$1 \times 10^8 M^{-1} sec^{-1}$	k_{4b}	$1.1 + 0.5 \times 10^7 M^{-1} sec^{-1}$
Q	$2.4 + 0.6 \times 10^2$	E^*_{ma3}	0.155 V
K_5	$2.0 \times 10^5 M^{-1}$	E_{mcu}	0.340 V
Q^*	3×10^2		
K^*_5	$1 \times 10^6 M^{-1}$		

The E^*_{ma3} is the E_m value for cytochrome a3 in mitochondria treated
with 6 mM ATP. In this model, the defined relative stoichiometric
ratio of the cytochrome c to cytochrome a3 and copper (2:1:1)
requires that the calculations be made for a final concentration
of 0.8 μM cytochrome c (0.4 μM cytochrome a3). This arises because
dilution changes the amount of membrane per unit total volume but
not the concentration of reactants within the membrane. The
fitting procedure has been to hold k_1, k_2, k_{4a}, E_{ma3} and E_{mcu}
constant at the indicated values while Q, K_5 and k_{4b} are adjusted
for optimum fit. The resulting variations are indicated in the
Table.
* These values are the values used in Figure 4 for intact cells
where the free Mg^{2+} concentration is near 1 mM, in contrast to
those for isolated mitochondria where the free Mg^{2+} is near zero.
In addition the constants in equation 4 must be changed to 0.8 M^{-1}
and $5 \times 10^3 M^{-1}$.

Figure 3

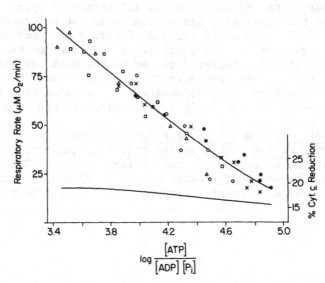

$$\log \frac{[ATP]}{[ADP][P_i]}$$

The dependence of the mitochondrial respiratory rate on [ATP], [ADP] and [Pi]. The simulated rate of mitochondrial respiration is plotted on the ordinate scale on left and the logarithm of the [ATP]/[ADP][Pi] is plotted on the abscissa. The reduction of cytochrome c as obtained from the curve fitting process is also plotted on the ordinate (scale on right). The respiratory rate data for suspensions of dog heart mitochondria as taken from Holian et al, 1977 are plotted for comparison. Each symbol is for data taken at a different phosphate concentration. The values are 1.6 mM (●), 3.2 mM (x), 5.1 mM (o), 7.0 mM (Δ), and 8.5 (□).

suspensions of well-coupled dog heart mitochondria at different [ATP]/[ADP][Pi]. A smooth curve has been drawn through the data points on the rate vs. log ([ATP]/[ADP][Pi]) curve. The values of points on this curve were then used in the equations of the model to generate the predicted cytochrome c reduction curve. On this basis, the model predicts that cytochrome c changes from approximately 20% reduced at low [ATP]/[ADP][Pi] (state 3) to approximately 15% reduced at high [ATP]/[ADP][Pi] (state 4). This is in good agreement with experimental measurements which show that under comparable conditions, cytochrome c was 19% to 22% reduced in state 3, and 14% to 18% reduced in state 4. The changes involved were too small for detailed experimental analysis of the dependence on [ATP]/[ADP][Pi], but they are qualitatively correct.

Application of the Model to the Respiration of Intact Cells and Tissue

The model yields a good mathematical fit to the behavior of suspensions of isolated mitochondria and it was therefore tested for its fit to their function in vivo. In intact cells the intra-mitochondrial $[NAD^+]/[NADH]$ can be accurately measured by the equilibration with substrate couples for which the enzymes are

Figure 4

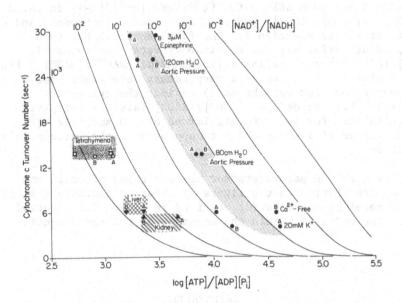

Fit of the experimental data for intact cells and perfused rat heart to the mathematical model. The total concentrations of cytochromes a_3 and c and the respiratory rate were measured in each case. For the isolated cell suspensions (Tetrahymena pyriformis, isolated liver cells and cultured kidney cells) the cellular [ATP], [ADP] and [Pi] were measured as well as the 3-OH-butyrate and acetoacetate. The latter were used to calculate the intramitochondrial $[NAD^+]/[NADH]$. The data was then plotted as the turnover number of cytochrome c against the intramitochon-drial $[NAD^+]/[NADH]$ (points labeled A) or against the cellular [ATP]/[ADP][Pi] (points labeled B). The perfused rat heart was similarly treated except that the cytosolic [ATP]/[ADP] was calculated assuming near equilibrium of creatine phosphokinase. Figure taken from a manuscript submitted for publication by Erecińska, Wilson and Nishiki.

exclusively located in the matrix space (3-OH-butyrate dehydrogenase, glutamate dehydrogenase). We can therefore make use of the
near equilibrium observed for the first two phosphorylation sites
(Erecińska et al., 1974; Wilson et al., 1974a,b; see also pp. 271-
278, this book):

$$NADH + 2c^{3+} + 2ADP + 2Pi \rightleftarrows NAD^+ + 2c^{2+} + 2ATP$$

$$K_{eq} = \frac{[NAD^+]}{[NADH]} \left(\frac{[c^{2+}]}{[c^{3+}]}\right)^2 \left(\frac{[ATP]}{[ADP][Pi]}\right)^2$$

The $[NAD^+]/[NADH]$ refers to the intramitochondrial pool while
$[ATP]$, $[ADP]$ and $[Pi]$ refer to the extramitochondrial pool.
Equation 3 has been solved for $[c^{2+}]$ and $[c^{2+}]/[c^{3+}]$ in terms
of $[NAD^+]/[NADH]$, $[ATP]/[ADP][Pi]$ and total cytochrome c and these
substituted into equation 1. The final equation has three
independent variables; the respiratory rate, the cytosolic
$[ATP]/[ADP][Pi]$ and the intramitochondrial $[NAD^+]/[NADH]$. Figure
4 is a plot of the calculated respiratory rate (expressed as the
turnover number for cytochrome c) against the cytosolic
$[ATP]/[ADP][Pi]$ at defined $[NAD^+]/[NADH]$ values. The plots
are calculated for an intracellular pH of 7.0 and free Mg^{2+}
concentration of 1 mM in order to approximate the intracellular
conditions.

The measured parameters for various types of cells and
tissues are plotted on the figure in order to indicate the fit
of the model to the behavior observed in vivo. The observed
fit of the model is within the accuracy of the experimental
data.

REFERENCES

Chance, B., Erecińska, M. and Chance, E.M. (1973) Oxidase and
Related Redox Systems II, (T.E. King, H.S. Mason and M. Morrison,
eds.) Univ. Park Press, p. 851-866.

Chance, B., Saronio, C. and Leigh, J.S.Jr. (1975) J. Biol. Chem.
250, 9226-9237.

Erecińska, M., Veech, R.L. and Wilson, D.F. (1974) Arch. Biochem.
Biophys. 160, 412-421.

George, P. (1965) in "Oxidases and Related Redox Sytems" (T.E. King,
H.S. Mason and M. Morrison, eds.) Vol. 1, John Wiley, N.Y. p. 3-33.

Gibson, Q.H. and Greenwood, C. (1964) J. Biol. Chem. 239, 586-590.

Greenwood, C., Wilson, M.T. and Brunori, M. (1974) Biochem. J. <u>137</u>, 202-215.

Holian, A., Owen, C.S. and Wilson, D.F. (1977) Arch. Biochem. Biophys. <u>181</u>, 164-171.

Lindsay, J.G. and Wilson, D.F. (1974) FEBS Letters <u>48</u>, 45-49.

Lindsay, J.G., Owen, C.S. and Wilson, D.F. (1975) Arch. Biochem. Biophys. <u>169</u>, 492-505.

Orii, Y. and King, T.E. (1972) FEBS Letters <u>21</u>, 199-202.

Owen, C.S. and Wilson, D.F. (1974) Arch. Biochem. Biophys. <u>161</u>, 581-591.

Wilson, D.F. and Brocklehurst, E.S. (1973) Arch. Biochem. Biophys. <u>158</u>, 200-212.

Wilson, D.F., Erecińska, M., Lindsay, J.G., Leigh, J.S.Jr. and Owen C.S. (1975) Proc. 10th FEBS Meeting, p. 195-210.

Wilson, D.F., Erecińska, M., and Owen, C.S. (1976) Arch. Biochem. Biophys. <u>175</u>, 160-172.

Wilson, D.F., Owen, C.S. and Holian, A. (1977) Arch. Biochem. Biophys., August issue.

Wilson, D.F., Stubbs, M., Oshino, N. and Erecińska, M. (1974 b) Biochemistry <u>13</u>, 5305-5311.

Wilson, D.F., Stubbs, M., Veech, R.L., Erecińska, M., and Krebs, H.A. (1974 a) Biochem. J. <u>140</u>, 57-64.

This research was supported by U.S.P.H.S. Grant GM21524. M.E. is an established investigator for the American Heart Association.

IN VIVO STUDIES OF MITOCHONDRIAL RESPIRATION

G. Austin, W. Schuler, and J. Willey

Loma Linda University   Section of Neurological Surgery

Loma Linda, California   U.S.A.

In the course of an investigation of adding new collateral blood flow to the cortex of ischemic patients, the point was raised as to whether an increase in cortical oxygen tension would lead to improved oxygen utilization and energy production. If so, this might at least partially supply an explanation for improved neurologic function. The work on isolated mitochondria is firm in stating that there is no decrease in O_2 utilization until less than 0.1 mmHg ambient PO_2 (Chance et al, 1955, 1973). On the other hand, recent work on in vivo mitochondria suggest that they may respond differently, i.e., changes in cortical mitochondrial respiration may occur at a much higher brain PO_2 (Rosenthal et al, 1975 & Austin et al, 1975). To investigate this problem, the authors used cats anesthetized similarly to humans undergoing microanastomosis surgery. Previous reported studies by others had shown the cytochrome a_3 end of the respiratory chain to be more responsive to changes in O_2 concentration. In the present study, the authors have added measurements of relative cortical PO_2 (bPO_2), relative cortical O_2 utilization ($b\dot{P}O_2$), and a power spectral analysis of the cortical electrical activity to obtain a measure of functional brain metabolism. Although numerous models of cortical oxidative metabolism have been published, in this presentation, the authors have adhered to the simplified Lehninger model of mitochondrial respiration (Lehninger, 1973).

METHODS: Cats were anesthetized with N_2O and O_2 in a 2:1 mixture after preliminary Ketamine. Immobilization was achieved by I.V. injections of Flaxedil. Relative cortical bPO_2 or O_2 availability at the electrode tip was measured by the Polarographic technique using a 25μ platinum teflon coated electrode inserted into the cortex. When the cortex was in good condition, the bPO_2 responded to changes in

FiO$_2$. bPO$_2$ was approximated by briefly occluding both common carotid arteries in the neck (CCO). The slope of the decline of bPO$_2$ during the first 3 seconds of CCO was measured as an index of relative bPO$_2$. Blood pressure was constantly monitored by means of a femoral artery catheter and maintained at a mean of greater than 100 mmHg by a femoral I.V. drip of physiologic saline. An estimate of functional brain activity was measured by a monopolar cortical recording, transformed from the time to the frequency domain using the Fast Fourier Transform technique and then plotting as a power spectral analysis. Cortical energy production in terms of oxidative phosphorylation was approximated by measuring the redox state of cytochrome a,a$_3$ (ox. cyt. a,a$_3$) by a noninvasive optical technique. This approach appeared to be valid as long as there was no evidence of uncoupling. This technique was a modification by (Jöbsis et al, 1976; after the original model of Chance, 1951) from the principal that the cytochromes in their reduced form absorbed light at specific wavelengths. Changes in the steady state cytochrome reduction level occur depending on the rate of O$_2$ utilization. This is heuristically true and also has been found true by measurement of O$_2$ utilization in isolated mitochondria by Chance and his coworkers (Chance et al, 1973). In essence a monochromatic light at "sample" and "reference" wavelengths alternately illuminate an area (3 mm diam.) of exposed cortex at a frequency of 60 Hz. The "sample" wavelength was 605 nm which is the maximum absorption spectrum of reduced cyt. a,a$_3$. The "reference" wavelength (590 nm) is a so-called equibestic point for Hb, determined by the fact that the Hb absorption changes at 590 nm are equal to those at 605 nm during shifts from Hb to HbO$_2$. All measurements are made in a darkened room to avoid ambient light. The signals arising from the light scattered differently out of the cortex at the two wavelengths are subtracted electronically and the difference is recorded. Light from the epi-illuminator is angled on to the cortex to further avoid specular reflection.   Arterial samples were frequently done at various FiO$_2$ levels and found to be roughly linearly proportional to FiO$_2$. The relative bPO$_2$ was changed by bilateral CCO, by altering FiO$_2$, by briefly changing the blood pressure before autoregulation occurred, and by abruptly producing anoxia through the use of 100% N$_2$ or stopping the heart by injection of KCl.

RESULTS: Fig. 1 shows a typical change in bPO$_2$ and ox. cyt. a,a$_3$ with CCO of 10 sec. duration. Fig. 2 shows the changes in cortical ECoG plotted as a power spectral analysis. These figures indicate that a brief 10 sec. period of CCO produces a drop in bPO$_2$, and decreased ox. cyt. a,a$_3$ followed by a burst of increased cortical electrical activity in the 3-10/sec. range. Fig. 3A&B show typical changes in bPO$_2$ and ox. cyt. a,a$_3$ with changes in blood pressure. Fig. 4A shows typical changes in bPO$_2$ and bPO$_2$ and Fig. 4B changes in ox. cyt. a,a$_3$ with altered FiO$_2$. Only in conditions when the cortex was in poor condition due to low blood volume and consistently low blood pressure, did the cortex fail to respond to altered FiO$_2$ between 10%

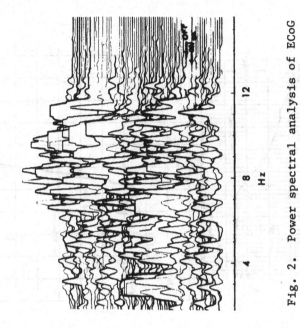

Fig. 2. Power spectral analysis of ECoG

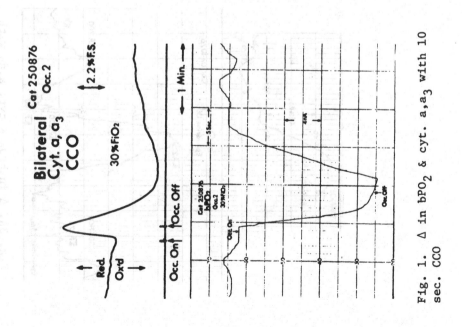

Fig. 1. Δ in bPO₂ & cyt. a,a₃ with 10
sec. CCO

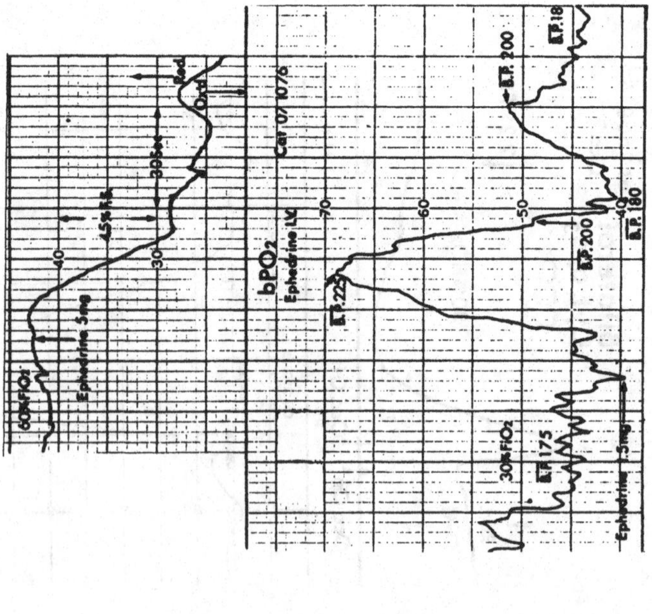

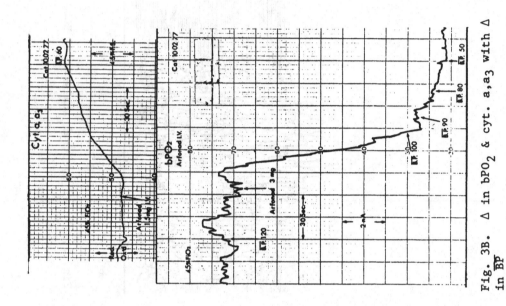

Fig. 3B.   Δ in bPO₂ & cyt. a,a₃ with Δ
in BP

Fig. 3A.   Δ in bPO₂ & cyt. a,a₃ with
Δ in BP

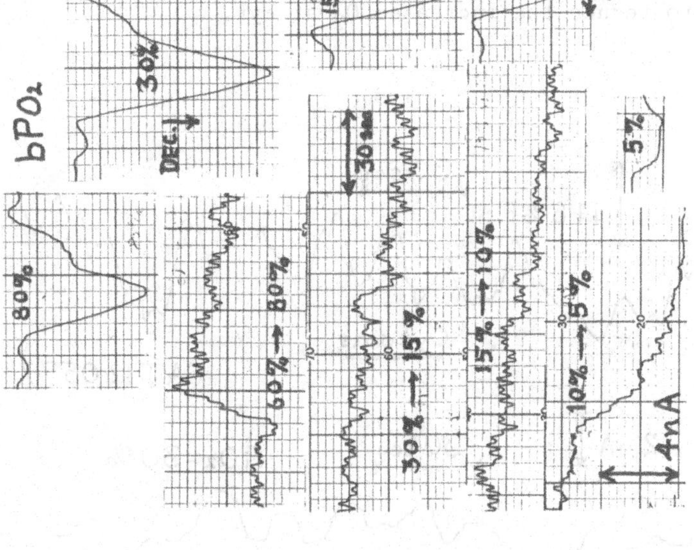

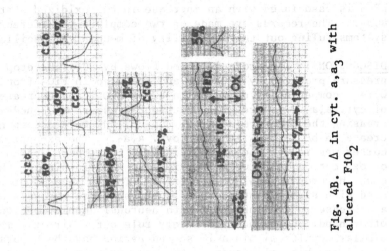

Fig. 4A. Δ in bPO₂ and bṖO₂ with altered FiO₂

Fig. 4B. Δ in cyt. a,a₃ with altered FiO₂

and 80%.   Fig. 5 shows oscillatory activity occasionally encountered due to an unstable cyt. a_3-O_2 system.   The oscillatory increase in bPO_2 is associated with an increase in the oxidized state of cyt. a,a_3.   The records are made on two completely different recording systems ruling out the possibility of mechanical oscillations.

DISCUSSIONS: The drops in blood flows by CCO, the drop in blood pressure produced by Arfonad, and the drop in FiO_2 from 30% to 15% were accompanied by decrease in bPO_2, bPO_2, and decreased oxidation of cyt. a,a_3.   Increasing the blood pressure by Ephedrine, and increasing the FiO_2 progressively up to 100% were accompanied by an increase in bPO_2, bPO_2, and ox. cyt. a,a_3.   The exception was when the cortex was in very poor condition and then there was no change in bPO_2 or ox. cyt. a,a_3 between FiO_2 10% and 100% inspite of the aPO_2 changing proportional to the FiO_2.   The 10 seconds of CCO were associated with significant changes in the spectral analysis assumed due to a decrease in available ATP with neuronal depolarization.   On the other hand, one cannot completely rule out a direct membrane effect. Similar results within a 10 second period have been obtained by Siesjo and his colleagues in the rat with a measured decrease in cortical ATP after 5-10 seconds of carotid occlusions (Nilssen et al, 1975; Nordberg et al, 1975).

The data we have presented suggest a significant difference in mitochondrial respiration in the cortical in vivo preparation compared to isolated mitochondria.   Current in vitro models fail to explain the sources of additional electrons that would have to be available to reduce the increased O_2 at cyt. a_3.

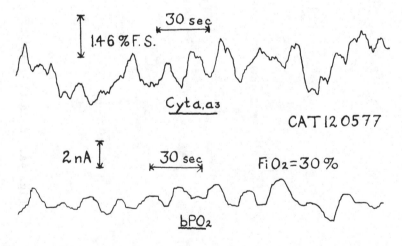

Fig. 5.   Oscillatory activity of bPO_2 & cyt. a,a_3

REFERENCES

1) Austin, G., Schuler, W., Haugen, G., Willey, J., La Manna, J., and Jöbsis, F. (1976) in "Contemporary Aspects of Cerebrovascular Disease" p. 46   (ed. Austin, G.M.)   Dallas, Texas, USA.

2) Chance, B. (1951) Rev. Sci. Instr. 22, 634.

3) Chance, B., Oshino, N., Sugano, T. and Mayevsky, A. (1973) in "Oxygen Transport to Tissue", p. 227, (ed. Bicher, H.I. & Bruley, D.F.) Plenum Press, New York.

4) Chance, B. and Williams, G.R. (1955) J. Biol. Chem. 217, 383.

5) Jöbsis, F.F., Keizer, J., LaManna, J., and Rosenthal, M. (1976) J. Appl. Physiol. (IN PRESS)

6) Lehninger, A.L. (1973) Bioenergetics. Benjamin Publishers, California.

7) Nilsson, B., Norberg, K., Nordström, C-H., and Siesjö, B.K. (1975) 93, 569.

8) Norberg, K., Quistorff, B., and Siesjö, B.K. (1975) Brain Res. 95, 301.

9) Rosenthal, M.J., LaManna, J.C., Jöbsis, F.F., Levasseur, J., Kontos, H., and Patterson, J. (1976) Brain Res. 108, 143.

REFERENCES

INDUCTION BY HYPOXIA OF A NEW HAEMOGLOBIN-LIKE PIGMENT

I. S. Longmuir, A. Young and R. Mailman

Department of Biochemistry, North Carolina State
University, Raleigh; and Division of Neuropharmacology,
University of North Carolina, Chapel Hill, NC, U.S.A.

Substances which bind strongly to cytochrome P-450 change the
kinetics of the uptake of oxygen by rat liver slices. The relationship between the respiration rate and ambient P_{O_2} of liver
slices from untreated rats is generally of the form of Michaelis-
Menten kinetics. Slices from animals after exposure to piperonyl
butoxide, metyropone or diazinon follow Warburg's equation
(Longmuir *et al.*, 1971). The mechanism postulated to explain these
findings is that normally the transport of oxygen through tissue is
facilitated by cytochrome P-450. When this latter pigment is bound
in the oxidized state to certain xenobiotics, it can no longer
react with oxygen and facilitate its transport. Since cytochrome
P-450 is bound to the endoplasmic reticulum, it cannot act as a
mobile carrier as proposed by Wittemberg (1959) but might act as a
"bucket brigade" carrier according to Scholander's model (1960).
Curran and Gold (1975) have considered the consequences of partial
deletion of carrier in the case of the general model. We have
applied a method of partial binding of cytochrome P-450 to determine
the effect this has on the kinetics of tissue oxygen uptake as a
function of cytochrome P-450 concentration in mice and rats. The
levels of this pigment were increased by exposure to hypoxia,
hyperoxia, phenobarbitone and 3-methylcholanthrene.

METHODS

The fraction of oxygen carried by facilitated diffusion was
measured by the method of Longmuir (1976) and the concentration of
cytochrome P-450 was measured by the method of Pashko and Longmuir
(in preparation).

Mice and rats were exposed to 100 Torr of oxygen for three and seven hours, respectively, and mice to 1500-3000 Torr for one hour.   These treatments both produced a 100% increase in mouse liver cytochrome P-450 but a smaller increase in the case of the rats.   The animals were exposed to phenobarbital by supplying them *ad lib* with a 0.1% solution as drinking water for five days. 3-methylcholanthrene dissolved in corn oil was administered by i.p. injection of 25 mgms/kilo daily for five days.   The animals were killed by cervical dislocation and the livers removed and sliced in the McIwain Buddle slicer; P-450 levels were determined before and after each experiment.· Since the actual determination of ΔP_{O_2}, the increase in P_{O_2} needed to maintain constant respiration rate after addition of nicotinamide, is measured near the end of the run; this value was correlated with the latter measurement of P-450.

Microsomes were prepared after perfusion of the livers and the Δ O.D. spectra determined on an Aminco D.W. 2 spectrophotometer.

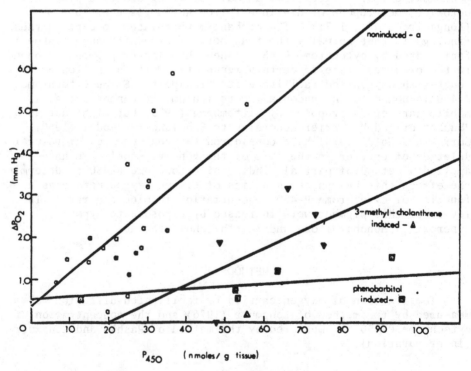

Fig. 1. Least Squares Regression Lines for Correlation Between P_{450} and ΔP_{O_2} in Rats.

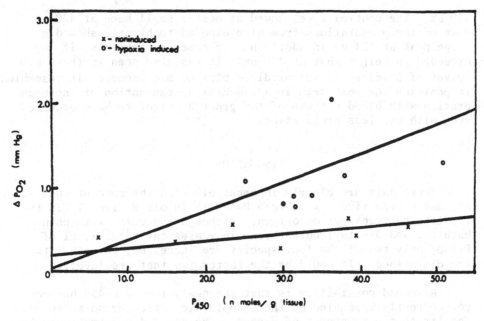

Fig. 2. Least Squares Regression Lines for Correlation Between P_{450} and ΔP_{O_2} in Mice.

RESULTS

Plots of ΔP_{O_2} against cytochrome P-450 for rats and mice are shown in Figs. 1 and 2, respectively.

The upper curve in Fig. 1 is a plot of the results obtained in rats both untreated and those exposed to hypoxia. It shows a correlation between ΔP_{O_2} and cytochrome P-450 (r = 0.61, significant difference from chance P = .005). The lower curves show that in the case of phenobarbital-treated animals the correlation is almost completely lost and reduced in those treated with 3-methylcholanthrene.

However, when the exposure to the inducers was continued for three weeks, the points then approached the uninduced line.

In the case of mice on the other hand, Fig. 2, only the livers from those exposed to hypoxia showed facilitated diffusion (r = 0.66, significant difference from chance P = .05).

The Δ O.D. curve of reduced versus reduced plus CO microsomes from livers of both groups of mice showed the expected peak at

450 nm. The control mice showed at most a small bump at 420 nm. Most of the preparations from mice exposed to hypoxia showed a large peak at 424 nm in addition. In some preparations, it exceeded in height that at 450 nm. It was also seen in the Δ O.D. curves of oxidized versus oxidized plus CO microsomes. It resembled in position the peak seen in accidental contamination of the preparation with blood but was of too great a height to have occurred even with careless preparation.

DISCUSSION

These data are clearly incompatible with the concept that all or most of the liver cytochrome P-450 is involved directly in the facilitated transport of oxygen. Although induction with phenobarbital and 3-methylcholanthrene increases the total level of P-450, only two of the four species are increased; the other two are diminished. It could be the latter two that are involved.

A second possibility is that the newly formed P-450 has not yet correctly assembled on the endoplasmic reticulum so as to facilitate the transport of oxygen. The new P-450 seems to be lost more readily, and the results of prolonged exposure support this hypothesis.

A third possibility is that the carrier is a haemoglobin-like pigment which sometimes increases pari passu with cytochrome P-450.

ACKNOWLEDGMENT

This paper is a contribution from the Department of Biochemistry, School of Agriculture and Life Sciences and School of Physical and Mathematical Sciences. Paper no. 5332 of the North Carolina Agricultural Experiment Station, Raleigh, North Carolina 27607.

REFERENCES

Curran, T. C. and Gold, H. (1975) J. Theor. Biol. 50, 503.

Longmuir, I. S. (1976) Adv.Exp.Med.Biol.75, 217.

Longmuir, I. S.; Martin, D. C.; Gold, H. J. and Sun, S. (1971) Microvasc. Res. 3, 125.

Scholander, P. F. (1960) Science 131, 585.

Wittemberg, J. B. (1959) Biol. Bull. 117, 402.

MYOGLOBIN-O_2-SATURATION PROFILES IN MUSCLE SECTIONS OF CHICKEN GIZZARD AND THE FACILITATED O_2-TRANSPORT BY Mb[+)]

V. Schwarzmann and W.A. Grunewald

Institut of Physiology, University of

8400 Regensburg, GFR

Using the cryomicrophotometric method developed by GRUNEWALD and LÜBBERS (1975, 1976) the local myoglobin-O_2-saturation was determined in muscle sections of chicken gizzard in the form of so-called myoglobin-O_2-saturation profiles (MbsO$_2$-profiles). Because of its high affinity towards oxygen, myoglobin is an excellent indicator for oxygen, especially for small PO_2-values as they may occur in the tissue. From the MbO$_2$-profiles quantitative results on the O_2-transport in the tissue can be derived.

In Fig. 1 a summary of the method is given. A 2000-μm-thick muscle section is placed into a gas-chamber and both sides are exposed to a nitrogen/oxygen gas mixture with known PO_2, and then rapidly frozen in liquid nitrogen. Following this, the frozen muscle sample is sectioned into 50-μm-thick slices at -60°C in a cryotom. These slices are placed in a microscope-cryostat at -100°C which lies between condensor and objective of the double-beam photometer UMSP 1 (C.Zeiss, Oberkochen). The local light-absorption of Mb is measured over the wavelength range of 520 to 620 nm. The MbO$_2$-spectra are evaluated according to the multi-component analysis of LÜBBERS and WODICK (1969, 1972). The premise for this analysis is that a measured Mb spectrum is a linear combination of so-called basic spectra. The MbO$_2$-saturation is calculated from the coefficients of the basic spectra by a Least Squares Fit. The local MbO$_2$-saturation measured along the oxygen

[+)] supported by Volkswagen-Stiftung

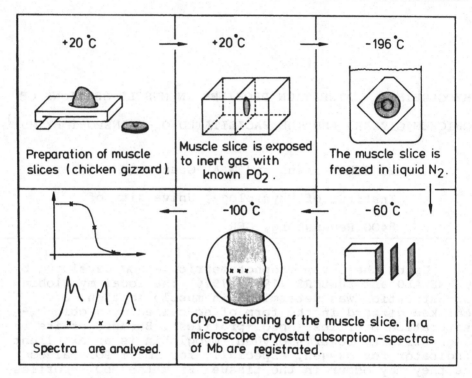

+20 °C   →   +20 °C   →   -196 °C

Preparation of muscle   Muscle slice is exposed   The muscle slice is
slices (chicken gizzard).   to inert gas with   freezed in liquid N_2.
                                known PO_2.

                          -100 °C   ←   -60 °C

Spectra are analysed.   Cryo-sectioning of the muscle slice. In a
                                microscope cryostat absorption-spectras
                                of Mb are registrated.

Figure 1
Summary of the method

diffusion pathway from the edge to the middle of the
muscle slice represents the MbO_2-saturation profile.
The basic spectra for this analysis are shown in Fig. 2.
They are the absorption spectra at $-100°C$ of oxygenated
and deoxygenated as well as of the artificial and almost
dehydrated deoxy-Mb.

A $MbsO_2$-profile can be obtained in the steady state
or in the non-stationary state. Three $MbsO_2$-profiles in
boundaries of the muscle sections a PO_2 of 144 mmHg was
applied for 3 min, 10 min and 30 min, at $23°C$. At this
temperature, the Mb is half-saturated with oxygen at a
PO_2 of 0.5 mmHg. Having applied the gas mixture for
3 min, we find this PO_2 in a depth of 100 µm, after
10 min in 225 µm, and, finally, after 30 min in 325 µm.
The increase of penetration depth with time and the
shape of these profiles are predicted by Hill's "Advancing
Front Theory" from 1929: a region with full saturation,
a precipitous decline of MbO_2-saturation by 90% within
85 µm is followed by a region with zero-saturation, Fig. 3.

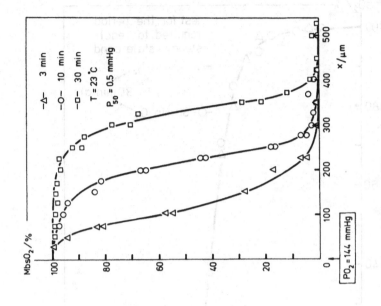

Figure 3

Myoglobin-O$_2$-saturation profiles after different times of oxygen diffusion.

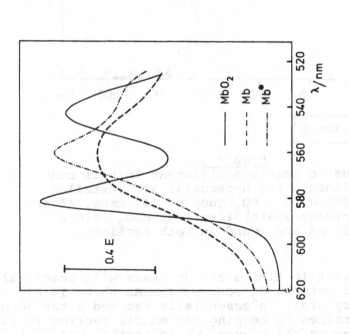

Figure 2

Myoglobin basic spectra at -100°C between 520 and 620 nm (E: extinction unit)
MbO$_2$: oxy-Mb spectrum,
Mb : deoxy-Mb spectrum,
Mb* : dehydrated deoxy-Mb spectrum

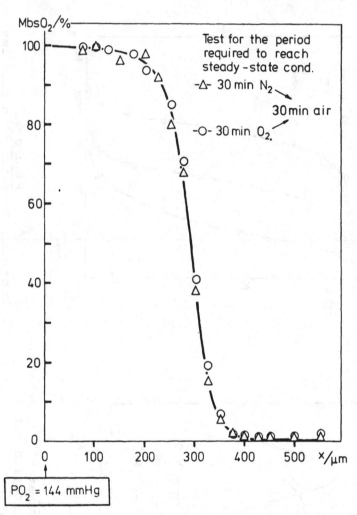

<u>Figure 4</u>
In two muscle sections different initial conditions (anoxia and hyperoxia) are installed
and submitted to a PO_2 jump of 144 mmHg. After
30 min (steady state) identical MbO_2 saturation profiles are found in both sections.

After a certain time a steady state will practically
be established between O_2-consumption.As shown in Fig. 4,
this stationary state is essentially reached after 30 min.
This was determined by keeping one muscle section in pure
nitrogen to remove all oxygen, while another was kept in
oxygen so as to be almost oxygenated. Both muscle sections
were subjected to a PO_2 of 144 mmHg for 30 min, and in

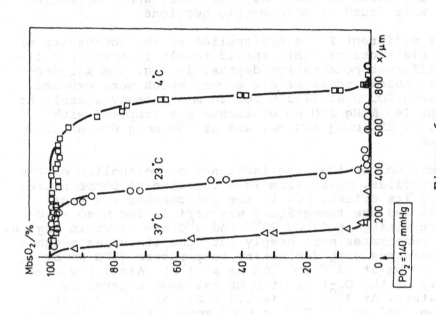

Figure 6

Steady state MbO₂-saturation profiles in tissue influenced by O₂-consumption which is a function of temperature.

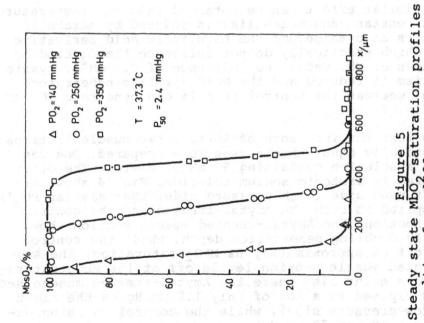

Figure 5

Steady state MbO2-saturation profiles resulting from different O₂ partial pressures at the boundaries of the muscle sections.

the steady state to same $MbsO_2$-profiles and penetration
depths were found in both muscle sections.

If different PO_2's are applied at the boundaries of
the muscle sections, this should result in $MbsO_2$-profiles
with different penetration depths. In Fig. 5 $MbsO_2$-pro-
files of muscle sections are shown, which were exposed
to various PO_2's at $37.3^{\circ}C$ for 30 min (steady state). At
a PO_2 of 140 mmHg 200 um of tissue are supplied with
oxygen, at 250 mmHg 400 um, and at 350 mmHg 600 um are
supplied.

Next we consider the influence of metabolism on the
$MbsO_2$-profiles. Metabolism is a function of temperature.
To study its effect, PO_2 in the gas-chamber was kept
constant and the temperature was varied. The $MbsO_2$-pro-
files resulting at $37^{\circ}C$, $23^{\circ}C$ and $4^{\circ}C$ are shown in Fig. 6.
Oxygen penetrates more deeply into the tissue as metabo-
lism decreases with decreasing temperature (200 um at
$37^{\circ}C$, 400 μm at $23^{\circ}C$ and 800 μm at $4^{\circ}C$). Also, the O_2-
affinity of the O_2-indicator Mb has been altered by
temperature. At $37^{\circ}C$ P_{50} is 2.8 mmHg, at $23^{\circ}C$ P_{50} is
0.5 mmHg, and at $4^{\circ}C$ P_{50} is 0.07 mmHg. Using the profile
at $4^{\circ}C$ we are able to determine the PO_2 in the steep part
of the profile with an accuracy better than 0.02 mmHg
(representing 10% MbO_2-saturation).

A similar effect can be obtained when the temperature
is kept constant and metabolism is reduced by metabolic
inhibitors as cyanide and the barbituric acid derivative
Amytal which practically do not influence the O_2-binding
properties of Mb. Under the influence of 0.1 mM of cyanide,
metabolism is reduced and the $MbsO_2$-profile penetrates
1050 um, whereas the control profile can penetrate 600 um
only, Fig. 7.

To test the influence of Amytal, two muscle sections
of practically equal thicknesses were prepared. One was
kept in a solution containing 50 mM of Amytal. The other
was stored in isotonic sodium chloride. Fig. 8 shows on
the left hand side (high pressure side) that similar PO_2's
were applied to both the Amytal-treated and the control
muscle section. The Amytal-treated muscle section shows
a roughly doubling penetration depth. While the control
levels off at approximately 0% MbO_2-saturation, the Amytal-treated muscle section levels off at 15% MbO_2-satura-
tion. This holds also where the Amytal-treated muscle section is exposed to a PO_2 of only 1.8 mm Hg on the right
side (low-pressure side), while the control is being exposed to a PO_2 of 72 mm Hg.

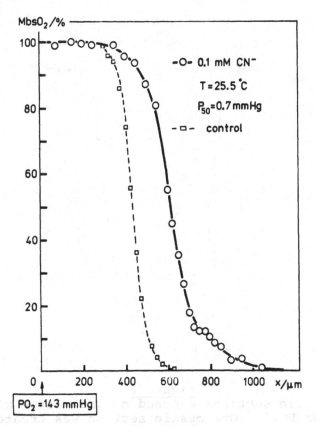

Figure 7

MbO$_2$-saturation profile influenced by 0.1 mM
of cyanide and control profile.

Finally we investigated the deviation from identity
of single point measurements by measuring the MbO$_2$-
saturation at various points equidistant from the boundary
of the muscle section. We found a mean deviation of $\pm$ 3%
MbO$_2$-saturation.

The MbO$_2$-saturation profiles were used to calculate
the facilitated diffusion of Mb. Fig. 9 shows measured
values as well as a profile calculated on the basis of
a mathematical model proposed by Hoofd (1977):

$$\alpha \ D_{O2} \ \frac{d^2}{dx^2} \ (PO_2 + P_f y) = M_{max} \ (PO_2 + P_f y)$$

$$\text{with} \qquad P_f = \frac{C_{Mb} \ x \ D_{Mb}}{\alpha \ D_{O2}}$$

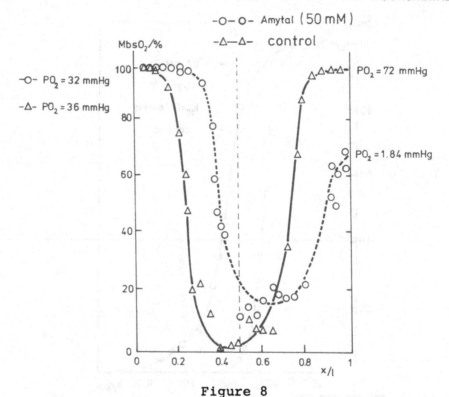

<u>Figure 8</u>

Two muscle sections exposed on both sides with
various PO_2's. One muscle section was treated
with a solution containing 50 mM of Amytal to
reduce metabolism, the other one is control.

Y = fractional MbO_2-saturation
C_{Mb} = Mb-concentration, D_{Mb} = diffusion coefficient of Mb.
$\alpha\ D_{O2}$ = oxygen permeability

The solution of the differential equation is:

$$\ln (PO_2 + P_f\ y) = A - \sqrt{\frac{M_{max}}{\alpha\ D_{O2}}}\ x$$

A Least Squares Fit showed that there is only a
facilitation of P_f = 1.6 mmHg. Similar P_f values are
obtained for the other $MbSO_2$-profiles shown before. For
a solution containing Mb in the concentration as it
occurs in chicken gizzard a P_f value of 28 mmHg is
expected. From this it is concluded that the mobility
of Mb in the muscle cell is greatly impeded and can
contribute to the oxygen transport only to a minor degree.

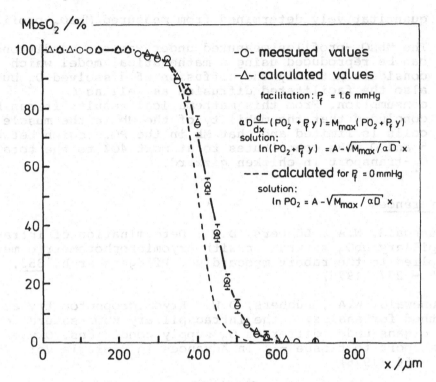

Figure 9

Facilitated diffusion of O$_2$ by myoglobin
diffusion in intact muscle can be calculated
using MbO$_2$ saturation profiles
(P$_f$ = 1.6 mmHg). A calculation without
facilitated diffusion (P$_f$ = O) is also given.

The same conclusion was reported by MOLL (1968) and
VAN HAREN (1975). Under favourable conditions, the oxygen
transport by Mb-diffusion may contribute a maximum of
40% of the diffusion of dissolved O$_2$-transport in the
PO$_2$-region of 5 - O mmHg and may increase the penetration
depth by approximately 50 µm, as can be derived from the
measured profile and a profile calculated without
facilitation.

Summary

It has been shown that the oxygen transport in intact
muscle can be quantitatively determined using Mb as an
oxygen indicator in the cryomicrophotometric method.

1) The influence of the parameters such as time, temperature, boundary PO$_2$ and metabolism on the oxygen
transport in sections of chicken gizzard could be

quantitatively determined from measured $MbsO_2$-profiles.

2) The $MbsO_2$-profiles measured under various conditions can be reproduced using a mathematical model which considers not only the diffusion of dissolved O_2 but also the facilitated diffusion as well as O_2 consumption. From this mathematical results it can be concluded that the mobility of the Mb in the muscle cells is limited and that Mb in the PO_2-region between 5 and O mmHg contributes to at most 40% to the total O_2-transport in chicken gizzard.

References

Grunewald, W.A., Lübbers, D.W.: Determination of intra-capillary HbO_2-saturation with cryomicrophotometric method applied to the rabbit myocardium. Pflügers Arch. 353, 255 - 277 (1975)

Grunewald, W.A., Lübbers, D.W.: Kryomicrophotometry as a method for analyzing the intracapillary HbO_2-saturation of organs under different O_2 supply conditions. Oxygen Transport to tissue -II in Advances in Biologie Vol. 75, 55 - 64 (1976)

Van Haren, R.: Diffusion of oxygen and oxygenated myoglobin myoglobin in the respiring smooth muscle of the chicken gizzard. Internal Report of the University of Nijmegen, The Netherlands (1975)

Hill, A.V.: The diffusion of oxygen and lactic acide through tissue. Proc-Roy Soc. Ser. B 104, 39 - 96 (1928/29)

Hoofd, L.C.: Personal communicution (1977) Dep. med. Physiol. Univ. Nijmegen, The Netherlands.

Lübbers, D.W., Wodick, R.: The examination of multi-component systems in biological materials by means of a rapid scanning photometer. Appl. Optics 8, 1055 - 1062 (1962)

Lübbers, D.W., Wodick, R.: Spektrophotometrische Analyse von Mehrkomponentensystemen bei Überlagerung von unbe-kannten Störkomponenten. Naturwissenschaften 8, 362 (1972)

Moll, W.: The diffusion coefficient of Myoglobin in muscle homogenate. Pflügers Arch. 299, 247 - 251 (1968)

SIMULTANEOUS MEASUREMENT OF GLUCOSE AND O_2 CONSUMPTION IN CELL SUSPENSIONS WITH MINIELECTRODES

B.T. Storey, K. Olofsson, W. Crowe and L. Mela

University of Pennsylvania School of Medicine

Philadelphia, Pennsylvania 19104, U.S.A.

Separation procedures which yield cell suspensions with homogeneous cell populations greatly facilitate the study of cell metabolism, but yield a limited amount of material. Multiple recording of metabolic parameters from minimum volumes is therefore useful. We have developed a method for the simultaneous recording of glucose and O_2 concentrations with polarographic electrodes in 0.26 ml suspensions of rabbit epididymal spermatozoa (RES). These cells are found "pre-separated" as a homogeneous population in the cauda epididymidis. They consume glucose and O_2 and produce lactate (Murdoch and White, 1967) and so provide a useful system to test the method as well as a system in which to study the effect of perturbations on aerobic glycolysis.

APPARATUS AND METHODS

The body of the polarographic electrode used for sensing both O_2 (Clark, 1956) and glucose (Clark and Clark, 1973) was sterling silver tubing, 1.5 mm O.D., 1.0 mm I.D. The sensor was Pt wire, 0.2 mm diameter. No effect of the copper content of the sterling on electrode operation was noted as compared to fine silver. Details of electrode construction are shown in Fig. 1. The electrode was connected to a polarographic amplifier constructed in the Johnson Research Foundation Sensitive Instrument Shop (University of Pennsylvania). For sensing O_2, the electrode was polarized at 0.72 to 0.82 V with Pt as cathode and 3 M KCl as conducting electrolyte (Clark, 1956); the tip was covered with 19 μm Teflon film held in place by an "O" ring cut from polyethylene tubing. For sensing glucose, the electrode was polarized at 0.90 V with Pt as anode (Clark and Clark, 1973); the tip was treated with a solution of

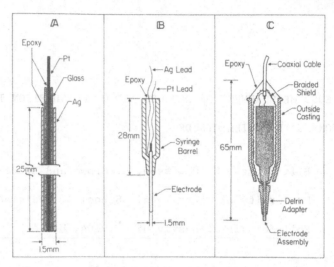

Fig. 1:   Diagram of polarographic electrode construction.
A: Electrode unit showing central Pt wire, with concentric layers
of epoxy resin, glass, epoxy, and Ag.   B: Electrode mounted in
bottom portion of 1 ml disposable tuberculin syringe barrel filled
with epoxy resin.   C: Complete electrode assembly.   The electrode
mounted as in B is surrounded by braided shielding, connected to a
RG-199 B/U Teflon-jacketed coaxial cable, and encapsulated by the
body of 1.5 ml polyethylene centrifuge tube (Eppendorf) with bottom
cut off.   The electrode shaft is inserted into a Delrin adapter for
mounting in the electrode chamber.   The protruding tip of the electrode allows mounting of the appropriate membrane.

glucose oxidase (Sigma Type VII) at 100 mg protein/ml and covered
with a membrane of CORIO brand edible sausage casing (kindly dona-
ted by Dr. L.C. Clark, Jr.).   The O_2 and glucose electrodes were
mounted in tapered Delrin adapters (Fig. 1C) designed to fit in the
top of the Plexiglas reaction chamber (Fig. 2A).   Delrin does not
adhere to Plexiglas, so that the electrodes could be removed to
cleanse the chamber of metabolic inhibitors with ethanol without
denaturation of glucose oxidase.

Spermatozoa were obtained from the caudae of excised rabbit
epididymides, as previously described (Storey, 1975).   Motility of
the samples was checked prior to use, and only those samples with
more than 80% of the cells moving were used.   Periodic checks on
different samples showed that sperm cells isolated and washed by
this method were intact, as shown by impermeability to Ca^{+2}
(Storey, 1975).   Reagents were used without further purification.
The inhibitor of oxidative phosphorylation, oligomycin, was
obtained from Sigma Chemical Company (St. Louis, Mo.); the

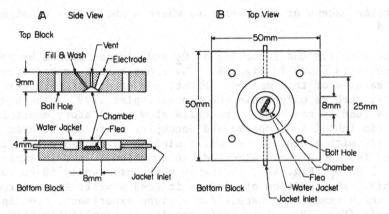

Fig. 2:   Side view and top view of electrode chamber. The
chamber is constructed from two blocks of Plexiglas 50 x 50 x 9 mm.
A: Section through the middle of the blocks. In the bottom block
is the chamber bottom and a surrounding water jacket for temperature control. In the top block is the conical chamber top with a
central vent, a channel for filling and washing, and a tapered hole
for the electrode with Delrin adapter. Chamber volume is 0.26 ml.
Bolt holes are omitted from bottom block for clarity. B: Top view
of the bottom block. In use, the two blocks are bolted together
with high vacuum silicone lubricant spread on the joined Plexiglas
surfaces which acts as a watertight gasket. The assembly is placed
on a magnetic stirrer. The twopiece design allows facile dismant-
ling for cleaning and the use of interchangeable tops for single or
multiple electrode recording. Up to four electrodes can be used
with a chamber of this volume.

uncoupler of oxidative phosphorylation, bis(hexafluoroacetonyl-
acetone), designated 1799, was kindly supplied by Dr. Peter Heytler
of E. I. du Pont de Nemours Inc. For measurement of glucose and
O_2 uptake, the cells were suspended in 150 mM NaCl/20 mM Tris Cl
buffer, pH 7.4, at 37°C containing 0.8 µM catalase. Reagents were
added as concentrated solutions with microsyringes in volumes less
than 1% of the reaction volume.

RESULTS AND DISCUSSION

The glucose electrode was found to be linear in response to
added glucose up to 5 mM, the highest concentration tested. The
response time to full scale is 1 to 2 minutes. The sensitivity of
the glucose electrode to O_2 concentration in the absence of glucose
was tested by using beef heart mitochondria and succinate to produce anaerobiosis. The electrode does not respond to change in O_2

consumption except at anaerobiosis, where a small loss of signal is observed.

The simultaneous recording of O_2 and glucose uptake by rabbit sperm cells is shown in Fig. 3A. The experimental trace illustrates three features of this method. First, the effect of metabolic perturbants, such as oligomycin and the uncoupler 1799, on both uptake rates is readily assessed. The cells show respiratory control: oligomycin inhibits O_2 uptake and uncoupler increases it over the basal rate with glucose. Second, a minimum O_2 concentration is required for the glucose electrode to function. In this experiment it was 62 μm O_2 (Fig. 4B); the range was consistently 60 to 70 μm O_2. Third, the addition of glucose induced a drift in electrode signal which remained constant for a given experiment, even in anaerobiosis (Fig. 3B). This drift results in anomalously high apparent rates of glucose consumption. In other experiments, the rate of drift ranged from negligible to more than 50% of the observed rate. When the rates of glucose consumption in the experiment of Fig. 3 were corrected for drift, the results shown in Table 1 were obtained.

The effect of lactate on the rate of aerobic glycolysis of rabbit sperm cells is shown in Fig. 4. Both the O_2 and the glucose uptake rates are increased on addition of lactate, although the latter slows down somewhat after the initial rate increase. The drift in anaerobiosis of the glucose electrode was negligible in this experiment, so no correction was required. These rates are summarized in Table 1.

Table 1:   RATES OF GLUCOSE AND O_2 UPTAKE BY RABBIT EPIDIDYMAL SPERM AT 37°

		Uptake, nmols/min-10^9 cells		% Glucose
Expt.	Additions	Glucose	O_2	Oxidized
Fig. 4	None	-----	3.1	---
	Glucose	35.7	8.5	4
	Oligomycin	14.2	4.9	6
	1799	35.7	15.5	22
Fig. 5	None	-----	3.1	---
	Glucose	9.1	4.9	9
	Lactate	14.1	7.9	---
	1799	44.5	14.4	---

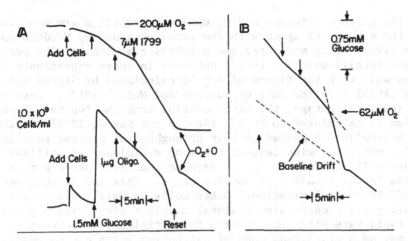

Fig. 3:   A: Simultaneous recording of O_2 and glucose concentrations in a suspension of rabbit epididymal spermatozoa (RES) in 150 mM NaCl/20 mM Tris buffer, pH 7.4, at 37°.   The top trace is O_2, the bottom trace is glucose.   B: Analysis of glucose trace, showing baseline drift corresponding to 62.5 nmol/min–10^9 cells and 62 µm O_2 cutoff for glucose electrode function.

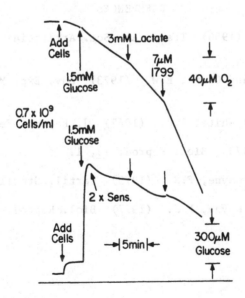

Fig. 4:   Simultaneous recording of O_2 (top trace) and glucose (bottom trace) in a suspension of rabbit epididymal sperm (RES) showing the effect of added lactate. Conditions as in Fig. 3. Only that portion of the experiment with O_2 concentration above 70 µM is shown.

The rates of glucose and O_2 uptake by rabbit sperm measured with the electrodes agree with the rates obtained by Murdoch and White (1967) using manometry and metabolite analysis. The percent glucose totally oxidized to CO_2 obtained in these experiments also agrees well with the figure of $6 \pm 1\%$ calculated by Storey and Kayne (1975) from the data of Murdoch and White (1967). Despite this small percentage, the mitochondrial contribution to ATP production is calculated to be 63% (Storey and Kayne, 1975). Sperm cell metabolism is geared to fast throughput of glucose to maintain ATP for motility, with less emphasis on efficiency of utilization. Lactate build-up does not occur because the cells are separate and diluted in the female reproductive tract. This can be considered as infinite vascularization. Other cells in well vascularized tissues – e.g., exercising skeletal muscle – also utilize glucose at a rapid rate with less concern for efficiency of combustion. This may be a widespread mode of metabolism which can be readily studied by the O_2/glucose electrode technique.

Supported by USPHS Grants HD-06274, HL-19737, GM-19867, GM-01540, GM-50318, and a grant from the Muscular Dystrophy Association, Inc.

REFERENCES

Clark, L.C. Jr.   (1956)   Trans. Am. Soc. Artificial Internal Organs 2, 41.

Clark, L.C. Jr. and Clark, E.W.   (1973)   Adv. Exp. Med. Biol. 37A, 127.

Murdoch, R.N. and White, I.G.   (1967)   J. Reprod. Fert. 14, 213.

Storey, B.T.   (1975)   Biol. Reprod. 13, 1.

Storey, B.T. and Kayne, F.J.   (1975)   Fertil. Steril. 26, 1257.

Storey, B.T. and Kayne, F.J.   (1977)   Biol. Reprod. 16, 549.

DENSITY DEPENDENT ENERGY CHANGES AND ADAPTIVE GROWTH IN POPULATIONS

OF MOUSE FIBROBLASTS IN VITRO

R.J. Werrlein

Department of Pathology
The Medical School
University of Bristol, Bristol, England

When a tissue is damaged due to pathological stress or wounding, recovery depends on the homeostatic mechanisms of the constituent cells to repair the damage and restore environmental constancy.
This infers that the integration of regulatory metabolism is activated and maintained through environmental feedback and requires
that populations of cells respond as a highly coordinated unit.
Adenine nucleotides and oxygen have been suggested as regulatory
parameters of metabolism (Atkinson, 1968; Holian et al, 1977;
Wilson et al, 1977a). On the strength of these suggestions their
combined energetics and homeostatic control over cell proliferation
and population density was investigated using a mammalian cell
culture system.

MATERIALS AND METHODS

Suspensions of WRL-10A cells (Glinos and Hargrove, 1965) were
maintained on Eagle's minimum essential medium containing 10% horse
serum, 1% L-glutamine, 100 units/ml of penicillin and 100 μg/ml of
streptomycin. The suspensions were grown in Erlenmeyer flasks,
stirred by a hanging magnetic bar and incubated at 35°C in an
atmosphere of 5% CO_2 in air. Experimental cultures were seeded
at 500,000 cells/ml and were maintained by daily medium renewal,
hemocytometer count and dilution in a state of exponential proliferation for a minimum of three days prior to each experiment. The
cultures were subsequently allowed to grow without dilution and
populations of these cells were prepared at intervals for combined
polarographic, enzymatic and spectrophotometric analyses according
to the methods of Wilson et al (1977b). Prepared samples were
drawn into a modified polypropylene syringe and were inserted into
a dual wavelength spectrophotometer (Chance, 1951) which had been

specially adapted for the analyses.   Cell samples were maintained
in suspension throughout the analyses by a magnetic stirrer and bar.
Respiratory rates were determined from the rate of oxygen depletion
by each sample with a Clark type O_2 electrode (Clark, 1956).
Duplicate samples withdrawn from the syringe were assayed for ATP
by the method of Lamprecht and Trautschold (1963) and for ADP and
AMP by the method of Adam (1963).   A cytochrome window to the
sample was aligned at right angles to the light path between the
light source and photomultiplier tube so that cytochrome C (cyt-C)
content and redox state could be determined from absorbancy
changes at 550-540 nanometers by the method of Wilson et al (1974).

RESULTS

Respiratory rates from 3 populations were determined and
grouped in ranges according to increasing population density.   In
Table 1 the average of these values shows that at low densities of
1-2 and 2-4 x 10^6 cells/ml mean respiratory rates were 1.81 and
1.52 x 10^{-11} ml O_2/cell/min.   At intermediate densities of 4-8 x
10^6 cells/ml mean respiratory rate had decreased by 48% to 0.93 x
10^{-11} ml O_2/cell/min. and at densities of 10 x 10^6 cells/ml and
greater it had dropped to 0.65 for an overall 64% decrease in
mean respiratory activity.

Adenine nucleotide concentrations were determined in 7 experiments and average ATP, ADP and AMP values were examined as a
function of increasing population density.   The histogram (Fig. 1)
shows that at ranges of 1-2 and 2-4 x 10^6 cells/ml average ATP
concentrations were relatively high at 6.57 and 5.22 f.mol/cell.

Table 1 : Respiratory rate as a function of increasing
          population density.

Population density ranges x 10^6 cells/ml.	1.0-2.0	2.0-4.0	4.0-8.0	8.0-10.0	10
Respiratory rate x 10^{-11} ml O_2 / cell/min.	1.53	1.49	1.22	0.91	0.84
	2.06	1.61	0.91	0.72	0.50
	1.84	1.91	1.00	0.72	0.62
	–	1.28	0.60	0.70	–
	–	1.28	–	0.81	–
	–	1.86	–	0.75	–
	–	1.24	–	–	–
Mean respiratory rate	1.81	1.52	0.93	0.77	0.65

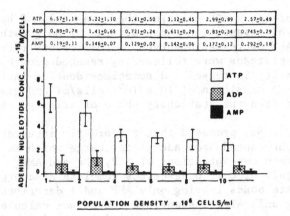

Fig. 1. A histogram of the average adenine nucleotide content per
cell determined in ranges of increasing population density.

At densities of 4-6 x 10^6 cells/ml the average ATP concentration
had decreased by 48% to 3.41 f.mol/cell.   This and subsequent ATP
decreases mirror almost exactly the density dependent changes
observed in mean respiratory rate.   By comparison ADP and AMP
content remained low and nearly unchanged throughout the profile.

Population growth curves (Fig. 2) revealed that at densities
of 1-4 x 10^6 cells/ml there was exponential proliferation in all
cultures and population density doubled or nearly doubled every day.

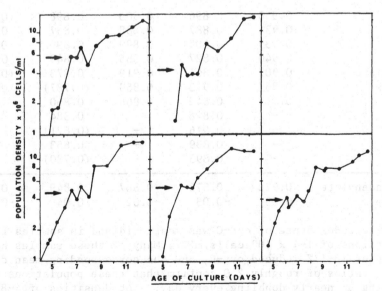

Fig. 2. Growth curves showing the kinetics of population growth
from low to high cell densities.

At densities of 4-6 x 10^6 cells/ml there was a 24-48 hour period of
no growth.   This transition phase plateau of no growth was coincid-
ent with the 48% decreases observed in respiratory rate and ATP
levels.   The plateaus were followed by renewed growth during which
population density increased and sometimes doubled in less than 24
hours.   At high densities of 10 x 10^6 cells/ml and greater all
populations entered the stationary phase of arrested cell growth.

    Atkinson (1968) proposed that the orderly integration of
metabolism might depend upon adenylate charge which he described as
a balance between concentrations of ATP, ADP and AMP.   In his
scheme on a scale of 0-1, 0 describes complete discharge of high
energy phosphate bonds leaving only AMP and 1 describes a full
charge leaving only ATP.   Adenylate charge was calculated for the
WRL-10A cells and grouped into ranges of increasing population
density (Table 2).   In ranges of 1-2, 2-4 and 4-8 x 10^6 cells/ml
adenylate charge was relatively high with mean values of 0.922,
0.876 and 0.887 respectively.   At 8-10 x 10^6 cells/ml and greater,
mean adenylate charge decreased to 0.849 and 0.838 with 30% of the
samples having pronounced overall decreases of up to 18%.

Table 2 : Population density and adenylate charge

Population density ranges x 10^6 cells/ml	1.0-2.0	2.0-4.0	4.0-8.0	8.0-10.0	10
	0.958	0.896	0.903	0.898	(0.777)
	0.934	0.887	0.888	0.837	0.851
	0.939	0.905	0.889	0.899	0.880
	0.940	0.827	0.885	0.849	0.832
Adenylate	0.907	0.861	0.919	0.873	(0.812)
charge	0.867	0.913	0.858	(0.787)	0.877
	0.911	0.849	0.866	0.860	-
	-	0.848	-	0.884	-
	-	0.916	-	(0.821)	-
	-	0.839	-	0.853	-
	-	0.893	-	(0.780)	-
Mean adenylate charge	0.922 $\pm$0.03	0.876 $\pm$0.03	0.887 $\pm$0.02	0.849 $\pm$0.04	0.838 $\pm$0.04

    The redox state of cyt-C was most oxidised in samples from
populations of 1-4 x 10^6 cells/ml.   Many of these samples had as
little as 10-17% reduced cyt-C, and the corresponding mean daily
growth ratios of roughly 2.0 confirm that these populations were
doubling or nearly doubling every day.   At densities of 4-8 x 10^6
cells/ml the percent of reduced cyt-C increased and individual

samples were largely between 24-34% reduced while the mean daily
growth ratios of the populations in this density range decreased to
1.2.   Three samples prepared from populations in the range of the
'transition phase plateau' had an unusually high percentage (48-86%)
of reduced cyt-C in spite of an ample supply of oxygen in the test
samples.   While these represent only 10% of the samples from that
range they suggested the possibility of a density and energy
dependent synchronization of cell growth and metabolic activity.

Total cyt-C determinations on two growing populations lend
additional support to the idea of density dependent synchronization
of metabolic activity and growth.   Table 3 shows that cyt-C content
in population 1 decreased from a high of 56 f.mol/cell, at a density
of 2.75 x 10^6 cells/ml on day 5, to a low of 22 f.mol/cell at a
density of 8.99 x 10^6 cells/ml on day 9.   On day 10 following two
days of no growth, there was a three fold increase in cyt-C to 64.5
f.mol/cell and within 9 hours the population density increased from
9.4 to 12.8 x 10^6 cells/ml while cyt-C content decreased to 23 f.
mol/cell.   In population 2 on day 8, after two days of limited
growth, population density increased from 4.22 to 10.22 x 10^6 cells/
ml in less than 11 hours and there was a simultaneous decrease in
cyt-C from 37 to 24 f.mol/cell.

Table 3 : Cyt-C concentrations per cell determined as a function
of increasing density in two populations of WRL-10A cells.

Age of culture (days)	Population (1) density x 10^6 cells/ml	Cyt-C x 10^{-15} M/cell	Population (2) density x 10^6 cells/ml	cyt-C x 10^{-15} M/cell
4	1.72	35.0	1.65	42.9
5	2.75	56.0	2.75	48.5
6	3.40	36.0	3.80	31.2
7	3.56	39.6	3.95	37.2
8	5.14	-	4.42	37.2*
8	7.33	26.5	10.22	24.3
9	8.99	26.3	9.44	28.8
9	8.99	22.3	10.74	27.3
10	9.40	64.5*	11.73	-
10	12.82	23.3	11.82	-

SUMMARY

Growth control, wound repair and differentiation in populations
of cells requires an orderly and purposeful integration of environmental feedback and metabolic activity.   In summary of the results
obtained the model presented in Fig. 3 proposes for further testing
that (1) at low population densities, where environmental conditions
are suitable for proliferation, there is exponential growth and the

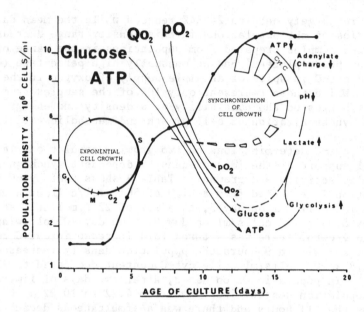

Fig. 3: A working model for study of population kinetics, environmental feedback and metabolic sequences in growth control, wound repair and cellular differentiation. Arrows down indicate known decreases and up indicate suspected increases.

cells of a population become randomly distributed in various stages of the growth cycle; (2) at intermediate densities (4-6 x 10^6 cells/ml) when the demands for continued exponential growth exceed the support of the environment (a) PO_2 decreases and oxygen availability becomes rate limiting; (b) respiratory rate (QO_2) decreases and the populations energy demand is shifted toward glycolysis causing (c) a sharp decrease in ATP concentration per cell. As a result of this energetic decline, overall metabolic activity which requires ATP, decreases; growth is temporarily delayed in the 'transition phase plateau' and there is concomitant synchronization of cell growth and metabolic activity. Populations of cells thus synchronized could respond to environmental feedback as a highly co-ordinated unit which is an essential feature of growth control and cellular differentiation. Synchronization could also account for the pronounced changes observed in energy charge, cyt-C redox state, cyt-C content per cell and recently in pH of the medium. It is felt that such changes are phenotypic expressions of the homeostatic mechanisms by which cells adapt to the special demands of their environment, and it is suggested that profiles of these population kinetics and temporal changes may help decipher regulatory sequences and transition phase events essential for growth, differentiation and wound repair.

REFERENCES

Adam, H. (1963) In 'Methods of Enzymatic Analysis' p.573 (ed. Bergmeyer, H.U.). Academic Press, New York.

Atkinson, D.E. (1968) Biochem. 7, 4030.

Chance, B. (1951) Rev. Sci. Instr. 22, 634.

Clark, L.C. (1956) Trans. Am. Soc. Artif. Internal Organs 2, 41.

Glinos, A.D. and Hargrove, D.D. (1965) Exp. Cell Res. 39, 249.

Holian, A., Owen, C.S. and Wilson, D.F. (1977) Arch. Biochem. Biophys. 181, 164.

Lamprecht, W. and Trautschold, I. (1963) In 'Methods of Enzymatic Analysis' p.543 (ed. Bergmeyer, H.U.). Academic Press, New York.

Wilson, D.F., Stubbs, M., Oshino, N. and Erecinska, M. (1974) Biochem. 13, 5305.

Wilson, D.F., Owen, C.S. and Holian, A. (1977) Archiv. Biochem., Biophys. In Press.

Wilson, D.F., Erecinska, M., Drown, C.W.R. and Silver, I.A. (1977b) Amer. J. Physiol. In Press.

DIRECT DETERMINATION OF LOCAL OXYGEN CONSUMPTION OF

THE BRAIN CORTEX IN VIVO

E. Leniger-Follert

Max-Planck-Institut fur Systemphysiologie

46 Dortmund, West Germany

Oxygen consumption of the total brain or of parts of the brain has been indirectly determined under different conditions by multiplying the cerebral arterio-venous oxygen difference by the total or regional flow. By this procedure only the mean oxygen consumption of a large area is determined and local differences in oxygen consumption cannot be detected.

Because microflow varies markedly within the brain cortex at different measuring sites even under steady state conditions, and as we assume that local metabolic differences could account for this behaviour, (Leniger-Follert and Lübbers 1975) we determined the local oxygen consumption of the brain cortex simultaneously at several measuring sites under in vivo conditions by a special method.

In 1962, Davies and Grenell were the first to determine the local oxygen consumption of the brain cortex from the slope of the PO_2 decrease after local occlusion of the pial circulation. However, some methodological objections have to be raised to those results as these authors could not determine the oxygen pressures in the brain tissue quantitatively. Later on, Lübbers (1968) determined the local oxygen consumption of the rabbit's brain. He interrupted the oxygen supply to the rabbit brain by stopping the blood flow by means of a cuff put around the neck of the animal. However, total cerebral ischaemia cannot be achieved by this procedure in all cases as shown by Opitz and Schneider (1950).

In the following report we describe a method to determine the

local oxygen consumption of the brain cortex quantitatively from
the slope of the oxygen pressure decrease recorded during a few
seconds of complete cerebral ischaemia.

PRINCIPLE AND METHODOLOGY

If the circulation of an organ is completely arrested, local
tissue PO_2 decreases.   The slope of the PO_2 decrease is a direct
measure of the local oxygen consumption of the tissue provided
that no chemically bound oxygen is released from haemoglobin.   To
be independent of haemoglobin, local tissue PO_2 can be elevated to
above 100 Torr.   Thus, local oxygen consumption can be calculated
from the slope of the PO_2 decrease, $\frac{\Delta PO_2}{\Delta t}$, multipled by the
solubility coefficient, for oxygen in the tissue, α_{O_2}, that is

$$\dot{V} = \frac{\Delta PO_2}{\Delta t} \cdot \alpha_{O_2} \cdot 100 \cdot 60$$

where, $\dot{V}$ = the local oxygen consumption in ml/100g/min.

Experiments were performed on cats which were anaesthetized
with Nembutal (30 mg/kg body weight), relaxed with Flaxedil and
ventilated mechanically.   Arterial blood pressure and arterial
blood gases were in the normal range when the experiments   started.

Local tissue PO_2 was recorded on the superficial layers of the
gyrus suprasylvius with a multiwire PO_2 electrode (Clark principle)
with eight individual PO_2 cathodes of 15 μm in diameter each
(Kessler and Lübbers 1966).   Only those electrodes were used which
had a response time of about 2 to 3 seconds for the 90% value.
The time courses of PO_2 changes during arrest of circulation and
after the end of ischaemia were determined and the oxygen
consumption for each second during ischaemia was calculated by an
electronic evaluation method.

During the experiment unipolar recordings of the electrocorticogram were made near the PO_2 measuring site and analysed by a
Fourier transformation.   Complete ischaemia of the brain was
produced by intrathoracic clamping of the innominate and left
subclavian arteries after ligation of both internal mammary arteries
as described by Hossmann and Sato (1971).   The time of ischaemia
ranged from 20 seconds to a maximum of 1 minute.   The disappearance
of the ECoG was used as the criterion for the completeness of
ischaemia.   ECoG disappeared totally about 20 seconds after the
beginning of ischaemia, if there was no collateral circulation.
In some experiments we recorded a microflow by means of the local

hydrogen clearance to determine whether total ischaemia was really achieved.   An additional criterion for completeness of ischaemia was the PO_2 overshoot after reperfusion which occurred only in those cases where ischaemia was complete.

To achieve independence from the chemically bound oxygen, the animals were ventilated with 100 vol.% of oxygen or carbogen.   Thus, tissue PO_2 values between 376 Torr and 100 Torr were reached. Records of corrected NADH-fluorescence revealed that the administration of pure oxygen or carbogen did not change the redox state of NADH/NAD of the brain cells and therefore the oxygen consumption.

RESULTS

1.   Within 0.1 seconds of the beginning of ischaemia, local tissue PO_2 decreased at all measuring sites.   Fig. 1 shows an original recording of the PO_2 measured simultaneously at 7 sites during and after a short period of complete ischaemia.   After reperfusion, a distinct overshoot of local PO_2 occurred although PO_2 had not reached zero Torr at the end of ischaemia.   The PO_2 overshoot was caused by local hyperaemia as shown by local hydrogen clearance. When ischaemia was not complete, local PO_2 returned to the initial value after reperfusion without an overshoot.

2.   Calculation of local oxygen consumption for each second during the period of complete ischaemia showed an apparent increase from zero to a maximum value during the first 2 to 3 seconds after the beginning of ischaemia.   This increase was due to the response time of the electrodes and the change of PO_2 gradients.   Then O_2 consumption remained constant for a few seconds (2-12 seconds) at different locations.   After this short period, oxygen consumption decreased continuously although tissue PO_2 values were rather high and had not reached the region of the haemoglobin dissociation curve (Fig. 2).   Recording and analysis of ECoG revealed that parallel to the decrease of the oxygen consumption the amplitude and frequency of ECoG decreased and disappeared totally some seconds later at about 15 to 20 seconds after the beginning of ischaemia although the brain cortex still contained oxygen.

3.   The rate of local oxygen consumption during the 'constant' period varied considerably at different measuring sites.   It ranged from 1 to about 9 ml/100 g tissue/min.   The mean value amounted to 3 ml/100 g/min. $\pm$ 1.5 (n = 100).

The results showed that it was possible to determine local oxygen consumption of the brain cortex in vivo immediately after complete circulatory arrest if an electrode with a short response time was used.   The calculation of oxygen consumption for each

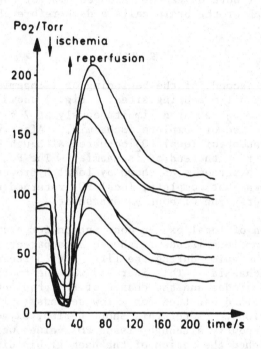

Fig. 1. Original traces of local tissue PO_2 recorded simultaneously
         at 7 measuring sites during and after a short period of
         complete ischaemia.   Note the PO_2 overshoot during
         reperfusion.

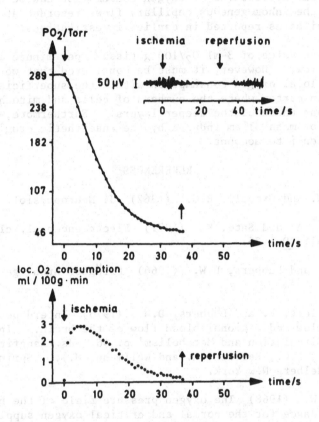

Fig. 2. Upper Part – PO_2 decrease measured at another site.
Lower Part – Local oxygen consumption.
In this case local oxygen consumption is constant only
until the 6th second.

second revealed that it remained constant only for a few seconds.
The decrease of O_2 consumption was possibly caused by the
accumulation of H^+ ions which could not be washed out (see Urbanics
et al, this symposium).   This may be a protective mechanism of
the brain to delay the onset of O_2 deficiency.

The local differences of oxygen consumption can be directly
related to the inhomogeneous capillary flows recorded at different
measuring sites as reported in earlier investigations.

The mean value of 3 ml O_2/100 g tissue per minute is
relatively low.   However, it must be considered that we only
determined local oxygen consumption within the superficial layers
of the brain cortex where the numbers of cells and mitochondria
are less than those of the deeper layers.   Furthermore, a
depression of metabolism induced by the anaesthetic drug (Nembutal)
must be taken into account.

REFERENCES

Davies, P.W. and Grenell, R.G.   (1962) J. Neurophysiol. 25, 651.

Hossmann, K.-A. and Sato, K.   (1971) Electroencephal. clin.
Neurophysiol. 30, 535.

Kessler, M. and Lübbers, D.W. (1966) Pflügers Arch. ges. Physiol.
291, R 32.

Leniger-Follert, E. and Lübbers, D.W.   (1975) Interdependence of
capillary flow and regional blood flow of the brain.   In
'Cerebral Circulation and Metabolism' p. 46 (eds. Langfitt, T.W.,
McHenry Jr., L.C., Reivich, M. and Wollmann, H.).   Springer-Verlag,
Berlin-Heidelberg-New York.

Lübbers, D.W.   (1968) The oxygen pressure field of the brain and
its significance for the normal and critical oxygen supply of the
brain.   In 'Oxygen Transport in Blood and Tissue' p. 124 (eds.
Lübbers, D.W., Luft, U.C., Thews, G. and Witzleb, E.).
Georg Thieme Verlag, Stuttgart.

Opitz, E. and Schneider, M.   (1950) Ergebn. Physiol. 46, 126.

STUDY OF TISSUE OXYGEN GRADIENTS BY SINGLE AND MULTIPLE INDICATORS

Britton Chance and Bjørn Quistorff*

Johnson Research Foundation, School of Medicine
University of Pennsylvania, Philadelphia, Pa 19194 USA
*Department of Biochemistry A, University of Copenhagen
Blegdamsvej 3, 2200 Copenhagen, Denmark

There are two types of naturally occurring oxygen indicators.
The first includes myoglobin and some soluble enzyme systems and may
be uniformly distributed in low concentration over the cytosol: the
second is localized and concentrated either in discrete organelles
about a micron in diameter such as the mitochondria or the peroxisomes (Weibel 1969), or in more extended organelles such as the
endoplasmic reticulum (Claude et al. 1947). In both cases, differing
resolutions and sensitivities are possible.

The measurement of gradients of oxygen concentration requires
determinations at two points sufficiently close together that they
are on a gradient of oxygen concentration (a "two-point method".
See e.g. Millikan 1936), or two closely spaced indicators that
respond to different PO_2's or oxygen concentrations (a "two-indicator
method. See e.g. Chance 1965, Oshino et al. 1975, Sies 1977a, b).
The two methods have in common the requirements for distance resolution and oxygen sensitivity: either the two points or the two indicators must be separated by an appropriate small distance. Granted
that these requirements can be fulfilled, the two methods would
seem to give identical information, but this paper suggests that the
two-indicator method may be more suitable for providing average
tissue oxygen gradients over a large tissue volume. Furthermore,
the two-point method is technically more difficult to execute since
spatial resolution of the oxygen gradient itself may require apertures as small as a few microns. In fact, apertures of 1.5 microns
(Thorell & Chance 1960) provide readily measurable optical signals
with the mitochondrion which contains localized high concentrations
of oxygen indicators (Thorell & Chance 1960). The two-indicator
method, on the other hand, demands that the indicators be close
enough to register PO_2's within the oxygen gradient (Weibel 1969);

however, in this case, larger signals are obtained since they are
derived from all indicators in the tissue volume.

Heterogeneity of the tissue, particularly liver (Pette and
Brandan 1966), can make interpretation of the results difficult.
For example, the two points of the two-point method may not be in
a homogeneous diffusion gradient need to be measured in order to
obtain appropriately averaged values. However, the two-indicator
method automatically averages all gradients within the span of the
two indicators; the only basic assumption is that the two indicators exist at an appropriate average spacing in all cells in
which gradients are to be measured. Such gradients may, however,
vary in steepness due to tissue heterogeneity and a corresponding
distribution will be obtained.

RESULTS

The results presented below decribe some chosen examples of
application of the two-point and two-indicator methods for determination of oxygen gradients in cells and tissues.

Two-Point Method

Three-dimensional studies of oxygen gradients in a model
cardiac infarct. In a Langendorf perfusion, a small branch of a
coronary artery of a rat heart was ligated to produce an ischemic
area in the wall of the left ventricle, 3 to 4 mm^2. The heart was
gently freeze-clamped, and the ischemic area located on the surface
of the frozen tissue - the general location can be determined by
UV illumination and visual observation. Following the transfer of
the sample to the low temperature redox scanner, a series of eight
consecutive scans was recorded from the myocardium at depths
between 100 μ and 1100 μ. In each scan, the fluorescence intensity
of reduced pyridine nucleotide (PN) and oxidized flavoprotein (Fp)
was measured at 3600 single points over an area of 36 mm^2. All
eight scans were vertically aligned and it was therefore possible
to obtain a three-dimensional representation of the ischemic area
in the myocardium by combining the data from the eight two-
dimensional scans.

Figure 1 shows a two dimensional display of the scans, i.e.
the ratio between Fp and PN fluorescence is displayed as a gray-
scale image employing suitable clipping functions. Reduced (low
Fp/PN areas) appear black, and oxidized areas appear light. The
same gray scale was used for all scans. The shape of the infarct
changes with depth, reflecting the perfusion pattern of the ligated
artery.

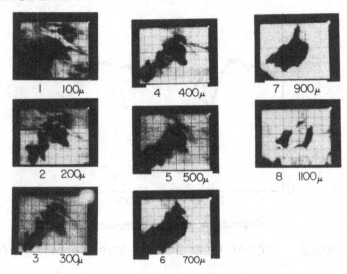

Figure 1: 2-D redox scans of freeze-trapped rat heart with model infarct. Sections are cut away every 100 μ.

At a depth of 1100 μ, the ischemic area starts to disappear, indicating that the endocardium has been reached. A striking feature of these images is the very sharp transition between oxidized and reduced tissue, which may be observed in all layers of the myocardium. As shown in Fig. 2, the transition involves a change in the Fp/PN ratio by a factor of five to ten which is achieved in most locations within 60 to 100 μ, i.e. the oxygen tension decreases sufficiently rapidly within 100 μ to cause a complete reduction of the mitochondria (see Quistorff, this volume). In isolated pigeon heart mitochondria, Sugano et al. (1974) found that a similar transition required a decrease in oxygen concentration from 5×10^{-7} M to less than 10^{-8} M, a difference of about 0.1 torr, or a gradient of at least 0.1 torr/100μ.

Two-Indicator Method

Cardiac tissue. In the studies of Fig.3, the two indicators are the mitochondria and the cytosolic myoglobin. In vitro, the experimental use of a suspension of mitochondria and myoglobin gives a clear-cut difference between the two indicators, as shown by the concavity of the cytochrome response vs. the myoglobin response. If the experiment is now repeated in the perfused heart, the concavity disappears and no difference in the responses of the two indicators can be detected; no observable amount of deoxymyoglobin or oxidized cytochrome exists in the in vivo system. Thus, the gradient is so steep that it cannot be measured by these two

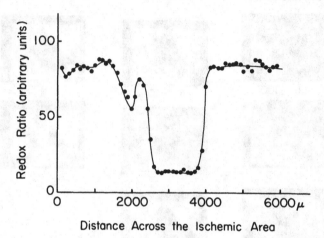

Figure 2: Typical redox profile across a model infarct.

indicators, whose spacing and P_{50}'s are too close together to be useful at normal respiration rates of perfused cardiac tissue. The difference of P_{50}'s is small, 1 torr, because of the high affinity of myoglobin for oxygen. The dimensions of the gradient are also small, possibly of the order of the intermitochondrial distance of 1μ. Therefore, the gradient may be greater than 1 torr/μ. Clearly, the myoglobin-cytochrome couple would be more appropriate for a tissue such as resting skeletal muscle or antimycin A-inhibited cardiac tissue, where the respiration rate is slower than in the perfused heart.

Mitochondria and peroxisomes. A variety of experiments are now vailable on rat liver in which the first indicator is the peroxisome and the second is the mitochondrion. The data considered for analysis are from Oshino et al. (1975) presented in their original form in Fig. 4. The two traces represent the responses of mito- chondrial cytochrome c as measured by direct spectrophotometry (solid circles), and $\overline{H_2O_2}$ generation (open circles), which was measured by peroxisomal catalase H_2O_2 and computed as the rate of production of H_2O_2 by the methanol titration method (Oshino et al. 1975). This approach depends upon equations that show that the H_2O_2 generation rate and the free H_2O_2 concentration can be precisely calculated from the molar concentration of an alcohol (methanol) which causes the concentration of the catalase H_2O_2 compound to decrease to half its maximal value. The H_2O_2 generation is thus sharply localized in the peroxisomes. In this experiment, H_2O_2 was generated by glycollate oxidase, which is also largely localized in the peroxisomes.

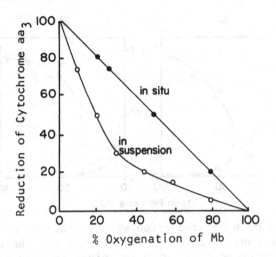

Figure 3: A plot of the relative response to oxygen of cardiac
myoglobin and cardiac mitochondria in suspension and in situ.

The profiles A and B represent titrations for two rates of mitochondrial respiration: A, uninhibited, and B, antimcyin A-blocked.
It can be seen directly from the graphs that the difference between
the titration curves for peroxisomal H_2O_2 and cytochrome c oxidation
is small, and maximal in the region of 50% oxygen in the perfusate.
The amplitude of the difference is somewhat truncated, due to the
fact that even before the peroxisomes achieve the reduced state,
P_R, some of the mitochondria do likewise (M_R). Thus, Panel A
corresponds to a steep tissue oxygen gradient, where the roughly
200 torr difference of K_M of the two systems occurs within the
average separation of peroxisomes and mitochondria, so the gradient
is of the order of several hundred torr per micron.

In Panel B, the oxygen gradient is decreased by slowing the
respiration of the mitochondria and leaving that of the peroxisomes
more or less constant. The extent of the decrease of the tissue
oxygen gradient will have to be determined by decreasing the flux
of the glycollate oxidase.

A feature of the profile of Panel B is that the glycollate
oxidase profile shows an extension towards lower PO_2's in the
presence of antimycin A than in its absence, which is attributed to
a decrease of the oxygen gradient. This allows faithful reproduction
of the in vitro profile for glycollate oxidase at the lower tissue
oxygen gradient. In fact, the K_m for glycollate oxidase in vitro
and in the tissue is approximately the same (300 μM or 190 torr).

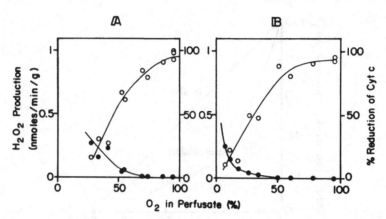

<u>Figure 4</u>:   Rates of H$_2$O$_2$ production with various O$_2$ concentrations
measured from methanol titrations (o) plotted vs. the extent of
reduction of cytochrome <u>c</u> (●) with 1mM glycollate as substrate.
A, in the absence of Antimycin A; B, with 8 μM antimycin A
(Oshino et al. 1975, reproduced with permission).

      Experiments with samples similar to those of Fig.4 employed
urate as substrate. The estimated value of the gradient for urate
oxidation is somewhat steeper, but still readily detectable by the
two-indicator method.

      If a peroxisomal substrate is omitted, there is a small resi-
dual H$_2$O$_2$ generation from the mitochondria, whose P$_{50}$ must match
that of cytochrome <u>c</u>. The maximal rate of this H$_2$O$_2$ generation is
only 4% of that obtained from the peroxisomes with glycollate as
substrate, so it is not a quantitative factor in the determination
of the H$_2$O$_2$ gradient.

      In a similar series of experiments, Sies has measured the
actual consumption of urate in a flow-through liver perfusion
(Sies 1977b), instead of the peroxisomal H$_2$O$_2$ generation. PaO$_2$
values are not available. Fig.5 shows a plot of the peroxisomal
signal vs. the mitochondrial signal for Sies's experiment (solid
triangles and compares it with data on the perfused organ under
nearly identical conditions with glycollate as the peroxisomal
substrate (open squares). In addition, data for hepatocytes (open
circles) are included (Jones et al. 1977). The averaging problem
is more severe with the flow-through studies, since the flow-
through averages the H$_2$O$_2$ generation in all lobes of the liver,
while the spectroscopic method for cytochrome measures its
response in a particular part of the lobe under observation.
Also, Sies used cytochrome <u>a</u> instead of cytochrome <u>c</u>. While it
would seem that the two methods should have given the same result,
they are in fact rather different (solid triangles); no difference

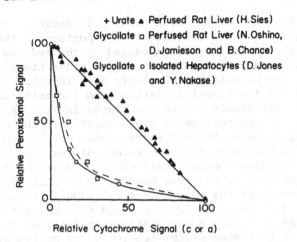

Figure 5: A plot of the peroxisomal signal (ordinate) vs. the mitochondrial signal (abscissa) for a variation of PaO_2 in urate-perfused liver by Sies (1977b) (▲); glycollate-perfused liver by Oshino et al. (1975) (■); and in a suspension of hepatocytes with glycollate as substrate by Jones et al. (1977 (o).

signal from the two indicators was detected in the normally respiring liver. It seems highly unlikely that the titration for cytochrome c would have been altered by the change of procedure, and so a reasonable assumption is that the flow-through method has detected portions of the liver that are less well-perfused than those under direct spectroscopic observation of the cytochrome c and catalese in the work of Oshino et al. (1975). The agreement of the cell and tissue data support the idea of intracellular oxygen gradients in the hepatocyte.

In summary, it is preferable to measure the two indicators in the same portion of an organ than to rely upon the assumption that the total organ would be as well-perfused as the parts under observation.

DISCUSSION

These experimental observations and analyses suggest a new approach to the detection of tissue oxygen gradients by the two-indicator method. The method requires perfusion of the organ with a variety of PaO_2's and an adjustment of the K_m's of the indicators so that they appropriately scan the tissue oxygen gradient and thus give a maximal difference signal (cf Fig.4) or an appropriate curvature of the plot of peroxisomal vs. mitochondrial signals (Fig. 5). The latter indicates the presence of a steep

gradient by the approach of the plot towards linearity. In the
case of Figs.4 and 5 a crude estimate of the portion of the equivalent two dimensional Krogh model occupied by the reduced peroxisomes and the oxidized mitochondria - a mixed redox state of the
two indicators - can be obtained by simply assuming that this portion is given by the fractional deviation from linearity in Fig.5
or the fractional difference of the two traces in Fig. 4A. These
values are 58 and 52% respectively, i.e., about half the equivalent
Krogh model is occupied by "mixed" redox states of the two indicators. Simplifying the model from two to one dimensions, the linear
dimension of the gradient becomes half the length of the model from
arterial to venous end, or for most models, about half of 200μ or
100μ. The difference of the peroxisomal K_m ($\sim$200 torr) and the
mitochondrial K_m (0.1 torr) is 200 torr, and the gradient is $\sim$2
torr/μ. Obviously, a thorough mathematical analysis of the combined reaction and diffusion in the two-indicator system will lead
to an accurate calculation of the tissue oxygen gradient.

ACKNOWLEDGEMENT

The assistance of Benson Margules, Eric Benshetler, Wolfgang
Nadler and John Sorge is gratefully acknowledged as is the support
of NIH HL-18708 and NS-10939,

REFERENCES

Chance, B. (1965) J. Genl. Physiol. 49, 163-188.

Claude, A., Porter, A.R. and Pickels, E.G. (1974) Cancer Res. 7,
421-430.

Jones, D.F., Mason, H.S. Nakase, Y. and Chance, B. (1977) Federation Proc. 36 (Abstr. 1555).

Millikan, G.A. (1936) Proc. Roy. Soc. London B-120, 366-388.

Oshino, N., Jamieson, D. and Chance, B. (1975) Biochem. J. 146,
53-60.

Pette, D. and Brandau, H. (1966) Enzym. Biol. Chim. 6, 79-87.

Sies, H. (1977a) In Tissue Hypoxia and Ischemia (M. Roberts, R.
Coborn, S. Lahiri and B. Chance, Eds.) Adv. Expt. Med. 78, 51-66.

Sies, H. (1977b). This Volume, pp.

Sugano, T., Oshino, N. and Chance, B. (1974) Biochim. Biophys.
Acta. 340-358.

Thorell, B. and Chance B. (1960) Exptl. Cell Res. 20, 43-45.

Weibel, E.R. (1969), J. Cell Biol. 42, 68-91.

DISCUSSION OF PAPERS IN SESSION 4

CHAIRMEN: DR. H. SIES and DR. D.F. WILSON

PAPERS BY: DRS. ERECIŃSKA and WILSON and by DR. WILSON et al

Dr. Sies: Your experiments were carried out in hypothermia at 25°C, which explains the low values for O_2 uptake by the isolated hepatocytes. In calculating the $\Delta\Delta G$ values, did you use the equilibrium constants for 37°C or 25°C?

Dr. Erecińska: All our experiments were carried out either at 25° or 22°C. The equilibrium constants were always corrected for the appropriate temperature and pH value.

Dr. Chance: 1. In skeletal muscles we have observed large changes of NAD/NADH during stimulated contractions. This would seem to differ from the results you describe on the heart.

2. In liver, we detect redox heterogeneities that make it difficult to assign a particular redox state to this organ unless it is the average of rather large extremes.

Dr. Wilson: I assume you mean that large changes in pyridine nucleotide fluorescence were observed on stimulation of contractions. As you are well aware, it is very difficult to tell how much of the PN fluorescence change is due to that in mitochondrial NAD/NADH. Our data refer to mitochondrial NAD^+/NADH measured from the equilibrium in the GDH reaction.

2. The heterogeneity you observe is due to the peculiar characteristics of the Hb-free perfusion system of the liver. We use suspensions of hepatocytes in which ample O_2 supply ensures homogeneity of oxygenation and there is no reason to suspect any

339

differences in the redox states of various cells.

Dr. Sies: In your three dimensional plot (figure 4), the capital A and B values, in general, are off by an order of magnitude along the lines drawn for $[NAD^+]/[NADH]$. Could this result from the fact that you used total tissue data for $[ATP]/[ADP][P_i]$ instead of the true cytosolic concentrations? A correction for this probably would lead to a better fit.

Dr. Wilson: Yes, for liver, kidney and tetrahymena the cytoplasmic $[ATP]/[ADP][P_i]$ should be somewhat larger than the whole cell values used in the figure. This would move the points labelled B toward those labelled A. In the perfused heart, the cytosolic $[ATP]/[ADP]$ was calculated directly from the creatine-phosphokinase equilibrium and no correction should be necessary.

PAPER BY: AUSTIN et al

Dr. Goldstick: Suggested that the decrease of bPO_2 (the initial slope of bPO_2 decrease upon carotid occlusion) with bPO_2 (PO_2 availability at the tip of the oxygen electrode) observed by Dr. Austin might be due to damping by O_2 liberation from Hb (as proposed by Dr. Reneau for similar data).

Dr. Friedli: Wondered if control experiments with perfused Hb-free or CO poisoned preparations might offer a direct test for the possible effect of O_2-Hb dissociation.

Dr. Chance: Thought that hypovolemia or anaemia might be used as a control for haemoglobin interference.

PAPER BY: DR. LONGMUIR et al

Dr. Chance: Some years ago, at the ISOX Symposium we actively discussed the possible role of P_{450} in facilitated diffusion, and it was thought by some at that time that oxygen would dissociate too slowly from P_{450} for facilitated diffusion. I think this prediction has now been fulfilled. Do you agree? The presence of bound Hb in microsomes was studied (I think by Pogell) and it should have the CO band near that which you mention. Do you agree?

Dr. Longmuir: Yes.

Dr. Sies: Nicotinamide has been added to microsomal preparations in studies of cytochrome P_{450}-linked drug oxidations to inhibit 5'-nucleotidase, so I am surprised that you use it as an inhibitor for cytochrome P_{450}. What is the basis for this?

Dr. Longmuir: We needed an inhibitor which readily entered tissue slices. Nicotinamide does this but we use it at a concentration which binds a little over half the P_{450}. At this concentration, about 5 mM, nicotinamide does not inhibit any other system.

PAPER BY: DR. WERRLEIN

Dr. Lübbers: Did I understand you correctly that your results show that at the end of the growing phase the supply of oxygen becomes rate limiting in spite of rapid stirring of the culture?

Dr. Werrlein: I am proposing in the model, from the combined results, that at intermediate densities oxygen availability in the cultures may become both rate limiting for continued exponential proliferation and at the same time a factor in the synchronization of cell growth. In fact we know that in spite of continuous stirring the PO_2 of the medium of high-density WRL-10A suspension cultures decreases from 140 mmHg to critical levels of 1-2 mmHg within six hours after medium renewal. (Vail, R. and Glinos, A. (1974) J. Cell Physiol., 83, 425).

Dr. Lübbers: If that is so then increasing the oxygen capacity of the medium by addition of haemoglobin should improve the oxygen supply and influence your experimental data.

Dr. Werrlein: The use of haemoglobin is an excellent suggestion which Dr. Erecińska also recommended to me.

Dr. Hunt: Several mitogens or growth factors will cause fibroblasts to divide to unusual densities or to divide significantly faster than usual. Is there room in your theories for these growth factors?

Dr. Werrlein: Yes, it is well known that serum, insulin and other factors have a stimulatory influence on cell growth in density inhibited populations and that serum promotes an increased uptake of P_i by the cells. If the growth stimulating factors to which you are referring have a similar effect which might for example shift the $[ATP]/[ADP][P_i]$ ratio as reported by Dr. Wilson yesterday, then the energy state and regulatory metabolism of cell population might be shifted in favor of an increased growth rate and final density.

PAPER BY: DR. LENIGER-FOLLERT

Dr. Chance: If the tissue still contained, as it appears to according to your polarographic measurements, more than enough oxygen to permit mitochondrial ATP synthesis, it is odd that the ECoG disappears and reappears.

Dr. Metzger: 1. Isn't ischaemia too unphysiological a situation for measuring O_2 consumption?

2. Did you observe an arousal reaction at the beginning of ischemia which could cause an increase of the O_2 consumption?

3. Do you think that during ischaemia K^+-ions are important as well as H^+-ions?

__Dr. Leniger-Follert:__ 1. You will see that one of our figures showed that O_2 consumption is constant during at least some seconds.

2. We had no arousal.

3. We have made some potassium measurements and these do show an increase.

__Dr. Banchero:__ If the response time of your electrodes is about three seconds, do you account for this delay when plotting your data (PO_2 and VO_2) versus time. Not only that, when the dynamic response is long (three seconds) each reading, measured discreetly, may not be accurate unless corrections are introduced. Have you done this?

__Dr. Leniger-Follert__: The apparent increase of oxygen consumption from zero to the maximal value is really caused by the response time of the electrode used. If you use an electrode with a shorter response time, for example a PO_2 needle electrode with a tip diameter of about 1 µm, you will see that this first phase is shortened. I think it is not necessary to correct the later readings because the electrode then shows the actual slope of the PO_2 decrease.

PAPER BY: DR. CHANCE et al

__Dr. Lübbers:__ What did you mean by the expression "sharp" in relation to the border zone? We showed in our paper with Grossmann that the width of the hypoxic zone situated between the normoxic and the anoxic tissue region, depends on the K_m value in the hypoxic zone and the respiration rate in the "zero order" region. The volume of this zone depends additionally on the actual decrease of the PO_2 along the capillary which supplies the tissue. In arterial hypoxia, blood flow may increase several hundred per cent so that due to the oxygen dissociation curve of Hb and the flow increase, the PO_2 decrease in the capillary blood becomes small. I mean that under such conditions, the hypoxic zone has a width and a volume which cannot be neglected.

__Dr. Chance:__ The border zones surrounding the infarct in an artificial coronary occlusion in the __in situ__ dog heart (see fig. 1- experiments with Clyde Barlow and Andy Harken) is marked by the

abrupt transition from dark to light (mitochondrial fluorescence
is bright in anoxia and dim in normoxia). The freeze-trapped
tissue shows sharp, clear edges around most of the perimeter of
the infarct. The resolution of the photography is about 10-20 μm
and the border zone is approximately this value. I would term
this a sharp border characteristic of the heart.

Oxygen, Radiation, and Neoplasia

INCREASE IN BRAIN TISSUE OXYGEN AVAILABILITY INDUCED

BY LOCALIZED MICROWAVE HYPERTHERMIA

H. I. Bicher

Department of Radiation Medicine
Roswell Park Memorial Institute
666 Elm Street, Buffalo, New York   14263 USA

Oxygen supply to brain tissue is a carefully guarded function (1,2), inasmuch as the effects of hypoxia or hyperoxia are promptly compensated by counteracting changes in blood flow and neuronal function (1-6). This physiological "autoregulation" barrier, however, may constitute an impediment to the therapeutic delivery of O_2 to imperilled tissue areas under conditions of pathological cerebral ischemia.

In the present study, we undertook to evaluate the effect that localized hyperthermia, precisely delivered in the form of microwave energy, will have both on local oxygen levels and the ability of the microcirculation to deliver oxygen to brain tissue upon breathing of the gas.

METHODS AND MATERIALS

Methods

The experiments were performed on 40 cats anesthetized with sodium pentobarbital and under positive-pressure breathing. Femoral artery blood pressure and carotid artery blood flow were recorded on a Grass Model 7 polygraph chart recorder using standard transducers. Tissue pO_2 was determined as described below using oxygen electrodes. The different respiratory mixtures tested were administered through the artificial respiration pump (Harvard, Model 607), and all

solutions were injected into the cannulated femoral
vein. Results reported represent average values of
five experiments for each procedure or level of
hyperthermia.

The O_2 ultramicroelectrodes used were of the "gold
in glass" type as previously described (3), (6). This
probe is used as an "external reference" O_2 microelectrode. The electronic circuitry to measure the
polarographic current was provided by a Model 1200
Chemical Microsensor System (Transidyne General Corporation, Ann Arbor, Michigan), and the results were
recorded on a Model 7 Grass polygraph. The procedure
for electrode calibration was the same as previously
described (7). Cortical responses to O_2 and N_2
breathing were determined as in preceding papers (5).

In several experiments a platinum-iridium Teflon-
coated wire, 120 μm diameter, was used as the O_2 electrode. Although its calibration was not sufficiently
reliable to determine actual T_pO_2 values, it was found
that for measuring transients (RT and O_2 breathing) the
values obtained correlated well with those from microelectrodes.

Brain tissue temperature was also recorded using
a Copper-Constantan microthermocouple (tip diameter
30-100 microns) inserted into the prefrontal cortex
brain tissue in close proximity to the O_2 microelectrode. An Omega Eng. Model 250 Digital Voltimeter
amplifier was used as a link between the microthermocouple and the polygraph.

Microwaves in the frequency of 2450 MHz were
produced by a Raytheon Magnetron and delivered through
a specially designed 5 cm diameter circularly polarized applicator loaded with a low dose dielectric
material having a dielectric constant of 6.

RESULTS AND DISCUSSION

Effects of Local Hyperthermia on TpO_2: As can be
seen in Figure 1, there is a rise in TpO_2 that parallels
the application of the microwaves and follows, closely,
changes in tissue temperature. The response is very
fast, TpO_2 increasing shortly after the rise in temperature, and then decreasing as the brain cools off.

EFFECT OF HYPERTHERMIA ON T_pO_2

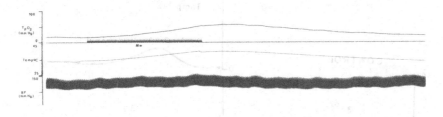

HYPERTHERMIA EFFECT ON T_pO_2 RISE DURING O_2 BREATHING

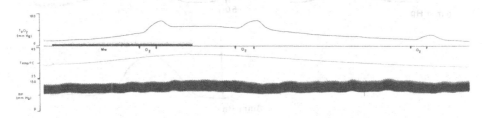

Figure 1 - From top: TpO_2, Tissue Temperature and B.P.
Mw irradiation when timer on. Time: 1 minute
O_2 breathing (see Figure 2). For explanation
see text.

There was also a small rise in blood pressure and
cerebral blood flow.

Effect of Localized Hyperthermia on the TpO_2
Response to O_2 Breathing: Breathing O_2 for one minute
usually causes a very small rise in T_pO_2 (Figure - 2
control). Local hyperthermia caused an increase in
this response that was proportional to the local brain
tissue temperature. The threshold was about 37.5°C
and a 40-50 mmHg increase could be recorded at 41°C.
No experiments were performed above 41°C.

The present studies clearly demonstrate that
localized microwave irradiation in the brain cortex
causes a rise in local TpO_2 which starts shortly after

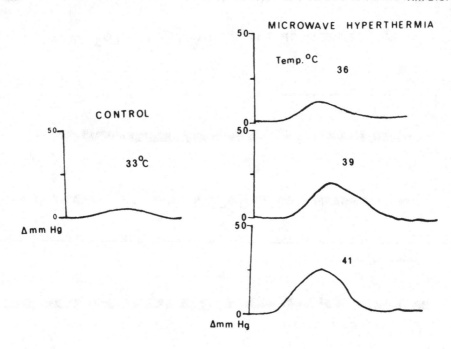

Figure 2 - TpO$_2$ records O$_2$ responses at different
         tissue temperature levels.

the rise in tissue temperature and follows closely the
time course of the hyperthermia.   During this time
there is also an increase in the local hyperoxia induced by O$_2$ breathing which also seems to be temperature dependent. The mechanism of this effect, either
through blood flow, metabolic or other changes (7),
remains to be elucidated.

     In previous publications we have described, and
others have confirmed a process of O$_2$ "autoregulation"
(1,2,4,5,6,8) which keeps TpO$_2$ within physiological
limits.   Local hyperthermia seems to be an effective
method to temporarily block this buffering process,
thereby increasing brain tissue oxygen levels.

SUMMARY

     The present experiments demonstrate by direct
measurements, that localized hyperthermia produced by

microwave irradiation increases the oxygen levels in brain tissue in a manner dependent on tissue temperature, with concomitant breaking of the oxygen autoregulation, thus allowing for an additional increase in TpO_2 upon O_2 breathing.

REFERENCES

1. Bicher, H.I. Brain oxygen autoregulation: A protective reflex to hypoxia? Microvas. Res. 8: 291-313, 1974.

2. Bicher, H.I., Reneau, D.D., Bruley, D.F.,et al Brain oxygen supply and neuronal activity under normal and hyperglycemic conditions. Am. J. Physiol. 224: 275-282, 1973.

3. Cater, D.B., Silver, I.A., Wilson, G.M. Apparatus and technique for the quantitative measurement of oxygen tension in living tissues. Proc. Roy. Soc. Lond. (Series B) 151: 256-276, 1959/1960.

4. Bicher, H.I., Bruley, D.F., Reneau, D.D., et al Effect of microcirculation changes on brain tissue oxygenation. J. Physiol. 217: 689-707, 1971.

5. Bicher, H.I., Knisely, M.H. Brain tissue reoxygenation demonstrated with a new ultramicro oxygen electrode. J. Appl. Physiol. 28: 387-390, 1970.

6. Bicher, H.I., Marvin, P. Pharmacological control of local oxygen regulation mechanisms in brain tissue. Stroke 7: 469-472, 1976.

7. Johnson, C.C., Guy, A.W. Non-ionizing electro-magnetic wave effects in biological materials and systems. Proc. IEEE 60: 692-699, 1972.

8. Leniger-Follert, E., Lubbers, D.W., Wrabetz, W. Regulation of local tissue PO_2 of the brain cortex at different arterial O_2 pressures. Pflugers Arch. 359: 81-95, 1975.

A PULSE-RADIOLYSIS STUDY ON ACTIVE OXYGEN

Hayashi, K., Lindenau, D.* and Tamura, M.

The Institute of Scientific and Industrial Research,
Osaka University, Osaka, Japan.
*Hahn-Meitner-Institut für Kernforschung Berlin GmbH,
Bereich Strahlen-chemie, D-1000 Berlin 39, Germany.

INTRODUCTION

The recent findings of the enzymic and non-enzymic generation
of the superoxide anion, O_2^-, and its scavenging enzyme, superoxide
dismutase, in living organisms may help to explain the molecular
mechanisms of oxygen toxicity and also the oxygen effect observed
in the radiation biology (McCord and Fridovich, 1968; McCord et
al, 1971). In this paper we focused our attention on the
reactions of O_2^- with certain haemoproteins such as myoglobin, haemoglobin, cytochrome c and peroxidase. The possible function of
myoglobin in protecting against O_2^- is also discussed. In the
present study, the pulse-radiolysis technique in combination with
the optical detection method was used with the nanosecond time-
resolution.

PRINCIPLE OF THE METHOD

When high energy radiation interacts with water, the hydrated
electron, e_{aq}^- is primarily formed (Chase and Hunt, 1975). In the
presence of oxygen, the hydrated electron reduces the molecular
oxygen to superoxide anion with the diffusion limited velocity.
Thus, with the short-pulsed irradiation, we can generate the
superoxide anion within less than few microseconds. The equations
1-a, b, c, describe the above.

$$H_2O \xrightarrow{\hspace{1cm}} e_{aq}^- \qquad 10^{-12} \text{ sec} \qquad\qquad \text{1-a}$$

$$e_{aq}^- + O_2 \xrightarrow{\hspace{1cm}} O_2^- \qquad 10^{-7} \text{ sec} \qquad\qquad \text{1-b}$$

$$O_2^- + Fe^{3+} -----> Product \qquad\qquad\qquad 1-c$$

In the absence of oxygen the reaction of eqn. 1-d occurs (Land
and Swallow 1971; Wilting et al 1974).

$$Fe^{3+} + e_{aq}^- -----> Fe^{2+} \qquad\qquad\qquad 1-d$$

where Fe^{3+}, Fe^{2+} designate the ferric and ferrous states of a
haemoprotein respectively.   The reactions of eqn. 1-c or 1-d can
be followed by the fast optical absorption spectrometry.

EXPERIMENTAL PROCEDURES

Human methemoglobin, sperm whale metmyoglobin, (for both of
which the iron atom is in the ferric state), horse radish peroxidase
(HRP) and cytochrome c from bovine heart were obtained commercially
and also prepared by the usual methods (Shannon et al 1966).
Sample solutions contained 5 to 20 μM proteins (on heme-basis),
50 mM phosphate buffer pH 7, and 0.1M methanol for scavenging the
hydroxyl and hydrogen radicals.   For anaerobic condition, the
solutions were bubbled with pure argon gas for longer than 30 min.

Pulse radiolysis experiments were carried out in the Hahn-
Meitner-Institut with 20 nsec pulse of 15 MeV provided by linear
accelerator.   The absorbed dose was measured by the Fricke dosimetry.

RESULTS

The reduction of ferric-haemoproteins by hydrated electron

Fig. 1 shows the disappearance of the hydrated electrons
measured by the absorption change at 650 nm due to the reaction with
ferrihorseradish peroxidase.   The reaction obeys the second order
kinetics as shown in Fig. 1-b and the rate constant for the reduction
by hydrated electrons can be estimated to be $3\sim4 \times 10^{10} M^{-1} sec^{-1}$,
which is almost a diffusion-controlled velocity.

Fig. 2 shows the absorption changes at 437 nm and 405 nm of
ferriperoxidase after irradiation in the absence of oxygen.   The
initial rapid absorption changes ($t_{1/2} \sim 5$ μsec) represents the
reduction process of ferric state to ferrous state, as verified by
the difference absorption spectrum taken at 20 μsec after pulse
(Fig. 2b).   Tbe spectrum is that of ferrous minus ferric states of
this enzyme (c.f. Fig. 4-c).   After completion of the reduction,
the relatively slow absorption change at 437 nm is seen, ($t_{1/2} \sim 70$
μsec) which probably arises from the conformational change of the
protein moiety.   This will be discussed elsewhere in more detail
(Hayashi and Tamura, unpublished).

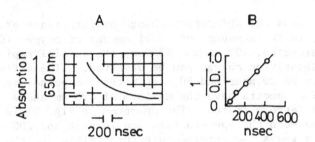

Fig. 1. A: Oscilloscope trace demonstrating the disappearance of
the hydrated electron in the presence of ferriperoxidase
by the absorption change at 650 nm; room temperature,
anaerobic condition.

B: The second order plot of the absorption change of the
hydrated electron obtained from Fig. 1A.

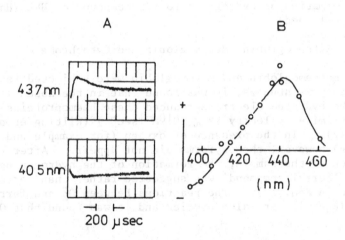

Fig. 2. Absorption changes of the peroxidase at 437 and 405 nm
after the radiation pulse under anaerobic conditions.

A: In the oscilloscope traces absorption increases in the
upward direction.

B: The difference spectrum obtained at 20 µsec after the
pulse. The normalized relative absorption intensity
is plotted against wavelength.

Pulse-radiolysis of ferriperoxidase in the presence of oxygen

Fig. 3 shows the absorption change of peroxidase after
irradiation, in the presence of small amount of oxygen (O_2; 10^{-5}M).
At both wavelengths, 400 nm and 435 nm, the initial rapid and the
later slow absorption change can be observed. The difference
spectra taken at 20 μsec and 30 μsec after the pulse are shown in
Fig. 4A. The spectra have the maximum of 420 nm and a shoulder
at 440 nm of ferrous state. The spectrum in Fig. 4B is the
difference between the spectra recorded 10 μsec and 200 μsec after
the pulse and shows the intermediate responsible for the slow
absorption change.

The 420 nm absorption can be identified as the oxyform ($Fe^{2+} \cdot$
O_2) of the HRP, named Compound III or oxyperoxidase (Tamura and
Yamazaki 1972). This is verified by the difference spectrum
between the oxyform minus ferric state shown in Fig. 4C. Thus
under this condition, the reduction of peroxidase and the formation
of the oxycompound is observed. Under air saturated conditions
(O_2, 2.5 x 10^{-4}M) the formation of the oxycompound is not seen.
This may arise from the disproportionation of O_2^- into H_2O_2 and O_2
with the formation of hydrogen peroxide compound of HRP (Hayashi
et al, unpublished).

Methemoglobin, Metmyoglobin and Cytochrome c

When methemoglobin and metmyoglobin were subjected to similar
pulse-radiolysis studies, it was found that in the absence of
oxygen, the hydrated electrons reduced these haemoproteins with the
diffusion-limited velocity ($k \sim 10^{10}M^{-1}sec^{-1}$) (Wilting et al, 1974)
see Eqn. (2). In the presence of oxygen (for example under air
saturation) however, the oxyforms did not appear. After the
irradiation of the sample, the formation of the hydrogen peroxide
compound, 'ferryl compound' was suggested rather than ferrous state,
as written in Eqn. (3). The reactions between O_2^- and ferricytochrome c (Eqn. 4) were also studied and it was found that O_2^- reduced

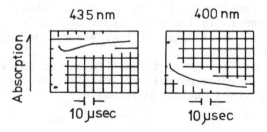

Fig. 3. Absorption changes at 435 and 400 nm of the ferriperoxidase
         after irradiation in the presence of 10^{-5}M oxygen.

ferricytochrome c with the second order rate constant of $\sim 10^5 M^{-1} sec^{-1}$ (Seki et al, 1976).

$$Fe^{3+}(MetHb \text{ or } MetMb) + e^-_{aq} \longrightarrow Fe^{2+}(Hb \text{ or } Mb) \qquad (2)$$

$$Fe^{3+}(MetHb \text{ or } MetMb) + O_2^- \longrightarrow Fe^{4+} \text{ (ferryl-Mb or -Hb)} \quad (3)$$

$$Fe^{3+}(cyt.c) + O_2^- \longrightarrow Fe^{2+} \text{ (cyt. c)} + O_2 \qquad (4)$$

DISCUSSION

Horseradish peroxidase was used in the present pulse-radiolysis experiments because reactions of this enzyme with hydrated electron or with superoxide anion, O_2^-, can easily be demonstrated. The rate constant for the direct formation of the oxycompound in the reaction

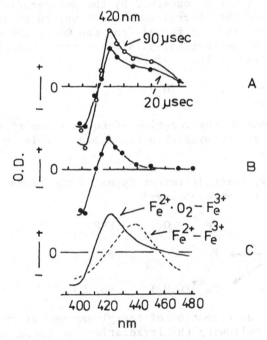

Fig. 4. A. The difference spectra obtained at 20 and 90 μsec after the pulse. The conditions were the same as those of Fig.3.
B. The difference spectrum between 10 and 200 μsec after the pulse.
C. The difference spectra of the ferrous minus ferric state (dotted line) and oxyform minus ferric state (solid line). All the spectra were normalized.

between ferric state and O_2^- (Equ. 5) can be estimated to be $k \sim 10^8 M^{-1} sec^{-1}$.

$$Fe^{3+} + O_2^- \longrightarrow Fe^{2+} \cdot O_2 \tag{5}$$

The alternative pathways depicted by Equ. (6) and (7) can be excluded because in both cases the reaction between oxygen and the ferrous state of the enzyme is the rate-determining step whose rate constant k of $4 \times 10^4 M^{-1} sec^{-1}$ (Tamura and Yamazaki, 1972) is much slower than the results derived from the curves of Fig. 3.

$$Fe^{3+} + O_2^- \longrightarrow Fe^{2+} + O_2, \text{ then } Fe^{2+} + O_2 \longrightarrow Fe^{2+} \cdot O_2 \tag{6}$$

$$Fe^{3+} + e_{aq}^- \longrightarrow Fe^{2+}, \text{ then } Fe^{2+} + O_2 \longrightarrow Fe^{2+} \cdot O_2 \tag{7}$$

With methemoglobin and metmyoglobin, however, the formation of oxycompound could not be observed by the pulse-radiolysis study. The appearance of the 'ferryl compound' instead of oxyform suggests that hydrogen peroxide is formed from the O_2^- by the disproportionation. It is noted that Eq. 5 is the reverse reaction of the well known autoxidation of the oxyform.

$$Fe^{2+} \cdot O_2 \longrightarrow Fe^{3+} + (O_2^-) \tag{8}$$

Thus, the absence of the reaction of Eq. 5 shows that both methemoglobin and metmyoglobin cannotplay a role in protecting against O_2^-.

In summary, three different types of reactions between O_2^- and ferrihemoglobins were observed.

$$Fe^{3+} + O_2^- \begin{cases} Fe^{2+} \cdot O_2 & \text{HRP} \\ Fe^{2+} & \text{cyt. c} \\ Fe^{4+}(H_2O_2) & \text{Hb, Mb} \end{cases}$$

Experiments on the formation of ferrylcompound of myoglobin in cardiac tissue following the irradiation are being planned in our laboratory.

ACKNOWLEDGEMENT

Most of the work was carried out at the Hahn-Meitner-Institute under the support of Prof. W. Schnabel to whom the authors express their many thanks.

REFERENCES

Chase, W.J. and Hunt, J.W.   (1975)   J. Phys. Chem. 79, 1975.

Land, E.J. and Swallow, A.J.   (1971)   Arch.Biochem.Biophys. 145, 365.

McCord, J.M. and Fridovich, I.   (1968)   J. Biol. Chem. 243, 5753.

McCord, J.M., Keele, B.B. and Friedovich, I.   (1971)   Proc. Nat. Acad. Sci. USA 68, 1024.

Seki, H., Ilan, Y.A., Ilan, Y. and Stein, G.   (1976)   Biochim. Biophys. Acta. 440, 573.

Shannon, L.M., Kay, E. and Lew, J.W.   (1966)   J. Biol. Chem. 241, 2166.

Tamura, M. and Yamazaki, I.   (1972)   J. Biochem. 71, 311.

Wilting, I., Raap, A., Braams, R., DeBruin, S.H., Rollema, H.S. and Janssen, L.H.   (1974)   J. Biol. Chem. 249, 6325.

LITERATURE

OXYGEN DIFFUSION CONSTANTS D AND K OF TUMOR TISSUE

(DS-CARCINOSARCOMA) AND THEIR TEMPERATURE DEPENDENCE

J. Grote, R. Süsskind and P. Vaupel

Institute of Physiology, University of Mainz

65 Mainz, FRG

To understand more thoroughly the tumor O_2 supply conditions, knowledge of O_2 diffusivity in tumor tissue is required. Since exact measurements of the O_2 diffusion constants of tumor tissue have not been carried out to date, previous investigations of tumor O_2 supply had to employ estimated values (6 - 8, 10). The results of these studies are in part contradictory.

Our study was designed to accurately determine the O_2 diffusion coefficient D and Krogh's O_2 diffusion constant K of DS-Carcinosarcoma tissue. This was accomplished through use of a method for investigating O_2 diffusion in tissue slices described by THEWS (1, 2,9). The investigations were conducted at temperatures between 20 and 40°C in order to describe the temperature dependence of tumor O_2 diffusivity. As test material, DS-Carcinosarcoma tissue, grown isolated in rat kidneys (11, 12), was used. The tumors were removed on the 9-11th day after implantation into the normal kidney parenchyma before tissue necrosis had set in. Because the presence of hemoglobin in the tissue slices as well as the O_2 consumption of the cells lead to an error in the measurements, immediately prior to removal, the tumor tissue was cleared of blood by means of a perfusion with Haemaccel[R] and tissue respiration was stopped by adding KCN to the perfusion solution. The possibility of very small quantities of blood remaining in lacuna-like tumor blood vessels must be considered. Under these conditions the determination of the O_2 diffusion constant K is not influenced, while the determination of the O_2 diffusion coefficient D must lead to values lower than the true constant. The results indicate, however, that this situation does not occur. Macroscopically visible tissue necrosis was not found in any of the kidney tumors investigated. Tissue water content was determined by freeze drying.

Results and Discussion

The mean values for the O_2 diffusion coefficient D and Krogh's O_2 diffusion constant K obtained from 73 investigations of O_2 diffusion in DS-Carcinosarcoma tissue conducted under temperature conditions of 20, 30, 37, and 40°C are summarized in Tab. 1. The mean weight of the tumors studied was 5.9 g and the mean water content 82.1 g%.

<u>Table 1:</u> O_2 diffusion constants D and K for tumor tissue (DS-Carcinosarcoma) under temperature conditions of 20, 30, 37, and 40°C. Values presented are mean values $\pm$ SEM.

Temp. (°C)	n	O_2 diffusion coefficient D $\cdot$ 10^5 ($\frac{cm^2}{s}$)	n	Krogh's O_2 diffusion constant K $\cdot$ 10^5 ($\frac{mlO_2}{cm \cdot min \cdot atm}$)
20	10	1.25 $\pm$ 0.05	19	1.7 $\pm$ 0.07
30	21	1.55 $\pm$ 0.06	18	1.75 $\pm$ 0.05
37	22	1.75 $\pm$ 0.04	20	1.9 $\pm$ 0.08
40	20	1.9 $\pm$ 0.07	16	2.0 $\pm$ 0.1

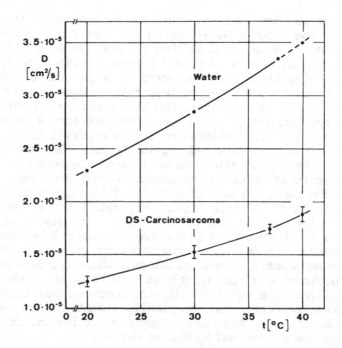

Fig. 1: Effect of temperature on O_2 diffusion coefficient D of tumor tissue (DS-Carcinosarcoma) and water (1) within the range 20-40° C.

The temperature dependence of the studied O_2 diffusion constants of
DS-Carcinosarcoma tissue is presented in Figs. 1 and 2. In the
temperature range 20 - 40 °C temperature variations in tumor tissue
cause changes in the O_2 diffusion coefficient D of 2.0 - 2.5 %/°C
and in Krogh's O_2 diffusion constant K of 0.5 - 1.5 %/°C.

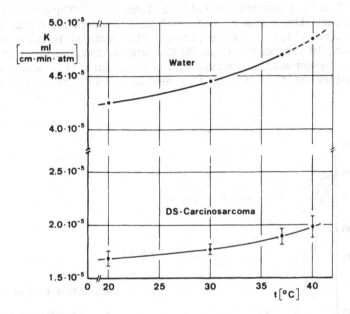

Fig. 2: Effect of temperature on Krogh's O_2 diffusion constant K of
tumor tissue (DS-Carcinosarcoma) and water (1) within the range 20-
40°C.

The determined values for the O_2 diffusion constants D and K
of DS-Carcinosarcoma tissue at 37°C fit well into the series of
comparable data obtained for different tissues (1-3, 9). When water
content is similar, there is no essential difference between the O_2
diffusion constants of normal tissues on the one hand and the
corresponding constants of tumor tissue on the other hand. The
demonstrated insufficient O_2 supply for DS-Carcinosarcoma of the
rat kidney cannot thus be attributed to extremely low O_2 diffusion
constants as postulated by RIEGER (6). The investigations of
THOMLINSON and GRAY (10) and TANNOCK (7,8) on the O_2 diffusion in
tumor tissue employed for the O_2 diffusion coefficient D values
which are larger than those measured under the temperature
conditions of 37°C.

The temperature dependence of the O_2 diffusion constants of DS-Carcinosarcoma tissue corresponds closely to findings for water, for muscle tissue and for pulmonary tissue (1,4).

A theoretical analysis of O_2 diffusion in DS-Carcinosarcoma tissue for the conditions of 37°C led to O_2 tension profiles at the venous end of the Krogh tissue cylinder model (5) as presented in Fig. 3. Here, the determined Krogh's O_2 diffusion constant K together with a O_2 consumption rate of 1.85 mlO_2/100g·min and the intercapillary distances as measured in comparable tumors of DS-Carcinosarcoma (11,13) were employed. The mean O_2 tension of the venous tumor blood measured in DS-Carcinosarcoma in the rat kidney during arterial normoxia and normocapnia (11) was used for the O_2 tension at the wall of the venous end of the tumor capillary.

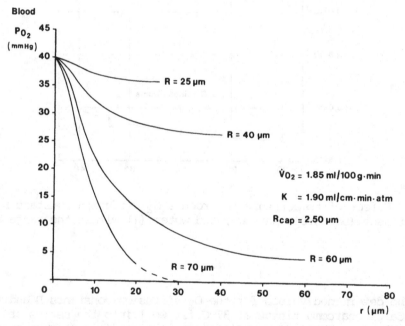

Fig. 3: Radial O_2 tension profiles at the venous end of the Krogh tissue cylinder in DS-Carcinosarcoma for the conditions of a cylinder radius of 25, 40, 60, and 70 µm.

As can be seen in Fig. 3, critical O_2 supply conditions in the DS-Carcinosarcoma tissue are to be expected when the distance between neighbouring capillaries exceeds 120 - 130 µm and the radius of the tissue cylinder correspondingly increases above 65 - 70 µm. Although the Krogh tissue cylinder model only approximately describes the actual O_2 supply conditions in the tumor tissue and although the employed value for the blood O_2 tension at the venous end of the capillary appears to be higher than the actual value; this result corresponds closely with the fact that necrosis could not be detected in DS-Carcinosarcoma tissue where the intercapillary distances did not exceed 130 µm. In older tumors presenting necrosis, the largest intercapillary distances attained values far in excess of this critical O_2 diffusion distance (11,13). The determined value for the tissue cylinder radius by which critical O_2 supply conditions are to be expected is comparable to results of TANNOCK (7,8) and VAUPEL (11).

References

1. GROTE, J.   (1967) Pflügers Arch. ges. Physiol. 295, 245-254
2. GROTE, J., THEWS, G. (1962) Pflügers Arch. ges. Physiol. 276, 142 - 165
3. KAWASHIRO, T., NÜSSE, W., SCHEID, P. (1975) Pflügers Arch. 359, 231 - 251
4. KROGH, A. (1918/19) J. Physiol.(Lond.) 52, 391 - 408
5. KROGH, A. (1918/19) J. Physiol.(Lond.) 52, 409 - 415
6. RIEGER, F. (1974) Arch. Geschwulstforsch. 43, 52 - 55
7. TANNOCK, I. F. (1968) Brit. J. Cancer 22, 258 - 273
8. TANNOCK, I. F. (1972) Brit. J. Radiol. 45, 515 - 524
9. THEWS, G. (1960) Pflügers Arch. ges. Physiol. 271, 227 - 244
10. THOMLINSON, R. N., GRAY, L. H. (1955) Brit. J. Cancer 9, 539 - 549
11. VAUPEL, P., (1974) In: Funktionsanalyse biologischer Systeme (ed. Thews, G.), vol. 1, Wiesbaden: Steiner
12. VAUPEL, P. (1976) Pflügers Arch. 361, 201 - 204
13. VAUPEL, P., GÜNTHER, H., GROTE, J., AUMÜLLER, G. (1971) Z. ges. exp. Med. 156, 283 - 294

INTRACAPILLARY HbO$_2$ SATURATION IN TUMOR TISSUE OF DS-CARCINOSARCOMA DURING NORMOXIA[+]

P. Vaupel[*], W.A. Grunewald[**], R. Manz[**], W. Sowa[**]

[*]Institute of Physiology, University of Mainz, FRG.

[**]Institute of Physiology, University of Regensburg, FRG.

Investigations on solid tumor tissue have shown that O$_2$ uptake by cancer cells depends largely on the supply conditions. The absence of sufficient neovascularization and a general rarefaction of the terminal vascular bed during tumor growth as well as reduced and inhomogeneous blood flow due to vascular stasis in neoplastic tissue prevent normal functions of the terminal vascular bed. In some areas of the tumor circulating blood is not visible despite the intactness of vessels. Stasis occurs since lacuna-like, sinusoidal and cystiform blood vessels cannot be drained completely because 'tissue-pressure' due to continuous cell proliferation can prevent efficient circulation. Thrombosis follows and results in the occlusion of the vessels (Vaupel 1977). In addition, a considerable portion of tumor blood crosses arterio-venous shunts instead of circulating through the vascular network. Furthermore, the acidic environment in tumors may reduce red cell deformability during tumor passage.

Due to these modifications a sharp increase in vascular flow resistance follows and an imbalance between O$_2$ consumption and O$_2$ supply to cancer cells results. The O$_2$ consumption is limited by the O$_2$ supply due to the modifications mentioned above, to the diminished O$_2$ transport capacity during progressive tumor anemia and to the impaired O$_2$ release by the acidosis-induced rigid red blood cells.

Mean tissue PO$_2$ values measured polarographically drop precipitously at the same time. PO$_2$ histograms reveal frequency distributions shifted to the left. The experiments provide

[+] Supported by Deutsche Forschungsgemeinschaft.

evidence that hypoxia and even anoxia occur in neoplastic tissue as the tumor increases in size, since critical diffusion ranges for O_2 are exceeded (Vauper 1974;   Vaupel et al, 1976;   Vaupel 1977).

According to these results one would expect that in solid tumor tissue very low intracapillary HbO_2 saturations predominate. In order to verify this assumption, HbO_2 saturations in tumor 'capillaries' were determined using the cryophotometric micromethod of Grunewald and Lübbers (1975,1976).

Methods:

Ascites cells of DS- carcinosarcoma were implanted into the left kidney of 10 rats where they were maintained 'tissue-isolated' (Gullino and Grantham, 1961;   Vaupel et al, 1971).   After an average of 10 - 13 days the infiltrating and destructively growing tumor cells completely replaced the kidney tissue, and the tumor mass was connected to the host by only a single artery and vein.   Afterwards the animals were anaesthetized by i.p. injection of pentobarbital sodium (30 mg/kg), and the left carotid artery was cannulated in order to record the arterial pressure using a Statham pressure transducer.   The abdomen was opened by an incision and the former left renal vein was exposed (further details concerning the operative procedure, blood flow measurements and monitoring of the mean arterial blood pressure have been described elsewhere (Vaupel et al, 1971;   Vaupel, 1974).

In order to determine HbO_2 saturations in tumor 'capillaries', the cryophotometric micromethod of Grunewald and Lübbers (1975, 1976) was employed.   Tissue samples (2 mm in diameter) of the tumors were removed in situ with precooled liquid nitrogen tongs. At a temperature of -60°C tissue slices of 15 μm were prepared from the frozen tissue specimens.   Intravascular Hb absorption spectra were measured within vessels of 3-8 μm diameter in the frozen tissue slices at -100°C in a vacuum isolated microscope cryostat and converted into intracapillary HbO_2 saturation values using a multicomponent analysis (Lübbers and Wodick, 1969). Immediately prior to removal of tumor tissue specimens, arterial and tumor-venous blood samples were taken in order to measure the parameters of respiratory gas exchange.   Details concerning the intracapillary cryophotometric micromethod have been presented elsewhere (Grunewald and Lübbers, 1975, 1976).

Results:

The results of 453 measurements on 13 tissue specimens from 10 tumors revealed that 67% of the measured values were in the range of 0-20% HbO_2 saturation (see Fig. 1).   53% of these values were in the range of 0 to 10% HbO_2 saturation.   Only 8% of the measured values exceeded 50% saturation when the animals were allowed to breathe air.   The mean HbO_2 saturation value during normoxia attained 17.4% saturation.   The median was 8.7% saturation, the modal class being 0-5% saturation.   The relevant parameters of

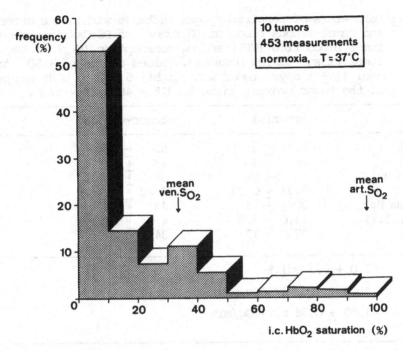

Fig. 1: Frequency distribution of measured HbO$_2$ saturation values
in tumor capillaries on 13 tissue specimens from 10 tumors.
Arrows indicate the mean arterial HbO$_2$ saturation and the
mean tumor-venous HbO$_2$ saturation, respectively.

respiratory gas exchange under these conditions are listed in Table I.
The frequency distributions of HbO$_2$ saturation values in various
tumors at the same stage of growth are presented in Fig. 2. It is
obvious that great   individual differences exist, the
smallest tumors showing relatively high HbO$_2$ saturations which are
found in superficial areas where   sufficient vascularization still
exists. In general, the frequency distributions are shifted to
lower HbO$_2$ saturation values and limited in variability. A mono-
tonous pattern of very low HbO$_2$ saturations predominates in the
tumor tissue of DS- Carcinosarcoma. Only relatively slight regional
differences can be found. In Fig. 3 the results of measurements at
different locations in the same tumor are shown. The measurements
demonstrate that very low HbO$_2$ saturations predominate in central
portions of the tumor tissue (upper panel), whereas great regional
differences can be found only in superficial, well supplied areas
(lower panel; this tissue specimen was taken from a depth of about
1 - 3 mm where the oxygenation of the red blood cells is not
affected by the diffusion of atmospheric oxygen into the tissue).

Table I: Parameters of respiratory gas exchange within the arterial
and tumor-venous blood of 10 tumors of DS-Carcinosarcoma,
tumor blood flow (TBF) and O_2 consumption ($\dot{V}_{O_2}$) of the
tumor tissue during normoxia. Values are means + SD. Tumor
age: 11 + 1 days, tumor wet weight: 5 + 2 g, body weight
of the tumor bearing animals: 318 + 46 g, T = 37°C.

	arterial	tumor-venous
Hb (g%)	8.1 + 3.5	8.2 + 3.1
Hct (%)	26 + 10	28 + 10
pO_2 (mm Hg)	98 + 29	36 + 9
pH	7.31 + 0.22	7.22 + 0.17
pCO_2 (mm Hg)	30 + 21	43 + 21
$[O_2]$ (vol.%)	11.0 + 4.8	4.0 + 3.9
S_{O_2} (%)	97 + 17	34 + 23

AvD_{O_2} = 7.0 + 2.3 vol.%

TBF = 15.0 + 7.0 ml/100g/min

V_{O_2} = 1.05 + 0,54 ml/100g/min

Theoretical analysis of the intercapillary pO_2 distribution in tumor tissue:

In order to calculate the intercapillary pO_2 distribution on
the basis of the measured intracapillary HbO_2 saturation values
the O_2 supply to tumor tissue is simulated by a digital model, the
tumor capillaries running rectilinear and parallel to one another.
The arterial inflows, and thus the blood flow direction within
tumor capillaries can thereby be varied as desired (GRUNEWALD and
SOWA, 1977). The following microcirculatory units were chosen to
represent the different variation possibilities:
1. concurrent capillary flow,
2. countercurrent capillary blood flow,
3. partial concurrent or countercurrent capillary blood flow, and
4. spirally arranged arterial inflows and venous outflows,
   shifted against one another by half the length of tumor
   capillaries (helix structure).
The occurrence of these four microcirculatory units was assumed to
be equal.

After simulating the intracapillary HbO_2 saturation values
obtained by the cryophotometric micromethod by means of the
various models, an intracapillary pO_2 (i.c. pO_2) frequency

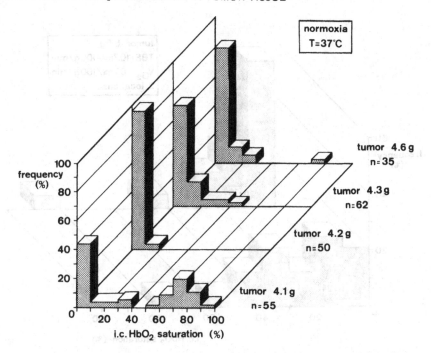

Fig. 2: Frequency distributions of HbO₂ saturation values in
various malignant tumors at the same stage of growth.

distribution can be calculated considering the O_2 dissociation
curve of Sprague- Dawley rats (BORK et al., 1975) as well as the
intracapillary pH alterations of the tumor blood during tissue
passage (see Fig. 4). On the basis of this i.c. pO_2 frequency
distribution, the tissue pO_2 values (tpO_2) in the intercapillary
regions can be computed using the parameters of respiratory gas
exchange and the data of morphometric analysis of the tumor
vascularization (see Table II).

The computation of the intercapillary pO_2 frequency distribution using the listed parameters shows that the frequency
distributions of the different microcirculatory units differ only
very slightly. For this reason the four frequency distributions
are averaged arithmetically and grouped into classes of 5 mm Hg.
In Fig. 5, the computed pO_2 histogram for the tumors having a mean
wet weight of 5.0 g is contrasted with a frequency distribution of
polarographically measured tpO_2 values in a tumor weighing 4.8 g
(measurements of tissue pO_2 values using gold- microelectrodes
see VAUPEL, 1974, 1977, VAUPEL et al., 1976). Comparison of the
polarographically measured histogram with the frequency distribution of tissue pO_2 values computed from the intracapillary
HbO₂ saturation values correspond sufficiently.

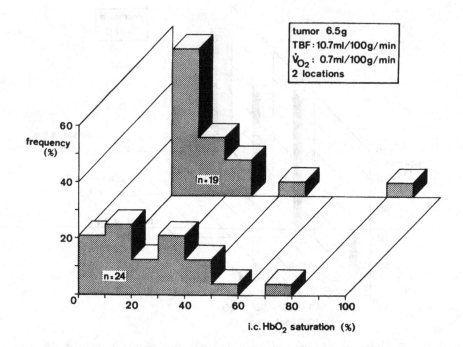

Fig. 3: Frequency distributions of HbO$_2$ saturation values at
different locations in the same tumor. Upper panel:
central portion of the tumor tissue; lower panel: superficial area with sufficient vascularization still existing.

Table II: Parameters of respiratory gas exchange and data of
morphometric analysis of tumor vascularization employed
for computing the intercapillary pO$_2$ distribution in
tumor tissue.

intercapillary distances	60 – 100 μm
length of tumor capillaries	62 – 120 μm
diameter of tumor capillaries	10 μm
arterial pO$_2$	98 mm Hg
venous pO$_2$ (effective)	6 mm Hg
shunt perfusion	30 %
pH	7.20
O$_2$ uptake	1.85 ml/100g/min
Hb concentration	8.15 g/100 ml
KROGH's diffusion constant	1.9 ml/cm · min · atm

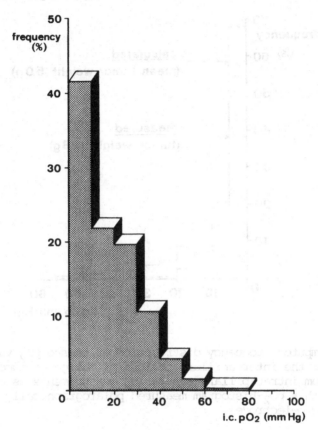

<u>Fig. 4</u>: Frequency distribution of computed intracapillary pO$_2$
values (i.c. pO$_2$). The computed data are derived from
intracapillary HbO$_2$ saturation values measured
cryophotometrically.

Summary:

The measurements of the intravascular HbO$_2$ saturation in tumor
capillaries using the cryophotometric micromethod reveal that very
low HbO$_2$ saturation values predominate in malignant tumors. Under
normoxic conditions only 8 % of the measured values exceed 50 %
saturation. 53 % of the intracapillary HbO$_2$ saturation values are
in the range of 0 - 10 % HbO$_2$ saturation. Great regional differences are seldom and can be found only in areas where a sufficient
vascularization still exists.

Taking into account the data of morphometric analysis of
tumor vascularization and the parameters of respiratory gas exchange, the measured frequency distribution of HbO$_2$ saturation

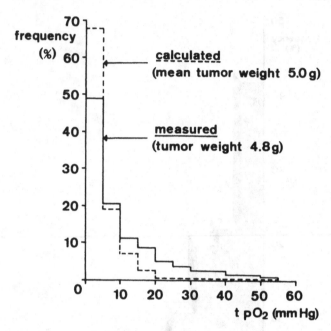

Fig. 5: Computed frequency distribution of tissue pO_2 values (tpO_2)
for the intercapillary regions of malignant tumors derived
from intracapillary saturation measurements as compared
with a pO_2-histogram measured polarographically using gold-
microelectrodes.

values in tumor capillaries is simulated by means of different
three-dimensional capillary structures. On the basis of these microcirculatory units, tissue pO_2 values are computed in the intercapillary regions. As a result of these calculations it can be
stated that the computed data derived from intracapillary HbO_2
saturations are in sufficient agreement with pO_2 values measured
polarographically using gold- microelectrodes.

References:

BORK, R., VAUPEL, P., THEWS, G.: Atemgas-pH-Nomogramme für das
        Rattenblut bei 37° C. Anaesthesist 24, 84 - 90 (1975)

GRUNEWALD, W. A., LÜBBERS, D. W.: Die Bestimmung der intra-
        capillären HbO$_2$-Sättigung mit einer kryo-mikrophoto-
        metrischen Methode angewandt am Myokard des Kaninchens.
        Pflügers Arch. 353, 255 - 273 (1975)

GRUNEWALD, W. A., LÜBBERS, D. W.: Cryomicrophotometry: A method for analyzing the intracapillary HbO₂ saturation of organs under different O₂ supply conditions. In: Oxygen transport to tissue - II. Eds.: Grote, J., Reneau, D., Thews, G.; New York, London: Plenum Press 1976

GRUNEWALD, W. A., SOWA, W.: Capillary structures and O₂ supply to tissue. Rev. Physiol. Biochem. Pharmacol. 77, 149 - 209 (1977)

GULLINO, P. M., GRANTHAM, F. H.: Studies on the exchange of fluids between host and tumor. I. A method for growing "tissue - isolated" tumors in laboratory animals. J. Nat. Cancer Inst. 27, 679 - 693 (1961)

LÜBBERS, D. W., WODICK, R.: The examination of multicomponent systems in biological materials by means of a rapid scanning photometer. Appl. Optics 8, 1055 - 1062 (1969)

VAUPEL, P.: Atemgaswechsel und Glucosestoffwechsel von Implantations-tumoren (DS-Carcinosarkom) in vivo. Wiesbaden: Steiner 1974

VAUPEL, P.: Hypoxia in neoplastic tissue. Microvasc. Res. 13, 399 - 408 (1977)

VAUPEL, P., GÜNTHER, H., GROTE, J., AUMÜLLER, G.: Atemgaswechsel und Glucosestoffwechsel von Tumoren (DS-Carcinosarkom) in vivo. I. Experimentelle Untersuchungen der ver-sorgungsbestimmenden Parameter. Z. ges. exp. Med. 156, 283 - 294 (1971)

VAUPEL, P., THEWS, G., WENDLING, P.: Kritische Sauerstoff- und Glucoseversorgung maligner Tumoren. Dtsch. med. Wschr. 101, 1810 - 1816 (1976)

OXYGEN LEVELS IN TUMORS IN C3H MICE DURING HYPERTHERMIA:

INITIAL DATA

H. W. Puffer, B. R. Wilson, and N. E. Warner

Department of Pathology, School of Medicine
University of Southern California
Los Angeles, California 90033, U.S.A.

Induction of tumor regression by hyperthermia has been reported since the late 19th century (Coley, 1893, Warren, 1935, Crile, 1962, and Pettigrew, 1975). These reports have generated renewed interest in the application of hyperthermia to cancer therapy. There seems little doubt that hyperthermia can increase damage to malignant cells without inducing unacceptable damage to normal tissue. However, the mechanism by which hyperthermia achieves these results remains unknown. It is known that oxygen levels in tumor tissue differs from that in normal tissue (Puffer, et al., 1976, and Vaupel, 1977). This study was undertaken to demonstrate whether changes in oxygen level occured in experimental mammary tumors in C3H mice during hyperthermia.

Materials and Methods

Female C3H mice were used throughout this study. This strain spontaneously develops a congenic type of RNA virus-induced mammary tumor with an incidence of approximately 90%. Once the tumors become palpable they increase rapidly in size. Tumors used in this study were approximately 0.5 cm dia. Prior to observation of oxygen levels, each mouse was anesthetized with pentobarbital 60 mg/kg, injected intraperitoneally. The hair was removed from skin overlying and a small incision made at the base of the tumor to permit placement of the electrode in the viable outer layer of neoplastic tissue. Placement of the electrode was observed using epi-illumination from an American Optical fiber optic illuminator model 11-80 and a Leitz stereomicroscope equipped with 3.8X objective and 12.5X eyepiece. Blood pO_2 in tissue was measured using Teflon encased, Hydron

coated, gold tissue electrodes (International Biophysics Corporation). A separate Ag/AgCl$_2$ anode was used as the reference electrode. The gold electrode was the cathode in the polarographic
system. Each gold tissue electrode was calibrated in isotonic
saline solution and the temperature coefficient was determined
for each temperature used during hyperthermia. The electrodes
were used in conjunction with a differential oxygen analyzer
model 630-001 supplied by International Biophysics Corporation.
Oxygen levels were expressed in mm Hg.

Whole-body hyperthermia was induced by submersing each mouse in a
constant temperature waterbath model MW-1120A-1 supplied by Blue
M Electric Company. Oxygen level was measured in tumor tissue of
each mouse at 37.5°C (body temperature), 38°, 39°, 40° and 42°C.
The mouse was allowed to equilibrate with the water bath for 30
minutes at each temperature before measurement of oxygen.

Results

The results are shown in Figure 1. Recorded oxygen levels in tumors ranged from 16-85 mm Hg. The data are divided into two
groups. In Group 1, oxygen levels ranged from 52 mm Hg at 37.5°C
to 85 mm Hg at 42°C. Calculation of the slope for Group 1 yields
a rate of 7.3 mm Hg of O$_2$/°C. In Group 2, oxygen levels ranged
from 16-20 mm Hg; the slope for this group was approximately 0.
Baseline O$_2$ levels varied significantly between the two groups.
The baseline O$_2$ level for Group 1 was 52 mm Hg and for Group 2
was 19 mm Hg.

Discussion

It is apparent from the results in Group 1 that oxygen levels in
tissue in experimental mammary tumors in C3H mice increase as temperature is increased during experimental hyperthermia by whole
body immersion in a water bath. Results with Group 2 animals do
not support these findings. The lack of adequate baseline oxygen
levels as well as failure of hyperthermia to effect oxygen levels
in this latter group is puzzling. Some difficulty was encountered
in the use of pentobarbital for anesthesia. We feel that this
may explain the lack of adequate oxygen levels in Group 2.

During preparation of this manuscript it was called to our attention that concurrent studies by Bicher and Vaupel (personal communications) have resulted in findings similar to that which we
are reporting for Group 1 animals. Bicher found that oxygen
levels in brain tissue increased as temperature increased during
hyperthermia induced by microwave irradiation. Vaupel found that
oxygen consumption in DS-carcinosarcoma tumors in rat kidneys at
39.5°C was significantly greater than at 37°C. These findings

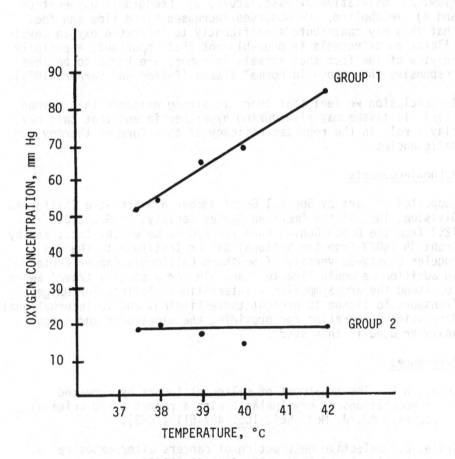

Figure 1.   Oxygen Levels in Tumor Tissue in Experimental Mammary Tumors in C3H Mice Undergoing Hyperthermia.

suggest that oxygen levels may play a role in the therapeutic efficacy of hyperthermia in the treatment of malignancies.

It is not clear what mechanisms may account for enhancement of oxygen levels during hyperthermia. Several factors may be involved and include the following: 1) increased rate of blood flow, 2) dilatation of vasculature, 3) hemoglobin oxygenation and 4) metabolism. We observed increased blood flow and feel that this may contribute significantly to increased oxygen levels. Dilatation of vessels is probably not that important, especially in view of the fact that vessels in tumors are known to be less responsive than those in normal tissue (Puffer and Warner, 1975).

In conclusion we feel that there is strong evidence that oxygen levels in tissue may rise during hyperthermia and that this may play a role in the reported efficacy of this form of therapy for malignancies.

Acknowledgements

Supported in part by Special Grant Number 626 from the California Division, Inc. of the American Cancer Society; by Grant DRG 1252 from the Damon Runyon Fund for Cancer Research, Inc.; and by Grant CA 14089 from the National Cancer Institute to the Los Angeles County-University of Southern California Cancer Center. In addition we would like to thank NIH for a partial travel award to attend the 3rd Symposium - International Society for Oxygen Transport to Tissue to present these findings and to International Biophysics Corporation for providing the electrodes and oxygen-analyzer used in this study.

References

Coley, W.B. The treatment of malignant tumors by repeated innoculations of erysipelas: with a report of 10 original cases. Am. J. Med. Sci. 105: 487-511 (1893).

Crile, G. Selective destruction of cancers after exposure to heat. Annals of Surg. 156: 404-407 (1962).

Pettigrew, R.T. Cancer therapy by whole body heating. International Symposium on Hyperthermia and Radiation, Washington, D.C., April 28-30 (1975).

Puffer, H.W., Warner, N.E., Schaeffer, L.D., Wetts, R.W., and Bradbury, M. Preliminary observations of oxygen levels in microcirculation of tumors in C3H mice in: Oxygen transport to tissue - II Eds. Grote, Reneau, and Thews, Adv. in Exp. Med. Biol. 75: 605-610 (1976).

Puffer, H.W., and Warner, N.E. Response of the microvasculature in experimental mammary tumors in C3H mice to selected vasoactive drugs. Proc. West. Pharmacol. Soc. 18: 133-135 (1975).

Vaupel, P. Hypoxia in neoplastic tissue. Microvascular Research. 13: 399-408 (1977).

Warren, S.L. Preliminary study of the effect of artificial fever upon hopeless tumor cases. Am. J. Roentgenology. 33: 75-87 (1935).

PREVENTION OF IONIZING RADIATION-INDUCED LIVER MICROCIRCULATION

CHANGES BY THE USE OF FLOW IMPROVERS

Bicher, H.I., D'Agostino, L., *Doss, L.L., Kaufman, N.
and Amigone, J.
Department of Radiation Medicine
Roswell Park Memorial Institute, *Ellis Fischel Hospital
Buffalo, New York and Columbia, Missouri, U.S.A.

Ionizing radiation causes destruction of mammalian tissue by two mechanisms (Kinzie et al, 1972): (1) inhibition of the proliferative capacity of rapidly dividing cells, and (2) irreversible damage to elements of the microcirculatory system. Organs such as liver, kidney and brain, not characterized by rapidly proliferating cells, exhibit a relatively pronounced radiosensitivity in spite of a very slow rate of cellular turnover. The radiosensitivity of the microcirculation could provide the reason for the radiosensitivity of the entire organ or tissue.

In previous publications (Bicher 1969; Bicher 1970; Bicher and Beemer 1967; Bicher and Beemer 1970; Bicher et al 1976) we have described microcirculatory damage to parenchymatous organs induced by intravascular platelet and red cell aggregation, as these processes tend to interfere with tissue oxygenation. The objective of this investigation was to elucidate the effects of flow improvers in preventing the above mentioned microcirculation damage.

METHODS AND MATERIALS

Oxygen Determination

The oxygen electrodes used in this series of experiments consist of a teflon coated Pt/Ir wire (120μ diam, 2 cm. long) that is advanced into the liver tissue through the lumen of a 26 G needle after the needle has penetrated the liver capsule. The electrode is allowed to 'float' with the normal respiratory excursions of the liver and is attached to the instrumentation by a 40μ gold wire which will not hamper this movement. The

electrodes are coated with Rhoplex AC 35 (a water carrying, highly
adhesive, oxygen pervious material, obtained from Rohm & Haas,
Philadelphia, Pa.) which is used to delay the 'poisoning' of the
electrode surface by protein electrophoresis.

The reference electrode is composed of a pure silver wire
coated with AgCl and encased in an agar-KCl bridge.   This reference
electrode is placed inside the abdominal cavity or subcutaneously.

The electrode is calibrated in vitro prior to insertion into
the liver using the technique developed by Silver (1963).

Reoxygenation times (RT, period of time required for TpO_2 to
return to its original level after a 60 sec. period of anoxic anoxia)
was determined as previously described (Bicher et al, 1971).   This
measurement has been found to be a good indicative parameter of the
ability of the microcirculation to deliver oxygen to tissue.   In
each experiment 5 determinations were made at 4 different locations
in the liver.

Determination of Platelet Adhesiveness and Aggregation

Photoelectric Method Platelet Aggregation.   The photoelectric
method to determine platelet aggregation in platelet-rich plasma
(PRP) has been described by Born (9).   Continuously stirred PRP is
placed in a transilluminated test tube, and the amount of light
transmitted is measured with a photocell.   Platelet aggregation is
induced by ADP.   The aggregates change the amount of light
received by the photocell, and can thereby be recorded.

To determine platelet reactivity to ADP in animals pre or post
irradiation, a dose response curve is carried out for a sample
from each animal, using increasing ADP concentrations from 0.1 μg
per milliliter to 10 μg per milliliter.   The concentration is
determined that gives a response midway between a minimum response
and a maximal response.   The ADP concentration giving a 'mean'
response is thus determined.

Rolling tube platelet adhesiveness test.   In this method,
previously described (Bicher 1970), a volume of 1.0 ml/tube of anti-
coagulated blood is placed in a series of 10 ml, 1.2 cm. diameter
non-siliconized test tubes containing no drug (control), and varying
concentrations of ADP and ATP.   These concentrations are less than,
equal to and more than the amount of ADP required for aggregation
as determined by the photoelectric method.   After rotation,
adhesive platelets adhere to the wall of the test tube, and those
remaining in the blood are counted.   The differences between the
platelet counts of the control and the tubes containing ADP
indicates percentages of platelet adhesiveness caused by the drug.

The effective dose of ADP to induce an increase in platelet adhesiveness is thus determined. A change in the required amount of ADP to induce this effect in an individual post irradiation animal as compared to that animal's pre irradiation requirement indicates the increase in platelet adhesiveness.

Histology, Liver Function Tests and Blood Chemistries

Tissue samples were obtained, fixed and stained using standard histological techniques for microscopy studies. Liver function tests and blood chemistries performed include LDH, SGOT, Bilirubin, Total Colloid, Serum Albumin, Total Serum Protein, A/G Ratio, Prothrombin Time, Alkaline Phosphatase, HCT, WBC, RBC, BUN, Na^+ and K^+. Standard methodology was used in all tests. Blood samples were drawn before and after radiation treatments for testing.

General Experimental Plan

The experiments were performed on female beagle dogs, 1 year old when treatment was started. All determinations were performed prior to radiation, and then again two weeks after radiation treatments ended.

Whole liver radiation was performed through parallel lateral opposing posts after radiological confirmation of field localization. The animals were treated to 4600 rads delivered in 23 treatments, total treatment time being 35 days. A Co^{60} Teletherapy HVL 11 pb unit at a SSD of 50 cm was used. Low molecular weight dextran (Rheomacrodex, Pharmacia), was infused (1 gm/kg), before each dose of radiation.

When determining TpO_2 the animals were under barbiturate anesthesia with tracheal intubation and cannulation of the femoral artery and vein. Blood samples for in vitro studies were obtained from the cannulated femoral vein. All surgical procedures were done under sterile conditions.

RESULTS AND DISCUSSION

At the present time, pre and post irradiation studies have been completed in 9 beagles.

Reoxygenation times: It was found that the normal reoxygenation time in the dog's liver is 2.14 minutes. This figure is larger than the RT in the cat's brain (0.68 min.) as previously reported (Bicher et al, 1975). Irradiation with the administration of Rheomacrodex provided an average reoxygenation time of 1.60 minutes. This is significantly less than the 3.26 minute reoxygenation time obtained after irradiation without the drug (see Fig. 1 and 2).

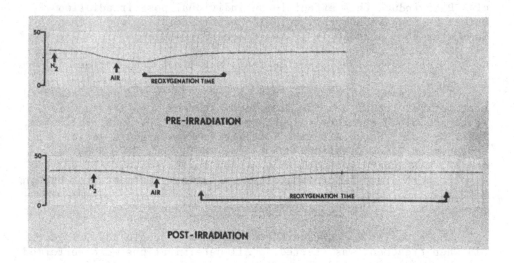

Fig. 1. Beagle Reoxygenation Times

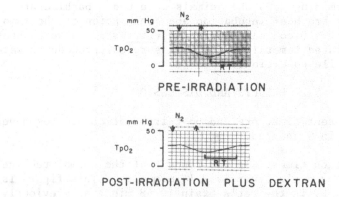

Fig. 2. Liver Reoxygenation Times

Platelet aggregation and adhesiveness: Both platelet aggregation and adhesiveness increased markedly after irradiation. The mean effective dose (MED) of ADP to induce 50% aggregation or adhesiveness decreased from 2.5 μg/ml to 1.3 μg/ml. The adhesiveness induced by the pre-irradiation MED was 46.6% before irradiation, 86.2% after irradiation, and 54.9% with irradiation plus Rheomacrodex (see Fig. 3).

Histology and Blood Chemistry: No significant changes were observed histologically in pre and post irradiation sections. The only significant changes in blood chemistry were: a decrease in albumin from 3.11 mg% to 1.91 mg% in 6 out of 9 dogs; alkaline phosphatase increased from 56 to 300 units in 7 out of 9 dogs. All other parameters were unchanged. The above parameters were unchanged in the group of beagles infused with dextran.

Recently Ingold (1965) demonstrated that the liver is not radio-resistant to ionizing radiation, but rather one of the more sensitive tissues. Ingold's studies indicated that the sensitivity of the liver is comparable to that of bone marrow, lymphoid tissue, germinal tissue and the kidneys.

Kinzie et al (1972) reported results which indicate that the prevention of intravascular coagulation (by heparinization) greatly reduced the impact of radiation upon the livers of rats. The

	NORMAL	RADIATED	RADIATED + RHEOMACRODEX
AVERAGE REOXYGENATION TIMES (MIN)	2.14	3.26	1.60
PLATELET AGGREGATION (MED DOSE ADP µg)	2.30	1.30	1.75
PLATELET ADHESIVENESS (%PLATELETS ADHERING)	46.6	86.2	54.9

Fig. 3. Microcirculation Changes-Liver Irradiation

apparent mechanism is the prevention of ischemia atrophic changes which would follow the post irradiation obliteration of the micro-circulation. Although these results would seem to indicate a principle of considerable importance in clinical oncology, additional information is not available.

The present studies clearly demonstrate that ionizing radiation induces profound deleterious changes in the ability of the microcirculation to oxygenate liver tissue. This is indicated by the marked prolongation in reoxygenation time, a sensitive para-meter of this function (Bicher 1974). The microcirculation disturbance could probably be mediated by increased intravascular blood cell aggregation, as indicated by the increase in platelet aggregation and adhesiveness hereby reported. The formentioned degenerative changes in the liver microcirculation can be prevented with the low molecular weight dextran, Rheomacrodex.

SUMMARY

Platelet aggregation and adhesiveness, as well as TpO_2 responses to hypoxia were measured as microcirculation parameters in beagle dogs subject to Co^{60} ionizing radiation to a dose of 4600 rads in 5 weeks. Simultaneously, changes in blood chemistry and coagulation were also determined. Marked changes in all studied parameters in the post radiation period lead to the conclusion that the radiation liver damage, which is at least in part mediated through microcirculation disturbances, can be prevented with the flow improver, Rheomacrodex.

This work has been supported by NIH Grant #CA 21033 01.

REFERENCES

1. Bicher, H.I. Prevention of sludge induced myocardial damage by an anti-adhesive drug. Bibl. Anat., 10: 202, 1969.

2. Bicher, H.I. Anti-adhesive drugs in thrombosis. Throm. et Diath. Haem., Suppl. 42: 197, 1970.

3. Bicher, H.I. Brain oxygen autoregulation: A protective re-flex to hypoxia. Microvasc. Res. 8: 291-313, 1974.

4. Bicher, H.I., Beemer, A.M. Induction of ischemic myocardial damage by red cell aggregation (sludge) in the rabbit. J. Atherosclerosis Res., 7: 409, 1967.

5. Bicher, H.I., Beemer, A.M. Prevention by an anti-adhesive drug of thrombosis caused by blood cell aggregation. Angiol., 21: 413, 1970.

6. Bicher, H.I., Dalrymple, G.V., Ashbrook, D., Smith, R., Harris, D. Effect of ionizing radiation on liver microcirculation oxygenation. 2nd International Conference for Society of Oxygen Transport to Tissue, 1976.

7. Bicher, H.I., Bruley, D.F., Reneau, D.D., Knisely, M.H. Effect of microcirculation changes on brain tissue oxygenation. J. Physiol. 217: 689-707, 1971.

8. Bicher, H.I., Marvin, P., Hunt, D.H., Bruley, D.F. Autonomic and pharmacological control of oxygen autoregulation mechanisms in brain tissue. ISOTT Symposium, Mainz, Germany, 1975. (To be published by Plenum Press, New York).

9. Born, G.V. Quantitative investigations into aggregation of blood platelets. J. Physiol. 162: 67, 1962.

10. Ingold, J., Reed, G., Kaplan, M.D. Am. J. Roentgenology 93: 200, 1965.

11. Kinzie, J., Studer, R.K., Perez, B., Potcher, E.J. Non-cytokinetic radiation injury; anticoagulants as radioprotective agents in experimental radiation hepatitis. Science 175: 1481, 1972.

12. Rubin, P. The radiographic expression of radiotherapeutic injury. An overview. Seminars in Roentgenology 1: 5, 1974.

13. Silver, I.A. A simple microelectrode for measuring pO_2 in gas or fluid. Med. Electron. Biol. Eng. 1: 547, 1963.

DISCUSSION OF PAPERS IN SESSION 5

CHAIRMEN: DR. I.A. SILVER and DR. H.I. BICHER

PAPER BY: DR. BICHER

Dr. Metzger: 1. What is the temperature dependance of your PO_2 sensor?

2. If you destroy autoregulation during hyperthermia, is the process reversible?

Dr. Bicher: The temperature dependance of the sensor is small enough to be negligible.

2. The autoregulation seems to be able to recover. We don't have hard evidence on this and don't know what time factor is involved.

PAPER BY: DR. GROTE et al

Dr. Goldstick: Your diffusion coefficients in water appear to be about 20% higher than those measured by myself and others. How did you measure D and K?

Dr. Grote: Our O_2 diffusion constants determined for water at 37°C (Pflügers Arch. (1967) 295, 245)correspond to the findings of various other groups, e.g. Hummielblau (1964). Diffusion of dissolved gases in liquids. Chem. Rev. 64, 527-550; Vaupel (1976) Pflügers Arch. 361, 201. The diffusion constants D and K of tumor tissue were determined by means of an experimental device for investigating O_2 diffusion in biological media as described by Thews (1960) Pflügers Arch. 271, 227.

391

PAPER BY: DR. VAUPEL et al

<u>Dr. Metzger:</u> Did you calculate the size of the hypoxic zone?

2. Are Michaelis-Menten kinetics included in the calculation of your tissue PO_2 values?

<u>Dr. Vaupel:</u> No, we didn't calculate the size of the hypoxic zone but we did include Michaelis-Menten kinetics in our calculation of PO_2.

Oxygen Transport in Disease

OXYGEN TRANSPORT IMPAIRMENT INDUCED BY THREE MAJOR CARDIOVASCULAR RISK FACTORS

Jørn Ditzel, Per Jæger and Jørn Dyerberg

Department of Medicine and Clinical Chemistry
Aalborg Regional Hospital, Denmark

INTRODUCTION

This paper is a report on examinations of the oxygen affinity of hemoglobin in subjects with diabetes mellitus, with hyperlipoproteinemia and in smokers, indicating the presence of a fluctuating disorder in the oxygen unloading from the erythrocytes in these conditions known as cardiovascular risk factors. Since these states may also be associated with an impairment in microcirculatory flow, the synergistic effects of these factors may lead to serious consequences for the oxygenation of tissues, particularly in those with a poor microcirculation as in the arterial walls.

MATERIAL AND METHODS

Forty diabetic children were examined twice in the morning, firstly during fasting prior to insulin and secondly in the forenoon 3-4 hours after a light breakfast and the usual morning insulin dose. None of the children showed signs of retinopathy or nephropathy and none were acidotic. None of the children were smokers and none had anemia. Forty-four subjects with hyperlipoproteinemia were examined in the morning after 12 hrs. of complete fasting. According to lipoprotein electrophoresis 4 had Type I hyperlipoproteinemia (HLP), 7 Type IIA, 15 Type IIB, 11 Type IV and 7 Type V HLP. Nineteen smokers (defined as healthy subjects who smoked more than 8 cigarettes per day) and 24 non-

smokers; all normal weighted men, twenty years of age
was selected from a military establishment in a blind
study. The individuals were examined in the fasting
state in the morning.

Arterial blood samples were drawn anerobically and
assayed within 15 min. for pH, pO_2, pCO_2, standard bicarbonate in a BMS-3 blood gas system (Radiometer A/S,
Copenhagen). Venous blood was collected into heparinized syringes and measurements of oxyhemoglobin dissociation curves (ODC) were performed at 37° and constant pCO_2 of 40 mmHg by the dissociation curve analyzer (Type DCA-1, Radiometer A/S, Copenhagen) providing a continuous print out of the ODC of whole blood
(Duvelleroy et al, 1970).

	P_{50} act pH mmHg
Diabetic children (before insulin)	27.1 ± 1.2
Diabetic children (after insulin)	25.9 ± 1.1*
Healthy children (n = 30)	27.3 ± 1.3
Subjects with HLP Type I	19.9 ± 1.6*
Subjects with HLP Type IIA	25.8 ± 1.2
Subjects with HLP Type IIB	24.8 ± 1.8**
Subjects with HLP Type IV	24.3 ± 2.0*
Subjects with HLP Type V	20.4 ± 1.6*
Healthy adults (n = 24)	26.2 ± 0.8
Smokers	25.2 ± 1.4*
Non-smokers	26.2 ± 0.8

Statistical differences between the respective group
and its control group

 *: p-value below 0.001
**: p-value below 0.005

Table 1: Mean values and SD of P_{50} act pH in diabetic
children before and after insulin, in subjects with
various types of hyperlipoproteinemias, and in smokers
as compared to control groups.

RESULTS

Diabetes mellitus

As can be seen from Table 1 the mean value of P_{50} of the ODC in the diabetic children was not significantly different from that of healthy children when studied in the morning prior to insulin, but was significantly lowered 3-4 hours after the insulin administration (p < 0.001).

Hyperlipoproteinemia

Likewise it can be seen from Table 1 that the mean P_{50} of the ODC was significantly lowered in Type I, IIB, IV and V HLP. P_{50} was particularly low in Type I and V HLP (p < 0.001).

Smoking

P_{50} was significantly lower among the 19 smokers as compared to that of the 24 non-smokers (p < 0.001).

DISCUSSION

The abnormality in oxygen transport in diabetes mellitus, in hyperlipoproteinemia and by smoking is related to biochemical aberrations in the blood, but the underlying mechanism leading to the increased oxygen affinity of hemoglobin differs in these conditions. Although juvenile diabetics have a significantly higher content of red cell 2,3-diphosphoglycerate (2,3-DPG) (Ditzel, 1976b) which should have shifted the ODC to the right a significantly increased oxygen affinity was observed postprandially following insulin. The mechanism for this phenomenon may be that diabetics, like smokers, form larger proportions of a hemoglobin (Hb A_{Ic}) with increased affinity for oxygen. The transient decrease in the oxygen unloading capacity induced by insulin administration may at least in part be due to a lowering of the red cell 2,3-DPG content in response to decreases in the concentration of plasma inorganic phosphate (Ditzel, 1976a). The investigation of the P_{50} in different types of hyperlipoproteinemia indicates that high concentrations of chylomicrons and very low density lipoprotein, i.e. the triglyceride-rich lipoproteins adversely affect the ODC (Ditzel and Dyerberg, 1977a,b). Previously a highly significant negative relationship has been found between the logaritmic value of the triglyceride concentration and the P_{50} (Ditzel,

1976a). In smokers carbon monoxide in red cells will
form carboxyhemoglobin (COHb). The presence of even a
small percentage of COHb will shift the ODC of the remaining normal hemoglobin to the left so that it less
readily releases its oxygen to the tissues.

A relatively new discovery in our understanding of
atherogenesis is the realization that probably the most
important cell in the development of the atherosclerotic
lesion is the myointimal cell (Wissler, 1974; Ross and
Glomset, 1976). If cell cultures of arterial smooth
muscle cells taken from human aorta are exposed to hypoxia, these cells will proliferate and the amount of
lipids being taken up by the cells will increase, while
lipid degradation will decrease. The cells may be quickly transformed into foam cells. Thus the arterial smooth
muscle cells seem highly sensitive to hypoxia (Robertson, 1968; Albers and Biermann, 1976). If a similar
hypoxia occurs in the aortic wall in vivo it is reasonable to assume that the atherosclerotic process would
be accelerated. Our investigations have shown that diabetes, hyperlipoproteinemia and smoking all impair red
cell oxygen unloading. Other investigations have shown
that these conditions also affect the microcirculatory
hemoglobin flow. A decrease in the calibers of the
microvessels have been observed in diabetes following
insulin (Ditzel, 1962, 1975), an impairment in the microcirculation has been demonstrated in hyperchylo-
micronemia (Kroeger, 1970; Kroeger et al, 1970), and a
nicotine induced arteriolar constriction occurs following smoking (Asano and Brånemark, 1970). If severe
atherosclerosis is considered to be a consequence of a
complex metabolic process, particularly involving disturbed lipid degradation in the arterial wall, these
defects in the oxygen supply may be of major importance
in atherogenesis.

SUMMARY

Diabetes mellitus, hyperlipoproteinemia and smoking are
three epidemiological factors known to increase the
incidense of atherosclerosis. It is demonstrated that
these factors all may lead to an impairment in oxygen
transport by changing the position of the oxyhemoglobin
dissociation curve and by affecting the microcirculatory hemoglobin flow.

REFERENCES

Albers, J.J. and Biermann, E.L. (1976) Biochem. Biophys. Acta. 424, 422.

Asano, M. and Brånemark, P.-J. (1970) In 'Advances in Microcirculation' p.125 (ed. Harders, H.) S. Karger, Basel, New York.

Ditzel, J. (1962) The conjuctival vessels in diabetes mellitus. Scand. Univ. Books, Munksgaard, Copenhagen.

Ditzel, J. (1975) In 'The Eye and Systemic Disease' p. 179, (ed. Mausolf, I.A.) C.V. Mosby Co., St. Louis.

Ditzel, J. (1976a) In 'Microcirculation 2. Transport Mechanisms Disease States' p. 88 (eds. Grayson, J. and Zingg, W.) Plenum Press, New York.

Ditzel, J. (1976b) Diabetes 25, 832.

Ditzel, J. and Dyerberg, J. (1977a) Metabolism 25, 14.

Ditzel, J. and Dyerberg, J. (1977b) J. Lab. Clin. Med. 89, 573.

Duvelleroy, M.A., Buckles, R.C., Rosenkaimer, S., Tung, C. and Laver, M.A. (1970) J. Appl. Physiol. 28, 227.

Kroeger, A. (1970) In 'Advances in Microcirculation' p.1 (ed. Harders, H.). S. Karger, Basel, New York.

Kroeger, A., Heiseg, N. and Harders, H. (1970) Klin. Wochenschr. 48, 723.

Robertson, A.L. Jr. (1968) Progr. Biochem. Pharmacol. 4, 305.

Ross, R. and Glomset, J.A. (1976) New Engl. J. Med. 295, 269.

Wissler, R.W. (1974) In 'The myocardium: Failure and Infarction' p. 155 (ed. Braunwald, W.). H.P. Publishing Co., New York.

OXYGEN PRESSURE VALUES IN THE ISCHEMIC MUSCLE TISSUE
OF PATIENTS WITH CHRONIC OCCLUSIVE ARTERIAL DISEASE

A. M. Ehrly and W. Schroeder

Dept. of Internal Medicine, Div. of Angiology
and Dept. of Physiology, Div. of Applied
Physiology, Medical School, University of
Frankfurt/Main, West Germany

Introduction

Quantification of muscle tissue blood flow is difficult, since morphological findings like stenoses or occlusions, or blood flow measurements like venous occlusive
plethysmography often do not reflect the clinical symptoms
of chronic occlusive arterial diseases. This is reasonable, since in a great number of elderly people without
clinical symptoms arteriosclerotic changes can be found
angiographically. Venous occlusive plethysmography on the
other hand is a measure for the overall blood flow, but is
not a suitable method for determination of nutritional
capillary muscle blood flow.

Therefore, in 1974 we started measurements of tissue
oxygen pressure (pO_2) directly in the ischemic muscle of
patients with chronic occlusive arterial diseases (1).
Technical problems have been overcome by the development
of membrane-coated micro-Pt electrodes with tip diameters
of 1-3 µm by Kunze and Lübbers and Cater and Silver (2,3).
We now use this method for pathophysiological studies, as
a diagnostic criterion as well as for quantification of
the benefit of therapeutic measures.

Material and Methods

Measurements were performed in the tibialis anterior
muscles of recumbent human subjects with fixed legs.
After local anesthesia of the skin (0.5 ml Scandicain 1%)

in the middle of the lower limb, 15 mm lateral to the
tibia, a plastic injection needle (Braunule 1R) was inserted through the skin. After removal of the steel
needle, the plastic cover was cut 2 mm above the surface
of the skin and the pO_2 electrode was introduced 10 mm
into the muscle tissue. Immediately after insertion the
electrode was withdrawn by a motor-driven micromanipulator
at a speed of 33 μm/sec through the muscle tissue. The
recording of the pO_2 in the muscle tissue was started
simultaneously with the movement of the electrode (4).
From these records the pO_2 values can be determined. The
mean pO_2 ($\overline{pO_2}$) is the arithmetic mean of all individual
pO_2 values collected from the records.

The micro-Pt electrodes had tip diameters of 2-4 μm
and were coated with polystyrole.

Results

A) In former investigations, the following results were
   obtained:

   1) Muscle tissue pO_2 of patients with chronic occlusive
      arterial diseases (severe intermittent claudication)
      was found to be 13.3 ± 5.4 Torr and thus statisti-
      cally significantly lower than in a control group
      of healthy volunteers (27.2 ± 4.4) (1).

   2) Muscle pO_2 at various sites in the lower leg muscles
      of patients with chronic proximal arterial occlu-
      sions or stenoses are not statistically significant-
      ly different (5).

   3) When patients under steady state conditions of their
      disease remain untreated, there are no statistically
      significant differences between mean $\overline{pO_2}$ values re-
      corded at intervals of 1-2 hours or 3-6 weeks (5).

B) The method is now more and more used as an additional
   diagnostic and therapeutic measure. I will give you
   some examples:

   1) A patient with a pain-free walking distance of 30 m
      showed a pathological oscillogram, reduced ankle
      pressure values, and occlusions and stenoses in the
      angiogram. Conservative treatment was ineffective
      and an arterial reconstruction, i.e. bypass, was
      planned. Muscle tissue pO_2 was 18 Torr, which is
      not severely abnormal, so that his vascular disease

did not seem to be the limiting factor for his pains. Thereafter, a more exact examination of the patient detected discrete symptoms of a neuritis. The neuritis was treated and the patient then had a pain-free walking distance now due to muscle ischemia of 150 m.

2) Beneficial therapeutic effects can be clarified with this method. So after ileo-femoral bypass in patients with chronic arterial occlusions an increase in muscle tissue pO_2 (e.g., 12.8 Torr before, 30.2 Torr after operation) was found.

3) When Ancrod (Arwin®), a viper venom preparation, is used as drug treatment in patients with COAD, there is a statistically significant increase in muscle pO_2 during a 14 day treatment (from 12.1 ± 3.8 Torr to 22.9 ± 11.2 Torr) (p < 0.005). Ancrod is a rheologically active substance which lowers fibrinogen concentration, thereby decreasing blood viscosity and red cell aggregation. The pO_2 results (6,7) agree very well with the clinical effects and with the pain-free walking distance in spite of the fact that this drug does not influence ankle pressure values or change the stenoses or occlusions itself (8).

4) Now another drug (Pentoxifylline) was investigated and showed a statistically significant increase in pO_2 values during the first 2 hours after intravenous injection of 200 mg Pentoxifylline in patients with chronic occlusive arterial disease (severe intermittent claudication). The initial low values (10.8 ± 3.2 Torr) raised to 16.3 ± 5.5 Torr, 20.0 ± 6.2 Torr, 18.5 ± 8.8 Torr after 30, 60, and 120 min after the end of the injection (n = 9, p < 0.0025, 0.001, and 0.05) (Fig. 1). In another series of experiments muscle tissue pO_2 in 7 patients with severe intermittent claudication could be increased even by continuous infusion of small doses of Pentoxifylline (20 mg within 30 min); initial pO_2 values 7.6 ± 1.9 Torr; immediately after the infusion 10.9 ± 3.8 Torr (p < 0.01). Pentoxifylline is also a rheologically active drug which improves the red cell deformability by increasing ATP concentration in the erythrocytes. Thereby, the red cells may now pass more easily through narrow capillaries (9,10).

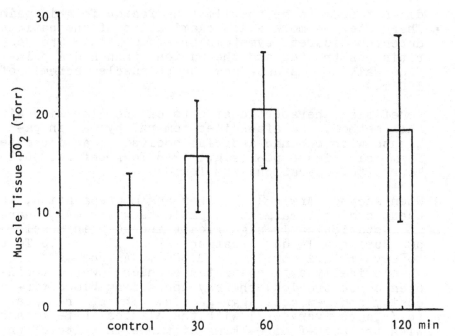

Fig. 1. Muscle tissue pO_2 in 9 patients with intermittent
claudication before and after intravenous injection of 200 mg Pentoxifylline.

Summary

     For 3 years tissue oxygen pressure has been measured
directly in the ischemic muscle of patients with chronic
arterial diseases. The measuring procedure is nearly
atraumatic, without pain, has no side effects, and can be
performed or repeated within 10 min. The present method
gives objective and quantitative data for oxygen supply to
tissue and therefore muscular microcirculation. It can be
used for pathophysiological studies, for diagnostic purposes, and for objective quantification of therapeutic
measures.

References

1) Ehrly, A.M., H.-J. Köhler, W. Schroeder, and R. Müller:
   Sauerstoffdruckwerte im ischämischen Muskelgewebe von
   Patienten mit chronischen peripheren arteriellen Ver-
   schlusskrankheiten. Klin. Wschr. 53, 687 (1975).

2) Kunze, K., and D.W. Lübbers: Die Messung des lokalen Sauerstoffverbrauches von Organen in situ mit der Platinelektrode. Plügers Arch. ges. Physiol. 247, 74 (1961).

3) Cater, D.B., and I.A. Silver: Electrodes and microelectrodes used in biology. In: Reference electrodes (eds. J.J.G. Ives and J.G. Janz), Academic Press, New York, 1961.

4) Schroeder, W., and W. Rathscheck: Investigation of the influence of acetylcholine on the distribution of capillary flow in the skeletal muscle of the Guinea pig by recording of the pO_2 in the muscle tissue. Plügers Arch. 345, 335 (1973).

5) Ehrly, A.M., and W. Schroeder: Sauerstoffdruckwerte im ischämischen Muskelgewebe von Patienten mit chronischen arteriellen Verschlusserkrankungen. Verh. Dtsch. Ges. Kreislaufforschg. 42, 380 (1976).

6) Ehrly, A.M., H.-J. Köhler, W. Schroeder, and R. Müller: Messung des lokalen Sauerstoffdruckes im ischämischen Muskelgewebe: Eine objektive Methode zur Beurteilung des Ischämiegrades bei Patienten mit peripherer arterieller Verschlusskrankheit. Jtg. Dt. Ges. f. Angiologie Köln 1975. In: E. Zeitler (Herausgeb.) Hypertonie G. Witzstrock-Verlag 1975, S. 201.

7) Ehrly, A.M., and W. Schroeder: Oxygen pressure in ischemic muscle tissue of patients with chronic occlusive arterial diseases. Angiology 28, 101 (1977).

8) Ehrly, A.M.: Therapy of occlusive arterial diseases with Ancrod (Arwin®), Artery 2, 98 (1976).

9) Ehrly, A.M.: The effect of pentoxifylline on the flow properties of hyperosmolar blood. IRCS Med. Science 3, 467 (1975).

10) Ehrly, A.M., and H.-J. Köhler: Altered deformability of erythrocytes from patients with chronic occlusive arterial disease. VASA 5, 319 (1976).

COMPUTER SIMULATION OF THE HUMAN THORACIC AORTA TO EVALUATE THE POSSIBLE ROLE OF SMOKING IN ATHEROGENESIS

Gary Schneiderman and Thomas K. Goldstick

Chemical Engineering Department
Northwestern University
Evanston, Illinois 60201   USA

An impaired oxygen delivery to arterial wall tissue has been implicated as one factor in the atherogenic process (Getz et al., 1969). The arterial wall has a precarious O_2 supply because its luminal side is completely avascular. Thus, the only supply of O_2 to the avascular tissue zone is by diffusion over rather long distances from two sources: (1) the arterial blood flowing within the lumen and (2) the blood flowing within the vasa vasorum, the micro-circulation of the outer portion of the wall.

Several possible mechanisms linking smoking and atherogenesis have been proposed and these were recently reviewed by Topping (1977). All of these are based on the increased levels of CO and nicotine found in smokers. The proposed mechanisms include impaired arterial wall metabolism and increased permeability caused by either CO-induced hypoxia as suggested by Astrup (1973) or direct CO-poisoning of mural cells. Astrup (1973) has found abnormally high levels of CO in the blood of smokers who inhale, up to 20% COHb. Partial saturation of blood with CO is known to result in an effective anemia and a leftward shift of the oxygen-hemoglobin equilibrium curve (OHEC) (Roughton and Darling, 1944). In Figure 1 this leftward shift is illustrated by comparison with the OHEC for a comparable simple reduction in O_2 carrying capacity (change in hematocrit only). The CO-induced effects impair the ability of the blood to carry and transport O_2 to the tissues of the body. Although it is unquestionable that CO inhalation produces a reduction in the O_2 supply to the tissue of the arterial wall, the degree of this effect is not known. This prevents a quantitative assessment of this particular mechanism. As a complementary step to experimental measurements, we have used a previously developed (Schneiderman et al., 1974a; Schneiderman, 1975) computer simulation of the O_2 supply to

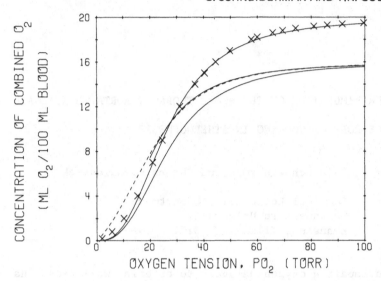

FIGURE 1: The OHEC: The symbols are from Severinghaus'(1966)
standard curve for humans. The line with these points is the normal OHEC used here. The dashed line is the calculated OHEC with
20% COHb and the line with it is the fitted OHEC used here. The
third line is the normal OHEC with 20% anemia.

the arterial wall to assess the extent of CO-induced mural hypoxia,
under various conditions, in a normal adult who suddenly increases
his blood CO level.

METHODS

The computer simulation consisted of numerical solutions of
appropriate partial differential equations describing arterial wall
O_2 transport including: (1) the composite, inhomogeneous nature of
the tissue O_2 transport and O_2 consumption parameters, (2) the O_2
supply from the vasa vasorum, (3) the O_2 diffusion and convection
(both dissolved and nonlinearly combined in the red cells) within
the lumen, and (4) a separate transport resistance for the thin,
cell-free plasma layer adjacent to the endothelial surface. The
effects of Womersley-type blood flow pulsatility and wall distensi-
bility have previously been considered (Schneiderman, 1975; Goldstick et al., 1977) and found to be negligible. The transmural PO_2
profiles predicted by this model are consistent with those measured
experimentally with microelectrodes (Schneiderman et al., 1974b;
Schneiderman, 1975). The effect of CO on the PO_2 profiles was found
by accounting for the effect of CO-induced arterial hypoxemia caused
by normal pulmonary shunting and the effect of CO-mediated shifts in

the OHEC acting on the O_2 transport systems of both the lumen and the vasa vasorum.

To carry out the simulation, it was necessary to know the OHEC, arterial PO_2 (P_a), and mean PO_2 of the outer, vascularized arterial wall tissue (P_o), all for different levels of blood CO. The normal (CO-free) OHEC was described by the Hill equation (Figure 1) which has two parameters: n, which determines the shape of the OHEC and P_{50}, the PO_2 at which one-half of all available hemoglobin sites are combined with O_2. In the presence of CO, the implicit computational method of Roughton and Darling (1944) was used and, to obtain an analytical functional relationship, a least squares fit of the calculated data ($22 < PO_2 < 100$ torr) was obtained using a model of the form of the Hill equation. For COHb levels of 0, 5, 10, and 20%, the calculated values of n and P_{50} are given in Table I.

Blood flowing through the pulmonary capillaries becomes equilibrated at the alveolar PO_2. However, a fraction of the systemic venous blood, α, is shunted and does not participate in the exchange process. This venous blood mixes with the oxygenated pulmonary blood to yield arterial blood at a PO_2 less than alveolar PO_2. By means of an O_2 balance, Brody and Coburn (1969) have shown that the final P_a will be decreased by shifts of the OHEC caused by CO in the blood. Such alterations in P_a have been observed experimentally in our laboratory and by others (e.g. Brody and Coburn, 1969). The P_a used in our simulation was calculated with their method using a normal P_a of 85 torr and an $\alpha = 0.06$ (which represents the sum of anatomical and physiological shunting).

The O_2 supply from the vasa vasorum was modelled by assuming a uniform PO_2 level (P_o) at the outer border of the avascular tissue annulus. For convenience, this value was assumed to be the same as the mixed venous PO_2 (P_v) as suggested by Forster (1970). P_v was computed by assuming an arteriovenous concentration difference of 5 vol %. To bound the actual physiological situation, two limiting cases for P_o were considered. Either the microcirculation of the arterial wall was considered to exhibit a perfect autoregulatory mechanism, thus maintaining P_o constant at the normal (CO-free) P_v, or no autoregulation, making P_o equal to the actual P_v.

RESULTS AND DISCUSSION

Transmural PO_2 profiles were calculated using O_2 transport parameters appropriate for a normal adult human thoracic aorta (Schneiderman, 1975). The effects of CO-induced mural hypoxia were calculated for individuals who smoked 20 to 40 cigarettes per day, corresponding to 5 to 10% COHb, and 40 to 60 cigarettes per day, corresponding to 10 to 20% COHb. Figure 2 shows an example of transmural PO_2 profiles calculated across the luminal blood flowing

G. SCHNEIDERMAN AND T.K. GOLDSTICK

TABLE I: Calculated values for the minimum tissue PO_2 (P_m) and endothelial PO_2 (P_e) for: Case I: P_a, P_o unchanged. Pulmonary shunt and vasa vasorum autoregulate for CO and maintain constant PO_2. Case II: Blood flow unchanged. P_a and P_o reduced by the effects of CO. Case III: Intimal thickening. Same as Case II but with intimal thickening of 25μ (to a total of 75μ). (The numbers in parentheses are the changes from Case I, 0% COHb. All PO_2's are in torr.)

		0% COHb	5	10	20
P_{50}		26.6	25.0 (1.6)	23.7 (2.9)	21.2 (5.4)
n		2.70	2.61	2.58	2.51
Cases II, III:	P_a	85.0	83.6 (1.4)	81.8 (3.2)	77.8 (7.2)
	P_o	37.4	34.8 (2.6)	32.3 (5.1)	27.5 (9.9)
Case I:	P_m	11.2	11.0 (0.2)	10.6 (0.6)	9.9 (1.3)
	P_e	64.7	64.0 (0.7)	63.2 (1.5)	61.5 (3.2)
Case II:	P_m	11.2	8.9 (2.3)	6.5 (4.7)	1.7 (9.5)
	P_e	64.7	62.8 (1.9)	60.6 (4.1)	55.7 (9.0)
Case III:	P_m	6.0 (5.2)	3.7 (7.5)	1.3 (9.9)	anoxic
	P_e	63.6 (1.1)	61.7 (3.0)	59.4 (5.3)	---

near the endothelium and across the adjacent avascular tissue region up to the vascularized portion of the media. The profiles were simulated at 20 cm from the entrance to the arterial segment of interest, but the results were essentially the same at either 10, 20, or 30 cm. The effects of COHb are illustrated in Table I in terms of the values of the minimum tissue PO_2 (P_m) and the PO_2 at the endothelial surface (P_e) which is the driving force for the luminal O_2 supply to the tissue.

In Case I, P_a and P_o were held constant at the normal values of 85.0 and 37.4 torr (no arterial hypoxemia effect and perfect autoregulation by the vasa vasorum). This case shows only the effect of the altered O_2 transport properties in the luminal blood. The effect of up to 20% COHb is small (Table I).

Figure 2 shows the results for Case II in which CO induced both hypoxemia in blood and uncompensated hypoxia in vascularized tissue. In Case II the effects are considerably larger than for Case I

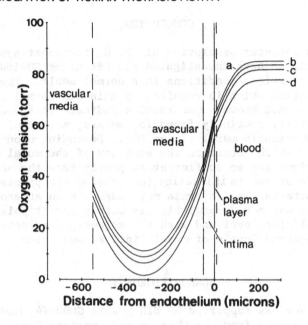

FIGURE 2: Transmural PO_2 profiles for Case II with: a. 0%, b. 5%, c. 10%, and d. 20% COHb.

(Table I). These effects are likely to be serious, especially for an avascular tissue presumed to be normally on the brink of hypoxia. The profiles indicate that it is the mid to inner media which is most likely to suffer hypoxic damage. This result is consistent with actual PO_2 profiles measured across the <u>ex</u> <u>vivo</u> rabbit thoracic aortic wall (Schneiderman et al., 1974b). Also, other investigators have shown that hypoxic damage in humans (Adams and Bayliss, 1969) and in experimental animals occurs in the mid to inner media of the aorta and other arteries.

In Case III, which was calculated for a modest increase in intimal thickness (from 50 to 75μ) with the other parameters from Case II, a level of 20% COHb was found to cause anoxia over a wide region within the inner media. A level of 10% COHb and a 75μ intima resulted in a tissue hypoxia as severe as that found for 20% COHb and a 50μ thick intima (Table I). Depending upon prevailing conditions, including the possible occurence of luminal blood flow disturbance (Schneiderman et al., 1977), even lower blood CO levels may be sufficient to precipitate the so-called vicious cycle of events leading to a more serious hypoxia. The actual mural PO_2 levels depend, in addition, upon changes in other arterial wall parameters which, taken together, determine the adequacy of the mural O_2 supply (Schneiderman, 1975).

CONCLUSION

Using a computer simulation of the O_2 transport system of the
arterial wall, we have investigated the extent of CO-induced mural
hypoxia under various conditions in a normal adult. The level of
mural oxygenation which is required to maintain normal arterial
wall health is not known. Our results indicate that moderate to
high COHb levels, routinely found in smokers, may result in a significant reduction in mural tissue PO_2. Depending upon the many
other factors which determine the adequacy of the mural O_2 supply,
these reductions may be sufficient to precipitate the so-called
vicious cycle of events initiating the atherogenic process. Thus,
CO-induced arterial wall hypoxia may indeed be an atherogenic
factor. This may act synergistically with a direct poisoning by
CO on the cellular level and with the adrenergic effects of nicotine
to cause dangerous levels of mural lipid accumulation.

ACKNOWLEDGEMENTS

This study was supported by NIH grants GM00874, HL01979, and
HL17517, and grants from the Chicago and American Heart Associations,
and Evanston Hospital. We gratefully acknowledge the valuable discussions with C.G. Ellis, H.E. Gutherman, Dr. L. Zuckerman, and
Dr. D.W. Cugell, and the technical assistance of Dr. E.A. Olson.

REFERENCES

Adams, C.W.M., and Bayliss, O.B. (1969) J. Athero. Res., 10, 327.
Astrup, P. (1973) Postgrad. Med. J., 49, 697.
Brody, J.S., and Coburn, R.F. (1969) Science, 164, 1297.
Forster, R. (1970) Ann. NY Acad. Sci., 174, 233.
Getz, G.S., Vesselinovitch, D., and Wissler, R.W. (1969) Am. J.
    Med., 46, 657.
Goldstick, T.K., Schneiderman, G., and Mockros, L.F. (1977) Fed.
    Proc., 36, 513.
Roughton, F.J.W., and Darling, R.C. (1944) Am. J. Physiol., 141, 17.
Schneiderman, G. (1975) Ph.D. Thesis, Northwestern Univ., Evanston.
Schneiderman, G., Goldstick, T.K., and Mockros, L.F. (1974a) Paper
    13d, 67th Ann. Meeting, AIChE, Washington, D.C.
Schneiderman, G., Goldstick, T.K., and Zuckerman, L. (1974b) Proc.
    27th ACEMB, 16, 283.
Schneiderman, G., Olson, E.A., Ellis, C.G., and Goldstick, T.K.
    (1977) Fed. Proc., 36, 513.
Severinghaus, J.W. (1966) J. Appl. Physiol., 21, 1108.
Topping, D.L. (1977) Atherosclerosis, 26, 129.

SYNCHRONOUS TRACER INJECTION FOR O_2 UPTAKE AND CO_2 PRODUCTION MEASUREMENT

J. S. Clark, F. L. Farr, A. H. Bigler, R. Jones,
C. A. Cutler, and E. J. Anderson
Primary Children's Medical Center
320 12th Avenue
Salt Lake City, Utah 84103

Existing methods for measuring O_2 consumption and CO_2 production require either air-tight connections to patients in the form of masks or nose pieces, or the patient is placed in a sealed box for monitoring expired gas volume and concentration.

Many patients, particularly infants and young children, don't tolerate such obtrusive interfacing to the monitoring equipment. The method described in this paper eliminates this requirement.

THEORY

In cases where CO_2 production is measured, alveolar ventilation is calculated using the relationship

$$\dot{V}CO_2 = \dot{V}_A F_A CO_2 \tag{1}$$

where $\dot{V}CO_2$ is CO_2 production, $\dot{V}_A$ is alveolar ventilation, and $F_A CO_2$ is the alveolar CO_2 fraction. Inspired CO_2 is assumed to be zero. O_2 consumption is a little more complicated since the calculation uses the inspired O_2 fraction and both O_2 and CO_2 alveolar fractions. The equation is:

$$\dot{V}O_2 = \dot{V}_A \left(FIO_2 \frac{1 - F_A O_2 - F_A CO_2}{1 - FIO_2} - F_A O_2 \right) \tag{2}$$

where $\dot{V}O_2$ is oxygen consumption, FIO_2 is the inspired oxygen fraction, and FAO_2 is the alveolar oxygen fraction.

Note that both $\dot{V}CO_2$ and $\dot{V}O_2$ are functions of $\dot{V}_A$ and gas

413

concentrations only, and it's the measurement of the $\dot{V}_A$ factor that requires the air-tight seal. The central idea of this new method is to obtain $\dot{V}_A$ without using such a seal. Once this is achieved, $\dot{V}O_2$ and $\dot{V}CO_2$ are obtained easily by knowing the inspired and expired gas fractions.

The alveolar ventilation is measured using helium as a tracer inserted as a bolus into the nostril synchronous with inspiration. The injection takes place early enough in the inspiratory phase so that all the tracer is carried into the alveolar compartment. After several breaths, a steady state condition is reached in which the rate of tracer injection equals the amount of tracer expired and is given by:

$$\dot{V}He = \dot{V}_A \cdot F_A He \qquad (3)$$

where $\dot{V}He$ is the rate of tracer injection (the product of known bolus volume and respiratory rate), and $F_A He$ is the steady state alveolar He fraction which is measured along with the alveolar O_2 and CO_2 gas fractions.

Equation 3 applies strictly to a hypothetical lung in which all alveoli have a common ventilation time constant. In a real lung and to a much greater degree in the diseased lung, a distribution of ventilation time constants exist. The degree to which equation 3 can estimate $\dot{V}_A$ depends therefore on the variance of the time constant distribution and the timing of the bolus injection with the inspiratory phase.

LUNG MODEL

By computer simulation of a lung model in which arbitrary distributions of specific airway conductance, specific compliance, and ventilation/perfusion ratio could be assigned, the associated error in measurement of $\dot{V}_A$, $\dot{V}O_2$, and $\dot{V}CO_2$ was calculated. With this simulation, the effects of varying the time of injection of the helium tracer bolus during inspiration and the time of sampling the expired gas during expiration could be studied and optimized for measurement accuracy.

The first model was designed to estimate the accuracy of measuring $\dot{V}_A$. In this model the distribution of perfusion was not a consideration since there is negligible transfer of helium between blood and gas. The model consisted of a lung of 10 compartments in which specific airway conductance and specific compliance can be arbitrarily assigned or can be distributed as log-normal with respect to lung volume (FRC) with varying mean and standard deviation. In addition, the dead space can be assigned for each compartment, or it can be distributed as a fixed

(specified) fraction of the compartmental FRC. The other parameters to be specified are the breathing frequency and the pleural
pressure amplitude. Pleural pressure was allowed to vary sinu-
oidally and was assumed to change uniformly throughout the lung.
The flow rates to and from the various compartments and their
tidal volumes depend on the individual R's and C's. The fraction
of a bolus of helium which goes to each compartment is just the
fractional flow rate to that compartment at the time the bolus
is injected into the inspired air stream. Alveolar helium concentration can be obtained from this fraction, from lung volume at
FRC, and from tidal volume. It is related to R, C, transpulmonary
pressure, and frequency of breathing. The mixed concentration
during expiration can be calculated from the individual alveolar
concentrations and the individual time-varying flow rates.

In applying this model, we found that the time curve of
expired He can vary markedly, depending on the type and degree of
inhomogeneity and the timing of the bolus injection. In addition,
different patterns apparently characterize R and C maldistribution
and therefore further development and refinement of these methods
may provide a valuable tool for clinical diagnosis. However, the
time curve of expired He concentration appears maximally flat
when the bolus is injected near mid inspiration and therefore,
we consider this timing to be optimal for estimating $\dot{V}_A$.

In the second model, the alveolar concentrations were
assumed to be governed by the individual $\dot{V}_A/\dot{Q}$ ratios, as is the
case for CO_2 and O_2. The alveolar concentrations were taken from
reference (1) as those resulting from a log-normal distribution of
$\dot{V}_A/\dot{Q}$ versus $\dot{Q}$ with mean $\dot{V}_A/\dot{Q} = 0.86$ and log standard deviation =
0.3. In addition, the parameters of model 1 were similarly
incorporated in this model. The test for the accuracy with which
a single sample taken during expiration can represent the mean
expired concentration as defined by equations 1-3, was performed
as follows: During a single exhalation the true amount of gas
expired was calculated by summing over the individual compartments.
This amount was then compared against values obtained using $\dot{V}_A$
and calculations of gas concentration taken at a point 80 percent
of the way through expiration, as recommended by Rahn and Farhi (2).
To reduce bias, the alveolar concentrations were randomly assigned
and the above calculation made 10 times; once for each of 10
shifts in these alveolar concentrations. The error was taken as
the mean of the absolute values of the 10 errors. Using a log-
normally distributed specific airway conductance with a mean of
0.4 and alveolar concentrations for O_2 for the log-normally
distributed $\dot{V}_A/\dot{Q}$ as described above and given in reference (1), the
error is 5 percent when the standard deviation of the log-normal
distribution of specific airway conductance is 60 percent of the
mean specific conductance. The results for CO_2 were almost

identical to O_2. We have tentatively chosen the 5 percent as
an upper limit to our error in estimating F_AO_2. Using equation
3, this gives a worst case error for $\dot{V}O_2$ of 14.5 percent.

EXPERIMENTAL METHODS

The technique used for comparing the STI method for measuring
$\dot{V}O_2$ and $\dot{V}CO_2$ with a standard using an air-tight seal is shown
in figure 1. Two small tubes are shown entering the nostrils of
a test subject, one supplying the helium bolus and the other
supplying the conduit for alveolar gas monitoring by a mass
spectograph. A fast responding thermister (referred to as a
thinnister) is also in a nostril connected to one of the tubes
to provide the timing reference for the bolus injection.

The standard is an O_2 consumption apparatus manufactured
by the Oxford Instrument Company, modified to measure CO_2 production and provide more accuracy by using the mass spectrometer
as the sensor for this instrument. The method employs the
Fick principle, using the differences in inlet and outlet gas
concentrations and flow. Flow was calibrated with a spirometer.
Although the test apparatus was designed to make simultaneous
comparisons, practical difficulties associated with multiplexing
the mass spectrograph and filtering its output forced the STI and

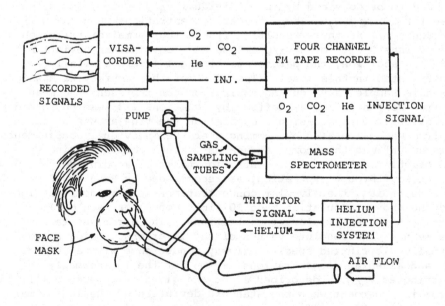

Figure 1: Block diagram of STI and Fick (standard) comparison
experiment

standard measurements to be alternated at few minute intervals.
Efforts were made to maintain the same physiological state for
comparisons; the subject was usually unaware of which method was
being employed.

EXPERIMENTAL RESULTS

Comparisons were made on seven normal adults and one adult
patient with advanced emphysema. Figure 2 shows the results of
a typical normal subject. The emphysema patient had considerable
difficulty tolerating the mask so that test protocol couldn't
be followed. His alveolar ventilation was very different depending on whether the mask was on or off.

Table 1 shows a tabulation of the mean values for the
subjects individually and the means and standard deviations of
all subjects collectively. Note that the data for normals shows
average means which differ insignificantly. Standard deviations
by both methods are about 6 percent.

A significant component of variance of the data appears to
be physiological in origin which points to the necessity of
improving the comparison technique to permit simultaneous
comparisons in order to determine the accuracy of the STI method
in patients with pulmonary disease. However, model predictions

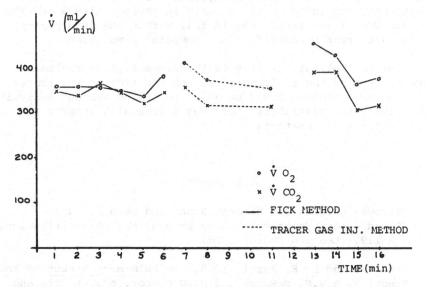

Figure 2: Comparisons of STI with Fick methods with a normal
subject (E.A.)

TABLE 1

	$\overline{\dot{V}O_2}$ (ml/min)			$\overline{\dot{V}CO_2}$ (ml/min)		
SUBJECT	FICK	STI	$\Delta\dot{V}O_2$	FICK	STI	$\Delta\dot{V}CO_2$
C.C.	333	336	-3	303	292	11
G.Y.	367	347	20	305	322	-17
B.J.	346	339	7	293	318	-25
K.L.	337	344	-7	304	305	-1
E.A.	373	375	-2	344	322	22
J.G.	426	426	0	414	396	18
J.M.	274	281	-7	252	249	3
*D.M.	412	449	-37	339	374	-35
AVERAGE (all data)	358±19	362±16	-4	319±18	322±19	-3

*patient with advanced emphysema

based on evidence provided by the flatness of the plateaus of the helium concentration curves during expiration, (which we have collected in several patients including babies, as well as the adult patient with advanced emphysema) indicate that the $\dot{V}_A$ measurement should be quite reliable in these patients and the $\dot{V}O_2$ and $\dot{V}CO_2$ measurements should fall within the 14.5 percent worst case error predicted by the computer simulation.

Future implications of this technique include the measurement of D_{LCO} by the addition of carbon monoxide to the tracer. Also, a new dimension could be added to helium washout analysis for identifying the distribution of lung volume with respect to ventilation time constants.

REFERENCES

1. Olszowka, Albert J., Hermann Rahn, and Leon E. Farhi., "Blood Gases; Hemoglobin, Base Excess, and Maldistribution," 118-119. Lea and Febiger, 1973.

2. Rahn, H. and L. E. Farhi, 1965. In Pulmonary Structure and Function, A.V.S. deReuck and M. O'Connor, eds. Little and Brown, Boston, p. 137.

MEASUREMENTS OF LOCAL OXYGEN PRESSURE IN SKELETAL MUSCLE OF PATIENTS

SUFFERING FROM DISTURBANCES OF ARTERIAL CIRCULATION

J. Hauss[1], K. Schönleben[1], U. Spiegel[1] and M. Kessler[2]

1. Chirurgische Universitäts-Klinik Münster,
   Allgemeinchirurgie, Münster, GFR
2. Max-Planck-Institut für Systemphysiologie,
   Dortmund 1, GFR

AIMS

It is well known that in modern highly developed countries most people, i.e. about 50% die of some kind of disturbance of the arterial circulation (Fig. 1). In 25% the cause of death is cancer and all other possible illnesses cause the death of the remaining part of the population. Until now the methods used for investigation in the clinic and also for the control of therapy are not very accurate, because most of them are based on subjective findings. The main aim of these investigations was therefore to find objective parameters for diagnostic orientation and for controlling the effect of our surgical or pharmacological therapy.

METHODS

The measurements were carried out in 52 patients using the oxygen multiwire surface electrode, which was developed by Kessler and Lübbers (1966). We chose the musculus quadriceps femoris as test organ. A 1-2 cm. wide incision of the skin and the muscular fascia is necessary, 15 cm. above the proximal patella edge. The electrode can be held in place on the muscular surface nearly without any weight.

RESULTS

Figure 1 shows one typical record which compares our preoperative and postoperative measurements. The histogram written before the operation was taken while the patient was resting in bed and it shows a mean value of 31.25 mmHg (Fig. 1).

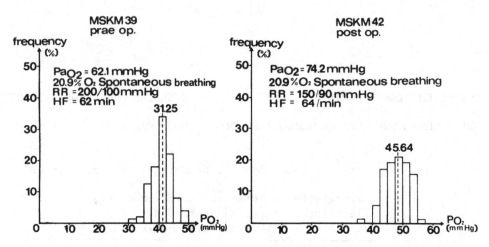

Fig. 1   Preoperative histogram of a patient with severe athero-
          sclerosis (left) and postoperative histogram after bypass-
          operation (right).

The configuration is normal, although significantly shifted to
the right as compared with a histogram of the musculus tibialis
anterior in healthy persons obtained with needle electrodes (see
also Kunze 1967).

Strikingly, even in the case of total occlusion of the large
vessels, anoxic values of local oxygen pressure were seldom
attained.   This result was disappointing but it was confirmed by
investigating other patients.   All these patients had no ischaemic
pain during rest.   The effect might be explained by the rigidity
of the vessel walls: they are no longer elastic and therefore
incapable of adaptation.   They seem to be fixed in a state of
non-vasoconstriction and perhaps this causes a 'luxurious' oxygen
supply during rest.   Another possible explanation may be that all
patients in the intensive care have their infusion programme.   So
this change of the volume may influence the microcirculation.
These are of course only careful attempts of interpreting this
phenomenon.

The postoperative histogram shows also a slight shift to the
right which means that the local oxygen pressure increased.   This
result was not unexpected.   Surprising was the effect of some
drugs we use in the intensive care unit.   For example at the
beginning of these investigations the effect of a drug which is
said to improve the rheologic qualities of the blood was studied.
A few drops of a derivative of Demethylxanthin called Pentoxifylin
which is usually added to an infusion, was put locally on the
surface of the muscle (Fig. 2.)

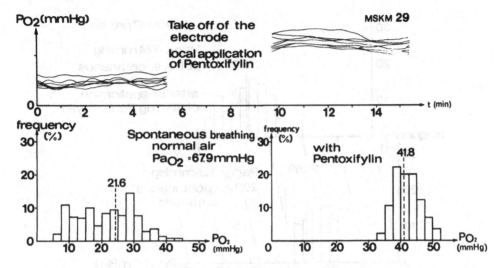

Fig. 2. The effect of local application of Pentoxifylin.
Continuous registration and histograms (below).

The comparison of the PO_2-histograms showed an obvious increase
of the local oxygen supply after application of this drug which does
not contain any substance causing hyperaemia.   In the upper part of
the illustration the continuous registration of the 8 wires of the
electrode is seen.   This measurement was monitored in a series of
12 patients (Fig. 3).

Figure 3 shows the histograms taken before and after intravenous application of Pentoxifylin.   An infusion containing 300 mg
of the drug was applicated and immediately a slight shift to the
right was registered.   The mean value rose from 25.59 up to 35.12
mmHg.   Other substances were also tested with respect to their
effect on PO_2.   These included: vasopressin, SNP, human albumin,
oxygen, glucose, laevulose and dopamin.   We think that this method
gives new information about the situation of the microcirculation
during clinical treatment.

CONCLUSIONS

1.   Surgical therapy like desobliteration or bypass operation
improved the local oxygen supply compared to the preoperative values.

2.   Preoperatively, even in the case of total occlusion of the large
vessels, anoxic or nearly anoxic values of local oxygen pressure
were not found.

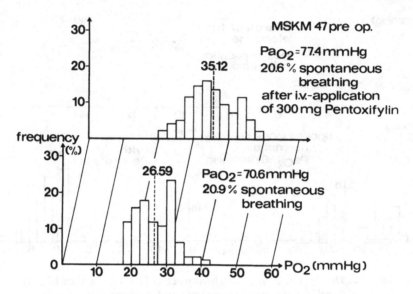

Fig. 3. Histogram before (left) and after (right) intravenous
        application of 300 mg Pentoxifylin.

3.   Conservative therapy i.e. administration of medicaments which
are said to change the rheologic properties of the blood, showed
significant effects, at least during infusion and up to two hours.

4.   The determination of the local oxygen pressure offers new
possibilities for the qualitative and quantitative control of
therapy to the clinician.

REFERENCES

Kessler, M. and Lübbers, D.W.   (1966) Pflügers Arch. ges Physiol.
291, R 82.

Kessler, M.   (1974) Microvasc. Res. 8, 283-290.

Kessler, M., Strehlau, R., Sinagowitz, E., Schönleben, K., Krumme, B.
and Bünte, H.   (1977) Microvasc. Res. (in print).

Kunze, K.   (1967) Das Sauerstoffdruckfeld im normalen und
pathologisch veränderten Muskel, Habilitationsschrift, Giessen.

Schönleben, K., Krumme, B., Bünte, H. and Kessler, M.   (1977)
Microvasc. Res. (in print).

INCREASED HEMOGLOBIN-OXYGEN AFFINITY IN PATIENTS WITH PANCREATITIS ASSOCIATED WITH TYPE I AND V HYPERLIPOPROTEINEMIA

Jørn Ditzel and Eigil Hess Thaysen,

Departments of Medicine and Clinical Chemistry
Aalborg Regional Hospital, Denmark

INTRODUCTION

It is now well established that one kind of pancreatitis is closely related to hyperlipemia and a lipoprotein electrophoretic pattern of Type I or V (Havel, 1969; Banks, 1971; Stum and Spiro, 1971; Farmer et al, 1973). In familial hyperlipoproteinemia (HLP) of these types acute pancreatitis may materialize when serum triglyceride levels are high (above 10 g/l), whereas remission occurs in response to a low fat diet. This association has led to the suggestion that the pancreatitis is caused by the disorder in lipid metabolism. The possible mechanism whereby hyperlipemia may predispose patients to attacks of pancreatitis remains poorly understood.

Recently we observed a considerable change in the oxyhemoglobin dissociation curve with increased affinity of hemoglobin for oxygen in subjects with familial fat induced lipemia (Ditzel, 1976; Ditzel and Dyerberg, 1977). It could be assessed that the oxygen unloading from the erythrocytes was diminished by approximately one third at medium pO_2, pertinent for many tissues in vivo. These observations suggest that hyperlipemia might affect tissue oxygenation by interfering with the delivery of adequate amounts of oxygen from blood to meet the requirement of tissues such as the pancreas.

Subject	Age/Sex yr	Total Lipids g/l	TG g/l	Chol g/l	Type	P$_{50}$ act pH mmHg	2,3-DPG umole/gHb	Hb g/100 ml
J.L.N.	43/F	55.15	51.48	8.87	V	21.8	13.0	12.6
W.W.P.	22/F	17.40	12.48	2.20	V	19.1	11.9	14.8
W.S.	48/M	45.72	40.36	5.40	V	22.3	13.8	15.5
J.R.B.	38/M	44.10	33.30	7.69	V	19.1	-	12.6
B.N.	15/M	38.80	38.06	3.30	I	20.9	14.3	12.1
D.N.	13/F	27.90	25.67	2.50	I	17.7	14.2	10.9
Controls		5.4* ±0.69	0.80 ±0.20	1.9 ±0.28	-	26.6 ±1.40	14.4 ±1.33	14.0 ±1.17

Table 1. Patients with Type V and I HLP with pancreatitis as compared to controls

*mean ± SD

In order to evaluate this possibility we decided to study the oxygen transport system of the red blood cells including the oxygen dissociation curve of blood from patients with acute or recurrent pancreatitis associated with familial or acquired Type I and V hyperlipoproteinemia.

MATERIAL AND METHODS

Six subjects with acute or recurrent pancreatitis and hyperlipoproteinemia were examined. Their data with respect to age and sex can be seen from Table 1. After an overnight fast venous blood was collected into heparinized syringes from a cubital vein. Total lipids, plasma triglycerides, serum cholesterol were done by routine laboratory procedures. Lipoprotein typing was done by an electrophoretic method of Dyerberg & Hjørne (1970). Red cell 2,3-diphosphoglycerate (2,3-DPG) concentration was determined according to Ericsson and de Verdier (1972). Measurements of oxyhemoglobin dissociation curves (ODC) were performed at 37° and constant pCO_2 of 40 mmHg by the dissociation curve analyzer (Type DCA-1, Radiometer A/S, Copenhagen) providing a continous print out of the ODC of whole blood (Duvelleroy et al, 1970). Arterial blood samples were drawn anaerobically and assayed within 15 minutes for pH, pO_2, pCO_2 and standard bicarbonate in a BMS-3 blood gas system (Radiometer A/S, Copenhagen).

RESULTS

In all 6 cases of pancreatitis (Table 1) the total plasma lipids and triglycerides (TG) were markedly elevated making the plasma creamy. Lipoprotein electrophoresis showed that the hyperlipoproteinemia was due to very high concentrations of chylomicrons, 4 cases were Type V and 2 cases familial Type I HLP. The ODC's in all patients were markedly shifted to the left with P_{50} at in vivo pH varying from 22.3 to 17.7 mmHg as compared to the normal mean value of 26.6 mmHg. The blood pH, oxygen saturation, MCHC and the concentration of erythrocytic 2,3-DPG were normal. The hemoglobin-concentration was slightly subnormal in 2 cases.

When washed red cells from the HLP patients were suspended in healthy plasma a tendency to normalization of the oxygen affinity of hemoglobin occurred, whereas the ODC was shifted to the left, when red cells

from a donor were suspended in lactescent plasma from
the patients.

The patients were treated with a low fat diet. In the
4 cases of HLP Type V there occurred a significant increase in the mean P_{50} values from 20.6 ± 1.7 to
25.1 ± 1.7 (p < 0.001) following a lowering of the
plasma lipid content.

DISCUSSION

The finding of a considerable change in oxyhemoglobin
dissociation in pancreatitis with hyperlipemia has not
previously been reported. The shift of the ODC cannot
be explained by a decrease in the concentration of red
cell 2,3-DPG or by alkalosis, as no alterations in
these quantities were found (Table 1). Since Types V
and I HLP are characterized by a massive accumulation
of chylomicrons, these lipoprotein particles may contribute to the changes observed in the hemoglobin affinity for oxygen. This contention is supported by the
observations of a shift to the left in the ODC when
healthy donor erythrocytes were suspended in lactescent
plasma from the patients, and conversely a shift to the
right when washed red cells from the hyperlipemic patients were incubated in homologous donor plasma.

Assuming a constant acidification of 0.1 pH at the
tissue level and that no adaptive changes take place in
the microcirculation, it can be calculated that the
amount of oxygen released from the erythrocytes at
medium pO_2 is diminished by approximately one third in
these cases. Peripheral oxygen supply is also governed
by local blood flow, and an impairment in the microcirculatory corpuscular flow could be another participating event in the reduction of peripheral oxygen delivery. Studies on the microcirculation in man and in experimental animals have indeed demonstrated that during hyperlipemia the capillary bed is overcrowded by
chylomicrons and that the corpuscular velocity in the
microvessels is markedly reduced (Kroeger, 1970). Furthermore, as in all generalized states of hypoperfusion (shock) the splanchnic circulation may be markedly affected by a compensatory vasoconstriction. The
resulting tissue hypoxia in the pancreas might lead to
cellular lysosomal rupture followed by release of pancreatic lipase into the capillaries (Fig. 1). This
causes hydrolysis of triglycerides carried by chylo-

microns, release of fatty acids, and microthrombus formation resulting in further local ischemia and pancreatitis. This concept for the development of pancreatitis, which is an elaboration of that of Havel (1969), explains why a low fat diet will favourably influence this kind of pancreatitis and might prevent further recurrence.

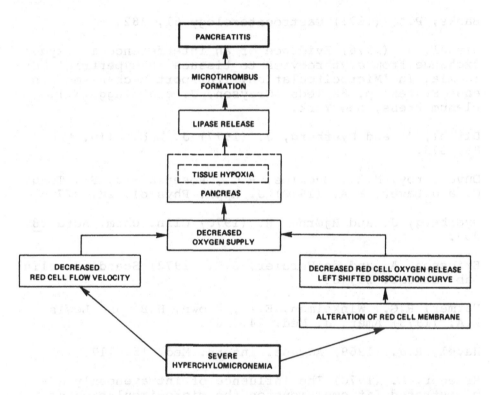

Fig. 1. Concept of mechanism leading to pancreatitis in hyperlipemia.

SUMMARY

Oxyhemoglobin dissociation curves were performed from blood of subjects with pancreatitis associated with Type V and Type I hyperlipoproteinemia. The hemoglobin-oxygen affinity was markedly increased with P_{50} varying from 22.3 to 17.7 mmHg. As the hyperlipoproteinemia subsided the clinical and laboratory signs of pancreatic affection disappeared. The increased hemoglobin-oxygen

affinity and decreased flow of red cells due to hyper-
chylomicronemia in the microcirculation may lead to
tissue hypoxia, which may act as a precipitating injuri-
ous factor leading to pancreatitis during severe hyperlipemia.

REFERENCES

Banks, P.A. (1971) Gastroenterology 61, 382.

Ditzel, J. (1976) Evidence of an interference in oxygen
exchange from erythrocytes to tissues in hypertriglycer-
idemia. In 'Microcirculation, Transport Mechanisms Disease States' p. 88 (eds. Grayson, J. and Zingg, W.).
Plenum Press, New York.

Ditzel, J. and Dyerberg, J. (1977) J. Lab. clin. Med.
89, 573.

Duvelleroy, M.A., Buckles, R.C., Rosenkaimer, S., Tung,
C. and Laver, M.A. (1970) J. Appl. Physiol. 28, 227.

Dyerberg, J. and Hjørne, H. (1970) Clin. chim. Acta 28,
203.

Ericsson, A. and de Verdier, C.H. (1972) Scand. J. clin.
Lab. Invest. 29, 85.

Farmer, R.G., Winkelman, E.I., Brown, H.B. and Lewis,
L.A. (1973) Amer. J. Med. 54, 161.

Havel, R.J. (1969) Advanc. intern. Med. 15, 117.

Kroeger, A. (1970) The influence of intravenously ad-
ministrated fat emulsions on the microcirculation of
pancreas and mesenteric adipose tissue. In 'Advances in
Microcirculation' p. 1 (ed. Harders, H.). S. Karger,
Basel, New York.

Kurz, G.H., Shakib, M., Sohmer, K.K. and Friedman, A.H.
(1976) Amer. J. Ophthal. 82, 32.

Stum, W.B. and Spiro, H.M. (1971) Ann. intern. Med. 74,
264.

EFFECTS OF CORONARY OCCLUSION ON MYOCARDIAL OXYGEN AND PULSATILE INTRAMYOCARDIAL PRESSURE

T. Koyama, T. Sasajima, T. Yagi, N. Miki and Y. Kikuchi

Res. Inst. Appl. Electr., Hokkaido University

060 Sapporo, Japan

When the coronary artery is occluded, both the myocardial tissue PO_2 and local contractile force decrease. However, the time courses of the decrease in PO_2 and contractile force seem to be different; the PO_2 of the inner portion of the ventricular myocardium decreases to 50% of the initial level in 30 seconds according to Winbury et al (1971), while the contractile force decreases to 40% of the control value in 10 seconds as seen in the figure shown by Theroux et al (1974). Since the relation between these two variables has not been studied systematically, we decided to investigate this by simultaneous measurements of the time courses of PO_2 in terms of O_2-availability (O_2 current through the platinum electrode) and pulsatile intramyocardial pressure (IMP) of the myocardium perfused by the left anterior branch of the coronary artery (LAD).

A small insulated piece of piezoelectric ceramic $Pb(Ti-Zr)O_3$ (2.0 x 1.0 x 0.4 mm), is placed in the inner wall of the left ventricular myocardium of anaesthetized open-chest dogs. When the ceramic is oriented parallel to the direction of myocardial fibres, the output signal represents one component of regionally inhomogeneous IMP (Koyama et al 1976). A bare tip platinum electrode (tip OD = 110 μm including glass insulation) is placed on the myocardial tissue close to the ceramic or mounted on the piece of the ceramic for simultaneous insertion.

An example of the actual measurements made in the ventricle having no visible collateral anastomoses is shown in Fig. 1, where the curves above and below indicate the pulsatile IMP and O_2-current, respectively. The small sections attached to the figure represent the high speed reproduction of ECG (above) and pulsatile IMP (below)

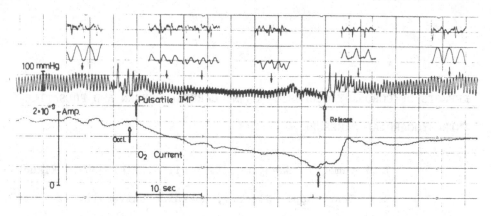

Fig. 1. Simultaneous recordings of local O_2-availability (O_2-current, below) and pulsatile intramyocardial pressure (pulsatile IMP, above). The sections attached above show the high speed reproduction of the pulsatile IMP pattern and ECG for the portions on the continuous recording indicated by the arrows.   The open arrows indicate the start and the end of the coronary occlusion.

of the corresponding portion of the continuous recordings.   On occluding the LAD, the pulsatile IMP decreases quickly and the positive wave which appears immediately after the R-wave of ECG disappears and is replaced with a negative wave in 5-10 secs. while the O_2-current decreases rather slowly.   At 5 and 10 seconds after the occlusion the positive wave of the pulsatile IMP is 50 and 20% of the control value and the O_2-current is 87 and 64% of the initial level, respectively.   In 20 seconds the IMP pattern becomes an irregular fluctuation.   On release of the occlusion the positive wave reappears and attains a height of 70% of the initial value in 5 seconds.   The recovery of the O_2-current is rapid for 10 seconds but very slow thereafter.   It returns to the initial level in 3 minutes.   In five measurements the pulsatile IMP and O_2-current at 10 seconds after the occlusion are 30.0 (SD = 12.4) % and 67.0 (SD = 11.2) % of the initial value on an average, respectively.

    To interpret the biological meaning of these observations we assume a model of Krogh's tissue cylinder in which O_2-consumption varies in direct proportion to pulsatile IMP, and coronary blood flow is reduced by LAD occlusion.   The PO_2 is calculated according to pseudodynamic method (Bruley and Knisely 1970) but using ADSL programme (computer room of our Institute and computer centre of Hokkaido University).   Furthermore, it is assumed that the capillary blood flows at a constant rate and the O_2-consumption shows no periodic oscillation.   The effect of deoxygenation velocity factor of blood, Fc', is not included in the calculation,

because it causes an almost uniform decrease of PO_2 in the tissue
by a few mmHg according to Mochizuki (this symposium) and probably
causes no serious errors for the analysis of the time courses of the
decrease in tissue PO_2.   Since Krogh's tissue cylinder for the
myocardium has the diameter of 14 μm (Thews 1962), the PO_2 at the
lowest corner is only 2 to 5 mmHg lower than the PO_2 of the venous
blood.   The calculated PO_2 at the boundary between capillary blood
and tissue along the capillary vessel is shown in Fig. 2, where the
blood flow velocity which is 1 mm/sec. under the normal condition
decreases by 1/5 and 1/10 because of the coronary arterial occlusion
and the O_2-consumption decreases by the rate of 1/2, 1/5 and 1/5,
1/10, respectively.   This figure shows that the rapid drop of
pulsatile IMP can reduce the rate of reduction in the local tissue
PO_2 to some degree, which agree qualitatively with the experimental
observations.

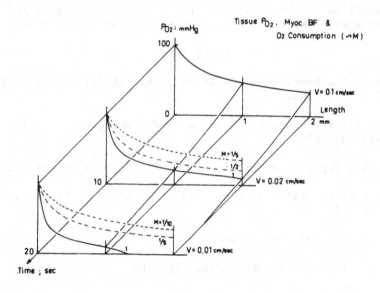

Fig. 2. The calculated PO_2 at the boundary between capillary blood
and myocardial tissue along the capillary length.   The blood flow
velocity v decreases from 1 mm/sec to 0.2 and 0.1 mm/sec, while the
O_2-consumption declines from 1.6×10^{-3} ml/ml/sec under the control
condition by rates of 1, 1/2, 1/5 and 1/10.   The values of the
constants employed for the calculation are as follows.   Radii of
the capillary vessel and tissue cylinder = 3.0, 14×10^{-4} cm,
diffusion coefficients in the capillary and tissue = 0.46, 1.0×10^{-5} cm^2/sec, O_2-solubility for blood and tissue = 2.4, 2.9×10^{-5}/mmHg, respectively, and O_2-capacity of capillary blood = 0.2
ml/ml.

Thus, we think that the local contractile force does not depend on the tissue PO_2 in the case of acute coronary occlusion and that the contractile force is modified by an unknown factor, so as to reduce an abrupt decrease of the local PO_2 during the transient acute occlusion of the coronary arterial branch.

SUMMARY

Local oxygen partial pressure in terms of O_2-availability and pulsatile intramyocardial pressure of the left ventricular myocardium of anaesthetized open-chest dogs have been measured simultaneously by means of a piezoelectric ceramic and a platinum electrode.   The tissue PO_2 decreases more slowly than the pulsatile intramyocardial pressure during a transient acute occlusion of the anterior descending branch of the coronary artery.   The slow decrease in the tissue PO_2 seems to be explicable by the assumption that the local myocardial contractile force decreases quickly due to an unknown factor during the acute coronary occlusion and that the O_2-consumption of the local myocardial tissue is reduced in accordance with the rapid decrease in the contractile force.

REFERENCES

Winbury, M.M., Howe, B.B. and Weiss, H.R.   (1971)   Pharmac. & Exp. Ther. 176, 186.

Theroux, V., Franklin, D., Ross, J. and Kemper, W.S.   (1974) Circ. Res. 35, 896.

Koyama, T., Yagi, T. and Kakiuchi, Y.   (1976)   Experientia 32, 1617.

Bruley, D.F. and Knisely, M.H.   (1970)   Chem. Eng. Progress, Symp. Series 66, 22.

Mochizuki, M.   This symposium.

Thews, G.   (1962)   Pflügers Arch. 276, 166.

HOMEOSTATIC RESPONSES TO INCREASED OXYGEN AFFINITY

Samuel Charache

Johns Hopkins University School of Medicine

Baltimore, Maryland   21205

Oxygen transport is probably normal in carriers of hemoglobins with altered oxygen affinity, as judged by the patients' lack of symptoms and by their excretion of normal amounts of erythropoietin (1-4). Possible adjustments to maintain homeostasis include changes in hemoglobin concentration; cardiac output, or its distribution; number of perfused capillaries (i.e., the capillary-cell distance); or oxygen utilization in the tissue (5-7). The choice between these adjustments varies from stress to stress (8); in the case of hemoglobins with altered oxygen affinity, a strong arguement was made that adjustments are almost entirely hematopoietic (9), and that mixed venous PO_2 ($P\bar{V}O_2$, a reflection of tissue PO_2) remains constant (10).

I have tabulated hemoglobin concentrations and P50's of carriers of high affinity hemoglobins which do not produce hemolytic anemia (Table 1). To normalize P50's to common conditions of measurement (37° C, pH 7.4, and pCO_2 40 mm Hg), I used:

$$\frac{x}{26.6} = \frac{\text{measured P50 of blood or hemolysate}}{\text{P50 of normal blood or hemolysate under experimental conditions}}$$

For hemoglobin Olympia the P50 calculated from properties of the hemolysate was 20.6 mm Hg, while the actual P50 of carrier's blood under standard conditions was 18.6 (36).

The hypothetical curve in Fig. 1 was calculated under the following assumptions:

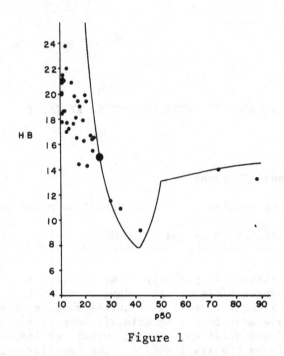

Figure 1

1) Arterial blood in normal persons, and in carriers of high affinity hemoglobins, is 98% saturated with oxygen. Arterial PO_2 may be low in persons with low P50 (21), but oxygen saturations are normal.

2) Mixed venous PO_2 is 40 mm Hg.

3) Using a modification of Hill's equation (52):

$$- n \log P50 + n \log PO_2 = \log \frac{S}{1-S} \qquad (1)$$

arterial oxygen saturation (S_{art}) is calculated from:

$$- n \log P50 + 2n = \log \frac{S_{art}}{1 - S_{art}} \qquad (2)$$

and venous saturation (S_{ven}) from

$$- n \log P50 + 1.602 \, n = \log \frac{S_{ven}}{1 - S_{ven}} \qquad (3)$$

4) Oxygen capacity is 1.34 ml O_2/gm Hb.

5) If adjustments are only hematopoietic, i.e. cardiac output, the distribution of blood flow and tissue PO_2 remain constant; and

arterio-venous oxygen difference is 4.3 m O_2/dl (normal 4.1-5.0 (53)); hemoglobin concentration in the blood must be

$$\frac{4.3}{1.34 \ (S_{art} - S_{ven})} \tag{4}$$

If one knows the hemoglobin concentration, S_{ven} can be calculated (Table 1) from equation (4), and mixed venous PO_2 can be determined from the dissociation curve, using the approximation in equation (3) if necessary.

Values of n used in the calculation were chosen to reflect values between PO_2's of 40 and 100 mmg Hg, and were assumed to be constant in that range:

P50	n	
10-15	2.5	
16-20	2.6	
21-30	2.7	
31-40	2.4	
41-50	2.4	1.1
51-75	1.1	1.0
75	1.0	

That assumption is probably incorrect, for n may vary widely across the dissociation curve of blood containing two hemoglobins with very different properties. Bellingham (54) used much lower n-values for blood containing high-affinity hemoglobins, but oxygen is transported primarily by the normal component in such samples, and n values between mixed venous and arterial pO_2 are consequently near-normal. Measured values of n at P = 40 mm Hg, for instance, were 2-2.5 in carriers of Hb Osler, McKees Rocks and Potomac (37,35,39).

Neville has stressed the importance of n in transport of oxygen by normal blood (55), but heme-heme interaction becomes even more important when a low-affinity hemoglobin is present. Reported values (some from hemolysates) for the mid-portion of the dissociation curve are:

Hb	P50	n	Reference
Hope	34	2.4	27
Hope	33	2.4	Unpublished data
	37	2.2	"
	41	2.6	"
Seattle	42	2.6	4
Kansas	70	1.1	30
Beth Israel	88	1.0	16

Table 1

Estimated Mixed Venous Oxygen Saturation and Pressure
in Carriers of Hemoglobins with Altered O_2 Affinity

Hemoglobin	HB (gm/dl)	$S\bar{v}O_2$ (%)	P50 (mm Hg)	$P\bar{v}O_2$ (mm Hg)	Method	Ref
Agenogi	11.5	69(ΔS = 27)	30	40	H	(11)
Alberta	19.4	82	15.5	36	C	(12)
Andrew Minneapolis	19.8	82	14	26	CC	(13)
Athens Ga.	14.3	76	20.7	31	CC	(14)
Bethesda	17.7	80	12,8	26	CC	(15)
Beth Israel	13.2	26(ΔS – 24)	88	40	C	(16)
Brigham	17.9	80	19.3	33	C	(17)
British Columbia	16.5	79	23.2	39	C	(18)
Chapel Hill	15.5	78	23	42	C	(19)
Chesapeake	19.9	82	20	35	C	(20)
Creteil	22	84	12.9	31	C	(21)
Heathrow	21	83	10.9	37	CC	(22)
Helsinki	16.4	79	23	35	C	(23)
Hirose	14.4	76	17.8	22	CC	(24,25)
Hiroshima	17	79	12.7	27	CC	(26)
Hope	10.9	64(ΔS = 29)	34	40	CC	(27)
J Capetown	16.3	79	19.7	14	CC	(28,29)
Kansas	14	37(ΔS = 23)	73	42	CC	(30)
Kempsey	21.3	85	10.6	30	CC	(31)
Little Rock	23.8	85	12.2	24	C	(32)
Malmo	18.4	81	10.9	34	CC	(33)
Malmo	21	83	11.4	37	C	(34)

Table 1 (con't)

Hemoglobin	HB (gm/dl)	S$\bar{V}O_2$ (%)	P50 (mm Hg)	$P\bar{V}O_2$ (mm Hg)	Method	Ref
McKees Rocks	17.8	80	10.3	30	C	(35)
Olympia	19.4	82	20.6	31	CC	(36)
Osler	20	82	10.3	33	C	(37)
Osler	20	82	10.3	33	C	(38)
Potomac	18.6	81	12.5	30	C	(39)
Providence	16.7	79	22	38	C	(40)
Radcliffe	18.6	81	11.6	27	C	(41)
Rahere	19	81	18	32	C	(42)
Rainer	21	83	10.9	34	C	(43)
San Diego	18.1	81	16.4	31	CC	(44)
San Diego	17.6	80	15.4	30	C	(45)
Seattle	9.2	80	15.4	30	C	(46)
Suresnes	16.5	79	16.9	32	H	(47)
Syracuse	21.5	83	11	38	CC	(48)
Vanderbilt	20.9	83	14.5	46	C	(49)
Wood	17.2	80	13.6	30	C	(50)
Yakima	18.6	81	12	32	C	(51)

See Appendix for calculation of mixed venous oxygen saturation from hemoglobin concentration. Oxygen pressures ($P\bar{V}O_2$) were obtained directly from dissociation curves (C), after the curves were corrected to standard conditions (CC) or calculated from Hill's equation (H). The hemoglobin concentration used for Hb J Capetown is from one family, and the corrected P50 is from another.

The poor fit of patients' hemoglobin concentrations to the calculated curve, and the low values calculated for $P\bar{V}O_2$, suggest that lowered tissue PO_2 may be an important mode of compensation for abnormal oxygen affinity, which is used to a variable extent from one patient to another.   That hypothesis can be evaluated with modern instrumentation, and if correct, mechanisms by which tissue PO_2 is lowered may be elucidated, and perhaps, exploited for treatment of patients with disorders more common than high-affinity hemoglobins.

ACKNOWLEDGEMENTS

Drs. G.R. Gray, S.B. Krantz, M. Mant, C. Poyart, D.M. Samson and F. Taketa provided unpublished data on the oxygen affinity of their patients' blood.   Mr. R. Kessler and Ms. I. Harris helped with programming, and Mrs. P. Hathaway and Miss M. Jessop provided technical assistance.

These studies were supported by research grant HL-02799 and Clinical Research Center grant RR-35, from the National Institutes of Health, United States Public Health Service.

REFERENCES

1.   Charache, S., Weatherall, D.J. and Clegg, J.B.   (1966)   J. Clin. Invest. 45, 813-822.

2.   Adamson, J.W., Parer, J.T. and Stamatoyannopoulos, G.   (1969) J. Clin. Invest. 48, 1376-1386.

3.   Adamson, J.W., Hayashi, A., Stamatoyannopoulos, G. and Burger, W.F.   (1972)   J. Clin. Invest. 51, 2883-2888.

4.   Stamatoyannopoulos, G., Parer, J.T. and Finch, C.A.   (1969) New Eng. J. Med. 281, 915-919.

5.   Finch, C.A. and Lenfant, C.   (1972)   New Eng.J.Med. 286, 407.

6.   Kety, S.S.   (1957)   Fed. Proc. 16, 666-670.

7.   Guy, C.R. and Eliot, R.S.   (1973)   Advances Cardiol. 9, 68-80.

8.   Balcerzak, S.P. and Bromberg, P.A.   (1975)   Seminars Hemat. 12, 353-382.

9.   Metcalfe, J. and Dhindsa, D.S.   (1972)   In 'Oxygen Affinity of Hemoglobin and Red Cell Acid Base Status' (eds. Astrup, P. and Rorth, M.) p.613-628.   Academic Press, New York.

10. Adamson, J.W. (1975) Seminars Hemat. 12, 383-396.

11. Castro, O., Winter, W.P., Doan, R.J., Lee, C.K. and Rucknagel,
    D.L. (1976) Clin. Res. 24, 630A.

12. Mant, M.J., Salkie, M.L., Cope, N., Appling, F., Bolch, K.,
    Jayalakshmi, M., Gravely, M., Wilson, J.B. and Huisman, T.H.J.
    (1976-77) Hemoglobin 1, 183-194.

13. Zak, S.J., Brimhall, B., Jones, R.T. and Kaplan, M.D. (1974)
    Blood, 44, 543-549.

14. Brown, W.J., Niazi, O.A., Jajalakshmi, M., Abraham, E.C. and
    Huisman, T.H.J. (1976) Biochim. Biophys. Acta. 439, 70-76.

15. Adamson, J.W., Hayashi, A., Stamatoyannopoulos, G. and Burger,
    W.F. (1972) J. Clin. Invest. 51, 2883-2888.

16. Nagel, R.L., Lynfield, J., Johnson, J., Landau, L., Bookchin,
    R.M. and Harris, M.B. (1976) New Engl. J. Med. 295, 125-130.

17. Lokich, J.J., Moloney, W.C., Bunn, H.F., Bruckheimer, S.M.
    and Ranney, H.M. (1973) J. Clin. Invest. 52, 2060-2067.

18. Jones, R.T., Brimhall, B. and Gray, S. (1976-77) Hemoglobin
    1, 171-182.

19. Orringer, E.P., Wilson, J.B. and Huisman, T.H.J. (1976)
    FEBS Letters, 65, 297-300.

20. Charache, S., Weatherall, D.J. and Clegg, J.B. (1966)
    J. Clin. Invest. 45, 813-822.

21. Poyart, C., Bursaux, E., Teisseire, B., Freminet, A.,
    Duvelleroy, M. and Rose, J. (1977) Submitted for publication.

22. White, J.M., Szur, L., Gillies, I.D.S., Lorkin, P.A. and
    Lehmann, H. (1973) Brit. Med. J. 3, 665-667.

23. Ikkala, E., Koskela, J., Pikkarainen, P., Rahiala, E-L., El-
    Hazmi, M.A.F., Nagai, K., Lang, A. and Lehmann, H. (1976)
    Acta. Haemat. 56, 257-275.

24. Yamaoka, K. (1971) Blood 38, 730-738.

25. Fujita, S. (1972) J. Clin. Invest. 51, 2520-2528.

26. Hamilton, H.B., Iuchi, I., Miyaji, T., Shibata, S. (1969)
    J. Clin. Invest. 48, 525-535.

27. Steinberg, M.H., Lovell, W.J., Wells, S., Coleman, M., Dreiling, B.J. and Adams, J.G. (1976) J. Lab. Clin. Med. **88**, 125-131.

28. Jenkins, T., Stevens, K., Gallo, E. and Lehmann, H. (1968) South Afr. Med. J. 2 Nov. 1151-1154.

29. Lines, J.G. and McIntosh, R. (1967) Nature **215**, 297-298.

30. Reissmann, K.R., Ruth, W.E. and Nomura, T. (1961) J. Clin. Invest. **40**, 1826-1833.

31. Reed, C.S., Hampson, R., Gordon, S., Jones, R.T., Novy, M.J., Brimhall, B., Edwards, M.J., Koler, R.D. (1968) Blood **31**,623.

32. Bromberg, P.A., Padilla, F., Guy, J.T., Balceryak, S.P. (1972) Chest **61** (Supp), 14S.

33. Boyer, S.H., Charache, S., Fairbanks, V.F., Maldonado, J.E., Noyes, A.N. and Gayle, E.E. (1972) J.Clin.Invest. **51**, 666-76.

34. Berglund, S. (1972) Scand. J. Haemat. **9**, 377-386.

35. Winslow, R.M., Swenberg, M.L., Gross, E., Chervenick, P.A., Buchman, R.R. and Anderson, W.F. (1976) J.Clin.Invest. **57**, 772-781.

36. Stamatoyannopoulos, G., Nute, P.E., Adamson, J.W., Bellingham, A.J. and Funk, D. (1973) J. Clin. Invest. **52**, 342-348.

37. Charache, S., Brimhall, B. and Jones, R.T. (1975) Johns Hopkins Med. J. **136**, 132-136.

38. Gacon, G., Wajcman, H., Labie, D. and Vigeron, C. (1977) FEBS Letters **56**, 39-42.

39. Charache, S., Jacobson, R., Brimhall, B., Murphy, E.A. Hathaway, P., Winslow, R.M., Jones, R. and Rath, C. (submitted for publication).

40. Charache, S., Fox, J., McCurdy, P., Kazazian, H. Jr. and Winslow, R.M. (1977) J. Clin. Invest. **59**, 652-658.

41. Weatherall, D.J., Clegg, J.B., Callender, S.T., Wells, R.M.G., Gale, R.E., Huehns, E.R., Perutz, M.F., Viggiano, G. and Ho, C. (1977) Brit. J. Haemat. **35**, 177-191.

42. Lorkin, P.A., Stephens, A.D., Beard, M.E.J., Wrigley, P.F.M., Adams, L. and Lehmann, H. (1975) Brit. Med. J. **4**, 200-202.

43. Adamson, J.W., Parer, J.T. and Stamatoyannopoulos, G. (1969) J. Clin. Invest. 48, 1376-1386.

44. Nute, P.E., Stamatoyannopoulos, G., Hermodson, M.A. and Roth, D. (1974) J. Clin. Invest. 53, 320-328.

45. Chanarin, I., Samson, D., Lang, A., Casey, R., Lorkin, P.A. and Lehmann, H. (1975) Brit. J. Haemat. 30, 167-175.

46. Stamatoyannopoulos, G., Parer, J.T. and Finch, C.A. (1969) New Eng. J. Med. 281, 915-919.

47. Poyart, C., Krishnamoorthy, R., Bursaux, E., Gacon, G. and Labie, D. (1976) FEBS Letters 69, 103-107.

48. Jensen, M., Oski, F.A., Nathan, D.G. and Bunn, H.F. (1975) J. Clin. Invest. 55, 469-477.

49. Paniker, N.V., Lin, K-I.D., Krantz, S.B., Flexner, J.M., Wasserman, B.K., Puett, D. (submitted for publication).

50. Taketa, F., Huang, Y.P., Libnoch, J.A., Dessel, B.H. (1975) Biochim. Biophys. Acta 400, 348-353.

51. Novy, M.J., Edwards, M.J. and Metcalfe, J. (1967) J. Clin. Invest. 46, 1848-1854.

52. Hill, A.V. (1910) J. Physiol. 40, IV-V.

53. Altman, P., Dittmer, D.S. (ed) Respiration and Circulation, Bethesda, Fed. Am. Soc. Exp. Biol. (1971) p. 139, 141, 319.

54. Bellingham, A.J. (1974) Clinics in Haemat. 3, 577-594.

55. Neville, J.R. (1977) Brit. J. Haemat. 35, 387-396.

HEMOGLOBIN-OXYGEN AFFINITY IN ORGANIC HEART DISEASE

J. R. Neville* and Terry Clemmer**

*Letterman Army Institute of Research
Presidio of San Francisco, CA 94129 U.S.A.
**1445 East Princeton Avenue
Salt Lake City, Utah U.S.A.

In a previous communication (Neville and Clemmer, 1975) we reported that the average P_{50} (7.4)≠ and n* values for the oxy-hemoglobin dissociation curve (ODC) in patients admitted to an intensive care unit were lower than those usually observed in healthy individuals. Only a few of the values that were obtained in this earlier study reflected a decreased hemoglobin-oxygen affinity despite the fact that many of these patients had heart disease (HD), a condition which, according to a number of investigators (Morse, et al., 1950; Metcalfe, et al., 1969; Woodson, et al., 1970; Kostuk, et al., 1973), is associated with an increased P_{50}. Decreased oxygen affinity has not been observed in HD by all investigators, however (see Discussion); therefore, our data (Neville and Clemmer, 1975) relating to the HD patients have been analyzed separately and the results are the subject of this report.

SUBJECTS AND METHODS

Blood from 65 patients admitted to an intensive care unit with known or suspected HD was analyzed for oxygen affinity and

---

≠ P_{50} (7.4) is the oxygen partial pressure at 50 percent saturation of hemoglobin, corrected to a pH of 7.4 using a Bohr factor of 0.53.

* This value (n) is the slope of the logarithmic plot of the Hill equation between 70 and 30 percent saturation. It is used as a measure of heme-heme interaction or cooperativity.

oxygen capacity. The original intention of this study was to canvass oxygen affinity in critically ill patients and there were no criteria applied to selecting this group other than their admission to the intensive care unit during the period of the study. There were 16 females and 49 males. The average age was 58.5 years. Many of the patients were being administered a variety of drugs, the most prevalent of which were digoxin, diuretics, and tranquilizers. The most common complaint was chest pain, and of 45 patients being observed or treated for myocardial infarction, 13 had positive clinical findings of infarction at the time of sampling.

Oxygen affinity and oxygen capacity were determined by our using the biotonometry technique (Neville, 1974). This technique offers several advantages: only a small blood sample is required; a complete and continuous record of the ODC is obtained; all measurements are done on a single sample; no extensive pre-equilibration or tonometry is required. Citrated samples were drawn from an antecubital vein and kept on ice until analyzed (usually within 30 minutes to an hour of sampling). The 10 transfused patients who had no known cardiac disease were hemorrhaging and had recently received an average of 9 units of stored whole blood or packed cells. The 10 normal controls were young, male laboratory personnel in good health.

RESULTS

Table 1 shows the mean values (±SEM) obtained for P_{50} and n in each of the three groups. Compared to normals, the HD and transfused groups showed statistically significant decreases of both P_{50} and n. The differences between the HD and transfused groups were not significant. Values for oxygen affinity in the normal group agree with those observed by others (Neill, et al., 1972; Metcalfe, et al., 1969). Stored blood rapidly loses 2,3-diphosphoglycerate (DPG) with a consequent decrease in P_{50}.

Table 1

P_{50} and n values (mean ± SEM) and Significance Estimates*

GROUP (N):	NORMALS (10)	HEART DISEASE (65)	TRANSFUSED (10)
P_{50}:	27.8 ± 0.1	24.5 ± 0.3 P<.001	22.8 ± 0.6 P<.001
n:	2.56 ± 0.05	2.31 ± 0.03 P<.01	2.13 ± 0.06 P<.001

*Compared to normals

Transfusion of such blood reduces the P_{50} of the ODC in blood
from the recipient (Valtis and Kennedy, 1953). Older red cells
likewise have a decreased heme-heme interaction (Edwards and
Rigas, 1967). Thus, in both the normal and transfused groups, the
results were consistent with expectations. The P_{50} and n values
for each of the 65 HD patients are plotted in Figure 1. For com-
parative purposes, the dashed lines in this figure indicate the
approximate ranges of P_{50} and n that are found in healthy subjects
when estimated with the biotonometry technique (Neville, 1974).
The plot characterizes the abnormal oxygen affinity that was observed in this group of heart disease patients. Figure 2 shows
dissociation curves representative of the approximate extremes of
the range of values indicated in Figure 1 (i.e., a high affinity
curve with P_{50} of 20 mm Hg and n=2.0, and a low affinity curve
with P_{50} of 30.0 mm Hg and n=3.0). These curves were constructed
with the Hill equation by using the indicated P_{50} and n values.

Figure 3 shows the hemoglobin-oxygen capacity as it related
to P_{50} in the HD patients in this series. Although an inverse relationship between these variables has been reported by others

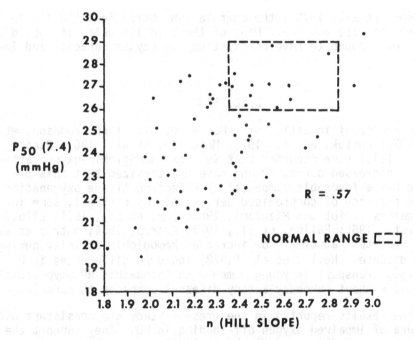

Figure 1. The position (P_{50} at pH 7.4) plotted against the shape
(n) of oxyhemoglobin dissociation curves found in 65 heart disease
patients.

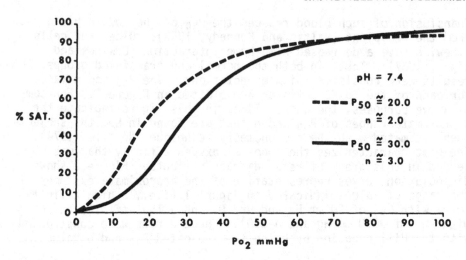

Figure 2. The approximate extremes of the oxyhemoglobin dissociation curves in 65 heart disease patients.

(Woodson, et al., 1970), the correlation coefficient (-0.17) in
the present case was low. Many of these individuals, it should be
noted, were found to have co-existing low oxygen capacity and low
P_{50}.

DISCUSSION

A number of investigators (Morse, et al., 1950; Woodson, et
al., 1970; Kostuk, et al., 1973; Metcalfe, et al., 1969; Daniel,
et al., 1975) have reported that *in vitro* hemoglobin-oxygen affinity is decreased during HD and have hypothesized that this decrease has a favorable compensatory effect on tissue oxygenation
in the presence of compromised perfusion. By contrast, some investigators (Eliot and Mizukami, 1966; Guy, et al., 1971; Eliot
and Bratt, 1969; Fallon, et al., 1973; Astrup, 1964; Astrup et al.,
1966) reported "abnormal" or increased hemoglobin affinity during
heart disease. Neill, et al. (1972) found no differences in P_{50}
or oxygen transport in young women with idiopathic HD (myocardial
ischemia without coronary artery disease) compared to normals.

The results reported in the present study are consistent with
the idea of impaired oxygen off-loading in HD. They support the
observations of Eliot and Mizukami (1966) and of Eliot and Bratt
(1969) with respect to cooperativity changes found in HD, a
measurement that has been less frequently reported for whole blood
than has the more common P_{50} index. The theoretical impact on

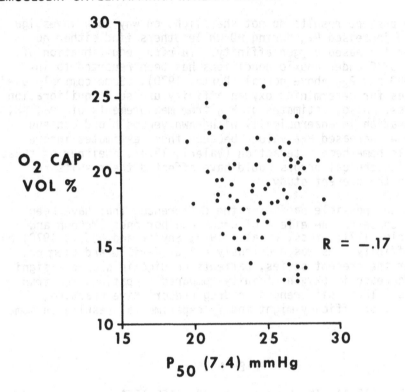

Figure 3. The oxygen capacity in relation to P_{50} at pH 7.4 in 65 heart disease patients.

oxygen transport of changes in n has recently been reviewed (Neville, 1977).

The studies of Astrup (1964), Astrup, et al. (1966), and Astrup, et al. (1967) have implicated carbon monoxide in the pathophysiology of atherosclerosis. Although the basis of this relationship is unclear, it is widely appreciated that carbon monoxide greatly alters the oxygen affinity curve and decreases the oxygen carrying capacity of hemoglobin. In this study, many HD patients who had left-shifted curves and low n values also had lowered oxygen capacity.

Thus, it is concluded that the altered oxygen affinity seen in these heart disease patients, particularly with anemia and/or partial saturation of hemoglobin with carbon monoxide could seriously alter the normal oxygen transport process and contribute to the development of hypoxia in the myocardium.

The present results do not shed light on why some investigators find increased P_{50} during HD while others find either no change or increased oxygen affinity. *In vitro* equilibration of blood at 37°C under anoxic conditions has been reported to increase DPG and P_{50} above normal (Rörth, 1970). Some commonly used techniques for determining oxygen affinity use such equilibration procedures. Also, estimates of P_{50} from measurements of PO_2, pH, and saturation in anaerobically withdrawn venous blood can spuriously show increased P_{50} values because these estimates ignore changes in heme-heme interaction (Valeri, 1974). Neither of these potential technical errors would have affected the results reported in the present study.

Another possible basis for the differences that have been reported concerns the effect of drugs and hormones (McConn and Del Guercio, 1971; Gross, et al., 1976; Snyder and Reddy, 1970) on oxygen affinity. As was previously noted (Neville and Clemmer, 1975) for the present series, patients on digoxin showed a significant decrease in oxygen affinity compared to patients on tranquilizers. Thus, differences in drug prescriptive practise, compliance, or efficacy might modify experimental results in some cases.

REFERENCES

Astrup, P. (1964) The Lancet, Nov 28, 1152-1154.

Astrup, P., P. Hellung-Larsen, K. Kjeldsen and K. Mellemgaard (1966) Scand. J. Clin. Lab. Invest. 18:450-457.

Astrup, P., K. Kjeldsen and J. Wanstrup (1967) J. Atherosclerosis Res. 7:343-354.

Daniel, J., M. A. Cohen, B. F. Lichtman, B. F. Schreiner and P. M. Shah (1975) Circulation, Suppl. II to Vols 51 and 52, II-131.

Edwards, M. J. and D. A. Rigas (1967) J. Clin. Invest. 46: 1579-1588.

Eliot, R. S. and H. Mizukami (1966) Circulation 34:331-336.

Eliot, R. S. and J. Bratt (1969) Am. J. Cardiol. 23:633-638.

Fallon, K. D., A. L. Malenfant, R. D. Weisel, and H. B. Hechtman (1973) Adv. Exp. Med. Biol. 37A:93-97.

Guy, C. R., J. M. Solhaug and R. S. Eliot (1971) Am. Heart J. 82:824-832.

Gross, G. J., D. C. Warltier and H. F. Hardman (1976) Eur. J. Pharmacol. 36:267-271.

Kostuk, W. J., K. Suwa, E. F. Bernstein and B. E. Sobel (1973) Am. J. Cardiol. 31:295-299.

McConn, R. and L. R. M. Del Guercio (1971) Ann. Surg. 174:436-448.

Metcalfe, J., D. S. Dhindsa, M. J. Edwards and A. Mourdjinis (1969) Circulation Res. 25:47-51.

Morse, M., D. E. Cassels and M. Holder (1950) J. Clin. Invest. 29:1098-1103.

Neill, W. A., M. P. Judkins, D. S. Dhindsa, J. Metcalfe, D. G. Kassebaum and F. E. Kloster (1972) Am. J. Cardiol. 29:171-179.

Neville, J. R. (1974) J. Appl. Physiol. 37:967-971.

Neville, J. R. and T. Clemmer (1975) Fed. Proc. 34:452.

Neville, J. R. (1977) Brit. J. Haematol. 35:385-393.

Rörth, M. (1970) Scand. J. Clin. Lab. Invest. 26:43-46.

Snyder, L. M. and W. J. Reddy (1970) J. Clin. Invest. 49: 1993-1998.

Valeri, C. R. (1974) Clin. Haematol. 3:656.

Valtis, D. J. and A. C. Kennedy (1953) Glasgow Med. J. 34:521-543.

Woodson, R. D., J. D. Torrance, S. D. Shappell and C. Lenfant (1970) J. Clin. Invest. 49:1349-1356.

The opinions or assertions contained herein are the private views of the authors and are not to be construed as official or as reflecting the views of the Department of the Army or the Department of Defense.

DISCUSSION OF PAPERS IN SESSION 6

CHAIRMEN: DR. J. DITZEL AND DR. R.E. FORSTER

PAPER BY: DR. DITZEL et al

Dr. Cain: Did the P_{50} changes have any functional consequence in terms of altered venous PO_2?

Dr. Ditzel: Mixed venous blood samples were not taken because there was no medical indication for cardiac catheterisation produres in these individuals. However, from the arterial blood samples, it was possible to calculate venous PO_2, assuming a constant uptake of 5 vol. % O_2 and, using each individual's oxygen dissociation curve (ODC), PaO_2, pH, etc. Such calculations indicate a statistically significant reduction in venous PO_2 associated with the leftward shift of the ODC.

PAPER BY: DRS. SCHNEIDERMAN and GOLDSTICK

Dr. Lübbers: In the carotid artery, a zone has been described in the wall which is almost impermeable to oxygen. Have you found such a thing in any of the arteries you have investigated?

2. Do you know if there are any DC changes in the arterial wall which might influence the PO_2 measurements?

Dr. Goldstick: We also were concerned about the possible presence of an oxygen barrier and we verified its absence in two ways.
1) we observed no discontinuities in the slope of the PO_2 profile;
2) we measured the PO_2 continuously at several points in the avascular layer following rapid changes in either the luminal or adventitial PO_2. At all points the PO_2 transients closely followed

the imposed changes, as would be predicted from simple diffusion in
a homogeneous medium without barriers. Of course, both of these
techniques are limited by experimental realities. In the first
case by the resolution of our profile and in the second by the
rapidity with which we could change the PO_2 at the two surfaces.
Therefore, we conclude that if there are barriers, they are very
small indeed. One would also think that it would be maladaptive
to have an oxygen barrier in a tissue where oxygen supplied by
diffusion is already over-extended.

As to your second question, the lack of discontinuities in the PO_2
profiles would also seem to indicate that if there are electrical
potential drops in the tissue, they must be of the order of only
a few millivolts. The plateau in our polarogram is sufficiently
flat that these do not appear to interfere with our measurements.
Of course, in more electrically active tissue (e.g. brain), one
should really put the reference electrode close to the measuring
tip as I know you have done.

Finally, our experimental PO_2 profiles were only meant to demonstrate that our simulated profiles have the correct general slope
and, most importantly, that the minimum PO_2 in the media which we
predict, does in fact exist. We did not attempt to adjust the
parameters in our simulation, which all came from the literature,
to fit our experimental curves. The main purpose of our simulation was to show the effect of COHb on the value of the minimum
PO_2.

Fetal and Maternal Oxygenation

MICROELECTRODE STUDIES IN THE BRAIN

OF FETAL RATS AND NEW BORN RATS

Wilhelm Erdmann

University of Alabama, School of Medicine
University Station
Birmingham, Alabama 35294

During the development of the fetus, differentiation of the nervous system is correlated to an increase of oxygen consumption of the brain. In response to the increased oxygen demand, the capillary network becomes more dense with the decisive decrease of the inter-capillary distance. This process is continued after birth such that the number of capillaries per volume unit of tissue in adults might be more than threefold compared to that of the newborn (Craigie 1955, Diemer 1968).

In the present study we investigated the influence of the described changes in oxygen consumption and inter capillary distance on the oxygen supply of the microarea of the brain cortex. Considering the grade of maturity of the newborn at birth two different groups had to be investigated.
1)   Newborns of mammalians which are born mature and have fully developed physical and neurological functions (so-called nest leavers). They show a fully developed capillary network at birth (Flexner 1953, Craigie 1955).
2)   Newborns of mammalians which are born rather immature, (so-called nest huggers). In immature newborns, the development of the capillary network reaches far into the post-natal life.

METHODS

Pre-natal measurements were performed in fetuses of pregnant rats (nest huggers) and in fetuses of pregnant guinea pigs (nest leavers). The oxygen partial pressure distribution was examined by insertion of oxygen microelectrodes (gold microelectrode system, Erdmann, 1972) which were inserted into the fetal brain through a small incision into the otherwise intact uterine wall. The head of the fetus was kept in position by three steel needles. The PO_2 electrodes were driven forward by means of a micromanipulator and the PO_2 values were registered each ten microns. The experiment was performed five, three and one day before calculated birthdate with more than fifteen fetuses in each group.

The investigation of the development of the oxygen supply pattern in the post-natal period was done in nest huggers. Because of their rather quick maturation and the speedy aging, mice were chosen for this experiment. The oxygen partial pressure distribution was examined in mice of three to four weeks of age, in mice of three months of age, six months of age, and one year of age. The animals were anesthetized with sodium pentobarbitol i.p. The heads of the animals were fixed in a micromanipulator system, the skull bone emaciated and the gold micro-electrodes inserted into the brain cortex through small bore holes drilled into the skull bone. The electrodes were driven through the cortex in steps of ten microns, and the oxygen partial pressure values statistically evaluated.

RESULTS

Calculation of the frequency of O_2 tension values demonstrates distribution characteristics of the adult cerebral cortex to be skewed to the left with fifty percent of the values below 5 mmHg and thirty-five percent below 2 mmHg (Rats). In contrary to these findings (Erdmann, 1972) the oxygen tension values in the fetal brain show relatively high mean values which decrease near term. Five days before birth seventy-five percent of the values were between 14 and 18 mmHg (Figure 1, left lower tracing). Three days before birth seventy-five percent of the values were between 10 and 16 mmHg (Figure 1, left middle tracing). On the day before birth the values were lower (Figure 1, left upper tracing), but still high in comparison with those of the adult rat.

The oxygen partial pressure distribution in guinea pigs' fetuses which are born very mature shows totally different disttribution characteristics. Five days before birth seventy-five percent of the tissue PO_2 values are found to be below 15 mmHg (Figure 1, right lower tracing), three days before birth seventy-five percent of the tissue PO_2 values are found to be below 13 mmHg (Figure 1, right middle tracing) and one day before birth seventy-five percent of the values are below 8 mmHg (Figure 1, right upper tracing).

The oxygen partial pressure distribution of mice three to four weeks after birth still shows rather high tissue PO_2 values compared to those of the adult. The peak of the distribution is to be found in the 7 to 8 mmHg PO_2 range (Figure 2, right tracing). In three months old mice the tissue PO_2 values have only fallen slightly compared to those measured in three-week-old mice and the peak distribution still is in the range of 6 to 8 mmHg (Figure 2, left tracing). A steep decrease of tissue PO_2 values is observed between the third month and the sixth months post-partum where more than fifty percent of the values are below 5 mmHg with a pronounced peak at 1 to 2 mmHg (Figure 3, right tracing). There is no decisive decrease of tissue PO_2 observed after the sixth month as to the registration of oxygen partial pressure distribution in the cortex of one-year-old mice (Figure 3, left tracing). A comparison of oxygen partial pressure distribution in different stages post-partum shows a significant shift of the frequency distribution of oxygen partial pressure to lower values from three weeks of age to three months of age and to six months of age while thereafter no further changes were observed.

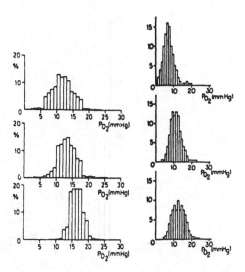

FIGURE 1:   Left Column: PO$_2$ distribution in the fetal brain of rats (nest huggers); 5 days before term (lower tracing), 3 days before term (middle tracing), 1 day before term (upper tracing).
Right Column: PO$_2$ distribution in the fetal brain of guinea pigs (nest beavers); 5 days (lower tracing), 3 days (middle tracing) and 1 day (upper tracing) before term.

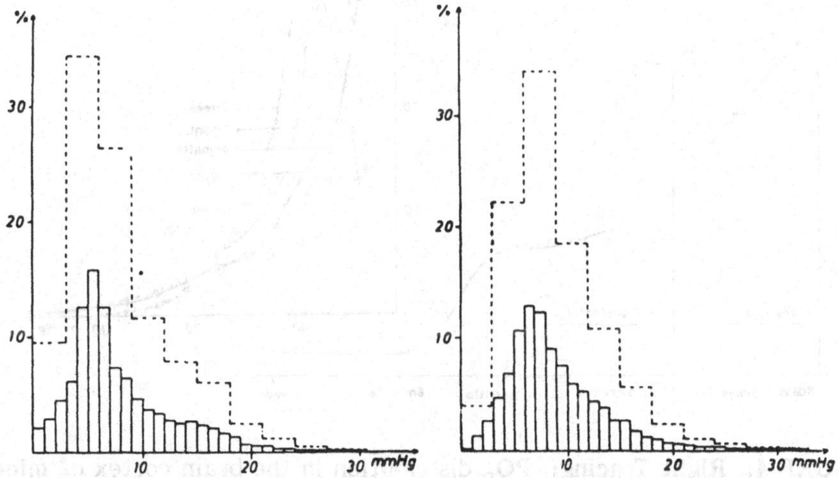

FIGURE 2:   PO$_2$ distribution in the brain cortex of mice 3-4 weeks of age (right tracing) and mice 3 months of age (left tracing).

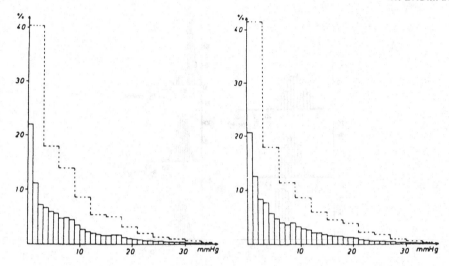

FIGURE 3: PO$_2$ values in the brain cortex of mice 6 months of age (right tracing) and 1 year of age (left tracing).

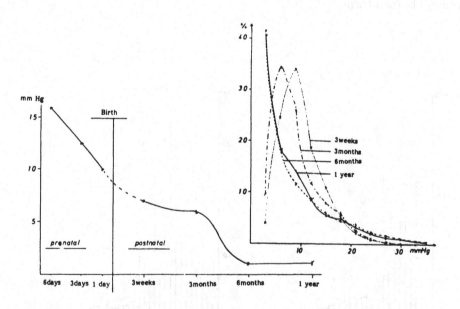

FIGURE 4: <u>Right Tracing</u>: PO$_2$ distribution in the brain cortex of mice 3 weeks, 3 months, 6 months and 1 year of age.
<u>Left Tracing</u>: Shift of the peak in the PO$_2$ distribution from the prenatal through the postnatal period of mice (nest huggers).

DISCUSSION

The shift of oxygen partial pressure distribution from high to low values in the last days of pregnancy can be explained by the known increase of the oxygen consumption of the brain assuming more functions. It is therefore understandable that this shift is more expressed in those fetuses (Guinea pigs) which are born with highly developed neurogenic functions at a mature stage.

The rat, and also the mouse, so-called nest huggers, are, compared to the guinea pig, so-called nest leavers, rather immature at birth. The neurogenic functions of rats and mice are underdeveloped at birth and comparable to those of the human being, also a nest hugger. Considering the shift of the oxygen partial pressure distribution from rather high values five to six days before birth to low values of the grown-up, two phases can be observed. The first rather steep slope in the last five days before birth, then a rather stable part of the curve in the first three months of life and another steep decrease of oxygen partial pressure values in the period between three and six months of age (Figure 5). Thereafter the final oxygen partial pressure distribution in the cortex has been reached. The increase of capillary density post-natal is observed in three phases: a primary slow phase, a secondary quick phase and a third slow phase. The quick phase of increase of capillary density has been defined by Flexner (1953) as critical phase. In this phase, the capillary density might be doubled in only a few days. This phase is characterized by the development of decisive cortical functions: the differentiation of neurons, the formation of neuro-piles, the functional differentiation of the brain and the final development of all cortical functions with a speedy increase of the oxygen consumption. While this critical stage is seen in the post-partum period in nest huggers, the critical phase in nest leavers already occurs prenatally.

The question after the cause of capillary growth seems to be explained by hypoxia experiments (Diemer 1965), and also by experiments in animals adjusted to living in high altitudes (Opitz and Palme 1944, Mercker and Opitz 1949, Valdiva 1958). The mechanism by which a chronic hypoxia effects capillary growth has been so far not yet explained. According to Diemer (1968) three possibilities have to be discussed: 1) production of vasopoietin under the influence of hypoxia; 2) continuously increased capillary perfusion, and 3) direct action of oxygen.

SUMMARY

Experiments have been performed on the tissue oxygenation of fetal brain during the last days of pregnancy in nest leavers and nest huggers. The follow-up of the oxygen partial pressure distribution in nest huggers was continued post natally. As experimental animals, guinea pigs were chosen as a typical example of nest leavers and rats and mice as typical examples for nest huggers who resemble in this respect the human being. The fetal PO_2 distribution has been evaluated at the fifth, third and first day before birth in rat fetuses and was compared to the ones in guinea pigs' fetuses. The oxygen partial pressure in rat fetuses shows a shift of oxygen partial pressure distribution from 70 to 80 mmHg five days before birth to 10 to 12 mmHg at birthday. In guinea pigs, the shift is even more significant with PO_2 values at birthday between 4 and 6 mmHg, thus the PO_2 distribution in newborn guinea pigs is similar to that in adult animals.

In the first three months after birth, the tissue PO_2 showed a very small drop between the third month of age and the sixth month of age, and a rather steep drop of tissue PO_2 values was observed when final adult values were reached.

The difference of the development of the PO_2 distribution between nest huggers and nest leavers was explained by the different stages of brain maturity at birth. The relatively little drop in tissue PO_2 in the first three months of age in nest huggers, despite a tremendous increase in oxygen consumption in the phase of development could be explained with an adequate increase of capillarization. In fact, in this period of neuronal, un-differentiation capillary density might double in just a few days. This phase was defined as critical phase and falls between the tenth and twenty-fifth day post-partum in rats. In the later stage of development, however, capillary growth does not seem any more to go along with increased oxygen consumption and thus explains the steep drop of oxygen partial pressure values beyond the third month of age.

With given density of the capillary mesh work the supply conditions of the maturing brain may furthermore be increased by changes of the diffusion parameters. Preliminary studies have shown that the shift of the oxygen diffusion coefficient and oxygen conductivity coefficient to lower values seem to be contradictive to the increasing demands of the cells. This shift is seen beyond the first three month period of age and seems to furthermore explain the PO_2 drop in the second half-year of life. This experiment needs further investigation and documentation.

REFERENCES

1. Craigie EH: Vascular pattern of the developing nervous system. In: Waelsh: Biochemistry of the developing nervous system. Academic Press, New York, 1955.
2. Diemer K: Der Einfluss chronischen Sauerstoffmangels auf die Capillarentwicklung im Gehirn des Saeuglings. Mschr. Kinderheilk. 113 (1965) 281.
3. Diemer K: Capillarisation and oxygen supply of the brain. In: Luebbers et al: Oxygen Transport in Blood and Tissue. Thieme, Stuttgart, 1968.
4. Diemer K, Henn R: Kapillarvermehrung in der Ratte unter chronischem Sauerstoffmangel. Naturwissenschaften 52 (1965) 135.
5. Erdmann W: Distribution of oxygen partial reserves pressures the cortex of fetal rat brain. A microelectrode study. In: Respiratory Gas Exchange and Blood Flow in the Placenta. DHEW Publication No. (NIH) 73-361, 1972.
6. Flexner LB: Physiologic Development of the Cortex of the Brain and its Relationsships to its Morphology, Constitution, and Enzyme Systems. In: Res. Publ. Ass. nerv. ment. Dis. Vol. XXXII, Metabolic and toxic diseases of the nervous system. William and Wilkins, Baltimore, 1953.
7. Mercker H, Opitz E: Die Gefaesse der Pia Mater hohenangepasster Kaninchen. Pfluegers Arch. ges. Physiol. 251 (1949) 117.

8.   Opitz E, Palme F: Darstellung der Hoehenanpassung im Gebirge durch Sauerstoffmangel. II. u. III. Mitteilung. Pfluegers Arch. ges. Physiol. 248 (1944) 298.

9.   Valdiva E: Total Capillary Bed in Striated Muscle of Guinea Pig native to the Peruvian Mountains. Amer. J. Physiol. 194 (1958) 585.

THE EFFECT OF ACIDOSIS ON RED CELL 2,3-DPG AND OXYGEN AFFINITY OF

WHOLE FOETAL BLOOD

P.D. Wimberley, M.D. Whitehead and E.R. Huehns

Department of Clinical Haematology

University College Hospital Medical School, London W.C.1

The aim of this study was to make sequential measurements on a series of premature infants with and without respiratory distress syndrome to assess the effect of acidosis and hypoxaemia on oxygen transport. 3 infants with an uneventful postnatal course (33 weeks gestation, birth weights 1325 gms, 1455 gms and 1484 gms) were compared with 6 infants who needed assisted ventilation for respiratory problems after birth (mean gestation 31.5 weeks, range 29 to 34 weeks; mean birth weight 1132 gms, range 800 to 1905 gms).

Haemoglobin, packed cell volume, foetal haemoglobin % (alkali denaturation rate method), red cell 2,3-diphosphoglycerate (Keitt, 1972), oxygen affinity, red cell pH, plasma pH, pCO_2 and pO_2 were measured on cord blood, at 24 hours, 72 hours, 1 week, 2 weeks and 4 weeks of age.

Because sequential measurements were being made on each infant, microtechniques were essential so that each set of measurements could be performed on less than 1 ml of whole blood. In order that oxygen affinity could be measured on 0.1 ml whole blood or less, a method was devised whereby percentage saturation was measured spectrophotometrically using a standard recording spectrophotometer, (Unicam SP1800) on a thin film of blood equilibrated to a known pO_2. Percentage saturation was calculated from the optical absorption spectrum by measuring optical density (O.D.) at two isobestic points for oxy- and deoxy-haemoglobin (507 and 570 nm) and two points of maximal difference in the same region of the spectrum (560 and 578 nm). Oxyhaemoglobin concentration of a partially saturated blood sample is proportional to either

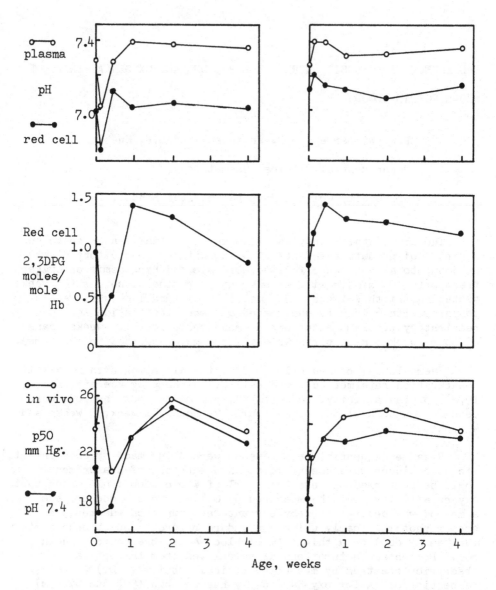

Fig. 1   (A) Postnatal changes
          in an infant of 31 weeks
          gestation with hyaline
          membrane disease.

          (B) Postnatal changes
          in an infant of 33 weeks
          gestation with an
          uneventful course.

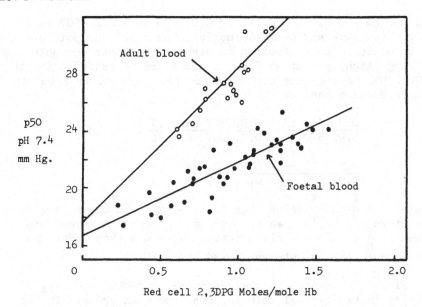

Fig. 2   p50 7.4 as a function of red cell 2,3-DPG for foetal
          blood (Hb-F > 85%). The regression line p50 (7.4) =
          5.24 DPG + 16.56 (r = 0.86, p < 0.001) is compared with
          that shown for adult blood (Hb-F < 1.0%) p50 (7.4) =
          10.51 DPG + 17.63 (r = 0.90, p < 0.001) (Bellingham
          et al., 1971).

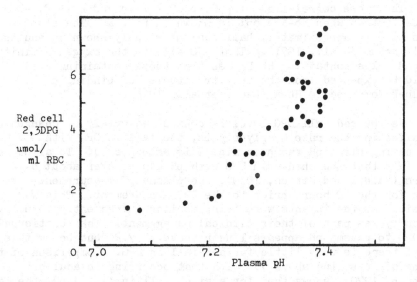

Fig. 3   Red cell 2,3-DPG as a function of plasma pH in foetal blood

O.D. 560 nm - O.D. 507 nm (X) or O.D. 578 nm - O.D. 507 nm (Y)
using total oxy- and deoxy-haemoglobin as reference points. As
the haemoglobin concentration between measurements on whole blood
may vary slightly, the Δ O.D.s X and Y are corrected using the
Δ O.D. (C) between the isobestic points. Percentage saturation
is then proportional to

$$\frac{\text{O.D. 560 nm - O.D. 507 nm}}{\text{O.D. 570 nm - O.D. 507 nm}} \quad (\frac{X}{C}) \quad \text{and}$$

$$\frac{\text{O.D. 578 nm - O.D. 507 nm}}{\text{O.D. 570 nm - O.D. 507 nm}} \quad (\frac{Y}{C})$$

Knowing the $\frac{X}{C}$ and $\frac{Y}{C}$ values for fully deoxy- and oxy-haemoglobin
percentage saturation can be calculated for any intermediate
values of $\frac{X}{C}$ or $\frac{Y}{C}$. The dissociation curve was then drawn from
4 or 5 measurements between 25 and 75% saturation.

Fig. 1 contrasts the changes in pH, 2,3-DPG, and oxygen
affinity in two typical infants, one from each group. In the
infant with respiratory distress there is a severe acidosis
immediately after birth associated with a marked fall in red cell
2,3-DPG concentration and a rise in oxygen affinity. In the
infant who remained normodotic, there is a clear rise in 2,3-DPG
level occurring within 24 hours after birth associated with a fall
in oxygen affinity. The same rapid postnatal increase in 2,3-DPG
has been shown in healthy full term infants (Versmold et al., 1973),
but the mechanism remains unknown.

The close correlation of p50, pH 7.4 with red cell 2,3-DPG
concentration when Hb-F > 85% is shown in Fig. 2. The slope of
this line is approximately half that previously shown in adults
(Bellingham et al., 1971). That DPG affects the oxygen affinity
of red cells containing Hb-F less than those containing Hb-A
would be expected from the in vitro studies of binding of 2,3-DPG
to Hb-F compared to Hb-A (Bauer et al., 1968).

As the red cell DPG level is controlled mainly by changes of
pH affecting the rate of glycolysis, the fall in DPG with
decreasing blood pH shown in fig. 3 is as expected. To allow for
the fact that the change in DPG with pH occurs over about 8-12
hours (Valeri and Hirsch, 1969), the plasma pH measurements are a
mean for the 12 hours prior to the DPG measurement. This was
possible as the infants were being monitored frequently (usually
4 hourly) as part of their clinical management. The relationship
of DPG to plasma pH appears linear above pH 7.2, but below this
level there is very little further fall in DPG. Comparison of the
slope of this line above 7.2 with that occurring in adults
(Astrup, 1970), shows that for a given fall in plasma pH, the fall

in foetal red cell DPG is almost twice that occurring in adult
red cells. Therefore, although the effect of DPG on Hb-F is less
than on Hb-A, the greater fall in DPG caused by a given degree of
acidosis suggests that like in adult blood, the oxygen affinity
change caused by the change in DPG level as pH alters, approximately
balances the Bohr effect.

References

Astrup, P. (1970) Red cell metabolism and function.
    ed. Brewer (Plenum Press) p.67.

Bauer, C., Ludwig, I. and Ludwig, M. (1968) Life Sciences, 7, 1,
    1339.

Bellingham, A.J., Detter, J.C. and Lenfant, C. (1971) J. Clin.
    Invest., 50, 700.

Keitt, A.S. (1972) Lab. Methods, 77, 470.

Valeri, C.R. and Hirsch, N.M. (1969) J. Lab. Clin. Med., 73, 722.

Versmold, H., Seifert, G. and Riegel, K.P. (1973) Resp. Phys.,
    18, 14.

OXYGEN AFFINITY CHANGES IN THE RED CELLS OF EMBRYONIC AND NEONATAL MICE

R.E. Gale, R.M.G. Wells and E.R. Huehns

Department of Clinical Haematology

University College Hospital Medical School, London W.C.1

The sequence of erythropoietic events occurring during normal development of an embryo to an adult is a useful system for demonstrating cellular differentiation in relation to function. In mice there are two generations of red cells. The first, the primitive erythroid cells, originate in the blood islands of the yolk sac from about 8 days gestation and enter the circulation at 9 - 10 days gestation. These are large nucleated cells which continue dividing after release, and synthesize the three embryonic haemoglobins, EI (x_2y_2), EII (α_2y_2), and EIII (α_2z_2). The second generation of red cells, the definitive erythroid cells, are produced in the liver and enter the circulation from about 12 days gestation. These are non-nucleated and contain only adult haemoglobin ($\alpha_2\beta_2$) (Fantoni et al., 1967).

We have studied the functional development of mouse red cells from 11 days gestation, through birth and on to adult life using a random bred strain of mice, CD-1. Blood was obtained from adults and newborn mice by decapitation. In order to obtain blood from unborn mouse embryos, the pregnant female was killed at known gestation, and the embryos carefully dissected out to avoid any contamination with maternal blood. Each litter was pooled in heparinized tubes containing cold isotonic NaCl and cut into small pieces to release the blood. After straining, the red cells were washed three times with saline. The oxygen affinity of the red cells suspended in various isotonic buffer solutions was determined as previously described (Huehns and Farooqui, 1975), and 2,3-diphosphoglycerate (DPG) was measured using an enzymic assay (Keitt, 1971).

The p50 of red cells suspended in a phosphate buffer at pH 7.4
and 37° was between 20.5 and 23.5 mm Hg in embryos, with a slight
rise in oxygen affinity just before birth, reaching a p50 of
18.5 mm Hg in the newborn. After this the oxygen affinity fell
gradually, p50 at 12 days after birth was 27.0 mm Hg, while in
adult mice it was between 29.5 - 32.0 mm Hg. Results at pH 7.0
followed those at pH 7.4. p50 for embryos was 31.0 mm Hg at
11 days gestation, there was some decrease in affinity to a
p50 of 35.0 mm Hg at 16 days gestation, followed by an increase
just before birth to a p50 of 31.5 mm Hg in the newborn. After
birth there was a gradual fall in affinity towards adult levels,
p50 between 44.5 - 48.5 mm Hg. Results at pH 6.7 showed a large
decrease in affinity between 11 and 13 days gestation, p50 at
11 days 22.5 mm Hg and at 13 days 42.5 mm Hg. A further decrease
gave a p50 of 56.0 mm Hg at 17 days gestation, which was followed
by a sharp increase in affinity at birth, p50 for newborn 46.0 mm Hg.
A gradual fall again brought the results to the adult value,
63.0 - 69.0 mm Hg.

DPG results showed that mouse adult red cells contain
approximately 2 μmoles DPG/μmole Hb, which is twice the relative
amount found in normal adult human cells. Embryonic mouse red
cells at 11 days gestation gave values of 0.6 and 1.0 μmoles DPG/
μmole Hb. A gradual decrease brought the levels to 0.1 μmoles
DPG/μmole Hb at 18 days gestation and in the newborn, but they
steadily rose again after birth to the adult level.

The results show that all mouse foetal red cells studied have
a higher oxygen affinity than adult red cells. This is similar
to the relationship of adult to foetal red cell oxygen affinity
in all mammalian species, and presumably helps the transport of
oxygen from the maternal to the foetal blood. Before a true
circulation is established and before the placenta is fully
developed, the embryo must obtain its oxygen supply from the
maternal interstitial fluid. No details of gas transport, either
CO_2 from or O_2 to the embryo are known. It is at this period of
development that the red cells contain embryonic haemoglobins,
and they also have higher oxygen affinities than red cells from
adults, the difference being of the same order as that between
newborn and adult mice above pH 7.0.

Below pH 7.0 the difference in oxygen affinity between
embryonic and adult red cells is much greater. The reverse
Bohr shift of mouse adult and human adult and foetal haemoglobins
commences at pH 6.0, which is outside the physiological range.
Mouse embryonic haemoglobins show a reverse Bohr shift commencing
around pH 7.0, a value which could well be reached intracellularly,
particularly before the placenta is fully formed, when the acid
products of metabolism may not be removed from the embryonic

circulation as quickly as would be the case later on in development. If the Bohr shift was the same as in adult mice, then the oxygen affinity would fall to very low levels, and oxygen transport at the range of pO_2s involved would be virtually impossible. The reverse shift which starts at pH 7.0 would therefore help to keep the oxygen affinity high enough at the lower pH values to maintain sufficient oxygen transport to the embryo. A similar result was reported by Bauer et al (1975) using haemolysates from mouse embryos at 12.5 days gestation.

Results from DPG estimations show that in the adult there are 2 molecules of DPG for every molecule of haemoglobin. These presumably lower the oxygen affinity of the cell by binding to haemoglobin, as well as by their effect, via the Bohr effect, in lowering the intracellular pH. Embryonic cells also contain DPG. Bauer et al. (1975) concluded that sufficient DPG was present in the embryonic cells to produce a significant decrease in oxygen affinity. They found that the maximal effect of DPG on oxygen affinity was similar for adult and embryonic haemoglobins when expressed in terms of shift in p50, but the intrinsic oxygen affinity of embryonic cells was higher. In our study the lowest DPG values were found at birth, at 18 days gestation and in newborn mice, which correlates with the high oxygen affinity found at this time. It is possible that this high affinity is needed for the period of relative hypoxia occurring during delivery and shortly afterwards.

The specific reverse Bohr shift below pH 7.0 and the presence of DPG allow modulation of the oxygen affinity of embryonic blood to maintain adequate oxygen transport, even when there is marked acidosis in the embryo.

References

Bauer, C., Tamm, R., Petschow, D., Bartels, R. and Bartels, H. (1975) Nature, 257, 333.

Fantoni, A., Bank, A. and Marks, P.A. (1967) Science, 157, 1327.

Huehns, E.R. and Farooqui, A.M. (1975) Nature, 254, 335.

Keitt, A.S. (1971) J. Lab. Clin. Med., 77, 470.

TEMPORAL CORRELATIONS BETWEEN PLASMA OVARIAN STEROID HORMONE

LEVELS AND INTRAUTERINE OXYGEN TENSION IN THE GUINEA PIG

David R. Garris and J. A. Mitchell

Department of Anatomy, Wayne State University

School of Medicine, Detroit, Michigan   48201   U.S.A.

INTRODUCTION

Oxygen is essential for blastocyst survival. Since, prior to implantation, the blastocyst has no direct connection with the maternal vasculature, a supply of oxygen sufficient to meet its metabolic needs must be available within the uterine lumen. In vitro studies indicate that mouse blastocysts require at least 7 mmHg of oxygen to sustain development (Auerbach and Brinster, 1968). While in vitro experiments have provided considerable information concerning conceptus metabolism and development, the environmental conditions to which the blastocyst is subjected during culture are different from the environment provided by the uterine lumen. Thus, until in vivo conditions are determined, the extent to which in vitro environments duplicate that in which blastocyst development and implantation normally occur, remains unknown.

To date the only systematic in vivo studies of intrauterine oxygen tension (pO_2) have been conducted in the rat (Mitchell and Yochim, 1968a,b and Yochim and Mitchell, 1968). It was found that estrogen and progesterone exert profound effects on intrauterine pO_2 via modification of uterine morphology, vasculature and metabolism. Furthermore, an oxygen tension gradient develops between the uterine lumen and the antimesometrial capillary plexus at the time of implantation. Thus, in the rat, ovarian steroid hormones are a major determinant of intrauterine pO_2 and may therefore play a significant role not only in blastocyst development but also in the process of implantation. Whether or not estrogen and progesterone modulate intrauterine pO_2 and are involved in the process of implantation in other species remains to be determined.

Experimental evidence for the possible involvement of intrauterine pO_2 in implantation has been obtained in the rabbit and
guinea pig. The existence in the rabbit of a hemotrophic relationship between uterine capillaries and the site of trophoblast attach-
ment has been elegantly demonstrated by Boving (1963). In the
guinea pig, cyclic changes in uterine vasculature occur (Markee,
1929), and hyperemia restricted to the antimesometrial endometrium
near the midpoint of each uterine horn has been reported (Bacsich
and Wyburn, 1939). Since the blastocyst normally implants on the
antimesometrial surface, a relationship between the localized hyperemia and implantation was suggested. The present study was
undertaken to determine intrauterine oxygen tension throughout the
estrous cycle and pre-implantation period in the guinea pig and to
determine the temporal correlations between plasma ovarian steroid
hormone levels and intrauterine oxygen tension.

MATERIALS AND METHODS

Animals: Adult virgin guinea pigs (English Short Hair: Camm
Research Institute) weighing 600-900 gms were housed under a controlled photoperiod of 14 hrs. light/day. Food and water were
available ad libitum. Vaginal smears were taken during the period
of vaginal patency; a predominance of cornified cells in the lavage
was used to denote estrus (Day 0). All animals exhibited at least
two normal cycles prior to use.

Measurement of pO_2: Intrauterine oxygen tension was measured
with an oxygen microelectrode-Microsensor-potentiometric recorder
assembly (Transidyne Co., Ann Arbor) on Days 0,2,6,8 and 12 of the
cycle. The electrode was calibrated in 0:100%, 5:95% and 20:80%
$O_2:N_2$ physiological saline solutions and the calibrated values corrected for guinea pig body temperature (39°C) and barometric pressure.

The tubal end of the uterus was exposed by a flank incision
in Innovar anesthetized animals (1 ml/kg body wt.). A Riley needle
was inserted into the uterine lumen through a scissor cut at the
utero-tubal junction and the needle held in place by a clamp assembly. The calibrated oxygen electrode was inserted into the Riley
needle and a record of intrauterine oxygen tension made for two
twenty minute periods interrupted by an electrode calibration check.
Recordings with calibration deviations exceeding ± 3 mmHg were re-
jected. Records (Fig. 1) were analyzed for minute-to-minute changes
in pO_2, and mean oxygen tension (maximum + minimum pO_2/2) was computed. All recordings were made between 1000 and 1500 hours on the
specified day of the cycle. Each uterine horn was used for only
one recording.

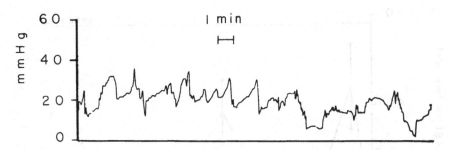

Figure 1: Chart recording of intrauterine pO_2 (mmHg). A typical rhythm may be observed with prominent increases and decreases in pO_2. Mean pO_2 levels were calculated following two 20-minute periods.

Arterial and venous pO_2: Arterial (A) and venous (V) pO_2 were measured by placing the tip of the calibrated electrode at the confluens of the renal vessels within the aorta and vena cava, respectively. Each recording was of twenty minutes duration.

Hormone levels: On Days 0,2,4,6,8 and 12, guinea pigs were lightly anesthetized with methoxyflurane, 2 ml of blood removed by intracardiac puncture and plasma collected. Plasma progesterone (P) was assayed by competitive protein-binding (Murphy, 1967). Plasma estradiol (E) was determined by double antibody radioimmunoassay (England et al. 1974).

RESULTS

Arterial and venous pO_2 remained constant throughout the estrous cycle (58 and 18 mmHg, respectively: Fig. 2). By contrast, significant cyclic differences were observed in intrauterine pO_2 (Fig. 2). A peak in intrauterine pO_2 of 44.0 ± 10.5 mmHg was observed on Day 0 of the cycle (p<.01: Day 0 vs. venous). By Day 2, intrauterine pO_2 had fallen to near venous levels (15.8 ± 6.0 mmHg) and remained low through Day 4 (20.4 ± 5.8 mmHg). However, Day 6 values were elevated (38.9 ± 7.2 mmHg) and were significantly different from those observed on Days 2 and 4 (p< .01). The midluteal rise of intrauterine pO_2 was followed by a return to venous levels on Days 8 (20.5 ± 5.5 mmHg) and 12 (16.2 ± 4.0 mmHg). Thus, intrauterine pO_2 exhibits cyclic fluctuations, peaking at the time of ovulation (Day 0) and at the expected time of blastocyst implantation (Day 6).

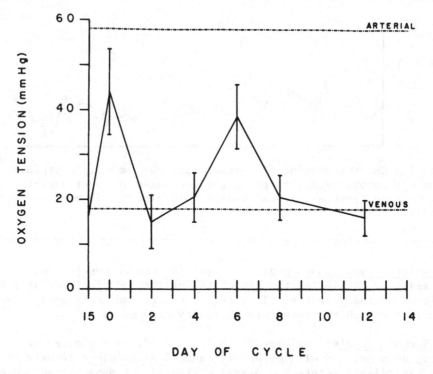

Figure 2: Intrauterine pO_2 (mean levels ±SEM) throughout the
estrous cycle (Day 0 = estrus). Arterial and venous levels are
denoted by dashed lines and were constant throughout the cycle.
(Number of animals per group = 5.)

        To determine if ovarian steroids participate in modulating in-
trauterine pO_2, cyclic fluctuations in plasma E and P were measured
for comparison with the cyclic changes observed in oxygen levels
(Fig. 3). Plasma P exhibited two surges, one on Day 0 consisting
of a transient increase followed by a decline to basal levels by
Day 1, and a second elevation extending from Days 2 through 6.
Plasma P exhibited basal values between Days 8 and 12. Similarly,
E exhibited two pronounced cyclic peaks. On Day 0, plasma E was
elevated but declined to basal levels by Day 2. Low levels were
maintained through Day 4 followed by a mid-luteal rise on Day 6.
By Day 8, E levels had again returned to basal levels which were
maintained through Day 12 of the cycle. Thus, the elevations observed in intrauterine pO_2 on Days 0 and 6 correspond temporally
with those observed in plasma E.

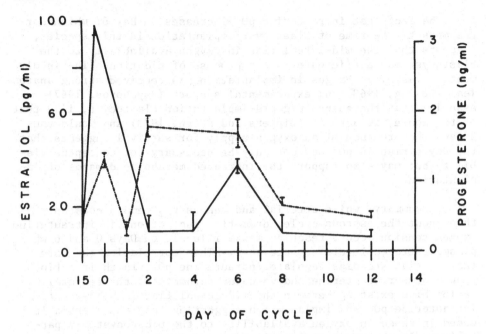

<u>Figure 3</u>: Cyclic fluctuations in mean (±SEM) plasma progesterone
(dashed line) and estradiol levels (solid line) are depicted. Day
0 and 6 E levels were significantly elevated (p<.01). (n = 3-8
animals per group.)

DISCUSSION

     The results of this study suggest that intrauterine oxygen
tension in the guinea pig is regulated, at least in part, by the
actions of ovarian steroid hormones. Cyclic fluctuations in intrauterine pO_2 parallel those of plasma estrogen and are reciprocal
to plasma progesterone levels except on Day 6. If, in fact, E
increases while P suppresses intrauterine pO_2, the presence of E
with elevated P levels on Day 6 may indicate that estrogen can
override the suppressive effects of progesterone during the mid-
luteal phase of the cycle and thereby increase oxygen availability
to the blastocyst at the time of implantation. The low levels of
pO_2 during the remainder of the cycle suggest that the factors
regulating oxygen availability are very sensitive to low levels of
circulating P which, in the absence of E, results in intrauterine
oxygen tension being equivalent to that of venous blood.

The fact that intrauterine pO_2 increases on Day 6, which corresponds to the time of blastocyst implantation in this species, suggests that the mid-luteal rise in oxygen availability to the blastocyst may participate in the process of nidation. The involvement of vascular changes in implantation has received strong anatomical (Boving, 1963) and experimental support (Psychoyos, 1967). Assuming that the guinea pig pre-implantation blastocyst, like that of the mouse, is aerobic (Biggers and Stern, 1973) and would thus demand the presence of an oxygen supply for survival suggests that the Day 6 rise in pO_2 may not only be necessary for conceptus viability but may also support the increased metabolic demands of implantation.

In summary, while arterial and venous pO_2 remain constant throughout the estrous cycle, dramatic fluctuations in intrauterine oxygen tension occur, reaching maximal levels on Days 0 and 6 when plasma estrogen levels are elevated. This correlation suggests that ovarian steroids regulate intrauterine pO_2 via their actions upon a number of uterine and vascular parameters, the temporal relationships existing between the mid-luteal rise in plasma estrogen, intrauterine pO_2 and implantation suggesting that the steroid induced increase in oxygen availability to the blastocyst may participate in the process of implantation in the guinea pig.

REFERENCES

Auerbach, S. and Brinster, R. (1968) Nature 217, 465.
Bacsich, P. and Wyburn, G. (1939) Trans. Roy. Soc. Edin. 60, 79.
Biggers, J. D. and Stern, S. (1973) Adv. Reprod. Physiol. 6, 1.
Boving, B. G. (1963) Implantation mechanisms. In 'Conference on Physiological Mechanisms Concerned with Conception.' Pergamon Press, Oxford.
England, B., Niswender, G. and Midgley, A. (1974) J. Clin. Endocr. Metab. 38, 42.
Markee, J. E. (1929) Am. J. Obstet. Gynecol. 17, 205.
Mitchell, J. A. and Yochim, J. (1968a) Endocrinology 83, 691.
Mitchell, J. A. and Yochim, J. (1968b) Endocrinology 83, 701.
Murphy, B. P. (1967) J. Clin. Endocr. Metab. 27, 973.
Psychoyos, A. (1967) Adv. Reprod. Physiol. 2, 275.
Yochim, J. M. and Mitchell, J. A. (1968) Endocrinology 83, 706.

OXYGEN CONSUMPTION AND DIFFUSION IN ISOLATED HUMAN

TERM PLACENTAL LOBULES PERFUSED IN VITRO

Andrée Guiet-Bara

Université Pierre et Marie Curie,
Biologie de la Reproduction (Pr. M. Panigel)
7 Quai St Bernard, 75230 Paris Cedex 05, France

An in vitro model has been perfected to perfuse maternal and foetal circulations in the isolated lobule of term human placentae. The present paper gives the results obtained using this experimental model to investigate   placental oxygen consumption and oxygen diffusion from the maternal to the foetal placental circulation.

MATERIAL AND METHODS

A hundred placental lobules have been subjected to the dual perfusion technique in a constant temperature room (37°C) immediately after natural delivery or cesarean section. On the foetal side, plastic tubings are introduced into the branches of the umbilical blood vessels on the chorial plate and advanced until they reach the arterial and venous cotyledonary stem vessels. On the maternal side, a fine glass cannula is introduced into the opening of a uteroplacental spiral artery or used to perforate the basal plate. The perfusion of the physiologic fluid is then initiated in a special chamber, both on the maternal and the foetal side (fig. 1).

The perfusion medium is Earle's physiological salt solution equilibrated with one of the following gas mixtures: A (5% O_2+ 5% CO_2+ 90% N_2) or B (95% O_2+ 5% CO_2). Mixture A, poor in oxygen, imitates the oxygen concentration in the foetal blood circulating in the umbilical arteries and mixture B, rich in oxygen, imitates the oxygen concentration of the maternal blood spurting from the uteroplacental arteries.

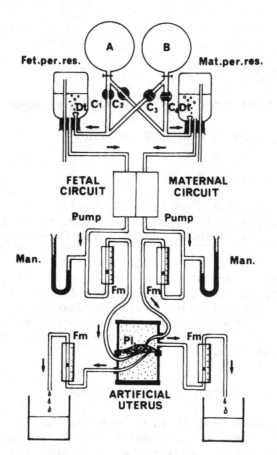

Figure 1. Perfusion system : A = gas mixture with 5% O_2, 5% CO_2 and 90% N_2; B = gas mixture with 95% O_2 and 5% CO_2; C_1, C_2, C_3, C_4 = two ways stop-cocks; Dt = gas dispersion tube; Fet. per. res. = foetal placental perfusion fluid reservoir; Fm = flow-meter; Man. = manometer; Pl = placenta; Mat. per. res. = maternal placental perfusion fluid reservoir.

To evaluate oxygen consumption of the placental tissue, only the foetal placental circulation of the lobule is perfused (single perfusion). Half an hour later, samples are taken from the inflowing and outflowing of perfusion media in the foetal coty-ledonary vascular circuit.

To evaluate oxygen diffusion from the maternal to the foetal side of the placenta, we have used the dual perfusion technique. After beginning the perfusion of the foetal placental circulation using Earle's solution equilibrated with A, we proceed, in some lobules, to the simultaneous perfusion of the uteroplacental circulation using Earle's equilibrated with B to produce a trans-placental PO_2 gradient. After a dual perfusion lasting 15 minutes (and every 15 minutes during one hour)we sample the perfusates flowing in and out of the foetal circuit.

The sampling is done under paraffin oil to determine the p H, the PO_2 and the PCO_2.

RESULTS

I Placental Oxygen Consumption

1) $\underline{PO_2\text{ changes in the foetal cotyledonary circulation.}}$ There is a fall of PO_2 in the perfusion medium during its circu-lation from the arterial to the venous side of the foetal coty-ledonary circuit. This arteriovenous PO_2 difference (ΔPO_2) appears to be more pronounced when Earle's + B is used: the ΔPO_2 averages 104±29 mm Hg for 15 placentae. Using Earle's + A , the ΔPO_2 averages 34±5 mm Hg for 43 placentae.

2) $\underline{\text{Oxygen utilization coefficient}}$

$$= \frac{\text{O}_2\text{ content of cotyledonary artery perfusate} - \text{O}_2\text{ content of venous cotyledonary perfusate}}{\text{O}_2\text{ content of cotyledonary artery perfusate}} \times 100$$

The oxygen utilization coefficient reaches 26±7% for 15 placentae when Earle's + B is used. The coefficient of oxygen utilization corresponding to the perfusion of Earle's + A is higher : 30±4% for 43 placentae.

3) $\underline{\text{Placental tissue oxygen consumption}}$. O_2 consumption is considered as the product of perfusion flow by the difference in the O_2 content of the arterial and the venous perfusates. The O_2 consumption given is the one used by one kilogram of pla-cental tissue.

For 14 placentae, O_2 consumption amounts to the average of 0.38±0.15 ml/min/kg when Earle's + A is used at a perfusion flow reaching 500 ml/min/kg. Using Earle's + B at an average flow rate of 500 ml/min/kg the average O_2 consumption reaches 1.9±1.2 ml/min/kg. This O_2 consumption reaches 3.3 ml/min/kg for a flow of 1000 ml/min/kg and 6.5 ml/min/kg for a perfusion flow of 2 500 ml/min/kg.

O_2 consumption is about 5 times higher with Earle's + B

than with Earle's + A when the average perfusion flow reaches 500 ml/min, this difference is highly significant ($p < 0.01$). There is a close relationship between the amount of O_2 consumption and the amount of O_2 supplied ($y = 0.223 \, x + 0.04$; $r = 0.98$; $p < 0.001$).

II Oxygen Diffusion from Uteroplacental to Foetal Placental Circulation (taking into account the placental oxygen consumption)

1) <u>PO_2 changes in the foetal cotyledonary circulation</u>. A single perfusion of Earle's + A, is performed on the foetal side of the placental lobule. The venous cotyledonary PO_2 is lower than the arterial cotyledonary PO_2 due to O_2 consumption by the placental tissue. For 33 placentae, arteriovenous difference $(\Delta PO_2)_1$ averages 33 ± 1 mm Hg. This value is not significantly different from 34 ± 5 mm Hg which corresponds to the average for all cases. Due to the variability of arterial cotyledonary PO_2, it seems preferable to express the cotyledonary arteriovenous PO_2 difference in arterial cotyledonary PO_2 %. This gives the average of $29 \pm 1\%$. For each placenta, the values thus determined under these conditions are the control values. When the foetal cotyledonary circulation is being perfused using Earle's + A, we start the uteroplacental perfusion using Earle's + B. The venous cotyledonary PO_2 increases and reaches a value superior to the arterial cotyledonary PO_2 (fig. 2). For each placenta, a new cotyledonary arteriovenous PO_2 difference is calculated as the $(\Delta PO_2)_2$. When a t test for paired observations is done, it is demonstrated that the mean of $(\Delta PO_2)_1$ $-(\Delta PO_2)_2$ is significantly different from 0 ($p < 0.01$). This demonstrates the existence of O_2 diffusion from uteroplacental to foetal placental circulation.

The venous cotyledonary PO_2 increase due to the diffusion related to the arterial cotyledonary PO_2 (taking into account the PO_2 variations due to the control placental tissue O_2 consumption) averages $53 \pm 2\%$ for 33 placentae. In the majority of cases, the diffusion of O_2 reaches a maximum after 1/4 to 1/2 h dual perfusion then it diminishes.

2) <u>Factors affecting the venous cotyledonary PO_2 during dual perfusions</u>. There is a significant correlation between the cotyledonary venous PO_2 and the arterial uteroplacental PO_2 ($y = 0.30 \, x + 20.30$; $r = 0.60$; $p < 0.001$). The correlation appears even closer between the ratio of uteroplacental to foetal placental flow and the cotyledonary venous PO_2 ($y = -4.55 \, x + 164.93$; $r = -0.67$; $p < 0.02$).

3) <u>Amount of oxygen which diffuses from the uteroplacental</u>

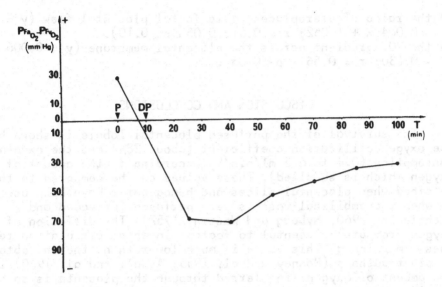

Figure 2. Arteriovenous PO₂ difference (PFa O₂ - PFv O₂, in mm
Hg) during the perfusion of the foetal side of a placental lobule: PFa O₂ = foetal placental arterial PO₂, PFv O₂= foetal placental venous PO₂, T = minutes of perfusion, P =sampling of
perfusate during the perfusion of the foetal circulation alone
(single perfusion) using Earle's + A, DP = starting of the maternal placental perfusion using Earle's + B while the foetal placental perfusion continues (dual perfusion).

to the foetal placental circulation. The placental oxygen con
sumption is first measured when only the foetal circulation is
perfused using Earle's + A. The oxygen consumed reaches an average of 0.42±0.17 ml/min/kg (for 11 placentae).

     When perfusion is initiated later on the maternal side
using Earle's + B, the amount of oxygen which is transferred
across the placenta averages 0.51±0.36 ml/min/kg (for 11 placentae). To this amount, one must add the oxygen which has diffused
and has been consumed by the placental tissue. Thus, the oxygen
diffusion reaches 0.93±0.38 ml/min/kg.

     4) Factors affecting the transplacental diffusion of oxygen.
We have mainly studied the part of flows and of uteroplacental
and foetal placental arterial PO₂. There appears a significant
correlation between the amount of oxygen which is transferred
and:
a) the cotyledonary flow (y = 0.0018 x + 0.1284; r = 0.70, p<
   0.010).

b) the ratio of uteroplacental to foetal placental flow (y = - 0.064 x + 1.052; r = 0.51; 0.05 < p < 0.10).
c) the PO_2 gradient across the placental membrane (y = 0.006 x - 0.830; r = 0.56 ; p ≤ 0.05).

DISCUSSION AND CONCLUSIONS

The survival of the perfused placental lobule is shown by the oxygen utilization coefficient (about 28%) and the oxygen consumption (0.4 to 6.5 ml/min/kg according to the amount of oxygen which is supplied). These values can be compared to those obtained when placental slices and homogenates have been used or when the umbilical vessels were perfused (Friedman and Sachtleben, 1960; Nyberg and Westin, 1957). The diffusion of oxygen from uteroplacental to foetal placental circulation reaches 1 ml/min/kg. This value is much lower than the one obtained by other authors (Romney and al, 1955; Assali and al, 1960) if the amount of oxygen transferred through the placenta is to be considered equal to the oxygen consumed by the foetus. Indeed, the physiological salt solution used as perfusion media have a much lower oxygen content than human blood; moreover foetal blood contains more hemoglobin than maternal blood and has a higher affinity to oxygen. In our in vitro experiments, the foetus has no longer to be taken into account. The present experimental model in which respiratory gas exchange continuously takes place will be perfected when oxygen carriers are added to the perfusion media. Hopefully, this will allow a better understanding of the complex mechanisms regulating physiologic transfer across the human placental membrane.

REFERENCES

Assali, N.S., Rauramo, L. and Peltonen, T. (1960) Am. J. Obstet. Gynec. 79, 86.

Friedman, E.A. and Sachtleben, M.R. (1960) Am. J. Obstet. Gynec. 79, 1058.

Nyberg, R. and Westin, B. (1957) Acta Physiol. Scand. 39, 216.

Romney, S.L., Reid, D.E., Metcalfe, J. and Burwell, C.S. (1955) Am. J. Obstet. Gynec. 70, 791.

HEMODYNAMICS AND OXYGEN DIFFUSION IN THE COTYLEDON OF THE HUMAN PLACENTA

L. Heilmann, C. Mattheck and W. Wiemer

Frauenklinik und Institut für Physiologie,

Universitätsklinikum, Essen, Fed. Rep. Germany

Due to the scarcity of available physiological data, our functional concept of placental insufficency is still very much dependant on theoretical considerations. The following paper deals with a model for the oxygen transport from the spiral artery to the villous capillary based on the cotyledon concept of the human placenta by Freese (1968).

The aspect to be considered first was the homogeneity of the <u>pressure distribution in the central space</u> of the cotyledon (ICS, fig. 1). The space into which the spiral artery opens was idealized as a funnel, which seemed justified on the basis of corrosive and angiographic studies by Freese (1968) and Borell et al. (1958). The Navier-Stokes equation was solved for small Reynolds numbers in spheric coordinates. For stationary conditions it takes the form

$$\eta \left(\frac{\partial^2 v}{\partial r^2} + \frac{2}{r} \frac{\partial v}{\partial r} + \frac{1}{r^2} \frac{\partial^2 v}{\partial \theta} + \frac{\cot \theta}{r^2} \frac{\partial v}{\partial \theta} - \frac{2v}{r^2} \right) = \frac{\partial p}{\partial r}$$

where ρ is the density of the blood, v the velocity, η the viscosity ($0,03$ g $\cdot$ cm^{-1} $\cdot$ s^{-1}), r the distance from the entry of the blood into the funnel, p the pressure, α the angle between the symmetry axis and the mantle, θ the angle between the symmetry axis and the velocity vector. The funnel thus represents a diffusor into which the blood is injected at a rate of Q = 0.1 cm^3 $\cdot$ s^{-1}. The latter value was obtained by dividing total placental blood flow by the number of cotyledons (Metcalfe et al., 1955). The resulting solutions for the distribution of velocity and pressure in this space were

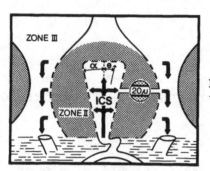

Fig. 1: Scheme of
the cotyledon

and

$$v(r,\theta) = \frac{Q}{4\pi r^2} \left(\frac{3(\cos^2\theta - \cos^2\alpha)}{2\cos^3\alpha - 3\cos^2\alpha + 1} \right)$$

$$p(r,\theta) = \frac{Q\eta}{2\pi r^3} \left(\frac{3\cos^2\theta - 1}{2\cos^3\alpha - 3\cos^2\alpha + 1} \right) + Const$$

For apertures of α = 15° or 45° - the normal range
as indicated by the results of Borell et al. (1958) and
Freese (1968) - these functions yielded a nearly homogenous distribution of pressure, and a parabolic velocity
profile (fig. 2). The average velocity of the maternal
blood appeared to be relatively low (0.3 cm/s at r = 0.5
cm), furnishing no indication of a socalled jet effect,
not even at angles of α = 15°. This homogeneous distribution of pressure warrants the conclusion that the intervillous space lateral to the ICS is perfused evenly
- provided the predecidual venous space has a similarly
homogeneous pressure profile.

On the basis of this parabolic velocity distribution
we could assume a laminar flow in the central space of the
cotyledon, and calculate the distribution of the O_2 concentration by diffusion. The diffusion equation in spherical coordinates takes the form.

$$\frac{\partial^2 C}{\partial \theta^2} + \cot\theta \, \frac{\partial C}{\partial \theta} - \frac{v_0}{D} \frac{\partial C}{\partial r} = 0$$

The solution is

$$C(r,\theta) = \sum_\ell A_\ell \, e^{\frac{-D\ell(\ell+1)r}{v_0}} P_\ell(\theta) + C_b$$

with

$$A_\ell = (C_i - C_b) \left(\frac{2\ell+1}{\ell(\ell+1)} \right) \left(\frac{d P_\ell(\cos\alpha)}{d\ell} \right)^{-1}$$

where l represents the roots of the equation P_1 (cosα)=0,
and P_1 the solutions of the differential equation of
Legendre. C_i is the O_2 concentration at the inflow
(assumed to be constant), C_b the concentration at the

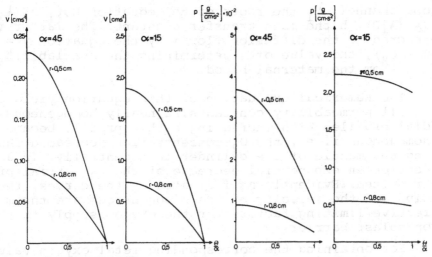

Fig. 2: Distribution of velocity (left) and pressure
(right) in the ICS-diffusor, for overall injection angles
(2 α) of 90° and 30°, and distances of 0.5 and 0.8 cm
from the mouth of the spiral artery. Abscissae: Distance
from the symmetry axis (relative angle θ/α).

mantle of the funnel. The evaluation of this equation
yielded a homogeneous distribution of concentration along
the flow axis. Consequently, a constant O_2 concentration
at the point of inflow into the intervillous channel
could be assumed, yielding the initial condition for the
following diffusion model.

The diffusion in the intervillous space was considered under the assumption that the maternal blood flow
in circular cylinders from the central space to the periphery (fig. 1). The solution of the stationary diffusion
equation

$$\frac{\partial^2 C}{\partial r^2} + \frac{1}{r}\frac{\partial C}{\partial r} - v\frac{\partial C}{\partial z} = 0$$

takes the form

$$C(r,z) = \frac{C_B - C_K}{R} 2 D h \sum_{1}^{\infty} \frac{J_0(\lambda_i r) e^{-\frac{D}{v}\lambda_i^2 z}}{(D^2\lambda_i^2 + h^2) J_0(\lambda_i R)} + C_K$$

where J_0 represents the Bessel function of zero order,
D the diffusion constant, C_B the O_2 concentration of the
maternal blood at the beginning of the cylinder, C_K the
O_2 concentration in the umbilical artery, R the radius
of the cylinder (normally 10 μ), z the length of the
cylinder (total length assumed to be $5 \cdot 10^3 \mu$), r the
radial distance from the axis of the cylinder within the

blood channel, λ_i the roots of the equation $D\lambda_i\ J_i(\lambda_iR) = h\ J_O\ (\lambda_iR)$, h the mass transfer constant. The latter is connected to the diffusion flow j by the equation $j = h(C_B- C_K)$, the value of j determining the availability of O_2 from the maternal blood.

The numerical evaluation of this equation yielded, at small permeability constants, a nearly homogeneous radial profile. With increasing h this profile became inhomogenous i. e., the O_2 concentration decreased faster along the mantle of the cylinder than centrally. In axial direction an exponential decrease of the O_2 partial pressure resulted. Evidently as indicated by the curves, the radius and the velocity of the blood stream are the most effective limiting factors for the oxygen supply to the trophoblast barrier.

For obtaining the corresponding fetal oxygen values we used a simple transformation of our model to cartesian coordinates. By solving the diffusion equation for stationary conditions the oxygen concentration in the maternal blood was found to be

$$C_1(y,z) = \frac{2j}{\ell D} \sum_1^{\infty} \frac{(-1)^i}{\lambda_i^2} e^{-\frac{D}{v}\lambda_i^2 z} \sin \lambda_i y - \frac{j}{D} y + C$$

and the oxygen concentration in the fetal blood, with y = L

$$C_2(y=L,z) = \frac{2j}{\ell D} \sum_1^{\infty} \frac{(-1)^i}{\lambda_i^2} e^{-\frac{D}{v}\lambda_i^2 z} \frac{[\sin(S_i y) + \cot(S_i L)\cos(S_i y)]}{\sin(S_i \ell) + \cot(S_i L)\cos(S_i \ell)} - \frac{j}{D} y + C$$

where y is the coordinate vertical to the flow axis, L the distance from the axis of the maternal capillary to the inner surface of the fetal capillary, and l the diffusion distance in the maternal blood. The villi were assumed to line the entire length of the maternal channel, the umbilical artery supplying these villi at the same, constant oxygen concentration. Each villus was thought to contact the maternal blood across the fetomaternal diffusion barrier (normally 6μ) over an average length of 70μ. The blood from these capillaries, possessing different oxygen concentrations depending on the respective position along the maternal cylinder, then merged in the umbilical vein (fig. 3). Oxygen partial pressures were calculated with the aid of the nomograms by Thews (1971).

According to these results, in the central portion of the intervillous space (flow distance about 2 mm) fetal end-capillary oxygen pressure decreases only little

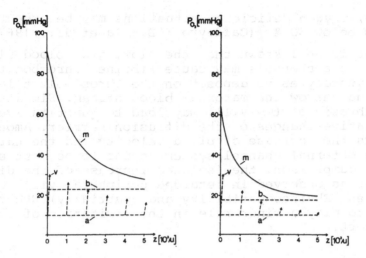

Fig. 3: Oxygen pressures of the blood passing through
the villous zone. m = maternal blood; a = pO_2 of the
blood in the umbilical artery; v = pO_2 of the endcapilla-
ry blood from individual villi along the maternal blood
stream (at distances of 1000μ and contact length of
70μ); b = pO_2 of the blood in the umbilical vein.
Abscissae: Distance from ICR. Left diagram: Normal pla-
centar perfusion conditions Right: Blood velocity
decreased by 30 %, and diffusion barrier doubled to 12μ.

(fig. 3). In this portion saturation values of the fetal
blood remain relatively high. In contrast in the periphery of the cotyledon, the oxygen pressure falls considerably. In this region, values of the fetal blood partly
approach the critical level for trophoblast cells which,
according to Longo (1972), ranges between 10 and 15 mm Hg.
Any further decrease of the oxygen supply by a decrease
of blood velocity, or width of the maternal channel
system, should cause the oxygen pressure to drop below
this critical level, since the values for the trophoblast
layer are intermediate between maternal end-intervillous
and fetal end-villous pressures. Our results also indicate that the oxygen exchange takes place at a relatively low average pressure gradient. Nevertheless, the mean
oxygen pressure resulting from the confluence of different
fetal capillaries in the umbilical venous blood is relatively high, amounting - according to our model - even
at unfavourable perfusion conditions (v = 300μ · s^{-1};
diffusion distance = 12μ) to 17.1 mm Hg, or a saturation
of 35 %. As animal experiments and clinical evidence in-

dicate, oxygen deficiency situations may be expected at values below 30 % (Caldeyro - Barcia et al., 1967).

It is well known that the slowing of blood flow distal to a stenosis may cause fibrine, thrombocytes and erythrocytes to deposit on the throphoblast layer, and thus narrow the maternal blood stream. Simultaneously, fibrosis of the villi may lead to quantitative and qualitative changes of the diffusion barrier. Among these factors the decrease of blood velocity and the narrowing of the maternal channel system appear to be most effective. In comparison, the isolated increase of the diffusion barrier as observed in retarded peripheral villi under diabetes, Rh-incompatibility and (partially) EPH gestosis seems to play a minor role in the limitation of oxygen transport.

REFERENCES

Borell, U., Fernström, J. and Westmann, A. (1958) Geburtsh. Frauenheilk. 18, 1

Caldeyro-Barcia, R., Casacuberta, C., Bustos, R., Giussi, G., Gulin, L., Escarcena, L. and Mendez-Bauer, C. (1967) Correlation of intrapartum changes in fetal heart rate with fetal blood oxygen and acid-base state. In'Diagnosis and treatment of fetal disorders' p. 205 (ed. Adamsons, K.) Springer-Verlag, New York

Freese, U. E. (1968) J. Reprod. Med. 1, 161

Heilmann, L., Mattheck, C. and Wiemer, W. (1977) In preparation

Künzel, W. and Moll, W. (1972) Z. Geburtsh. Perinat. 176, 108

Longo, L. D. (1972) Disorders of placental transfer. In 'Pathophysiology of gestation' p. 1 (ed. Assali,N.S.) Academic Press

Mattheck, C., Heilmann, L. and Wiemer, W. (1977) Z. Geburtsh. Perinat. In press

Metcalfe, J., Romney, S. L., Ramsey, L. H., Reid, D. E. and Burwell, C. S. (1955) J. clin. Invest. 34, 1632

Thews, G. (1971) Nomogramme zum Säure-Basen-Status des Blutes und zum Atemgastransport. Springer-Verlag,Berlin

This presentation was supported by grants from the DFG (SFB 114 and H 1010-1). Detailed reports are in preparation (Heilmann et al., 1977; Mattheck et al., 1977).

RESPIRATORY GAS TRANSPORT IN BLOOD DURING PREGNANCY
WITH HEMOGLOBIN CONCENTRATIONS BELOW 12g/100ml

J. Grote, D. Koch, G. Hermesdorf and
A. Abdelhamid

Institute of Physiology, University of Mainz

During pregnancy the conditions for respiratory gas transport in blood and respiratory gas exchange differ from that of non-pregnant healthy women. The hemoglobin concentration and, consequently, the O_2 capacity of blood decreases. The arterial CO_2 tension falls between the 10th and the 40th week of gestation to values of about 30 mmHg, while the pH of the arterial blood during the same period was found to be nearly constant at an elevated level (7). Investigations of blood O_2 affinity during pregnancy led to non-uniform results. Several investigators found no significant change whereas others described a significant decrease of blood O_2 affinity in pregnant women and a mean P_{50} value of about 31 mmHg. Among the factors which are considered to influence the O_2 affinity of blood, the intraerythrocytic 2,3-diphosphoglycerate concentration, in particular, increases during pregnancy (11).
The aim of this study was to investigate the influence of a reduction of blood hemoglobin concentration below 12g% on the conditions for respiratory gas transport in blood of pregnant women.

Methods

In venous blood samples taken from 67 pregnant women with hemoglobin concentrations below 12g% the O_2 dissociation curve was determined at 37 $^\circ$C and PCO_2= 40 mmHg by means of the method of Niesel and Thews (10). In

491

order to correct the obtained P_{50} values for the
conditions of pH 7.40, a Bohr factor of $\Delta PO_2/\Delta pH=-0.48$
was used. The hemoglobin concentration was measured
photometrically after the conversion of hemoglobin into
cyanmethemoglobin. Blood PCO_2 - pH dependence was
determined at SO_2 = 100% and 0% using the Astrup micromethod (1). ATP concentration in blood and the plasma
concentration of inorganic phosphate were measured by
conventional methods using Boehringer test combinations.
Additionally, in some cases plasma concentration of
inorganic phosphate was determined according to Gerlach
and Deuticke (4). Intraerythrocytic 2,3-DPG concentration
was determined enzymatically (9). All blood samples
were heparinized and stored at 4 $^{\circ}$C. Analyses were
completed within 3 hours after withdrawal.
The results of studies on blood samples of 7 non-
pregnant healthy women served as control values. For
comparison of the obtained O_2 dissociation curves and
$logPCO_2$ - pH equilibration curves with the corresponding
curves of non-pregnant women, results of previous
investigations were used (5).

Results and Discussion

In Tab. 1 the measured and calculated data of 67 pregnant
and 7 non-pregnant women are summarized. As can be seen
from the obtained mean values, during pregnancy from
the 21st to the 43rd week of gestation with decreasing
hemoglobin concentration there is a decrease in blood
O_2 affinity and an increase in the intraerythrocytic
concentration of 2,3-DPG. Simultaneously, the blood ATP
concentration and the concentration of inorganic
phosphate in plasma remained unchanged. The P_{50} value
determined in blood samples with a mean hemoglobin
concentration of 11.5g% and taken at the end of
pregnancy is comparable to the findings of Bauer et al.
(2). The obtained values for the concentration of 2,3-
DPG and the concentration of inorganic phosphate
correspond to those of Rörth and Bille Brahe (11);
however, an increase of the intraerythrocytic 2,3-DPG
levels during pregnancy could not be found when
hemoglobin concentration was below 12g%. Bauer et al.
(2) measured slightly elevated ATP concentrations in
blood at the end of pregnancy. The significantly
decreased O_2 affinity of the blood samples with low
hemoglobin concentrations (Fig. 1) cannot be fully
ascribed to the increased 2,3-DPG level in the red
blood cells. Other factors such as the concentrations

Table 1: Hemoglobin concentration, P_{50} at 37°C and pH 7.40, intraerythrocytic 2,3-DPG concentration, blood ATP concentration and plasma concentration of inorganic phosphate. Given are mean values ± SD, number of samples in parenthesis. I Hb < 11g%, II Hb=11-12g%, A gestation week 21-35, B gestation week 36-43, C control

	g.w.	Hb (g%)	P_{50} (mmHg)	2,3-DPG (mmol/1RBC)	ATP (mmol/1)	Pi (mmol/1)
C	–	13.6 (7) 0.6	(26.7) (1.6)	4.53 (7) 0.25	0.52 (6) 0.06	0.98 (6) 0.15
I A	30 5	10.2 (12) 0.7	33.8 (6) 3.9	5.98 (12) 0.50	0.47 (5) 0.03	1.01 (5) 0.16
B	39 2	10.6 (14) 0.4	34.1 (6) 1.8	5.77 (14) 0.40	0.54 (7) 0.09	1.08 (5) 0.14
II A	30 4	11.5 (17) 0.3	32.6 (6) 1.3	5.63 (17) 0.28	0.49 (8) 0.08	1.07 (8) 0.16
B	39 2	11.5 (25) 0.2	30.9 (15) 2.5	5.47 (25) 0.44	0.51 (11) 0.05	1.11 (10) 0.26

of cations or carbonic anhydrase, which are known to be
increased during pregnancy (2,7), may additionally be
responsible for the changings of the blood O_2 affinity.

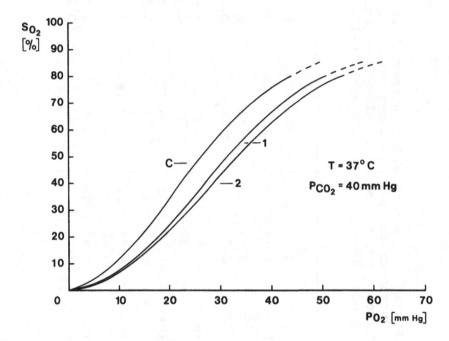

Fig.1: O_2 dissociation curve in blood of pregnant and non-
pregnant women at PCO_2 = 40 mmHg and t = 37°C. C: control
subjects, 1: pregnant women with mean Hb = 11.5g%,
2: pregnant women with mean Hb = 10.4g%.

     In the PCO_2 range 20 - 60 mmHg the $logPCO_2$ - pH
dependence of the investigated blood can be described
for the conditions of SO_2 = 100% and t = 37°C by the
following equations:

I   (Hb = 11.5g%) $logPCO_2 = -1.535pH + 12.96$

II   (Hb = 10.4g%) $logPCO_2 = -1.487pH + 12.60$

     The negative slope of the $logPCO_2$-pH equilibration
curves of the blood samples under investigation decreases
with decreasing hemoglobin concentration. Comparable results are obtained from blood of anemic patients as well
as from blood samples in which the hemoglobin concentration was decreased by adding plasma (6,8). The values
for base excess were within the normal range.Both findings

are in agreement with results of Duhm (3) which show
that total buffering capacity of the bicarbonate and
non-bicarbonate buffers of normal blood is not
significantly different from blood with elevated
intraerythrocytic 2,3-DPG concentrations.

The influence of O_2 saturation changes on plasma
pH of the blood samples was reduced in comparison to
normal blood. As can be seen from Fig. 2 the pH difference
between oxygenated and deoxygenated blood as determined
at PCO_2 = 40 mmHg and t = 37 $^{\circ}$C decreases significantly
with decreasing hemoglobin concentration.

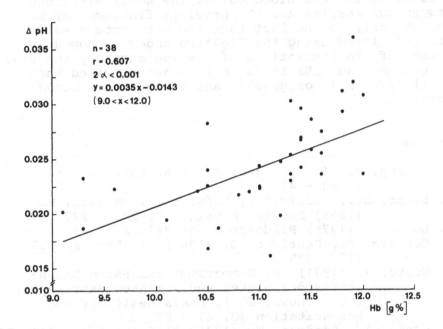

Fig.2: Influence of hemoglobin concentration on the pH
difference between oxygenated and deoxygenated blood
of pregnant women at PCO_2 = 40 mmHg and t = 37 $^{\circ}$C.

For the Haldane coefficient calculated for the
conditions of PCO_2 = 40 mmHg, pH = 7.40 and t = 37 $^{\circ}$C,
a mean value of
    0.017 meq/l per g/l Hb or
    0.27 meq/l per mmol/l Hb_m
was found. The change in base concentration during
deoxygenation of the investigated blood can be described

by the equations:

I $\Delta BE = 0.17Hb (1 - SO_2)$ (Hb given in g%) or

II $\Delta BE = 0.27Hb_m (1 - SO_2)$ (Hb_m given in mmol/l).

Both constants are indentical with the values determined in blood samples of anemic patients (6); they correspond to those found in normal blood (0.019, 0.31) (12). With respect to findings of Siggaard-Andersen (12) at plasma pH >7.1, an increase of the Haldane coefficient is to be expected with elevated 2,3-DPG concentrations in the red blood cells. The small difference between our results and the previous findings may be due, in part, to the fact that the base excess values were calculated using the Siggaard-Andersen nomogram. Because of the limitations of reading accuracy inherent in the nomogram, Δ BE tends to be underestimated when pH differences in oxygenated and deoxygenated blood are small.

References

1. Astrup, P. (1956) Scand. J. clin. Lab. Invest.
          8, 33 - 43
2. Bauer, Ch., Ludwig, M., Ludwig, I., Bartels, H.
          (1969) Respir. Physiol. 7, 271 - 277
3. Duhm, J. (1976) Pflügers Arch. 363, 61 - 67
4. Gerlach, E., Deuticke, B. (1963) Biochem. Z. 337,
          477 - 479
5. Grote, J. (1971) In: Nomogramme zum Säure-Basen-
          Status des Blutes und zum Atemgastransport
          (ed. Thews, G.), Anaesthesiology and
          Resuscitation 30, 47 - 83
6. Grote, J., Söndgen, W. (1976) Pflügers Arch. 365, R22
7. Lucius, H., Gahlenbeck, H., Kleine, H.-O., Fabel, H.,
          Bartels, H. Respir. Physiol. 9, 311 - 317
8. Mengden, H.-J. v., Schultehinrichs, D., Thews, G.
          (1969) Respir. Physiol. 6, 151 - 159
9. Michal, G. (1970) In: Methoden der enzymatischen
          Analysen (ed. Bergmeyer, H. U.) 2nd ed.
          1478 - 1483
10. Niesel, W;, Thews, G. (1961) Pflügers Arch. ges.
          Physiol. 273, 380 - 395
11. Rörth, M., Bille Brahe, N. E. (1971) Scand. J. clin.
          Lab. Invest 28, 271 - 276
12. Siggaard-Andersen, O. (1974) The acid-base status of
          the blood, 4th ed., Munksgaard, Copenhagen

DISCUSSION OF PAPERS IN SESSION 7

CHAIRMEN: DR. W. ERDMANN and DR. M. SILVER

PAPER BY: DR. ERDMANN

Dr. Chance: Was concerned as to how well the decrease of PO_2 with time would correlate with the increase in the number of mitochondria in the brain, and Dr. Silver asked what anaesthetic was used in the foetal experiments and also whether the mothers were given oxygen.

Dr. Erdmann: Replied that the anaesthetic was sodium pentobarbitone in both the pregnant and the neo-natal studies. Tracheotomy was performed but no extra oxygen was given and he relied on spontaneous respiration.

Dr. Lübbers: 1) Did you make your measurements in the gray or white matter?

2) The PO_2-Histogram of the brain cortex of your 1 year old mice shows a large proportion of low values. In other animals such as rats, guinea-pigs, dogs, cats, monkeys etc. I would consider such a histogram a sign of hypoxia. Do you think that in mice such a shift to the left is normal?

Dr. Erdmann: 1) The measurements were supposedly performed in the gray matter of the brain.

2) There might be insignificant hypoxia due to barbiturate anesthesia. I consider the shift of PO_2 values to the left as being within the normal range.

PAPER BY: DRS: WIMBERLEY and HUEHNS

Dr. Silver: When does the foetal haemoglobin change to the adult form?

Dr. Wimberly: In normal babies, the change to the adult form begins at or near birth, but in the premature, abnormal (acidotic) babies, the changeover is at the time when it would have been born, i.e. around 40 weeks. There thus seems to be an inbuilt mechanism which is timed to occur at the end of normal gestation and which controls the form of haemoglobin present.

Dr. Gardiner: 1) Was the acidosis in infants with respiratory distress syndrome primarily metabolic or respiratory, and was the type of acidosis important?

2) Did these infants all have comparable percentages of foetal haemoglobin?

Dr. Wimberley: 1) In most cases, the acidosis was mixed metabolic and respiratory. CO_2 data on these infants exists but has not yet been analysed. This is important as there is a separate effect of CO_2 on oxygen affinity which may be different in foetal blood compared to adult blood.

2. Yes, at birth all infants studied had HbF levels above 85%. These levels declined very slowly until the infants reached 40 weeks gestation, or equivalent, when a rapid switch from HbF to HbA occured.

PAPER BY: DR. GALE et al

Dr. Silver: 1) How long does the yolk sac last in mice and does it continue to produce embryonic haemoglobin?

2) Have any measurements of foetal or embryonic blood or plasma pH been made in vivo?

Dr. Gale: 1) The yolk sac placenta is functional for approximately eight days and produces only one batch of embryonic haemoglobin and no more.

2) No.

PAPER BY: DRS: GARRIS and MITCHELL

Dr. Silver: Where were the venous PO_2 measurements made? One would expect uterine venous PO_2 to rise if there is a marked increase in vascularity or blood flow through the tissue under the influence of oestrogen.

<u>Dr. Garris:</u> Measurements of venous PO_2 were made from the inferior vena cava. It was not possible to measure uterine venous PO_2 but it it probably would rise during oestrous and implantation.

<u>PAPER BY: DR.   GUIET-BARA</u>

<u>Dr. Silver:</u> If the perfusion fluid was aqueous (without protein or colloid) and the rate of flow was very high, was there tissue oedema at the end of a perfusion period? Did you make any histological examination of the tissue after the experiments and did you notice oedema or other abnormalities?

<u>Dr. Guiet-Bara:</u> The tissue was examined and some oedema was present.

Hypoxia, Ischemia, Shock

RELATIONSHIP BETWEEN ERYTHROPOIETIN LEVELS AND INTRARENAL

OXYGENATION DURING ANURIC HEMORRHAGIC SHOCK

Rex Baker, John D. Bray, and José Strauss
Division of Pediatric Nephrology
Department of Pediatrics
University of Miami School of Medicine
Miami, Florida 33152, USA

It has been shown that the kidney plays a major role in the production (Jacobson and Krantz, 1970) and perhaps inactivation (Fisher et al, 1968a) of erythropoietin (erythropoietic stimulating factor, ESF). Although most investigators believe that the renal cortex is the site controlling ESF production (Jacobson and Krantz, 1970), the evidence is not conclusive. Increase in ESF levels has been observed under a variety of stimuli including production of renal infarcts (Abbrect et al, 1966), constriction of the renal artery (Fisher et al, 1968b; Fisher and Samuels, 1967), infusion of vasopressors (Fisher et al, 1968b), hypoxic hypoxia (Murphy et al, 1971), and normovolemic anemia (Naets, 1959). However, this increase is not always present after renal arterial constriction (Murphy et al, 1967a) and hemorrhage (Murphy et al, 1967b). In addition, tissue oxygenation measurements have brought further questions about the relationship between hypoxia and ESF production (Hardwick et al, 1963). The present study was undertaken to evaluate the relationship between intrarenal oxygen availability (O_2a) and consumption ($\dot{V}O_2$) and serum ESF levels during anuric hemorrhagic shock in rabbits.

METHODS

Twelve experiments were performed in two groups of six unanesthetized male New Zealand rabbits weighing 3.08 ± 0.37 kg. Experiments were done on two groups of animals in order to measure different sets of variables. In group 1, a renal arterial occluder (Beran et al, 1968) and O_2-sensitive electrodes (Strauss et al, 1968; Strauss et al, 1974) were implanted and arterial blood samples were drawn for PO_2, PCO_2, pH, and hematocrit. In group 2, arterial blood samples were obtained for ESF determination.

The experimental design consisted of a one-hour control period followed by bleeding at the rate of 10 ml/5 min until a systolic central arterial pressure (CAP) of 60 mm Hg was attained (to produce interruption of glomerular filtration) (Munck, 1962; Strauss et al, 1971), two hours of shock (maintained at 60 mm Hg systolic CAP by withdrawing or reinfusing blood), reinfusion of shed blood at the rate of 10 ml/5 min, and finally one-hour postreinfusion period. During the shock period the shed blood was stored on ice in heparinized, capped syringes.

The O_2-sensitive electrodes (Pt, active, 175µ diameter; Ag-AgCl, reference, 500µ diameter) were implanted at least two weeks prior to the experiment. All reference electrodes were placed in the cortex (C), and the uninsulated sensing surface of the active electrodes in C, outer medulla (OM), inner medulla (IM), and papilla (P) of the left kidney.

In group 1, blood samples were taken and local O_2a and VO_2 index measurements were done at 60 and 30 minutes before bleeding, immediately after shock was established, at the end of the first and second hours of shock, and 30 and 60 minutes after reinfusion was completed. In group 2, blood samples for ESF were taken at the mid-point of the control period (30 minutes prior to beginning of bleeding), twice during shock (45 and 105 minutes after establishing shock), and at the mid-point of the postreinfusion period (30 minutes after completion of reinfusion). In groups 1 and 2, urinary volume was measured once during each period.

Prior to the experiment, animals were blindfolded and loosely wrapped in a sheet, and catheters were placed in the femoral artery and urinary bladder. The arterial catheter was used for sampling and monitoring CAP with a pressure transducer (Statham, model P23AA) connected to a recorder (Beckman, type R Dynograph). The bladder catheter was used for monitoring urinary flow rates. A thermistor probe connected to a Telethermometer (Yellow Springs Instrument Co., model 42SC) was placed in the deep subcutaneous back tissue for measuring body temperature. In group 1, previously implanted O_2-sensitive electrodes were connected to polarographs and the animal was allowed to stabilize for 30 minutes before the experiment began. The O_2a was measured polarographically in the four renal areas (Strauss et al, 1968; Strauss et al, 1974); VO_2 index was obtained from the slope of the fast linear portion of the O_2a-decay curve (ΔO_2a/sec) immediately following renal arterial occlusion (Strauss et al, 1969; Sinagowitz et al, 1976). After the experiment, O_2a and VO_2 index values were calculated and expressed as a percent of their own controls. Locations of the electrodes were confirmed by histologic examination after the experiments were completed and the animals were sacrificed.

Arterial blood PO_2, PCO_2, and pH were measured in a Blood
Micro System (Radiometer, model BMS-3b) and corrected for body temperature. Hematocrit was determined in blood centrifuged for five
minutes at 1,500 rpm. These values were used to calculate oxygen
content and capacity. Serum samples for ESF were immediately har-
vested and frozen at -75° C. They were sent frozen to Bio-Science
Laboratories (Van Nuys, Calif.) where determinations were performed
within six days of the experiment. Immunoassay of ESF was done with
an hemagglutination-inhibition technique (Jordan et al, 1969).

RESULTS

In group 1, mean local O_2a levels in all four areas of the
kidney fell in a drastic and parallel fashion during bleeding; they
reached their lowest points when a systolic CAP of 60 mm Hg was
first reached. During the two-hour shock the O_2a levels displayed
a gradual spontaneous increase; immediately after reinfusion they
overshot, then began to return toward control levels.

The intrarenal $\dot{V}O_2$ index response pattern to hemorrhagic shock
differed from that of O_2a in that in inner areas (IM and P), $\dot{V}O_2$
indices remained near control levels throughout the experiment while
in outer areas (C and OM) they fell after bleeding, continued to
fall gradually during shock, and returned to control after reinfusion
of shed blood. Outer area decreases in $\dot{V}O_2$ indices were less severe
than those in O_2a.

Arterial O_2 content fell with hemorrhage, continued to fall
gradually during shock, then returned toward control during reinfusion and postreinfusion. This O_2 content decrease was related principally to a decrease in hematocrit since PaO_2 increased during
shock.

In group 2, the mean ESF concentration in arterial serum fell
during hemorrhage and continued to fall during shock. After reinfusion of the shed blood, ESF levels began to climb toward control
levels but had not fully recovered by the end of the postreinfusion
period. The ESF response pattern to hemorrhagic shock most closely
followed that of outer renal (particularly cortical) $\dot{V}O_2$ index.

A drastically reduced or obliterated glomerular filtration
during shock could be demonstrated by cessation of urine flow
(anuria). Diuresis was re-established and began to return toward
control rate during the postreinfusion period.

DISCUSSION

It is generally agreed that serum ESF levels increase in response to stimuli which cause tissue hypoxia (Abbrect et al, 1966;

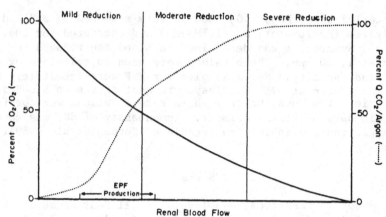

FIG. 1. Relationship between renal cortical metabolism and ESF (EPF) production during renal blood flow reduction [from Murphy et al (1967a) Invest. Urol. 4, 372].

Fisher et al, 1968b; Fisher and Samuels, 1967; Murphy et al, 1971; Naets, 1959), and that the renal cortex is a major site controlling ESF production (Jacobson and Krantz, 1970). However, preliminary data of our group have cast some doubt as to the existence of a constant relationship between decreased renal cortical O_2a and ESF levels under various hypoxia-inducing conditions (Hardwick et al, 1963). In addition, the data presented here show that ESF actually decreases during hemorrhagic shock in spite of local tissue hypoxia in all areas of the kidney and a significant decrease in arterial O_2 content. This indicates that other factors must also play a role in the erythropoietic response.

Jacobson et al (1957) have suggested that functioning renal tissue is necessary for ESF increases to occur. This idea has been further strengthened by Reissmann et al (1960) who found no ESF increase in rats after normovolemic and phenylhydrazine-induced anemia when previously poisoned with mercury bichloride. Since the latter selectively destroys renal tubular epithelium, it was suggested that tubular cells may normally be responsible for ESF increases by either removal of an ESF inhibitor or secretion of ESF (Reissmann et al, 1960). Another possibility is that an inactive extrarenally produced ESF precursor is normally activated by functioning tubular cells (Jacobson et al, 1957).

Murphy et al (1967a) found that renal structure was maintained but hormonal function such as ESF production was impaired when renal blood flow was reduced enough to decrease cortical respiration more than 37%. At this point, cortical anaerobic glycolysis was significantly activated (Fig. 1); however, medullary metabolic changes were variable and unrelated. These findings were confirmed in hemorrhagic shock experiments in dogs in which a mean aortic blood pressure of 50 mm Hg was maintained from one to five hours; after a critical point which correlated with the onset of anuria, ESF production apparently ceased (Murphy et al, 1967b).

In general, the results of experiments reported here are in agreement with those of Murphy et al (1967a and 1967b). Accordingly, we must conclude that a certain level of renal cortical respiration seems necessary for plasma ESF to increase in response to tissue hypoxia. Whether or not other factors play a role by themselves or by inducing changes in renal oxygenation or respiration needs to be clarified by further studies in experimental animals and in patients with renal diseases.

ACKNOWLEDGEMENTS

The authors thank Drs. J. Winkelman (Bio-Science Laboratories, Van Nuys) and B. J. Schmidt (Bio-Ciência/Lavoisier S.A., São Paulo) for their assistance in having the ESF determinations done.

REFERENCES

Abbrect, P.H., Malvin, R.L. and Vander, A.J. (1966) Nature 211, 1318.

Beran, A.V., Strauss, J., Brown, C.T. and Katurich, N. (1968) J. Appl. Physiol. 24, 838.

Fisher, J.W., Hatch, F.E., Roh, B.L., Allen, R.C. and Kelley, B.J. (1968a) Blood 31, 440, 1968.

Fisher, J.W. and Samuels, A.I. (1967) Proc. Soc. Exp. Biol. Med. 115, 482.

Fisher, J.W., Samuels, A.I. and Langston, J. (1968b) Ann. N.Y. Acad. Sci. 149, 308.

Hardwick, D.F., Strauss, J. and Misrahy, G.A. (1963) Am. J. Physiol. 205, 322.

Jacobson, L.O., Goldwasser, E., Fried, W. and Plzak, L. (1957) Nature 179, 633.

Jacobson, L.O. and Krantz, S.B. (1970) Erythropoietin and the Regulation of Erythropoiesis. The University of Chicago Press, Chicago.

Jordan, T.A., McDonald, T.P. and Lange, R.D. (1969) Am. J. Med. Technol. 35, 595.

Munck, O., Lassen, N.A., Deetjen, P. and Kramer, K. (1962) Arch. Ges. Physiol. 274, 356.

Murphy, G.P., Mirand, E.A., Johnston, G.S. and Schirmer, H.K.A. (1967a) Invest. Urol. 4, 372.

Murphy, G.P., Mirand, E.A., Takita, H., Schoonees, R. and Groenewald, J.H. (1971) Invest. Urol. 8, 521.

Murphy, G.P., Schirmer, H.K.A., Mirand, E.A., Benson, D.W. and Scott, W.W. (1967b) Invest. Urol. 4, 576.

Naets, J-P. (1959) Proc. Soc. Exp. Biol. Med. 102, 387.

Reissmann, K.R., Nomura, T., Gunn, R.W. and Brosius, F. (1960) Blood 16, 1411.

Sinagowitz, E., Baker, R., Strauss, J. and Kessler, M. (1976) Renal tissue oxygenation during hypoxic hypoxia. In 'Oxygen Transport to Tissue--II (Advances in Experimental Medicine and Biology, Volume 75)' p. 441 (eds. Grote, J. and Reneau, D.). Plenum, New York.

Strauss, J., Beran, A.V. and Baker, R. (1974) J. Appl. Physiol. 37, 988.

Strauss, J., Beran, A.V., Baker, R., Boydston, L. and Reyes-Sanchez, J.L. (1971) Am. J. Physiol. 221, 1545.

Strauss, J., Beran, A.V., Brown, C.T. and Katurich, N. (1968) Am. J. Physiol. 215, 1482.

Strauss, J., Beran, A.V., Katurich, N. and Brown, C.T. (1969) Renal regional O_2 consumption under "normal" and hemorrhagic shock conditions (Abstract). In 'Abstracts I. Free Communications. IVth International Congress of Nephrology' p. 351.

MODIFICATIONS OF SOMATOSENSORY EVOKED CORTICAL POTENTIALS DURING HYPOXIA IN THE AWAKE RABBIT

J. Manil, F. Colin and R.H. Bourgain

Laboratory of Physiology and Physiopathology V.U.B.
and Laboratory of Physiology U.L.B.
Eversstr. 2   —   B-1000 Brussels, Belgium

INTRODUCTION

Bicher et al. (1971, 1973) evidenced that the decrease of tissue pO_2 in the cortex of the cat under nitrogen breathing was followed by an increase of this pO_2. The phenomenon is accompanied by an increase in cerebral blood flow and a blocking of the action potentials registered at the prefrontal level of the cortex. Bicher (1974) postulated that the increase in tissue pO_2 is due to two compensatory autoregulatory mechanisms; firstly local vasodilation and secondly an active inhibition of the neuronal discharge which decreases the oxygen consumption by limiting the sodium influx into the cell and thus reducing the sodium/potassium pump energy expenditure, although it is generally admitted that oxygen deficiency causes a decrease of the activity of the pump with progressive cell membrane depolarization. It is well known indeed that the activity of the nervous system is rapidly abolished by anoxia. Lack of oxygen suppresses both the unitary discharge of the cells and even to a greater extent the synaptic transmission. In the present investigation the modifications of the somatosensory evoked potentials in the unrestrained awake rabbit were studied during hypoxia of the moderate (12 %) and severe (6.5 %) type.

MATERIALS AND METHODS

Rabbits were used as experimental animals; they present a lissencephalic structure of the brain which facilitates the interpretation of the electrical signals.

The electrodes are implanted under general anesthesia with
Hypnorm 0.5 mg/kg i.m. They are small silver discs (500 μm Ø) introduced through small holes drilled into the bone structure onto
the dura mater. A series of 4 electrodes is thus implanted 3 mm
from the midline and at a distance of 3 mm between each electrode.
The arrangement is made such that the second electrode starting
rostrally is located at the somatosensory area of the parietal
cortex. A reference electrode is inserted in the bulbus olfac-
torius.

An oxygen electrode kindly supplied by Bicher et al. is also
implanted. The different electrodes are all connected to a plug
and fixed to the bone structure by means of dental resin. The
hypoxia experiments were performed one week later. The control of
the gas mixtures used in the ventilation is performed by appropriate precision rotameters. The reference electrode for oxygen is a
silver-silver chloride electrode glued to the ear of the animal
and completely insulated with tissue glue (Cyanolit). The polaro-
metric current is measured over .65 volts through a 100 kΩ resistance and a 6.8 μF capacitor in parallel at the input of a DC Tek-
tronix amplifier. The tissue pO_2 is not measured in absolute
value but variations are easily detected.

The evoked cortical somatosensory responses are obtained by
stimulation of the contralateral forepaw at twice the motoric response value. The frequency of stimulation is one every two seconds. The evoked potentials are obtained by the averaging principle and represent the mean value of 5, 15 or 35 responses. EEG
recordings are continuously registered throughout the experiment
as well as the polarographic current.

RESULTS

In Figure 1 are indicated the results of two moderate hypoxic episodes (12 % oxygen) of short duration varying between 4
and 6 minutes. The tissue pO_2 curves are typical : their time-
constant values are identical and both demonstrate a beginning of
autoregulation. The evoked potentials are registered before (a),
during (b) and after (c) hypoxia. The potentials in (a) and (b)
are normal [positivity below baseline, amplitude peak-to-peak response (a) : 160 μV]. The normal characteristics were described
previously (Colin et al, 1975; Manil et al, 1975a, 1975b; Manil,
1976). During hypoxia the P_2 wave disappears and P_1 demonstrates
an increased duration. These modifications were found in all experimental animals. In order to investigate in detail those
findings longer episodes of moderate hypoxia were induced.

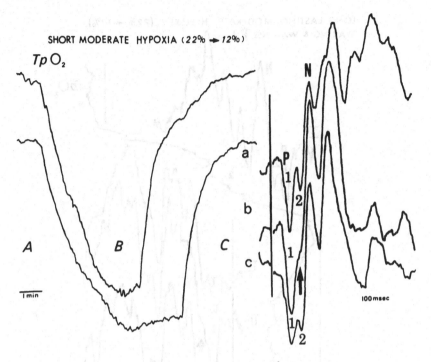

SHORT MODERATE HYPOXIA (22% → 12%)

Tp O₂

Figure 1 (see text)

Figure 2 demonstrates our findings (the tissue pO_2 is registered vertically). Four different phases can be distinguished :
(1) before hypoxia, (2) beginning of hypoxia, (3) maximal hypoxia,
(4) and (5) during autoregulation phenomena. In the control (1)
the evoked potentials (I) are normal demonstrating the typical
$P_1P_2N_2$ wave configuration. During phase (2) the potentials (II)
already show a decrease in P_2 which disappears in phase 3 (potentials III). During the compensatory mechanism (4) the evoked potentials (IV) show some regeneration of P_2 but when hypoxia continues (5) the autoregulation phenomena are less active and P_2
disappears while N_2 decreases in amplitude.

In Figure 3 the hypoxic episode lasts 20 minutes. The tissue
pO_2 can be divided into different phases : (1) prehypoxic, (2) beginning hypoxia, (3) and (4) maximal hypoxia, (5), (6) and (7)
autoregulation development and (8) → (21) stabilized autoregulation, (22) reoxygenation and (23) → (29) overshoot; 17 minutes
following the reoxygenation the tissue pO_2 is still above normal
level.

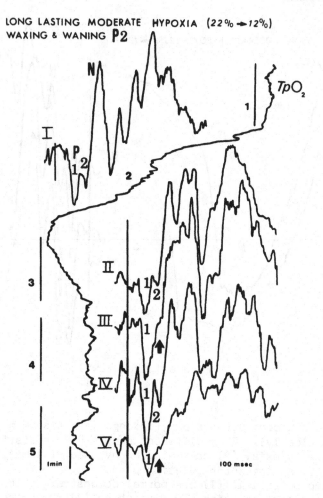

LONG LASTING MODERATE HYPOXIA (22% → 12%)
WAXING & WANING P2

Figure 2 (see text)

The compensation in this experiment is practically complete, the overshoot is very marked and of long duration. The evoked potentials were studied during this period at regular intervals as shown by the indicated figures. During the beginning and the maximal hypoxia, P_2 has disappeared completely as well as in the early phase of compensation. During the later phase of compensation P_2 waves wane and wax. During reoxygenation normalization of the evoked potentials occurs.

In Figure 4 a severe hypoxia (6.4 % O_2) is induced, no more autoregulation phenomena are evidenced except a very small overshoot phenomenon.

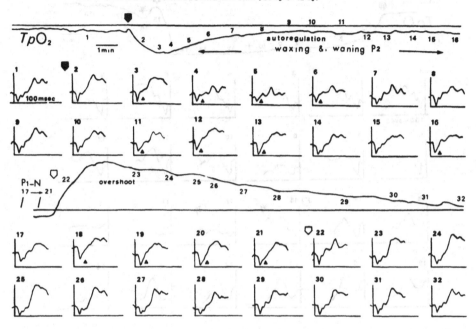

Figure 3 (see text)

During severe hypoxia the P_2 wave disappears completely, N_2 decreases in amplitude and P_1 increases in duration. During reoxygenation (15) normal complexes are evidenced but they are followed immediately (16), (17) and (18) by an electrical silence. Afterwards recordings of the anoxic agonic type are shown, very large P_1, no more P_2 wave at all and a decrease of N_2 although a normal tissue pO_2 was present at that time.

DISCUSSION AND CONCLUSIONS

The evolution of the tissue pO_2 during long lasting hypoxia shows the characteristic features described by Bicher. In our experiment the first manifestations of hypoxia are characterized by the disappearance of P_2 which normally originates in an associative area. This evidences that the cortical cells are not equally sensitive to oxygen. Certain areas are highly sensitive; this could be due to either increased metabolic needs, a different vascularity or both.

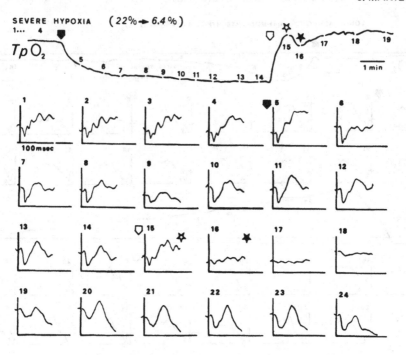

Figure 4 (see text)

When autoregulation sets in, P_2 reappears but with a great instability demonstrating a waning and waxing aspect. An increase in tissue pO_2 as a result of autoregulation does not restitute fully normal P_2 waves. This finding is not due to curare effect, as non-curarized animals showed identical results; furthermore, the EEG demonstrate an awake type of response.

In Figure 4 no autoregulation was observed and even during reoxygenation the complexes demonstrated permanent alterations. The animal had however been submitted to 6 previous hypoxic episodes before and it could well be that the autoregulation mechanisms were exhausted and the lack of compensation had resulted in permanent damage to the cortical cell function.

In conclusion, we can state that the evoked potentials do follow the evolution of the tissue pO_2 : P_2 disappears in the early phase and reappears during the autoregulation phase but remains very labile. When the hypoxia is of longer duration or more marked, N_2 decreases and can even inverse its polarity.

In our opinion the modifications of the evoked potentials do not reflect neuronal phenomena responsible for autoregulation. However, the evoked potentials are due to synaptic potentials and in future research the correlation between the modifications in the evoked potentials and the spontaneous firing of the neuron will have to be investigated.

REFERENCES

Amassian, E.V., Waller, H.J. and Macy, J., Jr. (1964) Ann. N.Y. Acad. Sci. 112, 5.

Baumgartner, G., Creutzfeldt, O. and Jung, R. (1961) In 'Cerebral Anoxia and the Electroencephalogram' p.5 (eds. Gastaut, H. and Meyer, J.S.). Charles C Thomas, Springfield, Ill.

Bicher, H.I. (1973) Autoregulation of oxygen supply to brain tissue. In 'Oxygen Transport to Tissue : Instrumentation, Methods and Physiology' pp.205-222 (eds. Bicher, H.I. and Bruley, D.F.). Plenum Press, New York.

Bicher, H.I. (1974) Microvasc. Res. 8, 291.

Bicher, H.I., Bruley, D.F., Reneau, D.D. and Knisely, M.H. (1971) J. Physiol. 217, 689.

Brooks, C. McC. and Eccles, J.C. (1947) J. Neurophysiol. 10, 349.

Colin, F., Manil, J. and Visser, P. (1975) Arch. Int. Physiol. Bioch. 83, 333.

Creutzfeldt, O., Bark, J. and Fromm, G.H. (1961) In 'Cerebral Anoxia and the Electroencephalogram' p.35 (eds. Gastaut, H. and Meyer, J.S.). Charles C Thomas, Springfield, Ill.

Creutzfeldt, O., Kasamatsu, A. and Vaz-Ferreira, A. (1957) Pflügers Arch. Ges. Physiol. 263, 647.

Creutzfeldt, O., Vaz-Ferreira, A. and Kasamatsu, A. (1955) Electroenceph. Clin. Neurophysiol. 7, 662.

Eccles, J.C., Kostyuk, P.F. and Schmidt, R.F. (1962) J. Physiol. 161, 237.

Ingvar, D.H. (1971) The focal cerebrovascular lesion. A survey of recent studies with isotope techniques and their clinical implications. In 'Cerebral Circulation and Stroke' pp.129-142 (ed. Zülch, K.J.). Springer Verlag, Berlin - Heidelberg - N.Y.

Kolmodin, G.M. and Skoglund, C.R. (1959) Acta Physiol. Scand.
45, 1.

Manil, J. (1976) Cerebrale somatosensorische geëvokeerde poten-
tialen bij het niet genarcotiseerde konijn. Thesis. Free University of Brussels (V.U.B.).

Manil, J., Colin, F. and Bourgain, R. (1975) Journal de Physiol.
71, 163A.

Manil, J., Colin, F. and Voogd, J. (1975) Arch. Int. Physiol.
Bioch. 83, 335.

Thomas, L.B. and Jenkner, F.L. (1952) Trans. Amer. Neurol. Ass.
77, 47.

ACKNOWLEDGEMENT

   We wish to thank Fernand Vereecke for his skilled technical
assistance.

TISSUE-PO$_2$ (P$_G$O$_2$) IN THE CAROTID BODY OF THE CAT AND TIDAL VOLUME (V̇) DURING NORMOVOLAEMIC HAEMODILUTION

R. Heinrich and H. Acker

Max-Planck-Institut für Systemphysiologie

46 Dortmund, West Germany

Although plasma expanders have been employed more and more often in clinical medicine, little is known about the function and reactions of the peripheral chemoreceptors under conditions of haemodilution. We have therefore studied how the peripheral chemoreceptors may be influenced by stepwise haemodilution, by investigating the behaviour of the tissue oxygen partial pressure (p$_G$O$_2$) in the carotid body of the cat and the ventilatory responses to hypoxia and hypercapnia. The experiments were done on 21 cats breathing spontaneously under sodium pentobarbital anaesthesia (40 - 65 mg/kg b.w.).

Fig. 1 shows the changes in haematocrit value (Hk), haemoglobin concentration (Hb), total arterial O$_2$-content total O$_2$, arterial blood gases and pH during stepwise haemodilution performed by administering Macrodex [R] (= Dextran, MW: 60000) in 30 ml units. After the infusion of Macrodex [R], Hk and Hb as well as total O$_2$ changed depending on the degree of dilution, whereas the arterial blood gases and pH remained unaltered. Changes of osmolarity were measured and values of 320 - 330 mOsmol/kg were found at extreme dilution values (to 4% Hk).

Fig. 2 shows a characteristic recording of p$_G$O$_2$, arterial blood pressure and (V̇) during haemodilution.

p$_G$O$_2$ remained constant down to a Hk value of 10-15%, and with further dilution it decreased slightly.

The average (V̇) was at about 900 ml/min and varied by 10% - 20% during haemodilution.

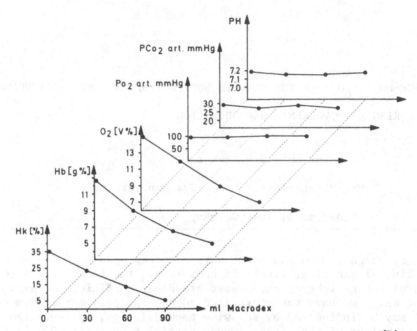

Fig. 1. Effect of stepwise haemodilution with Macrodex [(R)] on Hk, Hb, O_2-concentration of the arterial blood ($O_2[V\%]$), arterial pO_2, pCO_2 and pH.

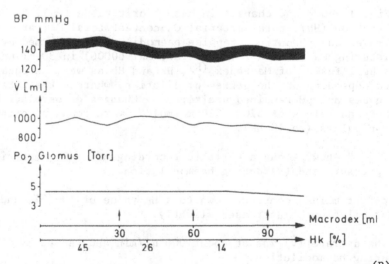

Fig. 2. Effect of stepwise haemodilution with Macrodex [(R)] on blood pressure (BP), tidal volume ($\dot{V}$) and tissue pO_2 (pO_2-Glomus) in the cat carotid body.

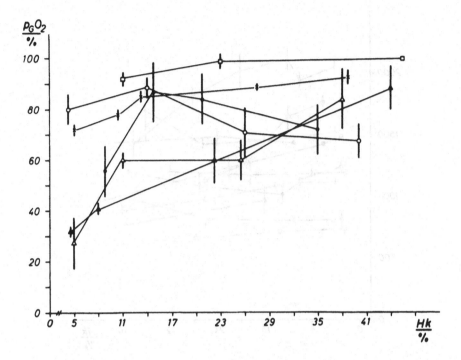

Fig. 3. Changes of tissue-PO₂ ($p_G O_2$) in the cat carotid body with
        haematocrit value (Hk).   (n = 6)

Figure 3 shows the results of 6 experiments in which the changes
of $p_G O_2$ in the carotid body were dependent on the degree of haemodilution, (i.e. the haematocrit value, Hk).   In five of the
experiments, $p_G O_2$ remained constant down to a Hk value of 10% - 15%
with a variation range of 10%.   With further dilution it decreased
to 20% of the original value.   In one experiment, $p_G O_2$ decreased
continuously during haemodilution.

Figure 4 shows the changes of ($\dot{V}$) during haemodilution.   The
figure shows a total of 11 experiments;   in six experiments $p_G O_2$ in
the carotid body was recorded as well.   The mean ($\dot{V}$) varied by
about 20% during haemodilution but no definite trend was observed.

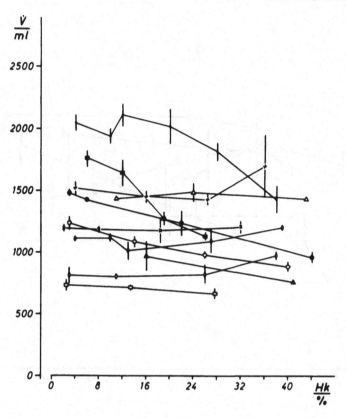

Fig. 4. Changes of tidal volume ($\dot{V}$) with haematocrit value (Hk).
       (n = 11).

Figure 5 shows changes in ($\dot{V}$) $p_G O_2$ and blood pressure (BP) under conditions of hypoxia and hypercapnia. In A, respiration of 5%
O_2 in N_2 led to an increase in ($\dot{V}$) and a simultaneous decrease in
$p_G O_2$, whereas the change in BP was not uniform. In B, respiration
of 6% CO_2 + 20% O_2 + 74% N_2 also increased ($\dot{V}$) while $p_G O_2$ and BP
were unchanged. To investigate the ventilatory response to different
degrees of haemodilution, the effects of hypoxia as well as hypercapnia were investigated at each step of dilution. The highest
ventilatory response was defined as 100%.

Fig. 6 shows the changes in the ventilatory response during
hypoxia (expressed as % maximum ventilation $\Delta V/\%$) with respect to Hk.
The values for $\Delta V/\%$ obtained during hypoxia were non-uniform: in
four experiments ΔV decreased by 10% to 50%, while in two an increase
of the maximum ventilatory response was noticed with decreasing Hk.

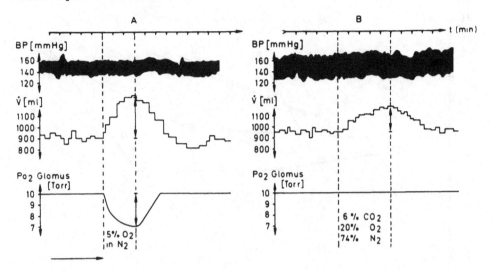

Fig. 5. Effect of A hypoxia, and B hypercapnia, on blood pressure
(BP), tidal-volume ($\dot{V}$) and tissue-PO$_2$ in the cat carotid
body (pO$_2$-Glomus) (Arrows indicate the maximum amplitude
of the change).

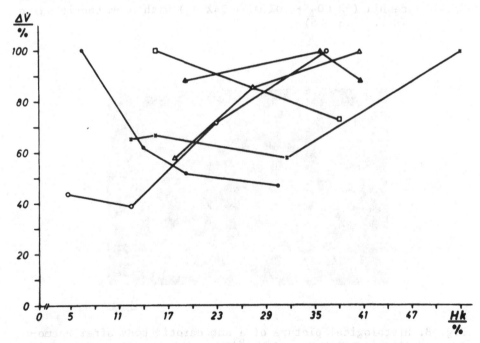

Fig. 6. Changes in the ventilatory responses ($\Delta V/\%$) during hypoxia
(5% O$_2$ in N$_2$) with haematocrit value, (Hk). (n = 6)

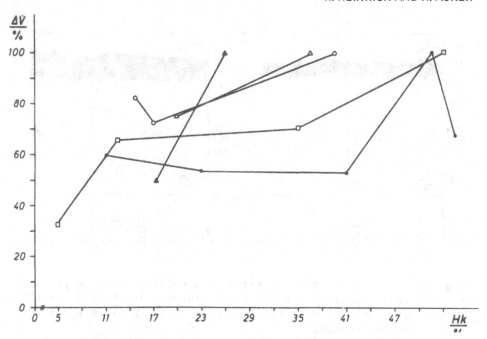

Fig. 7. Changes in the ventilatory responses ($\Delta V/\%$) during hypercapnia (6% CO_2 + 20% O_2 + 74% N_2) with haematocrit value
(Hk).   (n = 5).

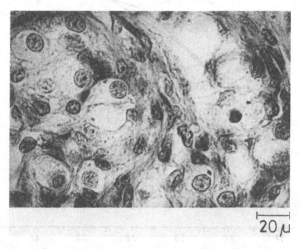

Fig. 8. Histological picture of a cat carotid body after haemodilution with Macrodex [R] to a haematocrit value of 4%.
(We thank Dr. E. Seidl, Max-Planck-Institut für Systemphysiologie, Dortmund, for this picture).

Figure 7 illustrates the change in $\Delta V/\%$ during hypercapnia with increasing haemodilution. The maximum ventilatory responses to hypercapnic stimulation decreased to 30% as Hk decreased in five experiments.

Normovolaemic haemodilution with Macrodex [R] to very low haematocrit values causes damage to the carotid body. Fig. 8 shows a histological picture of cat carotid body taken after haemodilution to a haematocrit value of 4%. Some areas are considerably damaged, as shown by disaggregation of glomus cells, slightly swollen Type-I cells, pyknotic nuclei located towards the border, cytolytic effects and vacuolization, and a general acidophilia indicating the beginning of destruction of the nuclei.

SUMMARY

During normovolaemic haemodilution with Macrodex [R], the basic respiratory activity is unchanged, while the ventilatory responses to hypoxia and hypercapnia generally decrease. The $p_G O_2$ in the cat carotid body remains constant down to an Hk of 10% to 15% and then decreases. This confirms the suggestion of Acker and Lübbers (1976) that increased plasma flow through the carotid body does not influence the oxygen supply to this organ, despite variations of both oxygen transport capacity and haemoglobin concentration.

The fine structure of the carotid body is partly destroyed by haemodilution with Macrodex [R] and this could account for the impaired chemoreception.

REFERENCES

Acker, H. and Lübbers, D.W. (1976) Pflügers Archiv. <u>366</u>, 241.

OXYGEN EXTRACTION IN SEVERELY ANEMIC DOGS AFTER

INFUSION OF NaHCO$_3$ OR HCl*

Stephen M. Cain

University of Alabama Medical Center

Birmingham, Alabama, U.S.A.

When anesthetized dogs were made acidemic or alkalemic during very severe hypoxic hypoxia, the slight but significant differences in mixed venous PO$_2$ were not associated with any significant differences in survival time, oxygen delivery, or oxygen uptake (Cain, 1976). Oxygen uptake was apparently dependent only on the total oxygen delivery ($\dot{Q}xCaO_2$). There were at least two reasons for the seemingly independent behavior of oxygen uptake from any Bohr shifts in dissociation curve position. One was the much shorter diffusion distances for O$_2$ as capillary beds were fully utilized. The second was the relative insensitivity of the oxyhemoglobin dissociation curve to Bohr effects at the lower extreme. This last reason would not apply in anemic hypoxia because, at low hematocrits near 10%, mixed venous PO$_2$ and saturation remained in the midrange even though O$_2$ delivery had become limiting to O$_2$ uptake in the whole animal (Cain, 1977). With normal arterial PO$_2$, a shift of the dissociation curve to the right as hemoglobin affinity for O$_2$ is decreased by acid infusion would not bother loading but could increase the PO$_2$ at which O$_2$ was unloaded at the tissues. These more recent experiments utilized HCl and NaHCO$_3$ infusions to alter pH during isovolemic hemodilution severe enough to decrease O$_2$ uptake in the anesthetized paralyzed dog ventilated adequately. The acid condition, which should have favored an increase in delivery PO$_2$, might reasonably have been expected to increase O$_2$ uptake. The results were opposite and the reasons more complex than that reasonable but simple expectation.

In figure 1, the experimental protocol can be readily perceived.

*Supported by Research Grant HL 14693, National Heart, Lung, and Blood Institute.

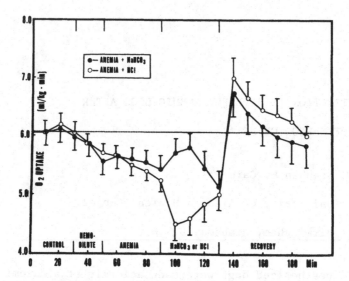

Fig. 1.   The O$_2$ uptake as dogs were made anemic and then either
alkalemic or acidemic

After the animal was stable with respect to blood gases and gas
exchange, control data were collected for 30 min.   During the next
20 min, blood was exchanged isovolemically with 6% dextran (MW=
70,000) in warm Tyrode's solution until O$_2$ uptake was lowered by 5
to 10% of the control value.   This occurred with about 87 ml/kg of
blood exchange and near an hematocrit of 9%.   The fact that O$_2$
uptake was limited by O$_2$ delivery was verified by the observation
of a steady rise in arterial excess lactate levels.   Data were
collected for 40 min more during this severe anemic period.   At
the end of that period, 3 ml/kg of 1.0 N NaHCO$_3$ was given IV in
one group and the same volume of 0.3 N HCl in the other.   There
were 10 animals in each group.   After an additional 40 min of
anemia with either NaHCO3 or HCl, homologous red blood cells were
returned to the animal and data were collected for a 1-hr recovery
period after appropriate correction of acid-base alteration.

O$_2$ uptake was decreased equally in both groups by hemodilution.
With time, there was a tendency for a continued decrease but during
the initial period of anemia, there was no significant difference
between the two groups nor should there have been.   With acid infusion, there was a marked further decrease in O$_2$ uptake which
gradually returned toward the preinfusion value.   With base infusion, on the other hand, there was a significant but transient
increase in O$_2$ uptake by the end of the experimental period.   When
red blood cells were reinfused, there was some overshoot of O$_2$
uptake and a return to the control value.

The change in hydrogen ion concentration is shown in figure 2.

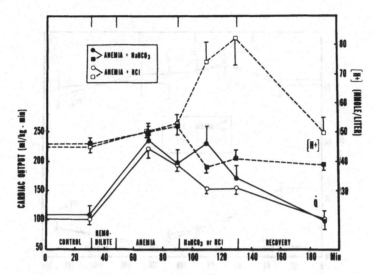

Fig. 2. Changes in cardiac output ($\dot{Q}$) and hydrogen ion concentration
[H^+] during anemia, $NaHCO_3$ or HCl infusion, and following
reinfusion of red blood cells.

In terms of pH, both groups went from about 7.35 during the control
period to about 7.28 at the end of the anemia period. Infusion of
acid lowered pH to about 7.1 and $NaHCO_3$ raised it to about 7.4.
Cardiac output, shown in this same figure, increase initially over
100% with hemodilution and then decreased with time. Infusion of
$NaHCO_3$ increased cardiac output transiently. This was not simply
a volume effect because the same volume of HCl tended to decrease
cardiac output. The changes in cardiac output were a smaller
mirror image of the changes in hydrogen ion concentration but were
parallel to the changes noted in O_2 uptake.

     The arterial and mixed venous PO_2, as shown in figure 3, were
not significantly different in the two groups even after infusion
of acid and base. Using a standard dissociation curve for dog
blood, the difference in pH created by the infusions was sufficient
to increase P_{50} by 10 torr in the acidemic animals. Mixed venous
PO_2 was not affected, however, and was lowered about the same amount
in both groups by hemodilution.

     Although the changes in O_2 uptake after severe hemodilution
seemed mostly related to the ability of the heart to maintain its
compensatory increase in output, another factor was also operative.
That factor was the ability of the periphery to extract more O_2
from the total transported after acid infusion, as can be seen in
figure 4. Inspection of the filled circles fitted by the dashed
line shows that O_2 uptake was not as well related to total O_2
delivery following $NaHCO_3$ infusion as it was following acid infusion,

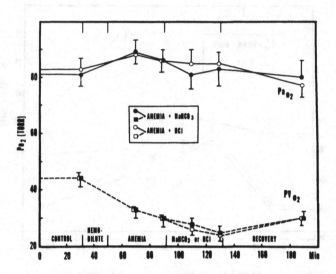

Fig. 3. Arterial (PaO$_2$) and mixed venous (P$\bar{v}$O$_2$) O$_2$ tensions
         following hemodilution, NaHCO$_3$ or HCl infusion, and
         reinfusion of red blood cells.

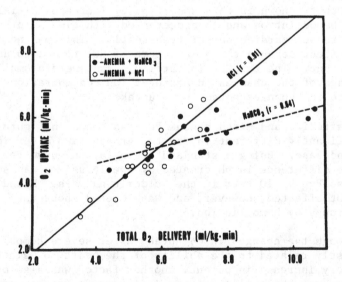

Fig. 4. O$_2$ uptake in relation to total O$_2$ delivery ($\dot{Q}$xCaO$_2$) during
         severe anemia following NaHCO$_3$ or HCl infusion.

represented by the circles fitted by the continuous line. After
bicarbonate, the linear regression showed a flat slope of 0.24
with correlation coefficient of 0.64. Following acid infusion, the
slope increased to 0.82 and the correlation coefficient went to
0.91. If the slopes of these lines are reduced to their physiologic
significance, they represent the extraction ratio for O_2. Following
acid, the strong dependence of O_2 uptake upon total O_2 delivery was
the result of more complete O_2 extraction. Bicarbonate infusion
actually did not change the degree to which O_2 was extracted from
the untreated anemic state. Figure 5 shows the data collected before acid or base were infused with respect to the linear relationships found afterwards. The bicarbonate line fits the untreated
data very well. On the other hand, almost without exception, the
untreated anemic data points fell below the line fitted to the data
obtained after acid infusion.

     There were two observations from these experiments that deserve
comment. When isovolemic hemodilution was carried to the point of
limiting whole body O_2 uptake, a highly critical factor was the
ability of the body to compensate by increasing cardiac output when
the heart itself was subject to O_2 limitations of energy production
(Von Restorff, et al, 1975). The effects of base infusion to increase output temporarily and of acid infusion to do the opposite
may have represented their respective actions to enhance and inhibit
glycolysis. The true benefit of base infusion can be questioned,
however, since cardiac output fell again and O_2 uptake fell more

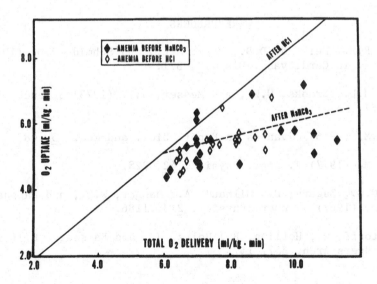

Fig. 5. O_2 uptake in relation to total O_2 delivery during severe
         anemia but before infusion of $NaHCO_3$ or HCl.

rapidly after their temporary increases. In experiments on rat heart muscle, Bing et al (1973) showed that the lesser mechanical performances of hypoxic heart muscle in an acid environment may actually have been protective in that contracture did not develop at acid pH but did at normal or alkaline pH.

The other noteworthy observation was the increased efficiency with which the periphery extracted O_2 after acid infusion. This was marked by a striking dependency of O_2 uptake upon total O_2 delivery. To achieve that highly correlated relationship required that regional blood flow to have been distributed in precise proportion to O_2 demand. Why should that have been more true in anemic hypoxia after acid infusion? If one hypothesizes that anemic hypoxia per se offered minimal stimulation to peripheral chemoreceptors, then there might have been a deficit of sympathetic tone relative to a similar degree of hypoxic hypoxia. Without strong vasoconstrictor tone, there might have been relative overperfusion of peripheral areas having lower O_2 demands. Acid infusions have been shown to increase plasma catecholamine levels (Nahas, et al, 1967) and may also have directly stimulated peripheral chemoreceptors (Abboud, et al, 1976). With a resultant increase in vasoconstrictor tone during anemic hypoxia, distribution of O_2 by way of blood flow was maintained in stricter proportion to regional needs. In any event, the possible effects of acid and base infusion upon position of oxyhemoglobin dissociation curves after severe anemia were negligible with respect to these other factors which affected tissue O_2 delivery.

REFERENCES

Abboud, R.M., Heistad, D.D., Mark, A.L., and Schmid, P.D. (1976) Prog. in Cardiovasc. Dis. 18, 371.

Bing, O.H.L., Brooks, W.W., and Messer, J.V. (1973) Science 180, 1297.

Cain, S.M. (1976) Advances in Exper. Biol. and Med. 75, 483.

Cain, S.M. (1977) J. Appl. Physiol. 42, 228.

Nahas, G.G., Zagury, D., Milhaud, A., Manger, W.M., and Pappas, G.D. (1967) J. Amer. Physiol. 213, 1186.

Von Restorff, W., Hofling, B., Holtz, J., and Bassenge, E. (1975) Pflügers Arch. 357, 15.

THE EFFECT OF DEXTROSE/INSULIN INFUSION ON THE DURATION

OF RESPIRATORY ACTIVITY IN THE ANOXIC RAT

R. G. Clark, G. Jackson Rees, and F. Harris

Departments of Pediatric Anaesthesia and Child Health
University of Liverpool
Liverpool, England

Intra-cellular brain glucose varies with the blood glucose
level in both newborn and adult animals (1). In the case of the
newborn, the brain/blood glucose ratio is much higher than that of
the adult, as is also the brain glycogen level in the newborn.
This difference in tissue carbohydrate level in the neonate is not
confined to the brain, and is true of many other tissues. The
period of time for which the neonatal heart will continue to beat
in the face of anoxia is directly related to the myocardial glycogen
content, and if this is reduced the tolerance to anoxia is reduced
proportionally (2). If, in this respect, the brain is analogous to
the heart, the high tolerance of the newborn brain to anoxia would
be related to the brain carbohydrate level, and if the relationship
between carbohydrate level and tolerance of hypoxia were causal,
it should be possible to increase the tolerance of the adult brain
to anoxia by increasing the carbohydrate content of the brain.

It has been reported that intra-cisternal injection of insulin
elevates the brain glycogen level in adult rats (3) (Table 1). This
effect is unlike that of systemically administered insulin which
results in a fall in brain glycogen levels, which is secondary to
the induced hypoglycaemia.

To test the hypothesis that systemic insulin, in the absence
of hypoglycaemia, will increase the energy reserves of the brain,
and thereby modify the response to anoxia, rats were studied following the administration of insulin and glucose. They were pre-
treated with glucose and insulin, and the duration of respiratory
activity in the face of anoxia was measured.

531

TABLE 1. Effect of intracisternal Insulin on metabolite levels in rat brain in vivo (after Strang & Bachelard).

Metabolite	No. of tests	Content (μmoles/g)	
		Control	Insulin*
Glycogen	9	1·40	2·06†
Glucose	9	0·99	1·00
Glucose 6-P	9	0·07	0·115†
Lactate	7	2·46	2·26
Glutamate	3	9·01	8·60
Glucose (muscle)	3	0·81	0·70
Glycogen (muscle)	5	13·6	13·7

*Insulin was administered intracisternally, 4·5 hr. before death by rapid freezing.
†Statistically significant (P< 0.00!) (Strang and Bachelard 1971).

METHODS

Adult male Wistar rats, weight 250–300 gms were infused with a solution of 5% Dextrose, 1 gram per kilogram per hour containing 0.75 I.U. soluble Insulin, for a period of two hours, under Halothane (0.5%)/air anaesthesia.

The rectal temperature, blood glucose, electrocardiograph and respiratory patterns were recorded, the latter by a strain gauge transducer attached to the chest wall.

The rats were subjected to cerebral anoxia by either exposure to an oxygen free atmosphere or by cardiac arrest induced by the intravenous injection of a 5 ml air bolus. Respiration showed the characteristic pattern of three phases, initial hyperventilation (r), sudden apnoea (s), a period of terminal gasping (t). The total duration of respiratory activity following the onset of anoxia was measured as 'The time to last gasp' (x) (Fig. 1).

The blood glucose was estimated by tail tip venous blood samples. The blood glucose level did not fall below 5 mmoles/litre or rise above 9 mmoles/litre in the dextrose/insulin treated rats during the period of the infusion.

Rectal temperature did not alter by more than 0.5°C in any animal during the period of anaesthesia.

The rats were divided into five groups of ten animals as set out in Table 2.

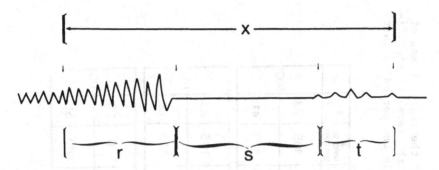

Fig. 1. Diagrammatic representation of the respiratory pattern
following the onset of hypoxia showing stage of hyperventilation
(r), primary apnoea (s), terminal gasping (t), and time to last
gasp (x).

The two groups infused with dextrose and insulin were matched
with two control groups likewise subjected to either an oxygen free
atmosphere or cardiac arrest by the intravenous injection of a bolus
of air.

The group infused with a 5% dextrose (without insulin) solution
at a rate of 1 gram per kilogram per hour for two hours prior to
exposure to an oxygen free atmosphere were matched to the same control group as those infused with glucose and insulin.

RESULTS

The respiratory pattern in those animals pre-treated with dextrose and insulin showed gross differences from the respective control groups (Fig. 2). The period of hyperventilation (r) following
the onset of cerebral hypoxia was of a similar duration in all five
groups, with the times in the cases of those animals exposed to an
oxygen free atmosphere being longer, representing the clearance
period of the lung.

A large increase in the duration of the period of primary
apnoea (s) was seen in those animals pre-treated with dextrose and
insulin as compared to the control groups. A similar difference
was seen in the persistence of terminal gasping. These changes can
be seen in Table 3, showing also the mean times to last gasp together with the standard deviation and level of significance.

The group infused with dextrose alone showed no significant
difference from the control group similarly exposed to an oxygen
free atmosphere (Table 3). There was no significant difference

TABLE 2. The procedure adopted in each of the five groups of 10 rats.

	GROUP	no. of rats
A	EXPOSED TO AN OXYGEN FREE ATMOSPHERE.	10
B	INFUSED WITH 5% DEXTROSE 1G/Kg/Hr. FOR 2 Hrs. PRIOR TO EXPOSURE TO AN O_2 FREE ATMOSPHERE.	10
C	INFUSED c̄ 5% DEXTROSE 1G/Kg/Hr. CONTAINING INSULIN 0.75 I.U./G. DEXTROSE PRIOR TO EXPOSURE TO AN O_2 FREE ATMOSPHERE.	10
D	EXPOSED TO CARDIAC ARREST BY I.V. AIR.	10
E	INFUSED AS IN GROUP C PRIOR TO CARDIAC ARREST BY I.V. AIR.	10
	TOTAL	50

TABLE 3. The duration of the three phases of respiratory activity and the level of significance of the difference in the period to last gasp in the five groups.

Group	$\bar{x}$ secs.	$\bar{s}$ secs.	$\bar{t}$ secs.	$\bar{x}$ time to last gasp	S.D. of $\bar{x}$	P
Anoxia Controls	38	52	15	105	23	
Anoxia Dextrose Insulin	31	99	53	176	41	<.001
Anoxia Controls	38	52	15	105	23	
Anoxia Dextrose	28	53	21	103	12	N.S.
Cardiac Arrest Controls	14	48	8	70	23	
Cardiac Arrest Dextrose Insulin	16	104	49	169	51	<.001

between the two groups infused with dextrose and insulin (Fig. 2)
demonstrating that the persistance of respiratory activity was not
attributable to an intact circulation and improved cardiac performance secondary to the effect of the infusion upon the myocardium.

CONCLUSION

The results demonstrate that the infusion of glucose and insulin
extends the period of respiratory activity in the face of hypoxia,
and that this effect is not produced by the infusion of dextrose
alone.

The mechanism whereby this effect is produced is uncertain.
The known effect of insulin on brain carbohydrate metabolism, and
the fact that newborn animals with high tissue carbohydrate levels
have a high tolerance of hypoxia, suggests that the effect of glucose and insulin infusion is the result of elevating the intracellular energy reserves.

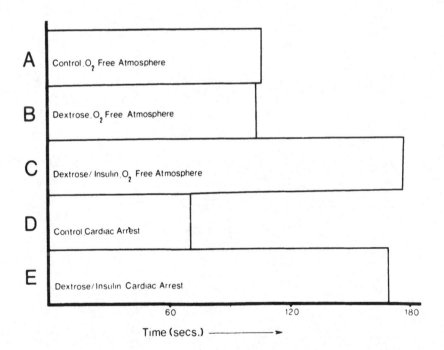

Fig. 2. The total period of respiratory activity following the
onset of anoxia in each of the five groups.

It will, however, be necessary to study the effect of glucose and insulin infusion on the levels and rates of change of brain substrates and metabolites during anoxia to establish that this is the mechanism by which the observed effects on respiration are produced.

REFERENCES

1. Mayman, C.I. (1968) Neurology 18, 294.

2. Dawes, G.S., Mott, J.C., and Shelley, H.J. (1959) J. Physiol. 146, 516.

3. Strang, R.H.C. and Bachelard, H.S. (1971) J. Neurochem. 18, 1799.

OXYGEN CONSUMPTION AND OXYGEN EXTRACTION OF THE FELINE

LIVER UNDER DIFFERENT TYPES OF INDUCED HYPOXIA*

Joachim Lutz and Hans-Gerd Schulze

Physiologisches Institut der Universitat

D-8700 Würzburg, BRD

Under normal blood flow extraction of O_2 by the liver is less than 40% of the oxygen supplied. This ratio of consumed to supplied O_2 increases drastically when O_2 supply diminishes with blood flow. For instance an O_2 extraction greater than 95% is reached during relative ischaemia (Lutz et al, 1975). The experiments reported below were performed to test the mechanism of this extremely high O_2 extraction, which is seen otherwise only in the coronary circulation.

METHODS

The livers of cats (2.5 - 3.5 kg body weight) anaesthetized with chloralose (60 mg/kg) - urethane (260 mg/kg) were perfused using regulated roller pumps (Lutz 1972) which produced either constant flow or constant pressure inputs to the hepatic artery and, via the superior mesenteric artery and the intestinal vessels, to the portal vein. Perfusion fluid was the animal's own blood, drawn from the lower aorta; filtered bovine blood was added to keep the haemoglobin concentration constant. Continuous measurements of PO_2 and pH were performed on the arterial, portal and hepatic venous blood by continually drawing blood from each vessel and pumping it through an assembly with PO_2 electrodes (Clark-type spherical electrodes, Lübbers and Windisch, 1962; Fa. Eschweiler, Kiel), and pH electrodes (Fa. Ingold, Frankfurt). After passing the electrodes, the blood was returned together with blood from the ligated inferior vena cava into the jugular vein. Oxygen saturation was calculated according to values for the cat given by

* Supported by a grant of the Deutsche Forschungsgemeinschaft.

Bartels and Harms (1959), using our own computer programmes (Lutz
and Schulze, 1975).   Figures derived in that way were more reproducible than those obtained by spectrophotometric determinations,
especially for very low saturations of hepatic venous blood.
Control measurements were done with a Lex-O_2-Con instrument
(Lexington Ltd., Mass.).   Haemoglobin content of blood was measured
at 30 min. intervals by a cyan-haemoglobin method.   Most values
were continuously recorded on two recorders with 6 channels each
(Fa. Linseis, Selb/BRD).

RESULTS

During a reduction of the total hepatic blood flow to nearly
60% of its control value the changes shown in Fig. 1 occurred. O_2
consumption decreased only from 5.94 $\pm$ 0.34 (S.E.M.) to 5.41 $\pm$ 0.35
ml O_2/(min $\cdot$ 100 g), (i.e. less than 10%).   This was possible
because of a marked increase of O_2 extraction.

The relation between the O_2 extraction and the O_2 supply[*] is
shown in Fig. 2.   It demonstrates that the normal O_2 consumption
rate of nearly 6 ml O_2/(min $\cdot$ 100 g) can be maintained within the
normal limits of $\pm$ 10% only if the O_2 supply is kept above about
10 ml O_2/(min $\cdot$ 100 g).   This is despite an increase of O_2
extraction of more than 50%.   Further increase in O_2 extraction
which accompanies the reduction of O_2 supply occurs with a decrease
of O_2 consumption: i.e. the increase of O_2 extraction can not
compensate completely for the decline of O_2 supply.   Although
theoretically, normal O_2 consumption could be maintained with an
O_2 supply of only 6 ml O_2/(min $\cdot$ 100 g) providing there was an
extraction of 95%, in practice the consumption fell, under these
conditions to less than 4.5 ml O_2/(min $\cdot$ 100 g).

The partial compensation of the diminished O_2 supply is
clearly revealed in Fig. 3.   Under a constant O_2 consumption the
O_2 extraction would follow the hyperbola.

$$O_2 \text{ extr.} = \frac{O_2 \text{ cons.}}{O_2 \text{ suppl.}}$$

---

*To show various interrelations in the following figures oxygen
supply instead of blood flow is plotted on the abscissa.   Thus,
the influence of animals and tests with different haemoglobin
contents is compensated.   The normal O_2 supply of the liver amounts
to 15 - 18 ml O_2/(min $\cdot$ 100 g) with an O_2 content of 15 g/dl, a
blood flow of 100 ml/(min $\cdot$ g), and an arterial blood flow fraction
of 30% - dependent upon the specific O_2 consumption of the
intestine.

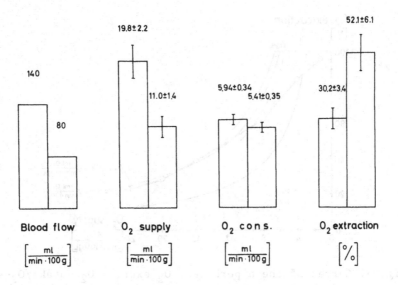

Fig. 1. Behaviour of the liver after blood flow reduction in
the normal range of regulation.

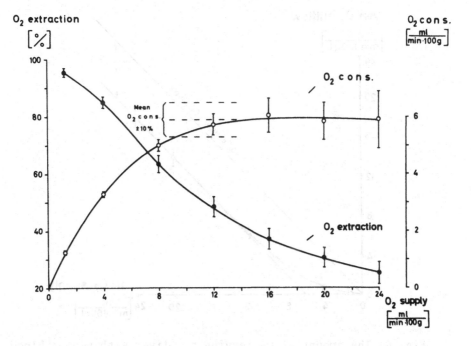

Fig. 2. O_2 extraction and O_2 uptake as a function of O_2 supply.

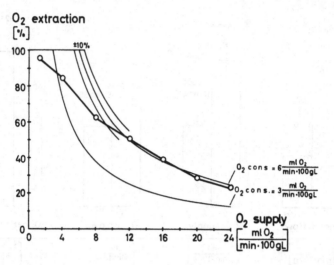

Fig. 3. Curves of the hyperbolae: O_2 extr. = O_2 uptake/O_2-supply
and the true extraction curve, which leaves the range of
normal O_2 uptake at about 60% O_2-extraction.
At 87% O_2 extraction the O_2 uptake is already reduced to
half.

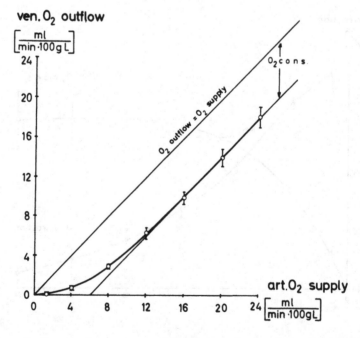

Fig. 4. The amount of O_2 leaving the liver with venous blood
showing a splay like that in curves from the kidney.

However, below an O_2 supply of about 10 ml O_2/(min · 100 g) the experimentally observed curve diverges from that of the hyperbola.   With further reduction of O_2 supply the steepness of the extraction curve diminishes, so that with an extraction of 87% the theoretical hyperbola for only 3 ml O_2/(min · 100 g) is intersected.

When venous O_2 outflow is plotted <u>vs</u> O_2 supply (Fig. 4) a similar decrease in the slope of the curve is seen at low values of O_2 supply.   In the absence of O_2 consumption, the values for the venous outflow would be on a straight line: venous outflow = O_2 supply.

The distance between the measured values and this line indicates the amount of O_2 consumption.   With decreasing O_2 supply the outflow curve turns off towards the origin instead of running rectilinear to an O_2 supply of 6 ml O_2/(min · 100 g).   This behaviour is similar to the splay which can be seen in data from the kidney, when the excretion of glucose is plotted as a function of glucose supply or concentration.   In both cases no definite threshold exists, above which a constant amount of oxygen or substrate is turned over.   The possible mechanism which explains this behaviour will be discussed later.

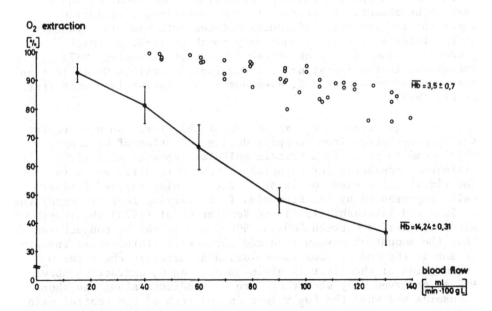

Fig. 5.   A high O_2 extraction does not presuppose small blood flow:
under haemodilution during normal blood flow extreme O_2
extractions also occur.

The finding of a very high O_2 extraction under conditions of low O_2 supply combined with very low blood flow rates may lead to the suggestion that these excessive values would only be produced by long contact times and under very low blood flow velocities. To test this, we chose a second type of hypoxia, anaemic hypoxia during haemodilution.

The haemoglobin content was reduced to 3.5 g/dl by infusion of dextran (Macrodex ^{R*}). The O_2 supply was markedly decreased by this procedure but the very high O_2 extraction values ($\sim$90%) observed above were also seen here even during flow rates within the range of about 100 ml/(min. $\cdot$ 100 g) (Fig. 5). Thus it is the low O_2 supply per se which determines the O_2 extraction, rather than the flow conditions.

DISCUSSION

In order to explain the effect of an early decrease of O_2 consumption with the contrasting late increase of O_2 extraction values to more than 90%, the following suggestions are made.

The capacity of the liver for highly efficient extraction of oxygen is due to a small diffusion resistance between parenchymal cells and blood stream where basement membranes are missing. Furthermore, morphologically predetermined functional O_2 shunts seem to be absent, in contrast to the intestinal circulation. There the intervascular distances between both vascular branches in the intestinal villi amount only to about 15-20 μm which produces a counter current system for oxygen (Lundgren 1967). Therefore, in the intestinal circulation the maximum O_2 extraction rises to not more than 75%, even during a relative ischaemia (Lutz et al, 1975).

The high rates of O_2 extraction of the liver can not prevent the O_2 consumption from dropping during reduction of O_2 supply. This seems to point to a certain cellular inhomogeneity with different thresholds for O_2 uptake. However, differences in individual cells need not exist. The vascular supply of liver cells represented by the sinusoids is of varying length: according to Suwa and Takahashi (1971) and Kessler et al (1973) the length of sinusoids varies between 200 and 500 μm. It can be conjectured that the amount of oxygen required for optimal turnover is insufficient at the end of long sinusoids, and therefore the total O_2 consumption of the liver is diminished. An O_2 extraction above 95% is observed only when there are O_2 gradients along the short sinusoids and when the PO_2 values in the area of the central vein are low.

---

* Kindly provided by Knoll AG, Ludwigshafen.

Distinct intercellular O_2 gradients along the sinusoids (in contrast to intracellular gradients) have also been suggested by Sies (1977) who found a similar O_2 dependence of urate oxidase and cytochrome oxidase in situ in contrast to the largely different O_2 affinities of the isolated enzymes.

REFERENCES

Bartels, H. and Harms, H. (1959) Pflügers Arch. ges Physiol. 268, 334.

Kessler, M., Lang, H., Sinagowitz, E., Rink, R. and Höper, J. (1973) In 'Oxygen Transport to Tissue' (eds. Bicher, H.I. and Bruley, D.F.) Plenum Press, N.Y., p.351.

Lundgren, O. (1967) Acta Physiol. Scand., Suppl. 303, 1.

Lutz, J. (1976) Pflügers Arch. 335, R89.

Lutz, J., Henrich, H. and Bauereisen, E. (1975) Pflügers Arch. 360, 7.

Lutz, J., Schulze, H.G. and Michael, U. (1975) Pflügers Arch. 359, 285.

Sies, H. (1977) In 'Hypoxia and Ischemia' (eds. Reivich, M., Coburn, R.F., Lahiri, S. and Chance, B.), p. 51, Plenum Press, N.Y.

Suwa, N. and Takahashi, T. (1971) Morphological and morphometrical analysis of circulation in hypertension and ischemic kidney. (ed. Büchner, F.) Urban and Schwarzenberg, München.

THE EFFECTS OF LOW O_2 SUPPLY ON THE RESPIRATORY ACTIVITY, REDUCED PYRIDINE NUCLEOTIDE FLUORESCENCE, K^+ EFFLUX AND THE SURFACE PO_2 AND PCO_2 OF THE ISOLATED, PERFUSED RAT LIVER

S. Ji, J. Höper, H. Acker and M. Kessler

Max-Planck-Institut für Systemphysiologie

Rheinlanddamm 201, 46 Dortmund, West Germany

The problem of oxygen transport to tissue may be analyzed in terms of three main fluxes and their conjugate thermodynamic forces, namely the convectional flux of oxygen through the vascular network driven by the perfusion pressure, the diffusional flux of O_2 from the capillary wall to the interior of cells driven by the PO_2 gradient, and the flux of O_2 through the redox chemical reaction network driven by the chemical affinity. Under physiological conditions, any one of the three fluxes will be affected by alterations in any one of the three forces. In the present study, we have investigated the metabolic and ionic effects of altering two of the three forces, the perfusion pressure at a constant arterial PO_2 and the arterial PO_2 at a constant perfusion pressure. The results obtained show that the main difference between "no flow" anoxia and "normal flow" anoxia (Kessler et al., 1974) involves a dramatic increase in the tissue PCO_2 and the activity of extracellular K^+ in the former but not in the latter. In addition, the extent of pyridine nucleotide reduction as judged from the NAD(P)H fluorescence increase is approximately twice as great in ischemia as in "normal flow" anoxia. These differences may underlie the interesting observation made by Höper et al. (1973) that "no flow" anoxia is much more detrimental to the preservation of ATP in perfused liver than "normal flow" anoxia.

METHODS

Albino Wistar rats (200 - 300 g) fed ad libitum were anaesthetized with Nembutal® (60 mg/kg). The isolated liver was perfused with the Krebs-Ringer bicarbonate solution (3.5 % albumin) at room temperature (22° - 23° C) using the perfusion setup shown schematically in Figure 1. The surface PO_2 was measured with a multi-wire pla-

tinum electrode (Kessler et al., 1976), the arterial and venous
PO_2 values with Clark-type Pt electrodes, the flow rate with an
electromagnetic flow meter (Statham), the surface K^+ activity with
a valinomycin electrode (Höper et al., 1976), and the surface PCO_2
with a membrane-covered Pt electrode newly designed by Lis et al.
(in preparation). The NAD(P)H fluorescence (F) and uv reflectance
(R) were measured with a micro-light guide coupled to a Johnson
Foundation DC fluorometer as described elsewhere (Ji et al., 1977).
The depth of penetration of the uv light (300 - 400 nm) into liver
tissue was estimated to be approximately 850 μ and the number of
liver cells monitored 10^3 to 10^4. The rate of O_2 uptake was calculated from the relation, ((arterial PO_2, torr) - (venous PO_2,
torr)) x (flow rate, ml/min/g liver w.w.) xα, where α is the solubility coefficient of O_2 in our perfusate taken to be 3.61 x 10^{-5}
per torr.

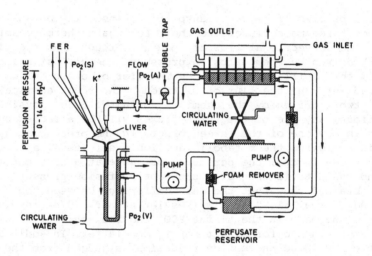

Figure 1. A schematic drawing of the perfusion setup (self-explana-
          tory).

RESULTS AND DISCUSSION

     In Figure 2 is shown the result of a typical experiment, where
the rate of O_2 supply was varied by changing the perfusion pressure
(Δflow experiment). The plot was obtained from data stored on a
magnetic tape (Solartron) using a computer-assisted plotter (Benson).
As the flow rate was decreased, both the surface and venous PO_2
traces decreased stepwise, the surface PO_2 reaching zero at the
flow rate of 1.0 ml/min/g. The venous PO_2 trace showed a transient
increase of 55 torr in 144 seconds. Out of 17 similar experiments,
we have observed 13 such venous PO_2 transients. In the particular

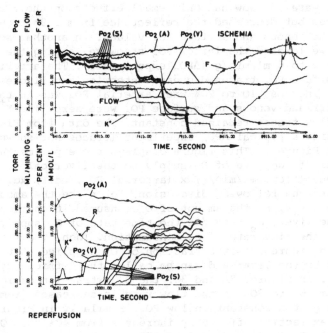

Figure 2. Continuous measurement of PO_2, NAD(P)H fluorescence, uv
reflectance, flow rate and surface PO_2 and K^+ activity
during a " Δ flow" experiment.

experiment shown, the transient venous PO_2 increase is probably
associated with the sixth flow change (from 1.9 to 1.0 ml/min/g)
and not with the seventh (from 1.0 to 0.37 ml/min/g), since the
effect of the latter flow drop is not expected to affect the venous PO_2 at least 110 seconds later. The mechanism underlying the
transient venous PO_2 increase is not known at present. The almost
simultaneous increase (24 %) in the NAD(P)H fluorescence observed
suggests that the venous PO_2 transient may be related to the reduction of some intracellular pyridine nucleotide pool, although such
a correlation between the local (fluorescence) and the global
(venous PO_2) measurements may not always hold. When ischemia is induced, the K^+ activity increased from 7.2 to 24 mM in 10 minutes
(the erratic K^+ trace after the first 10 minutes is probably due to
the separation of the K^+ electrode from the shrunken liver) and the
fluorescence trace showed a further increase (24 %) during the next
7 to 8 minutes. The reflectance trace remained unaltered during the
first 10 minutes of ischemia. At the end of 15 minutes of ischemia,
the inflow channel was opened and the liver was subjected to 2.3 cm
H_2O perfusion pressure for 5 minutes. This caused the flow to rise
from 0 to 0.8 ml/min/g, the fluorescence to decrease from 141 % to
99 %, and the K^+ activity to decrease from about 20 mM to 7.9 mM.

Further increase in flow had only small effects on the fluorescence
and K^+ traces but decreased the reflectance from 119% to 98% and
increased the venous and surface PO_2 values. In another set of experiments, we lowered the inflow PO_2 stepwise keeping the flow rate
constant at 5 to 6 ml/min/g (ΔPO_2 experiments). The arterial, venous and surface PO_2 traces decreased stepwise and fluorescence was
observed to increase 10 to 20% when arterial PO_2 was in the range
30 to 50 torr and venous and surface PO_2 were zero. The K^+, reflectance and flow traces remained constant. The data from Figure 2
and those from a typical ΔPO_2 experiment (traces not shown) are
compared in Figure 3. This figure displays the experimental data
as functions of the rate of O_2 supply to the liver calculated from
the relation, (flow, ml/min/g) x (arterial PO_2, torr) xα. In order
to facilitate the following discussion, let n_s be the amount of O_2
supplied to liver, n_c the amount of O_2 consumed in chemical reactions in the liver, $J_s = dn_s/dt$ the time rate of O_2 supply, and
$J_c = dn_c/dt$ the time rate of O_2 consumption. Then, the ratio
$J_c/J_s = n_c/n_s$ represents the fraction of O_2 supplied that has been
metabolized by the liver and can be called the "efficiency of O_2
extraction". In Figures 3A and 3C, the O_2 extraction efficiency increases from 36% to 80% as the flow rate is decreased from 7.5 to
zero ml/min/g at a constant inflow PO_2. Similarly in Figures 3B and
3D, the O_2 extraction efficiency increases from 40% to 100% as
the arterial PO_2 is decreased from 470 torr to zero at a constant
flow rate. The slope (dJ_c/dJ_s) of the O_2 uptake curve at a given O_2
supply rate can be interpreted as the fraction of an increment of
O_2 supply rate that contributes to the rate of O_2 uptake. In terms
of this quantity, we may divide an O_2 uptake curve into three regions A, B and C where, respectively, the following relations hold:
$dJ_c/dJ_s = 1$, $1 > dJ_c/dJ_s > 0$, and $dJ_c/dJ_s = 0$. A careful examination reveals that Figure 3C contains B region only and Figure 3D
contains both A and B regions.

Figures 3C and 3D show that decreasing the O_2 supply rate leads
to a decrease in O_2 uptake even when the venous PO_2 is still high.
This observation can be readily explained in terms of the inhomogeneous distribution of capillary lengths in the liver as pointed
out by Kessler et al. (1973). That is, the presence of short capillaries will account for high venous O_2 content, whereas the long
capillaries with their associated anoxic zones will explain the
decrease in O_2 uptake in the B region of the O_2 uptake curve. The
local measurements shown in Figures 3E through 3L, except for reflectance, register the difference between the two ways of altering
the O_2 supply rate. In 3G and 3H, the NAD(P)H fluorescence increases
maximally by 45% when the perfusion pressure is lowered but only
by 14% when the arterial PO_2 is lowered. Similarly, the extracellular K^+ activity increases by 17 mM only in the former case. The
surface PCO_2 is the third indicator capable of distinguishing

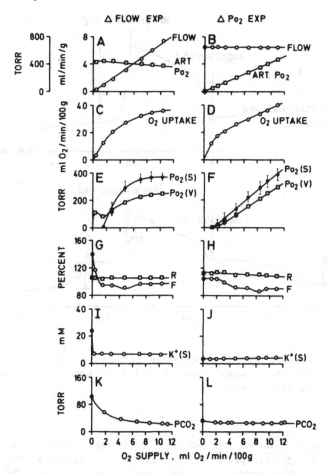

Figure 3. The effects of altering the O$_2$ supply rate on the O$_2$ uptake rate, NAD(P)H fluorescence, uv reflectance, surface PO$_2$ and PCO$_2$, venous PO$_2$ and interstitial K$^+$ activity. The data were obtained in three separate experiments (1 = A, C, E, G and I, 2 = B, D, F, H, J, and 3 = K, L).

between the Δ flow and Δ PO$_2$ experiments. Unlike the extracellular K$^+$ activity, however, the PCO$_2$ value changes continuously with the flow rate.

The relatively low fluorescence increase (15%) observed during the Δ PO$_2$ experiment as compared to the increase (45%) observed during the Δ flow experiment (compare 3H and 3G) could in principle be explained as a consequence of an incomplete tissue anoxia as might be suspected from the fact that the minimum arterial PO$_2$ value experimentally achieved by equilibrating the perfusate with 95% N$_2$

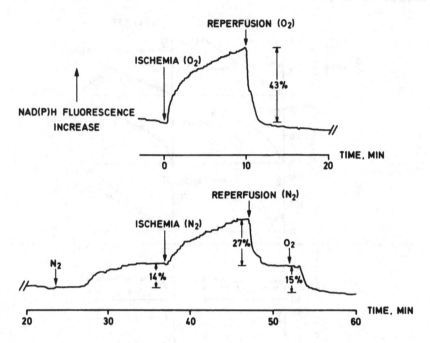

Figure 4.   The NAD(P)H fluorescence increase caused by a "sudden"
            ischemia (upper trace) and a ischemia preceded by N_2-
            anoxia (lower trace).

- 5% CO_2 for 5 minutes was 50 torr (see 3B). However, as alluded
to above, the global parameters such as the arterial PO_2 is a poor
indicator for the redox state of local tissue areas. The fact that
the fluorescence intensity in 3H has already reached the plateau
even at the arterial PO_2 value of 70 torr suggests that the tissue
site which was optically monitored with the micro-light guide was
anoxic when the arterial PO_2 fell below this value.

Perfusing the liver with a perfusate equilibrated with 95% N_2
- 5% CO_2 for over one hour usually caused 15 to 20% fluorescence
increases, indicating that the maximum fluorescence increment
achievable by N_2-anoxia is 15 to 20% under our experimental conditions.

The contrasting difference between the fluorescence increments
induced by "no flow" anoxia and "normal flow" anoxia is shown in
Figure 4. Ischemia caused a 43% increase in fluorescence in 10 minutes. Reperfusion decreased the fluorescence to slightly below the
pre-ischemic level in about 1.5 minutes. After 10 minutes of recovery, oxygen in the equilibrating gas mixture was replaced by nitrogen, which led to a 14% fluorescence increase in 15 minutes. The
subsequent ischemia caused a further increase in fluorescence in

the amount of 27% in 10 minutes. As can be seen, this step-wise increase in fluorescence is completely reversible. Therefore, the results show that, under our experimental condition, "no flow" anoxia causes 2 or 3 times as much fluorescence increases as "normal flow" anoxia. Brosnan et al (1970) demonstrated that a 5-minute ischemia in the rat liver in situ induced the cytosolic NADH/NAD$^+$ ratio to increase approximately twice as much as the mitochondrial NADH/NAD$^+$ ratio. Based on their data and on the fact that the mitochondrial electron transport chain is certainly completely reduced in "normal flow" anoxia, it is tempting to suggest that the N$_2$-induced fluorescence increase is due predominantly to the reduction of the mitochondrial pyridine nucleotide pool whereas the ischemia preceeded by anoxic perfusion leads to the reduction primarily of the cytosolic pyridine nucleotide pool. This suggestion, however, should be tested by direct biochemical analysis of appropriate redox couples. Regardless of the validity of this interpretation, Figure 4 clearly shows that the fluorescence increase induced by a "sudden" ischemia consists of at least two components, i.e., the O$_2$-sensitive component (14 to 15%) and the flow-sensitive component (27%). The latter component may be influenced by the high PCO$_2$ observed in the ischemic liver.

ACKNOWLEDGEMENT

We thank Ms. B. Bölling for her able technical assistance and Mr. R. Strehlau and his crew for their computer work.

1. Brosnan, J. T., Krebs, H. A. and Williamson, D. H. (1970) Effects of Ischemia on Metabolite Concentrations in Rat Liver. Biochem. J. 117, 91.

2. Lis, K., Acker, H. and Lübbers, D. W. (1977) A PCO₂ Surface Electrode based on the Principle of Electrical Conductivity (in preparation).

3. Höper, J., Kessler, M. and Starlinger, H. (1973) Preservation of ATP in the Perfused Liver. In "Oxygen Transport to Tissue" p. 371 (eds. Bicher, H. I. and Bruley, D. F.) Plenum, New York.

4. Höper, J., Kessler, M. and Simon, W. (1976) Measurements with Ion-Selective Surface Electrodes (pK, pNa, pCa, pH) During No-Flow Anoxia. In "Ion and Enzyme Electrodes in Biology and Medicine," p. 331 (eds. Kessler, M. et al). Urban & Schwarzenberg, München.

5. Ji, S., Chance, B., Nishiki, K., Smith, T. and Rich, T. (1977)
    Micro-Light Guides: A New Method for Measuring Tissue Fluores-
    cence and Reflectance. Am. J. physiol. (accepted for publica-
    tion).

6. Kessler, M., Lang, H., Sinagowitz, E., Rink, R. and Höper, J.
    (1973) Homeostasis of Oxygen Supply in Liver and Kidney. In
    "Oxygen Transport to Tissue" p. 351 (eds. Bicher, H. I. and
    Bruley, D. F.) Plenum, New York.

7. Kessler, M., Höper, J., Schäfer, D. and Starlinger, H. (1974)
    Sauerstofftransport im Gewebe. In "Mikrozirkulation" p. 36
    (eds. Ahnefeld, F. W. et al). Springer-Verlag, Berlin.

8. Kessler, M., Höper, J. and Krumme, B. A. (1976) Monitoring of
    Tissue Perfusion and Cellular Function. Anesthesiology 45, 184.

DISTURBANCES OF EXTRACELLULAR pK, pNa AND pH DURING NO-FLOW ANOXIA

J. Höper, M. Kessler, S. Ji, H. Acker

Max-Planck-Institut für Systemphysiologie

4600 Dortmund, Rheinlanddamm 201, GFR

Introduction

It has been known for many years that immediately after the onset of ischemia (no-flow anoxia) a fast depletion of cellular energy-rich phosphates occurs (Thorn et al., 1957; Brettschneider 1964, Brosnan et al. 1970, Chance et al. 1965, Schmahl et al. 1966, see Cohen 1973). In contrast to no-flow anoxia, a norm-flow anoxia (anoxic anoxia) is tolerated over a longer period of time (Höper et al. 1973, Kessler et al. 1974, 1976 a, b). Already in 1953 Opitz considered that during no-flow anoxia the acidosis caused by accumulation of lactic acid may be responsible for the irreversible cellular damage of the brain, but the cellular mechanisms which cause the cellular alterations have not yet been explained completely.

Methods

As a model for our investigations the isolated and hemoglobin-free perfused rat liver (perfusion temperature 22° C) was used (Kessler 1967, Lang 1970, Höper et al., in preparation). Measurements of tissue Po_2 were performed with multiwire Po_2-electrodes (Kessler and Lübbers 1966). NAD(P)H fluorescence was monitored with a micro-light-guide photometer recently developed by Ji et al. (accepted for publication). Extracellular ion activities were measured by means of ion-selective surface electrodes (Kessler et al. 1974 b, 1976 b, Höper et al. 1976). Pco_2 was recorded by a surface Pco_2 electrode according to Lis et al. (in preparation).

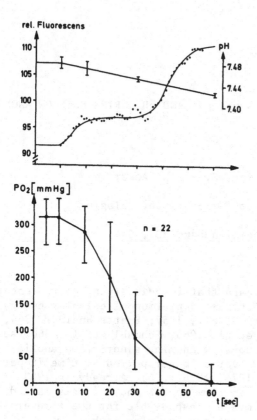

Fig. 1
Changes in tissue Po_2
(mean value, minimal and
maximal Po_2), surface pH
(mean value $\pm$ s.d.) and
NAD(P)H fluorescence
during the first 60 sec
after onset of no-flow
anoxia

Results

Fig. 1 shows the results of measured tissue Po_2, NAD(P)H fluorescence and extracellular pH (measured by a surface electrode) during
the first 60 sec after the onset of no-flow anoxia. As can be seen,
extracellular pH starts to decrease immediately while tissue Po_2
is still high and NAD(P)H fluorescence shows only slight change.
Estimations of the tissue lactate content indicate (Fig. 2) that
this decrease in pH during the first 60 sec of no-flow anoxia can
not be explained by the increase in lactic acid due to anaerobic
glycolysis. The lactate content increases during the first minute
of no-flow anoxia only from 366 ± 116 nmol/g tissue ^{w}/w to
599 ± 136 nmol/g tissue ^{w}/w.
Measurements of tissue Pco_2 show that immediately after inducing
no-flow anoxia there is an increase in the CO_2-partial pressure on
the liver surface (Fig. 3).
During this early phase of no-flow anoxia the ATP content
drops, even though oxygen is still available in the tissue (Fig. 4).

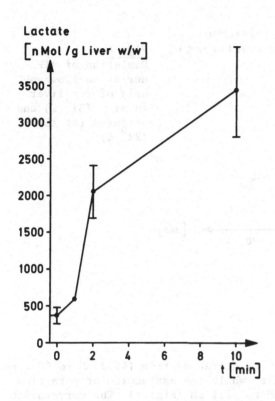

Fig. 2
Increase in lactate content in liver tissue (nmol/g liver ^{w}/w $\pm$ s.d., n=5, except the value one minute after the onset of no-flow anoxia (n=3)) during no-flow anoxia

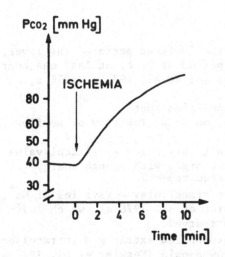

Fig. 3
Original trace of pCO_2 measurement at the liver surface during no-flow anoxia, performed by a pCO_2 electrode according to Lis et al. (in preparation)

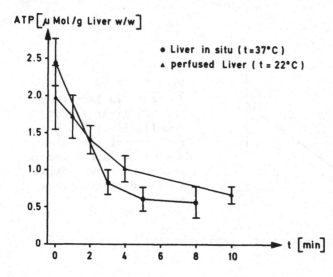

Fig. 4
Depletion of ATP
during no-flow an-
oxia of rat liver
in situ (37° C) and
perfused rat liver
(22° C)

The extracellular sodium activity decreases from 145.2 mM to 68.2 mM
during 9 min of no-flow anoxia, while the extracellular potassium
activity increases from 5.5 mM to 12.1 mM (Fig. 5). The correlation
between the initial ATP depletion and the decrease in extracellular
Na shows an almost linear relationship, suggesting that the initial
decrease in ATP may be caused by an activation of the sodium/potas-
sium pump (Kessler et al. 1976 b).

Discussion
If norm-flow anoxia is induced in the isolated perfused rat liver,
the organ can tolerate for a long period of time, at last one hour
(Höper et al. 1973, 1975, 1976, Kessler et al. 1974 a, 1976 a, b,
Ji et al. 1977).
This observation holds under the condition that:
1. microflow is not disturbed, i.e. no local low-flow or no-flow
   anoxia occurs,
2. extra- and intracellular pH do not fall below a critical value
3. anaerobic glycolysis provides the organ with enough energy to
   maintain the minimum metabolic requirements.
If these conditions are fulfilled extracellular activities of Na[+],
K[+], and Ca[+] remain unchanged (Kessler et al. 1976 a), which indicates that cellular integrity is preserved.
In contrast to norm-flow anoxia, pronounced extra- and intracellular acidosis develops during no-flow anoxia (Kessler et al. 1976 a,

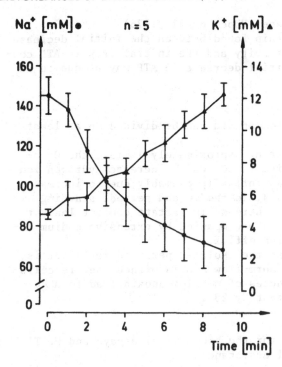

Fig. 5
Alterations in extra-
cellular activities of
Na$^+$ and K$^+$ after the onset of no-flow anoxia.
The measurements were
performed by ion-selec-
tive surface electrodes

b). The measurement of extracellular surface pH, as shown in Fig. 1,
indicates that protons are generated already during the first
60 sec. This initial decrease in pH as well as the changes in extracellular Na$^+$ (Fig. 5) and in ATP content (Fig. 4) occur although
oxygen is stiff available. NAD(P)H fluorescence starts to show a
pronounced increase not before tissue oxygen tension approaches
0 mm Hg. The early decrease in pH may be caused by an accumulation
of CO_2 generated from oxidative metabolism. The measurement of tissue
Pco_2 shown in Fig. 3 is in agreement with this supposition. Immediately after inducing no-flow anoxia the CO_2 tension is observed to
increase. A distinct increase in lactate occurs after tissue Po_2
reaches 0 mm Hg, which is obtained after 1 min. Therefore it is unlikely that an increase in lactic acid causes the increase in hydrogen ion activity during the first 60 seconds.
Williams et al. (1971) showed that increasing the CO_2 content of
the inspired air causes a rapid fall in hepatic cell resting potential. They suggested that this is due to an increased membrane permeability. As pointed out by Kessler et al. (1976 a) an increase in
hydrogen ion activity may lead to a protonation of the plasma membrane and cause the early changes in extracellular activities of
Na$^+$, K$^+$, and Ca^{++}. The changes in Na$^+$ and K$^+$ which are most likely
due to a sodium influx and a potassium efflux lead to the depolari-

zation of the plasma membrane (Höper et al. 1976).
The almost linear relationship found between the initial decrease
in extracellular sodium acitivity and the initial drop in ATP content suggests, that the initial decrease in ATP may be due to an
activation of Na/K ATPases.

Summary
The initial period of no-flow anoxia can be divided in at least
two parts.
During the first period lasting approximately 1 min., the O_2 a-
vailable in tissue gives rise to CO_2 which increases hydrogen ion
activity and may lead to Na^+ influx (presumably due to increased
membrane permeability to Na^+). In the second period, starting
after the first minute, the increase in lactate content leads to
further decrease in pH and is accompanied by extensive sodium influx and a distinct potassium efflux.
However, it is striking that the isolated perfused rat liver is
able to tolerate 1 hour of norm-flow anoxia without severe cellular damage, whereas two minutes of no-flow anoxia lead to a decrease in cellular ATP content by 28%.

Acknowledgement
We thank Dr. H. Starlinger for the biochemical assays and U. Tlolka
for the excellent technical assistance.

References

Bretschneider, H.J. (1964) Verhandlungen der deutschen Gesellschaft f. Keislaufforschung, 30. Tagung.

Brosnan, J.T., Krebs, H.A. and Williamson, D.H. (1970) Biochem.
J. 117, 91.

Chance, B., Schoener, B., Kregel, K., Rüssmann, W., Wesemann, W.,
Schnitger, H., Bücher, Th. (1965) Biochem. Z. 341, 325.

Cohen, M.M. (1973) Biochemistry, Ultrastructure and Physiology of
Cerebral Anoxia, Hypoxia and Ischemia. Monographs in Neutral
Sciences, Vol. 1. S. Karger, Basel.

Höper, J., Kessler, M. and Starlinger, H. (1973) In 'Oxygen
Transport to Tissue' Vol.37A, p.371. Plenum Publ.Corp. New York.

Höper, J., Schäfer, D., Starlinger, H., Tlolka, U. and Kessler, M.
(1975) Pflügers Arch. Suppl. 355, 80.

Höper, J., Kessler, M., Simon, W. (1976) In 'Ion and Enzyme
Electrodes in Medicine and Biology' p.331. Urban and Schwarzenberg,
Munich.

Ji, S., Chance, B., Nishiki, K., Smith, T. and Rich. T. Am. J. Physiol. (accepted for publication).

Ji, S., Höper, J., Acker, H and Kessler, M. This symposium.

Kessler, M. and Lübbers, D.W. (1966) Pflügers Arch. 291, 82.

Kessler, M. (1967) Habilitationsschrift, Marburg/Lahn.

Kessler, M., Höper, J., Schäfer, D. and Starlinger, H. (1974a) In 'Klin. Anästhesiologie und Intensivtherapie, Bd. 5: Mikrozirkulation', p.36. Springer, New York.

Kessler, M., Höper, J. and Simon, W. (1974b) Fed. Proc. 33, 279.

Kessler, M., Höper, J., Krumme, B. and Starlinger, H. (1976a) In 'Ion and Enzyme Electrodes in Biology and Medicine' p. 335, Urban and Schwarzenberg, Munich.

Kessler, M., Höper, J and Krumme, B.A. (1976b) Anesthesiology 45, 184.

Lang, H. (1970) Dissertation/Bochum.

Lis, K., Acker, H. and Lübbers, D.W. (in preparation)

Opitz, E. (1953) Verhdlg. d. deutsch. Gesellsch. f. Kreislaufforschung, 19. Tagung, p. 26.

Schmahl, F.W., Betz, E., Dettinger, E. and Hohorst, H.J. (1966) Pflügers Arch. 265, 34.

Thorn, W., Heimann, J., Müldener, B. and Gercken, G. (1957) Pflügers ARch. 265, 34.

Williams, J.A., Withrow, C.D. and Woodbury, D.M. (1971) J. Physiol. 215, 539.

CYTOCHROME OXIDASE AND URATE OXIDASE AS INTRACELLULAR O_2 INDICATORS IN STUDIES OF O_2 GRADIENTS DURING HYPOXIA IN LIVER

Helmut Sies

Institut für Physiologische Chemie, Physikalische Bio-

chemie und Zellbiologie der Universität München, Germany

SUMMARY

Results obtained from a new approach of investigating O_2 distribution in intact perfused liver under hypoxic conditions are presented. Based on the signals observed by organ absorbance spectrophotometry from two compartments with oxidases of markedly different O_2 sensitivity, the mitochondria and the peroxisomes, a distribution between high O_2 and zero O_2 zones is postulated, an intermediate border zone of O_2 concentrations between the $K_{0.5}(O_2)$ values being virtually absent(steep intercellular O_2 gradients).

INTRODUCTION

The pattern of distribution of oxygen between different hepatocytes("intercellular O_2 gradients") in the intact liver is not precisely known. The distribution of O_2 between cells will become of particular importance under limiting conditions, i.e. in hypoxic states.

Methods employed so far in studying this problem include polarography to measure localized O_2 tensions with microelectrodes(for reviews, see Lübbers, 1968; Kessler et al, 1976) on the one hand, and non-invasive methods such as fluorometry and photometry of intracellular signals on the other(Chance et al, 1973). A recent development in the application of the latter methods in the study of O_2 distribution was the simultaneous observation of two O_2-dependent parameters of different O_2 sensitivity("two-indicator method"), providing information on localized O_2 supply from the comparison of the O_2 pro-

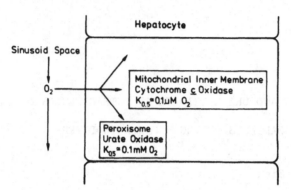

Fig.1. O_2 flow along liver sinusoids and into hepatocytes containing oxidases in different compartments

files as observed from the pigments in situ with those observed in vitro. This approach is based on certain assumptions(see below), it has been applied to the perfused heart(Chance, 1976) and to the perfused liver(Oshino et al, 1975; Sies, 1977a,b). The results obtained by this approach for the liver will briefly be outlined here with emphasis on current problems.

METHODS

The two indicator signals may be followed by organ spectrophotometry(see Sies & Schwab, this volume), or by a combination with simultaneous perfusate analyses for the second indicator(Sies, 1977a,b).

RESULTS AND DISCUSSION

Organ perfusion system versus isolated cell incubation. It is obvious that information on O_2 distribution in the intact organ must be obtained from the intact organ and not from the isolated cells which, however, may serve as useful controls. This apparently trivial statement underlines the fundamental difference in dynamic steady states in open and closed systems: while steady states in the organ are characterized by heterogeneous populations of metabolite profiles, those in cell incubations represent essentially homogeneous profiles. Fig. 1 serves to illustrate the situation in intact liver. O_2 as delivered to the tissue travels along the sinusoid from the portal to the central region of the liver lobule. Adjacent hepatocytes take up O_2 from the sinusoid for reduction by intracellular oxidases, thus creating a gradient (a) from the sinusoid to the cells and (b) along the length of the sinusoid. For the present considerations, the latter is denoted by "intercellular O_2 gradient".

Cytochrome c oxidase and urate oxidase as O_2 indicators. Mitochondria and peroxisomes contain these two terminal oxidases of sig-

Table 1. O_2 dependent parameters during hypoxia at half-maximal(50 %) reduction of cytochrome oxidase (or cytochrome c). References in parentheses: (1)Sies, 1977a;(2)Sies, 1977b;(3)Oshino et al, 1975;(4) this work.

System	Parameter	% of normoxic control
Perfused Liver	Rate of urate removal	50(1,2)
	Level of catalase Compound I	50(4)
	Rate of H_2O_2 formation from urate or glycolate(see text)	15-20(3,4)
	NAD^+ Redox potential(mito-chondrial and cytosolic)	50(2)
Isolated Hepatocytes	Rate of urate removal	<3(1,2)

nificantly different O_2 sensitivity: half-maximal O_2 concentration for cytochrome c oxidase reduction is of the order of 0.1 μM O_2, whereas half-maximal O_2 concentration for urate oxidase is of the order of 0.1 mM O_2.

In experiments with isolated hemoglobin-free perfused rat liver it was surprising to note--in view of the approx. 1,000-fold difference in O_2 sensitivity--that in hypoxia half-maximal restriction of urate removal occurred only at half-maximal reduction of cytochrome oxidase as indicated in Table 1. In contrast, in isolated hepatocytes half-maximal restriction of urate removal occurred at quite low

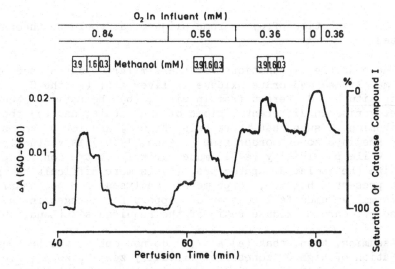

Fig.2. Organ spectrophotometric recording of catalase Compound I from perfused liver in presence of 2 mM glycolate.

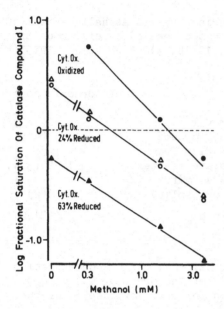

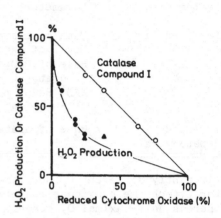

Fig. 3. Log-log plot of data from Fig. 2 for evaluation of H_2O_2 formation according to Oshino et al., 1973.

Fig. 4. Level of catalase Compound I and estimated H_2O_2 formation rate as related to redox state of cytochrome oxidase in perfused liver. Data from experiments like Fig. 2, open circles and triangles; from Oshino et al., 1975, full circles.

degrees of reduction of cytochrome oxidase, as would be theoretically expected.

The possible explanations for the similar O_2 dependence of cytochrome oxidase and urate oxidase in liver are: (a) the O_2 affinities in situ are different from in vitro; (b) the ratio of the two enzymes varies in different regions of the lobule; and (c) the O_2 distribution is such that there exist high O_2 and low O_2 zones while an intermediate zone("border zone"(Chance, 1976)) is virtually absent. While possibility (a) is made unlikely by the control experiment with the isolated hepatocytes, (b) is more difficult to rule out at present. However, morphometric analyses of mitochondrial and peroxisomal volumes fail to provide support for changes in the urate oxidase/cytochrome oxidase ratio of the required size(Loud, 1968).

Assuming, then, that (a) and (b) do not apply, the pronounced demarkation of high O_2 zones from virtually zero O_2 zones, i.e. very steep intercellular O_2 gradients, remains the plausible explanation. The border zone is defined here as the concentration range between the two $K_{0.5}(O_2)$ values, 0.1 µM and 0.1 mM.

Glycolate oxidase as second indicator. The half-maximal O_2 concentration for glycolate oxidase is about 0.3 mM O_2(Oshino et al, 1975), and H_2O_2 formation from glycolate has been estimated by Oshino et al(1975) to be halved at a degree of reduction of cytochrome c of only 10 %. The rates of H_2O_2 formation were estimated from measurement of the catalase-H_2O_2 complex(Compound I) during titration with added hydrogen donor, methanol, according to Oshino et al(1973). The apparent discrepancy between this observation and the above-mentioned data on urate oxidase was investigated(Fig. 2); the methanol titration of catalase Compound I is shown for three steady states of hypoxia, and the data are plotted in Fig. 3 in a log-log plot of fractional saturation of Compound I vs. methanol concentration. The results on H_2O_2 formation confirm those of Oshino et al(1975) but, in addition, they clearly indicate that the total level of catalase Compound I decreases parallel to the degree of cytochrome oxidase reduction(Fig. 4) and, secondly, that the slope in the log-log plot(Fig.3) is less than -1.0 under hypoxic conditions, being about -o.7. This indicates that increased amounts of endogenous hydrogen donor for catalase Compound I may be formed under the hypoxic condition, thus making the calculation of H_2O_2 formation subject to a correction.

Similar observations were obtained in methanol titrations of catalase Compound I when urate was used as a substrate instead of glycolate.

Cytochrome oxidase and NAD^+ redox indicators. It follows from the above that practically all O_2-dependent parameters should fall on a single curve. Thus, the redox indicator metabolite couples for the mitochondrial and cytosolic NAD^+ systems, ß-hydroxybutyrate/acetoacetate and lactate/pyruvate, respectively, follow the graded increase in cytochrome oxidase reduction by graded increases in their redox potential(Sies, 1977b).

How can the steep O_2 gradients during hypoxia be explained? While the question of the spatial organisation of the high and zero O_2 zones in hypoxia must be left open to topological studies, e.g. by histochemical methods, the alternative is, in principle, between (a) the demarkation occurring at a certain point along the length of the sinusoid, and (b) the regulation by microcirculatory control between different sinusoids(high flow vs. low flow).

It is known that the rate of electron flow in the respiratory chain is dependent on the phosphorylation potential(Klingenberg,1963) and that the perfused liver operates in a state near that defined for isolated mitochondria as ADP-controlled, or State 4(Chance & Williams, 1956),as shown by Sies et al(1969). Further, Wilson et al (1974) observed that the respiratory chain in perfused liver is in near-equilibrium with the phosphorylation potential; the approach has now been extended to an analysis under hypoxic conditions in cultured kidney cells(Wilson et al, 1977). These near-equilibrium relationships may, with the partial restriction of high-energy phosphate production in the hypoxic state, lead to a <u>localized</u> increase of O_2 uptake in the organ('State 4 to State 3 transition'), thereby contributing to a steepening of the intercellular O_2 gradient.

In closing, it is emphasized that the hemoglobin-free perfused liver may be a particularly suited experimental model to reveal and study the effects of steep O_2 gradients. Hemoglobin or other O_2 carriers in the perfusate may broaden the gradient(Sies, 1977a,b), and the extent of broadening can be followed in future applications of the concept of the two-indicator approach, in order to ultimately allow an extrapolation to the <u>in vivo</u> situation.

(Supported by Deutsche Forschungsgemeinschaft, SFB 51, Grant D/8).

REFERENCES

Chance, B. & Williams, G.R. (1956) Adv. Enzymol. <u>17</u>, 65.

Chance, B., Oshino, N., Sugano, T. & Mayevsky, A. (1973) In:Oxygen Transport to Tissue (eds. Bicher,H.I. & Bruley,D.F.)p.277,Plenum,N.Y.

Chance, B. (1976) Circulation Res. Suppl. I, <u>38</u>, 69.

Kessler, M., Höper, J., Krumme, B.A. (1976) Anesthesiology,<u>45</u>,184.

Klingenberg, M. (1963) Angew. Chem. <u>75</u>, 900.

Loud, A.V. (1968) J. Cell Biol. <u>37</u>, 27.

Lübbers, D.W. (1968) In:Biochemie des Sauerstoffs (eds. Hess,B. & Staudinger, H.J.) p.67, Springer Verlag, Heidelberg.

Oshino, N., Chance,B.,Sies,H.,Bücher,T.(1973)Arch.Bioch.Bioph. <u>154</u>, 117.

Oshino, N., Jamieson, D. & Chance, B. (1975) Biochem.J. <u>146</u>, 53.

Sies, H., Brauser, B. & Bücher, T. (1969) FEBS Lett. <u>5</u>, 319.

Sies, H. (1977a) In:Tissue Hypoxia and Ischemia (eds. Reivich, M., Coburn, R., Lahiri, S. & Chance, B.) p.51, Plenum Press, New York.

Sies, H. (1977b) Hoppe-Seyler's Z. Physiol. Chem. <u>358</u>, 1021.

Wilson, D.F., Stubbs, M., Oshino, N., Erecinska, M. (1974) Biochemistry <u>13</u>, 5305.

Wilson, D.F., Erecinska, M., Drown, C. & Silver, I.A. (1977) Amer. J. Physiol. In press.

FLOW STASIS, BLOOD GASES AND GLUCOSE LEVELS IN THE RED PULP OF THE SPLEEN

A.C. Groom, M.J. Levesque and D. Brucksweiger

Department of Biophysics, University of Western Ontario

London, Ontario. N6A 5C1 Canada

It is known that the membrane of the red blood cell loses its extreme deformability and becomes increasingly stiff at O_2 tensions below 30 mm Hg (LaCelle, 1970). Under certain conditions stasis of blood can occur within the red pulp of the spleen, and it is possible that the ensuing local hypoxia, if sufficiently severe, could lead to increased rigidity of the sequestered red cells and an acceleration of the process known as cell "conditioning" in the pulp (Griggs et al, 1960). This would be accelerated by substrate deprivation and these factors would together contribute to a shorter life-span of cells incubated within the spleen (Weed et al, 1969).

Much of what is commonly accepted about the conditions within the splenic pulp is based on indirect evidence only. Thus, because there is clear evidence for a slow-transit vascular pool in the spleen (e.g. Levesque and Groom, 1976a) and because the red cells in blood incubated in vitro at 37°C show deleterious changes (LaCelle, 1969; Murphy, 1967; Weed et al, 1969), the conclusion has been drawn that the environmental conditions for red cells in the splenic pulp must be similar to those which develop in incubated blood in vitro. In practice, it is very difficult to test this hypothesis, for the simple reason that it has not been possible to collect blood from the splenic pulp without contamination from blood in the rapidly-flowing parts of the splenic circulation (Prankerd, 1963; Jandl, 1967). This objection applies when blood is collected from the cut surface of the freshly excised spleen (Prankerd, 1960) and also when samples are withdrawn from the splenic pulp by tissue aspiration (Vaupel et al, 1973).

A splenic drainage procedure has recently been described
(Levesque and Groom, 1976a) which appears to avoid the above
objection and enable samples of blood from the slow-transit
vascular pathway to be obtained. Using this method it was shown
that under normal conditions the pH of blood in the splenic pulp
of cat is 7.20, but that during stasis this falls toward 6.8
(Levesque and Groom, 1976b). These results suggested, specifically,
that some revision of current views on intrasplenic pH (Murphy,
1967) appeared to be necessary. In the wider sense, however,they
indicated that a re-evaluation of blood gases and glucose levels
in blood from the red pulp, before and after stasis, would be in
order. The present paper reports the results of such an investigation.

METHODS

Cats were anesthetized with sodium pentobarbital (40 mg/kg,
intraperitoneally) and the spleen was surgically exposed and
isolated, the main splenic vessels being undisturbed. Side
vessels of the splenic inflow and outflow were cannulated, without
occluding the circulation through the organ, and the spleen was
left in situ throughout the experiment. By clamping the appropriate vessels the spleen was permitted, without prior stasis, to
empty its contents passively via the venous side branch cannula
into a series of graduated tubes. When the outflow ceased a small
quantity of noradrenaline (0.5 μg in 0.1 ml saline) was injected
via a polyethylene tube inserted through the arterial cannula to
the level of the arterial bifurcation. This was sufficient to
induce active contraction of the spleen. Further blood samples
were then collected until the outflow finally ceased. In some
experiments the entire inflow and outflow were occluded for periods
of either 20 or 60 min prior to drainage, and in these cases the
spleen was transferred to a bath filled with saline at 37°C for the
duration of occlusion and drainage.

Blood gas tensions were determined on all samples by means of
a Corning 165 blood-gas analyzer, glucose concentrations were
measured using an enzymatic/colourimetric procedure (GOD-Perid
method: Boehringer, Mannheim) and hematocrits were measured by a
Microhaematocrit centrifuge.

RESULTS

The total blood volume in the relaxed spleen of the cat is
0.51 ± .07 (SD) ml/g splenic wt and during drainage, after maximal
contraction of the spleen by 0.5 μg noradrenaline, a volume of
blood equivalent to 0.45 ± .03 ml/g (SD) is discharged from the

organ (Levesque and Groom, 1976a). In the present series of
experiments the splenic weight was not recorded in all cases; for
this reason we have plotted (Fig. 1) the values of haematocrit,
glucose concentration and gas tensions versus % total blood drained,
instead of versus ml/g. The mean value of the initial haematocrit
(34%) was not significantly different from that of femoral venous
blood (35.5%). After the first few milliliters, however, the
haematocrit rose steadily to a mean value of 79%.

   In fasting cats the glucose concentration in peripheral
venous blood lies in the range 60 to 100 mg/100 ml. We have
chosen to express the glucose concentration in each splenic blood
sample as a percentage of that in the animal's peripheral venous
blood immediately prior to splenic drainage. It is clear, from
Fig. 1, that in spleens whose blood flow was not interrupted until
drainage was begun the glucose concentration (solid triangles)
never fell below 60%, approx. When blood flow was stopped for 60
min the glucose concentration (solid circles) was zero in all
samples. After occlusion for 20 min the glucose concentration
(open circles) lay between 80 and 100% for the first quarter of
the total blood drained, then fell, progressively, reaching a
value of zero for the last quarter drained.

   Measurements of blood gases in splenic drainage samples
(Fig. 1: right) showed that, for spleens in which blood flow was
maintained until drainage was begun, the O_2 tensions (open squares)
fell very rapidly to 65 mm Hg, declining slowly thereafter to a
mean value of 54 mm Hg at the end of drainage. The corresponding
CO_2 tensions (solid squares) rose steadily from an initial value
of 47 to a final value of 64 mm Hg. Following occlusion of blood
flow for 60 min, however, the O_2 tensions (open circles) were
found to be near zero and the CO_2 tensions (closed circles) at 70
mm Hg throughout the first three-fifths of the total blood drained.
For the last two-fifths a steady rise of O_2 tension occurred, from
zero to a final value of 30 mm Hg, and this was accompanied by a
decline in CO_2 tension from 70 mm Hg to a final value of 60 mm Hg.

DISCUSSION

   The splenic drainage procedure made it possible for 90% of
the total blood content of the relaxed, feline spleen to be
examined. The mean volume of blood expelled from the spleen was
18 ml; instead of collecting this as one mixed sample, the outflow
was fractionated into successive 1 ml samples. The haematocrit of
the initial sample was in each case comparable to that of femoral
venous blood but, as drainage continued, the haematocrit rose
gradually to a mean final value of 79%. Compartment analysis,
based on the washout kinetics of red cells and ^{125}I-albumin from

the spleen, has shown that in the cat this organ contains two
distinct pools of blood (Levesque and Groom, 1976a). The smaller
of these (0.09 ml/g) contains blood of haematocrit 37% and is
perfused by 90% of the total flow; the mean transit time through
this compartment is therefore quite short. The larger pool (0.42

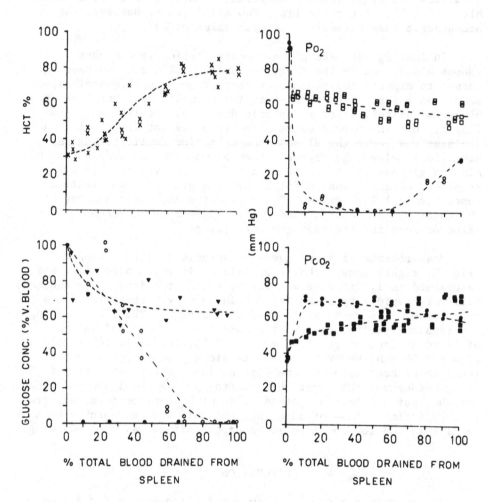

Fig. 1.   Haematocrit, glucose concentration (% of that in venous
          blood), P_{O_2} and P_{CO_2} in successive samples of blood
          collected from the spleen of cat, during drainage with
          the arterial inflow occluded (see text).
          <u>Abscissa</u>: cumulative volume of splenic blood drained
          (% of total) up to the point when each sample was taken.
          Spleens with no prior interruption of flow: glucose ▼ ,
          P_{O_2} ▫ , P_{CO_2} ■ . Occlusion for 20 min: glucose, ○ .
          Occlusion for 60 min: glucose ● , P_{O_2} ○ , P_{CO_2} ● .

ml/g) contains blood of haematocrit 75% and is perfused by only
10% of the total splenic blood flow; the mean transit time through
this compartment is consequently much larger (by a factor of almost
40) than that through the first compartment. Morphological studies,
at different stages of washout, have identified this second pool
as blood in the red pulp (Song and Groom, 1971). During splenic
drainage, therefore, expulsion of blood from the fast-transit pool
will be completed ahead of that of blood from the slow-transit
pool in the red pulp. The haematocrits of the initial and final
drainage samples would thus be expected to correspond to those of
blood in the fast and slow pools, respectively, as is the case.

The haematocrit data therefore suggest that the last samples
collected during splenic drainage are indeed representative of
blood from the red pulp, and this is borne out by the progressive
changes in gas tensions and glucose concentrations which are found
during drainage. The results obtained, from spleen autoperfused
until the moment when drainage was begun, suggest that the glucose
concentration and O_2 tension in the red pulp are normally not less
than 60% of the corresponding values in peripheral venous blood
(Fig. 1). These data, taken in conjunction with the fact that the
corresponding value for the pH of blood in the pulp is 7.20
(Levesque and Groom, 1976b), indicate that the commonly accepted
notion of a hostile environment for red cells in the pulp of the
normal spleen by virtue of the very low values of pH, P_{O_2}, and
glucose concentration which exist there is not, in fact, true.

The present investigation shows that when blood flow is
occluded, the glucose concentration in splenic blood falls very
rapidly indeed, the concentration in the pulp reaching zero in less
than 20 min. At the same time the O_2 tension falls, though much
more slowly; thus after occlusion for 60 min a rise in O_2 tension
from zero to 30 mm Hg was found in the last quarter of the total
blood drained from the spleen. This rise, plus the corresponding
decline of 10 mm Hg in CO_2 tension, bears out that the last sample
of blood collected was from an area of high haematocrit (and,
therefore, high O_2 availability) within the spleen. Taken together
with the fall in pH of blood in the pulp to 6.83 after 60 min
occlusion (Levesque and Groom, 1976b) these investigations show
clearly that under conditions when impairment of flow through the
red pulp occurs, a hostile environment for red cells does indeed
develop there very rapidly, the principal stress being substrate
deprivation.

There is good reason to believe that impairment of red cell
flow through the pulp can occur when abnormal cells become trapped
there. After injection of 2.5×10^9 heat-treated red cells into
the splenic artery of cat, it has been found (Levesque and Groom,
1977) that no less than 50% of the normal red cells in the splenic

pulp become immobilized. Vaupel and his colleagues (1973), using a microelectrode to measure O_2 tensions within rabbit spleens, showed that after injection of heat-treated cells a decline in O_2 tension by 20 to 25 mm Hg occurred. Clearly O_2 availability in the pulp was reduced, and it seems likely that marked changes in glucose concentration and a decline of pH must have occurred also. These findings therefore suggest that when abnormal cells are trapped in the splenic pulp a positive feedback system occurs, the local environment becoming more hostile to red cells and leading to more severe cellular damage.

REFERENCES

Griggs, R.C., Weisman, R. Jr. and Harris, J.W. (1960) J. Clin. Invest. 39, 89.

Jandl, J.H. (1967) Hereditary spherocytosis. In 'Hereditary disorders of erythrocyte metabolism' p.209 (ed. Beutler, E.). Grune and Stratton, New York and London.

LaCelle, P.L.   (1969) Transfusion 9, 238.

LaCelle, P.L.   (1970) Seminars in Hematol. 7, 355.

Levesque, M.J. and Groom, A.C. (1976a) Amer. J. Physiol. 231, 1665.

Levesque, M.J. and Groom, A.C. (1976b) Amer. J. Physiol. 231, 1672.

Levesque, M.J. and Groom, A.C. (1977) J. Lab. Clin. Med. (in press).

Murphy, J.R. (1967) J. Lab. Clin. Med. 69, 758.

Prankerd, T.A.J. (1960) Quart. J. Med. 29, 199.

Prankerd, T.A.J. (1963) Brit. Med. J. 2, 517.

Song, S.H. and Groom, A.C. (1971) Can. J. Physiol. Pharmacol. 49, 734.

Vaupel, P., Braunbeck, W. and Thews, G. (1973) Respiratory gas exchange and P_{O_2} distribution in splenic tissue. In 'Oxygen transport to tissue' p.401 (eds. Bicher, H.I. and Bruley, D.F.) Plenum Press, New York and London.

Weed, R.I., LaCelle, P.L. and Merrill, E.W. (1969) J. Clin. Invest. 48, 795.

INTESTINAL O_2 CONSUMPTION UNDER LOW FLOW CONDITIONS

IN ANAESTHETIZED CATS

J. Hamar, L. Ligeti, and A.G.B. Kovách

Experimental Research Department
Semmelweis Medical University
Budapest, Hungary

Since Wiggers' study on the 'Portal pressure gradients under experimental conditions, including haemorrhagic shock' (Wiggers et al, 1946) a number of observations have been carried out to clarify the role of the small intestine in various types of shock. The small intestine is regarded as a shock organ (Fine 1967), since its circulation quickly deteriorates and thus contributes to the irreversibility of the shock. However, the autoregulation of the intestinal blood flow during reduced perfusion has been repeatedly verified (Johnson 1960; Haglund and Lundgren 1972). A similar circulatory reaction of the small intestine was also found by Haglund (1973) during haemorrhage. These autoregulatory reactions are considered to maintain constant pressure within the exchange vessels of the intestinal circulation (Svanvik 1973).

We have studied the intestinal metabolic rate of oxygen ($IMRO_2$) during different types of hypoxia, in order to establish whether this contributes to the protection of the intestinal functions under these conditions.

Two sets of experiments have been made. Haemorrhagic hypotension was applied in the first series. The general consequences of the haemorrhage may overlap the mechanism which regulates the circulatory patterns within the small intestine. Therefore in another series the small intestine was locally hypoperfused. In the latter studies an attempt was made to mimic the changes in blood flow that occur during haemorrhage.

METHODS

Cats deprived of food for 24 hours prior to the experiments
were anaesthetized with Na Pentobarbital.

Shock studies

Arterial blood pressure was reduced to and maintained at 60
mmHg for 60 min. (B.I.) according to the method of Engelking and
Willig (1958).   The pressure was further reduced to 35-40 mmHg for
another bleeding period (B.II).   B.II lasted as long as there was
a 50% spontaneous reuptake of the maximal volume of the shed blood.
Venous outflow from the distal 2/3 of the small intestine, beginning
10 cm. distal to the duodeno-jejunal flexure, was directly measured.
Care was taken to avoid damage of the lymphatics and the nerves
running in the mesentery.

Perfusion Studies
(Fig. 1)

The superior mesenteric artery was perfused via a perfusion
pump (Watson-Marlow Ltd. type MHRE-88).   Arterial blood for the
perfusion was taken from the femoral artery.   Nerve fibres and
lymphatic vessels of the mesentery were left intact.   Venous outflow was collected and continuously returned to the femoral vein

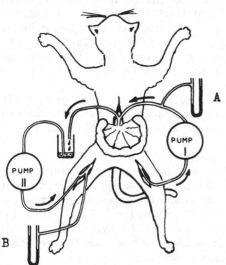

via another perfusion pump
(Harvard Instrument Co. type
1210).   The level of the
venous outflow was first
determined, then the arterial
perfusion pump was set at a
constant speed identical with
the venous outflow measured
before.   The rate of the
perfusion was later reduced
either by 25% and 50% or 50%
and 75% of the control flow.
The first hypoperfusion period
(either 25% or 50% of the
control flow) lasted 40-60
min.   The duration of the
second period (either 50% or
75% flow reduction) was 30-
40 min.

Fig. 1. Experimental model for the perfusion studies.   Pump I.
connected between the femoral and the superior mesenteric arteries;
Pump II. connected between the reservoir collecting the venous outflow and the femoral vein. Manometer A records the perfusion pressure
changes; Manometer B records blood pressure in the femoral artery.
Arrow indicates the direction of the blood flow.

Heparin (2 mg per kg body weight) was given to avoid blood clotting. The systemic arterial blood pressure and the perfusion pressure were continuously recorded.

Arterial and mesenteric venous blood samples were analysed for pH, pCO$_2$, haemoglobin (Hb) and oxygen saturation.   Intestinal metabolic rate (IMRO$_2$) was calculated from the Hb, O$_2$ saturation and blood flow values.

RESULTS

1.   Shock studies (Table I).

Resistance to blood flow decreased continuously throughout the two bleeding periods.   Venous outflow reached 71% and 55% of the control level by the end of B.I. and B.II. respectively.   At the same time of hypotension IMRO$_2$ values were 88% and 64% that of the prebleeding level.   The correlation coefficient of blood flow versus O$_2$ consumption did not differ significantly from zero during the control period and B.I.   It was however 0.787(p<0.001) at the end of B.II.

2. Perfusion studies (Table II).

Vascular resistance decreased by 20-25% that of the control value independently of the rate of the perfusion.   IMRO$_2$ decreased to 96%, 89% and 35% that of the control level when the blood flow was reduced by 25%, 50% and 75%, respectively.   Oxygen consumption became dependent on blood flow when the perfusion was reduced by 75% of the original value (r=0.635, p<0.01).

COMMENTS

Control blood flow values, especially those in the shocked group fell within the lower range of the 'normal' intestinal blood flow (see Folkow 1967).   The lower values can be attributed to the trauma caused by the operation.   This might result in a higher rate of sympathetic activity and, consequently in a lower rate of blood supply to the intestine (Folkow et al, 1964).

Venous oxygen saturation did not decrease below 60% in the perfusion studies nor below 50% in the shocked group.   This can be attributed to an intramural redistribution of the blood flow (including shunts) within the intestinal wall (Svanvik 1973). Mechanical perfusion itself may also change the vascular patterns of the small intestine (Wallentin 1966).

The 50% flow reduction in the perfusion studies resulted in blood flow values (12-14 ml/min/100 g tissue) which were similar to those obtained during B.I. in the shocked group.   In both hypoxic

TABLE I

Shock studies

Parameter	Control	B.I.	B.II.
Art. pres.	120	57	37
mmHg	5.0	0.9	0.7
Ven. outflow	17.7	12.6*	9.6*
ml/min x 100g	1.5	1.3	1.4
Resistance	7.76	5.16*	4.21*
	0.62	0.51	0.97
Ven. pH	7.30	7.24*	7.11*
	0.014	0.035	0.029
Art. pCO_2	32.0	21.2*	19.4*
mmHg	1.8	2.2	2.2
Ven. O_2 sat.	63.0	49.0*	49.6*
%	2.4	2.6	2.8
Art. Hb.	13.5	12.0*	10.6*
G/100 ml	0.58	0.43	0.47
O_2 consumpt.	1.09	0.92*	0.63*
ml/min x 100g	0.07	0.07	0.08
n	25	23	17

Numbers represent the means/first rows/$\pm$ S.E./second
rows.   Significant differences compared to control
values are indicated by *.   The dimension of the
resistance values: mmHg/ml/min x 100g tissue.

TABLE II

Perfusion studies

Parameter	Control	Flow reduction		
		25%	50%	75%
Perf. pres.	125.0	78.5*	55.3*	29.4*
mmHg	4.5	4.0	3.9	5.3
Flow	26.3	20.1	13.3	6.1
ml/min x 100g	1.29	1.13	0.71	0.73
Resistance	5.05	4.13*	4.31*	4.15*
	0.31	0.28	0.25	0.32
Ven. pH	7.25	7.22*	7.17*	7.12*
	0.018	0.016	0.019	0.046
Art. pCO$_2$	33.2	31.6	31.0	30.4
mmHg	1.35	3.12	2.38	2.57
Ven. O$_2$ sat.	75.3	66.5*	57.8*	65.8*
%	2.0	3.7	2.6	2.6
Art. Hb.	15.2	15.0	14.7	14.7
G/100 ml	0.59	0.57	0.47	0.52
O$_2$ consumpt.	1.08	1.15	0.96	0.34*
ml/min x 100g	0.11	0.10	0.08	0.06
·n	23	12	23	12

See the legend of Table I.

periods IMRO$_2$ decreased to a lesser extent than did blood flow. The autoregulatory reaction of the intestinal blood flow could also be observed in both types of studies, since the resistance to the blood flow decreased in each case.   This was accompanied by another mechansism which maintains the energy supply of the intestinal tissue at control level during hypoxia.   IMRO$_2$ however becomes dependent on blood flow if the hypoxia continues further (B.II) or the blood supply is very low (75% flow reduction in the perfused studies).

REFERENCES

Engelking, R. and Willig, F.   (1958) Pflügers Arch. ges Physiol. 267, 306.

Fine, J.   (1967) Gastroenterology 52, 454.

Folkow, B.   (1967) Gastroenterology 52, 423.

Folkow, B., Lewis, D.H., Lundgren, O., Mellander, S. and Wallentin, I. (1964) Acta. Physiol. Scand. 61, 445.

Haglund, U. (1973) Acta. Physiol. Scand. 89, 129.

Haglund, U. and Lundgren, O. (1972) Acta. Physiol. Scand. 84, 151.

Johnson, P.C. (1960) Amer. J. Physiol. 199, 311.

Svanvik, J. (1973) Acta. Physiol. Scand. 385.

Wallentin, I. (1967) Acta. Physiol. Scand. 68, 304.

Wiggers, C.J., Opdyke, D.F. and Johnson, J.R.   (1946)   Amer. J. Physiol. 146, 192.

TISSUE BLOOD EXCHANGE AND TISSUE OXYGEN TENSION IN RELATION TO TOTAL BODY OXYGEN CONSUMPTION IN EXPERIMENTAL SURGICAL SHOCK

Haglind, E., Dawidsson, I., Lund, N., Appelgren, L. and Gelin, L-E.
Kirurgiska kliniken I, Sahlgrenska sjukhuset,
University of Göteborg, S-413 45 Göteborg, Sweden

The purpose of this work was to study blood to tissue exchange by both flow and diffusion in skeletal muscle and to relate these local tissue variables to total body oxygen consumption in an intestinal shock model in dogs. Furthermore this shock model was used to evaluate the effectiveness and duration of different plasma substitutes in counteracting the experimental surgical shock.

MATERIALS AND METHODS

Sixty dogs were anaesthetised with ketamine chloride and pancurium bromide and ventilated on air. After appropriate cannulation the animal was allowed to stabilise and control measurements were made. Splenectomy was then performed (duration 20 min) and the small intestine was exteriorised for three hours. During this time the dogs developed hypovolaemia to 65% plasma volume, haemoconcentration (haematocrit = 59%) and a fall in arterial blood pressure to 95 mmHg. Measurements of muscle blood flow PO_2 and oxygen consumption were made before the intestines were replaced. The effects of infusion of different plasma substitutes were investigated after replacement of the intestines within the abdomen. A single infusion of 20 min. duration was given and measurements were made after 1, 2 and 4 hours. The colloids (Dextran 40) were given in a dose of 1.5 g/kg body weight in a 3.5% solution. Ringer's acetate was given in a volume 3 times that of the colloid solutions.

Muscle capillary blood flow and diffusion capacity was measured during the radioactive isotope clearance technique described by Appelgren. The diffusion capacity in skeletal muscle was expressed as a PS-value, which is a product of capillary permeability (P) and the capillary area open to metabolic exchange (S). Muscle tissue oxygen tension was measured with a PO_2-electrode inserted into the muscles.   The total body oxygen consumption was measured continuously according to Guyton.

RESULTS

Fig. 1A shows the muscle blood flow (Q_{Xe}) expressed in ml blood/min/100 g tissue, in relation to the PS-value (ml plasma/min/ 100 g tissue).   The position for each single dog is marked in the control and in the shock situation.   The lines around the control and shock states were drawn by hand to separate these two states. There is practically no overlap between control and shock in respect of the PS-value.   The muscle blood flow decreased in shock as compared to the control.   However there was a marked overlap in values between control and shock.

Fig. 1B shows that muscle PO_2 was higher in the control situation compared with that during shock.   The total body oxygen consumption during control and shock situations was also clearly separated as is seen in Fig. 1C.

In order to assess the results statistically a computer analysis was performed on the means, standard deviations and the regression coefficients for all observations in control and shock for all sixty dogs.

Fig. 1D, E, F shows the result of computer analysis.   The triangle is the mean of all sixty animals in the control situation and the black dot the mean in shock.   The ellipses drawn around the means represent one standard deviation from the mean and the slope of the ellipse is due to the regression coefficient.   Fig. 1D shows the PS-value, Fig. 1E the muscle oxygen tension, and Fig. 1F total body oxygen consumption, all in relation to the muscle blood flow.

The effects of infusion of Dextran or Ringer in the shocked animals can be assessed by a similar type of statistical analysis.

Fig. 2 shows the relationship between muscle oxygen tension and blood flow in the different groups of animals.   Fig. 2A shows the results of 8 untreated animals.   The ellipses represent all 60 animals in control and shock.   The black triangle and the black dot are now the means for the 8 untreated animals in control and shock respectively.   The circles with figures inside represent the means of these 8 animals, 1, 2 and 4 hours after replacement of the intestine.   Untreated animals remained in the shock area for at least 4 hours.   The total body oxygen consumption and the PS-value in the untreated group did not improve either.

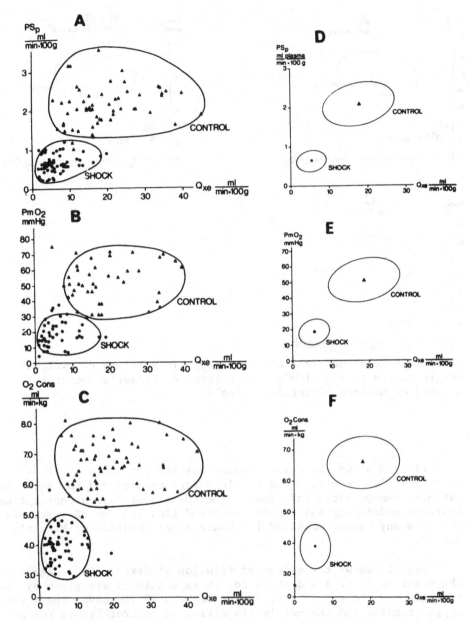

Fig. 1. The muscle capillary blood flow (Q_{xe}) in relation to capillary diffusion capacity (PSp), muscle oxygen tension (PmO_2) and to total body oxygen consumption (O_2-cons).   A, B and C are experimental results, D, E and F show the computer analyses.

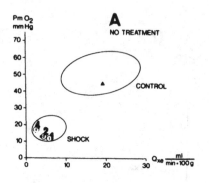

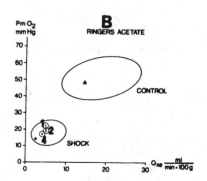

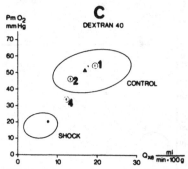

Fig. 2. Skeletal muscle blood flow (Q_{Xe}) in relation to skeletal muscle oxygen tension (PmO_2) for untreated, Ringer's acetate-infused or Dextran 40-infused animals.

Fig. 2B shows the corresponding results for animals infused with Ringer's acetate. The muscle oxygen tension did not show any definite change after infusion. The total body oxygen consumption improved moderately but the muscle blood flow and the PS-value did not show any change measured 1-4 hours after infusion of Ringer's acetate.

Fig. 2C shows the effect of infusion of Dextran 40. Again the means in control and shock for these 8 animals are given by the triangle and the dot. Infusion of Dextran 40 increased the muscle oxygen tension and the muscle blood flow to control levels for at least 2 hours. A corresponding restitution of total body oxygen consumption was seen for 4 hours and of the PS-value for 2 hours.

SUMMARY

This experimental shock model was well defined by the marked decrease in total body oxygen consumption, muscle PO_2 and diffusion capacity during shock. Infusion of large amounts of electrolyte solution did not lead to a restoration of muscle oxygen tension after 1-4 hours. Dextran 40 infusion however restored both local PO_2 and blood flow in the muscle as well as total body oxygen consumption.

REFERENCE

Appelgren, L. (1972) Acta. Phys. Scand. Suppl. 378, Göteborg.

SKELETAL MUSCLE PO$_2$: INDICATOR OF PERIPHERAL TISSUE

PERFUSION IN HAEMORRHAGIC SHOCK

Juha Niinikoski and Lauri Halkola

Department of Surgery and Cardiorespiratory

Research Unit, University of Turku, Turku, Finland

Reduced tissue perfusion, hypoxia and acidosis are essential features in the pathophysiology of haemorrhagic shock and their correction is the ultimate goal of the treatment. In the present work skeletal muscle oxygen tension and muscle surface pH were continuously recorded in lightly anaesthetized, tracheostomized male rabbits during graded haemorrhage and subsequent fluid management.

METHODS

Muscle PO$_2$ was measured by implanting a Silastic tube between the external and internal oblique abdominal muscles (Niinikoski and Hunt, 1972). The tube was perfused with hypoxic saline solution whose PO$_2$ equilibrated to the average PO$_2$ of the surrounding tissue because Silastic is extremely permeable to oxygen. The equilibrated fluid, whose PO$_2$ now indicated muscle PO$_2$, was directed to an O$_2$ electrode in a blood gas analyzer (Fig.1). Muscle pH was monitored with a use of a L-shaped muscle surface pH electrode implanted against the external oblique abdominal muscle. Arterial and venous pressures, arterial blood gases, acid-base status and arterial blood lactate concentration were serially recorded, and cardiac output and peripheral vascular resistance were assayed by means of impedance cardiography.

Haemorrhagic shock was induced by a graded 30 % blood loss. The rabbits were progressively bled in increments of 10 % of blood volume. After each bleeding a 15-minute stabilization period was allowed. At 30 % blood loss the mean arterial pressure was 20-30 mmHg. The subsequent fluid management was carried out

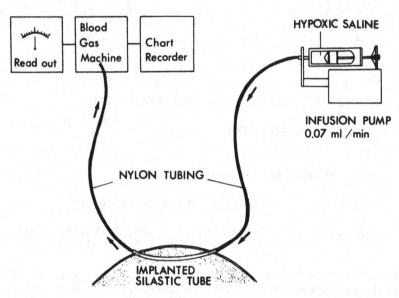

Fig.1. Technique of continuous monitoring of tissue PO_2 by means of an implanted Silastic tube.

according to three different protocols: 1) reinfusion of shed blood alone, or 2) volume correction with an equivalent volume of a plasma expander (Haemaccel[R], Behring Institut) and subsequent reinfusion of shed blood, or 3) massive infusions of a balanced salt solution, Ringer's lactate, averaging three times the volume of blood loss plus subsequent reinfusion of shed blood. Altogether 15 rabbits were used.

RESULTS

Baseline muscle PO_2 was $31 \pm SD$ 5 mmHg and the corresponding muscle surface pH $7.33 \pm SD$ 0.12. Muscle oxygen tension declined rapidly in proportion to blood loss and reached minimum values at 30 % blood loss. Reduction in muscle surface pH, blood pressure and cardiac output as well as increase in peripheral vascular resistance and blood lactate concentration lagged behind blood loss. Arterial blood PO_2 showed very little alterations during haemorrhage and subsequent fluid management.

In experiments where reinfusion of shed blood was the only treatment the increase of muscle surface pH lagged behind that of muscle oxygen tension (Fig.2).

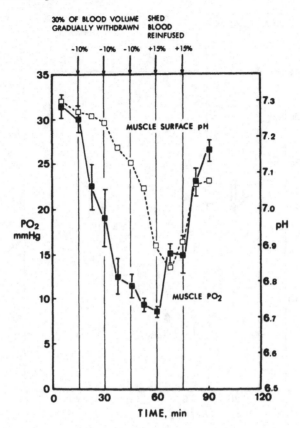

Fig.2. Skeletal muscle PO$_2$ and muscle surface pH in rabbits during graded haemorrhage and after subsequent reinfusion of shed blood.

Correction of hypovolaemia with an equivalent volume of plasma expander and thereafter with reinfusion of shed blood also returned the muscle PO$_2$ to normal despite marked haemodilution (Fig.3). Again, the response of muscle surface pH to the fluid management was slower.

Treatment of haemorrhagic shock with massive volumes of Ringer's lactate resulted in transient increases of muscle PO$_2$ after each injection probably because the administered fluid escaped quickly into the tissue interstitium that had undergone fluid loss during haemorrhage (Shires et al, 1973). After this extracellular

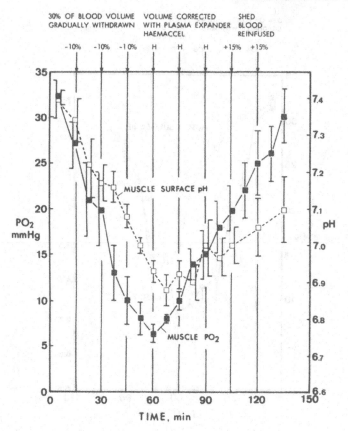

Fig.3. Skeletal muscle PO$_2$ and muscle surface pH in rabbits during graded haemorrhage and subsequent fluid management with an equivalent volume of a plasma expander, Haemaccel[R], in three phases and thereafter with reinfusion of shed blood. The figures indicate the mean ± S.E.M.

fluid deficiency had been corrected reinfusion of shed blood returned the muscle PO$_2$ to normal (Fig.4). Also in this group normalization of muscle surface pH was slower. Figure 5 shows a single experiment with massive infusions of Ringer's lactate: clear humps of muscle PO$_2$ and cardiac output after each administration of Ringer's lactate and response of various parameters to blood replacement. In these tests haemodilution was clearly smaller than

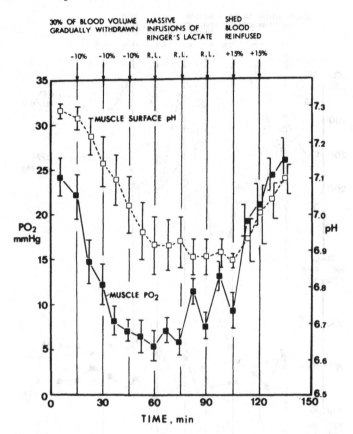

Fig.4. Skeletal muscle PO$_2$ and muscle surface pH in rabbits during graded haemorrhage and subsequent fluid management with large volumes of Ringer´s lactate and thereafter with reinfusion of shed blood.

in the aforementioned studies with a plasma expander. Central venous pressure remained below 5 cm H$_2$O throughout the fluid management.

Arterial blood lactate concentrations increased about four-fold after haemorrhage and declined gradually during subsequent fluid managements (Fig.6). It is probable that the slow response of muscle surface pH to the fluid managements was due to elevated lactate concentrations still present at the final phase of the experiments.

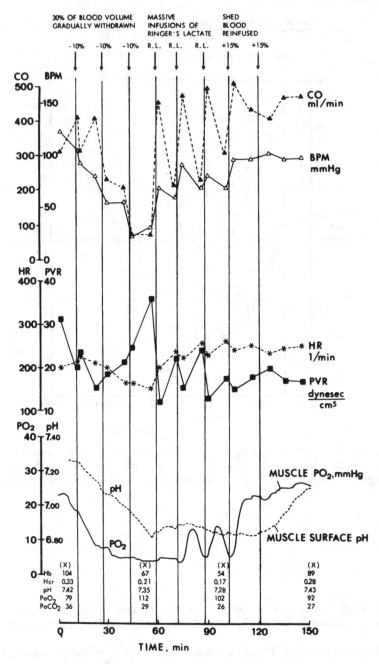

Fig.5. Parameters describing the circulatory status in one rabbit
during graded haemorrhage and subsequent fluid management with
massive infusions of Ringer's lactate and reinfusion of shed blood.

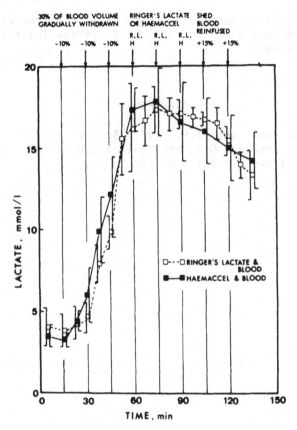

Fig.6. Arterial blood lactate concentrations in rabbits during
graded haemorrhage and subsequent fluid managements.

SUMMARY

The following conclusions can be made on the basis of this work:
1) Measurements of skeletal muscle oxygen tension provide an
excellent index of tissue perfusion in haemorrhagic shock.
2) Correction of cardiac output and arterial blood oxygen tension in haemorrhagic shock does not necessarily ensure normal
tissue oxygenation.
3) In haemorrhagic shock adequate replacement of blood loss
using a balanced salt solution in addition to blood replacement is
an integral part of the fluid management.
4) Correction of hypovolemia with an equivalent volume of a
plasma expander and subsequent reinfusion of shed blood also returns

tissue perfusion to normal. However, this treatment results in marked haemodilution and correction of extracellular fluid loss remains inadequate.

REFERENCES

Niinikoski, J. and Hunt, T.K. (1972) Surgery 71, 22.
Shires, G.T., Carrico, C.J. and Canizaro, P.Cι (1973) Major Problems in Clinical Surgery 8, 119.

MONITORING OF TISSUE PO$_2$ IN PATIENTS DURING INTENSIVE CARE

K. Schönleben, J.P. Hauss, U. Spiegel, H. Bünte,
M. Kessler*
Chirurgische Universitäts-Klinik, Allgemein-chirurgie,
Münster, West Germany
*Max-Planck-Institut für Systemphysiologie, Dortmund

The measurement of tissue-PO$_2$ with the multiwire surface electrode developed by Kessler and Lübbers is a well known method in the physiological research (Kessler et al, 1966). We, as clinicians, recognise the importance of local PO$_2$ measurement in determining a totally new parameter, which can not be obtained from any routine clinical investigation. The important information concerning microcirculation which can be obtained this way may, under some circumstances, be of crucial importance in survival of critically ill patients.

METHODS

The test organ was skeletal muscle, m. quadriceps femoris (for rationale see Sinagowitz 1974; Kessler 1974). Clinical studies and the evaluation of results were done as described by Schönleben et al (1977). The changes in local PO$_2$ were registered in the forms of histograms (for significance of those of Kessler 1977).

RESULTS

We would like to demonstrate the value of local PO$_2$ measurement in typical clinical examples selected out of a total number of 55 patients.

1. Early recognition of volume deficiency

Decrease in total blood volume leads in the first instance into displacement of blood from the periphery into the central circulation. Therefore ABP, CVP and hr, the three classic parameters of circulation, remain relatively constant for a certain

period of time.   The diminishing O_2 supply at the periphery is
being continuously registered by PO_2 monitoring electrodes and
provides an early signal of an imminent danger.

Fig. 1 shows a record of PO_2 obtained in a patient suffering
from an acute gastro-intestinal haemorrhage.   The continuous
decrease of local oxygen pressure after each shift of the electrode
to another measuring area indicates the beginning of haemorrhagic
shock.   At each measuring point the highest and lowest values of
the PO_2 recorded by 8 electrode wires are marked.   BP, CVP and hr
remained constant during that time period.   A quick blood transfusion could improve the condition.   Not earlier than one hour
after this treatment clinical symptoms of the haemorrhage were
observed.   The patient showed haematemesis.

2.   Control of inspiratory oxygen supply

In the clinic the analysis of blood gases is used to establish
whether artificial respiration and increased inspiratory oxygen
supply should be administered to the patient or not.   However
correct conclusions concerning the oxygen supply of the organs are
not always possible.   A low arterial PO_2 can nearly always be
corrected simply by increasing the inspiratory oxygen supply.   The
harmful effect of too high oxygen concentrations is not shown.
Kessler defines two sorts of perturbations of the PO_2 histogram:
(a) disturbances of microcirculatory patterns without anoxia, (b)
disturbances of microcirculatory pattern with anoxia.   Both are
shown in the next example (Fig. 2).

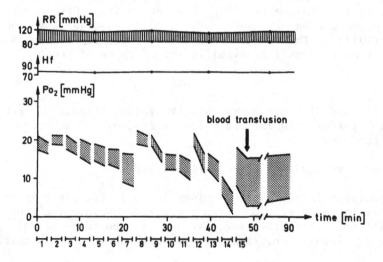

Fig. 1. Registration of a beginning of haemorrhagic shock.

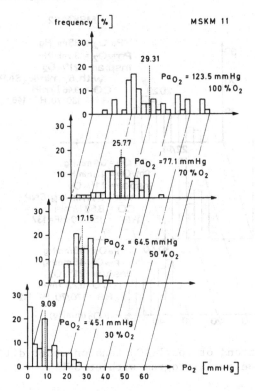

Fig. 2. Effect of different inspiratory O$_2$-concentrations on
the local oxygen tension.

In a polytraumatised patient with shock lung the assisted
respiration with an oxygen content of 30% was insufficient (see
lowest histogram and paO$_2$).   Here we found disturbances of microcirculatory pattern with anoxia.   By increasing the oxygen up to
50%, the local oxygen supply improved significantly: the histogram
became physiological.   An elevation to 70% O$_2$ gave even a better
paO$_2$, but in the tissue the number of hypoxaemic areas increased.
Pure oxygen then caused pathological changes in the local oxygen
supply.   There are very high and very low oxygen areas, which show
that breathing of pure oxygen caused a counterregulation of microcirculation.   Such a configuration of a histogram is typical for
disturbances of microcirculatory pattern without anoxia.   According
to the electrode measurement the inspiratory concentration of 50%
O$_2$ was optimal for this patient.   Findings in 22 other patients
were adequate.

3.   Control of pharmaco-dynamic changes of the local PO$_2$ tension

The qualitative pharmaco-dynamic effects of certain cardiovascular drugs on the different organs are theoretically known from

MSKM 52

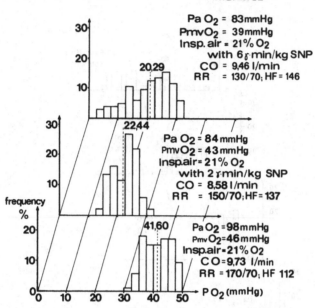

Fig. 3 Downward trend of local PO$_2$ tension under different dosages of SNP. Below: Histogram without SNP.

pharmacological studies.   At present there is no comparable method, which makes it possible to get a qualitative and quantitative analysis of the effects of those drugs on the microcirculation in the organs.   Example: Many observations suggest that administration of sodium nitroprusside yields to controlled hypotension. SNP diminishes selectively the tonus of the smooth vessel-muscles. We investigated a patient who received SNP because of a critical blood pressure rise after the operation of a subdural haematoma (Fig. 3).

Total of 48 mg SNP were applied within 3 hours, a very low therapeutic dosage, far below that assigned toxic dosage.   The desired therapeutic effect was soon obtained, the other parameters did not show any measurable changes.   Blood acidosis was not observed.   Nevertheless we found a decrease in local PO$_2$ tension dependent on the dosage of SNP which did not cause local anoxia. The reason for this effect of SNP remains unknown.   Perhaps redistribution of the blood within the single organ causes a diminution of PO$_2$ tension in skeletal muscle.   Alternately the SNP induced vasodilatation may have caused a change of the O$_2$ transport to the tissue.   Whatever the mechanism, it is important to point out that availability of a method for direct control of changes during the application of drugs is mandatory.

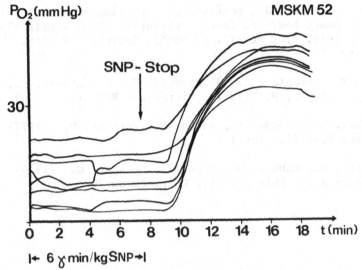

Fig. 4. Local PO$_2$ of skeletal muscle during and after the administration of SNP.

Fig. 4 shows that the effects of SNP on the PO$_2$ of the skeletal muscle disappear shortly after the infusion of this drug has
been stopped.

DISCUSSION

The aim of our contribution is to show what conclusions can be
drawn from monitoring tissue PO$_2$ in the clinical practice.   We
presented typical results from different investigated groups, which
however were confirmed by numerous other measurements.   The number
of investigated patients in the individual groups is still too
small and the sorts of illnesses are too different, that we could
present summarised statistically significant results.   The other
clinical parameters were mostly uncharacteristic.   We are sure,
that the PO$_2$-monitoring in the tissue is able to teach us about the
onset of pathological states of ventilation and volume changes
because compensating physiological regulations are checked.   The
conventional clinical measurements only show alterations when the
compensative mechanisms are extremely overloaded.   Skeletal muscle
surely is not representative for all organs, but we get a hint,
that in cases of persistent anoxia, there is serious danger for
vital organs.

REFERENCES

Kessler, M. and Lübbers, D.W.   (1966) Pflügers Arch. ges. Physiol.
R82, 291.

Kessler, M., Höper, J., Schäfer, D., Starlinger, H. (1974)
In 'Klin. Anaesthes. und Intensivtherapie, 5": Mikrozirkulation'
(eds. Ahnefeld, F.W. et al), p. 36-52, Springer, Berlin,
Heidelberg, New York.

Kessler, M., Strehlau, R., Sinagowitz, E., Schönlebel, K.,
Drumme, B., Bünte, H. (1977) Microvasc. Res. (in press)

Schönlebel, K., Krumme, B., Bünte, H., Kessler, M. (1977)
Microvasc. Res. (in press)

Sinagowitz, E., Rahmer, H., Rink, R., Kessler, M. (1974)
Langenbecks Arch. chir. suppl., Chir. Forum 301.

ENHANCEMENT OF CO_2-ELIMINATION BY INTRAPULMONARY HIGH FREQUENCY PRESSURE ALTERNATION DURING "APNOEIC OXYGENATION"

P.P. Lunkenheimer, H. Ising, I. Frank,
M. Scharsich, K. Welham, and H. Dittrich
Chirurgische Universitätsklinik, 44 Münster
Institut für Physiologie, 1 Berlin, West Germany
Hospital for Sick Children, London, Great Britain

Since 1973 we have explored an oscillatory modification
of "diffusion respiration" which, perhaps, may widen the
understanding of some particularities in the dynamics
of intrapulmonary gas flow.

During our search for a method to excite
the heart by pressure oscillations with
a view to test its dynamic strength as
an index for contractility, we finished
by using pulmonary airways as a pneu-
matic transmission element. From these
experiments, we learnt that the trans-
bronchial transmission of high frequency
pressure oscillations resulted in an
inhomogenous pattern of pressure amplitudes within the thoracic cage. The non
linear and distinctly different dynamic
elasticity of lung tissue, chest wall,
diaphragm and all associated organs
characterised the chest as a complex
damped harmonic system. This work led

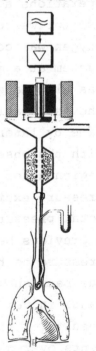

fig. 1

us to the supposition that intrapulmonary high frequency
pressure oscillation enhanced intrapulmonary gas-
mixing (2).

Methods: On 17 mongrel dogs of either sex weighing
between 12 and 27 kg anesthesia was induced by 10-15 mg/
kg Pentobarbital with 0,5 mg Atropin. Intubation was
performed after relaxation by Pancuronium bromide
(0,05 mg/kg every 20 minutes) and mechanical ventilation was sustained by a Dräger Pulmomat with O_2 and
nitrous oxide (1:2). Both femoral arteries and veins
were canulated for blood sampling, fluid substitution
and blood pressure control. Bloodgas controls were done
initially, and every 5 to 10 minutes, during the
period of oxygen insufflation. After these preliminary
operations a diaphragm pump driven by an electro-dynamic
exciter was connected to the endotracheal tube (fig. 1).
Oxygen was continuously insufflated into the closed
system at a mean pressure of 14 cm H_2O. Carbon-dioxide
was eliminated by an absorption cell. In this absorber
the oscillating gas volume came in contact with the soda
lime by lateral gauze filter perforations.

With the onset of oxygen insufflation, that is with the
beginning of "diffusion respiration", the periodical
pressure excitation at a frequency of 24 Hz and at a
total pressure amplitude of up to 50 cm H_2O was started.
A previous Dextran perfusion to adjust central venous
pressure to the elevated mean intrapulmonary pressure
has been shown to be necessary to compensate the impedance in venous return.

Results: (fig. 2) In 12 out of the last 15 experiments over a period of 1 to 5 hours CO_2-elimation could
be optimized such that the blood level of carbon dioxide could be kept rising at a distinctly lower rate

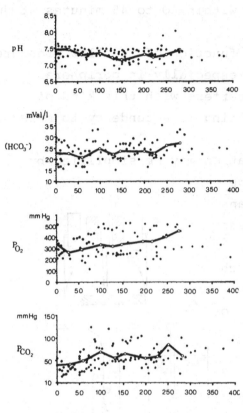

than in the classical method
of "apnoeic oxygenation"
described in 1904 by Vohard
(1, 3, 5, 6). Stabili-
zation of its partial
pressure to a fixed value
could never be obtained.
Yet, the reason for the
slow drifts in blood pCO_2
could not be determined.
Oxygenation in all cases
was more than sufficient.
The most important patho-
logical finding was an ever
present tendency to meta-
bolic acidosis which, for
variably long periods
could be controlled by the
administration of buffer-

fig.   2 Acid-base-balance   solutions such as Sodium-
        and blood gases   bicarbonate or Tris.
        during a 400 minutes
        period of activated
        diffusion respiration on 9 dogs.

Discussion: Modulation of the mean O_2-insufflation
pressure by high frequency pressure oscillations (4)is
apparently able to enhance intrapulmonary and intra-
bronchial gas mixing resulting in an alveolo-oral CO_2-
washout flow comparable to that found during normal
ventilation, whereas the classical method of "apnoeic
oxygenation" results in a tremendous increase in P_{CO_2}.
Kristofferson and Rattenborg found the 200 mm Hg

level of P_{CO_2} to be reached within 40 to 45 minutes at the latest (5).

Yet, severe disturbances in function of the "low pressure compartment" of circulation, especially in peripheral microcirculation seem to interfere with this kind of diffusion respiration, resulting in a tendency to metabolic acidosis.

The mechanism of CO_2 elimination may be simplified by considering the thoracic cage with all its associated organs to be likened to a stiff glass tube and a coupled elastic balloon (fig.: 3). When such a system is filled up with smoke, it shows no tendency to escape through the defined upper opening (leakage between piston and cylinder). In contrast, it settles down in the lower part of the system. With the beginning of the oscillatory pressure excitation by the connected piston pump, the smoke is rapidly mixed-comparable to an extremely enhanced diffusion- and is quickly driven to the opening for elimination within 5 to 15 seconds.

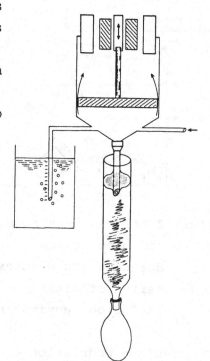

fig.: 3 Model of the thoracic cage as an oscillating system consisting of a stiffness (glas tube), an elasticity (balloon) and an exciter.

Arrows mark the leakage between piston and cylinder.

1. Draper, W.B., Whitehead, R.W.
   The phenomenon of diffusion respiration
   Anesth. Analg. 307 - 319, 1949

2. Frank, I., Noack, W., Lunkenheimer, P.P., Ising, H.
   Light - and electron microscopic investigations of
   pulmonary tissue after high-frequency positive-
   pressure ventilation (HFPPV)
   Anaesthesist 24, 171 - 176, 1975

3. Holmdahl, M.H.
   Pulmonary uptake of oxygen, acid-base metabolism.
   and circulation during prolonged apnoea
   Acta chir. scand. 111, 421 - 424, 1950

4. Jonzon, A., Öberg, P.A., Sedin, G., Sjöstrand, U.
   High-frequency positive-pressure ventilation by
   endotracheal insufflation.
   Universitetsforlaget I Aarhus, XLIII, Suppl.
   Uppsala 1971

5. Kristoffersen, M.B., Rattenborg C.C.
   Apnoische Oxygenation
   Anesthesist 17, 292 - 295, 1968

6. Volhard, F.
   Über künstliche Atmung durch Ventilation der Trachea
   und eine einfache Vorrichtung zur rhythmischen
   künstlichen Atmung
   Münch. Med. Wschr. 46 a, 2o9 - 211, 1908

CHANGES IN CEREBROCORTICAL pO_2-DISTRIBUTION, rCBF AND EEG DURING HYPOVOLEMIC SHOCK

N.WIERNSPERGER,P.GYGAX,W.MEIER-RUGE

Department of Basic Medical Research

Sandoz Ltd,Basel,Switzerland

The prevention of the onset of irreversible damages in the brain is the primary aim in the treatment of cerebral vascular disorders.Surprisingly,the influence of hemorrhagic shock on tissue oxygenation,though it was extensively studied on various organs (Sinagowitz et al.,1973) was seldom measured in the brain.For this reason,we decided to simulate a vascular insufficiency by using the model of hypovolemic shock.Changes in blood flow in the grey matter were correlated with their consequences on tissue pO_2 and EEG.In view of recent clinical results which demonstrate that disease states can disrupt the relationship between regional blood flow and oxidative metabolism (Raichle et al.,1976),we tried to improve the disturbed tissue oxygenation in two ways: a) by increasing the blood flow to the brain with a vasodilating drug (Papaverine) and b) by regulating the catecholamine metabolism with an α-adrenolytic drug,Dihydroergotoxine (Greenberg and Snyder,1977).

MATERIALS AND METHODS

All experiments were performed on cats (n=51),immobilized with Flaxedil and artificially ventilated.In order to avoid the protective effect of barbiturates on vascularly induced oxygen deprivation (Gygax et al.,1975a),the animals were anesthetized with an N_2O/O_2 mixture (70%,30%). The femoral artery was connected with a reservoir,which allowed blood to be withdrawn to achieve the hypovolemic

shock.This system was regulated by a manometer,permitting
the stabilization of the mean arterial blood pressure(MABP)
at any desired level.The femoral vein was catheterized for
administration of drugs.Body temperature,blood gases and
end-expiratory pCO_2 were monitored during the whole duration of the experiment.Measurements of physiological parameters occured in the exposed suprasylvian gyrus.
The regional cerebral blood flow (rCBF) was measured using
the local hydrogen clearance technique and data were analyzed on-line by a computer.Bipolar EEG-recordings were
achieved frontally and occipitally by insertion of silver
silver-chloride microelectrodes into the skull.The EEG
was quantified by means of Fourier transformation.
Oxygen partial pressures were obtained with gold microelectrodes (tip 1-2μ),whose construction and utilization
were described elsewhere (Wiernsperger et al.,1976).The
measurements were performed at a polarization voltage of
(-1000 mV) against a silver silver chloride reference
electrode.
Following a control period of 30 min,the hypovolemic shock
was induced by blood letting until a MABP of 45 mm Hg was
attained.This pressure was kept constant over the entire
period of hypotension,i.e.120 min.Twenty minutes after
the beginning of the oligemic phase,the drugs were administered in following doses:
- 0,9% NaCl solution (control animals,20 cats)
- 1 mg/kg Papaverine (17 cats)
- 0,08 mg/kg Dihydroergotoxine (14 cats)
The substances were each disolved in NaCl solution to a volume of 20 ml and infused over 20 min at a rate of 1ml/min.

RESULTS

It is well known that pO_2-recordings depend closely
on the measurement location within the tissue.For this
reason,the values obtained have to be examined in their
entirety.Consequently,we plotted the individual values
on a histogram,divided into 7 classes of 7 mm Hg each,
except the 7th class which contains all values higher
than 43 mm Hg.By this method,we obtained a frequency distribution similar to that of other detailed examinations
(Smith et al.,1977).The pO_2 distributions are presented
in Fig.1 at 4 stages during the experimental run:
a)at the end of the normotonic control period
b)in the hypotensive phase before drug administration
c)immediately after drug administration
d)at the end of the 120 min period of hypotension.

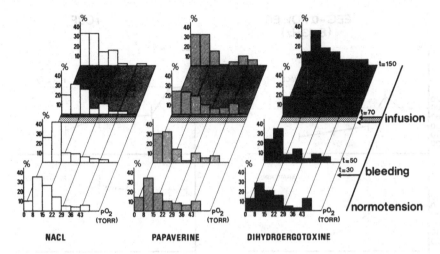

Fig.1.Cerebrocortical pO₂-distribution during hypovolemic
shock (NaCl,control,n=160) and its modification
by Papaverine (n=100) and Dihydroergotoxine (n=76)

    A few minutes after the onset of oligemia,the histogram
shows a shift to the left,as a consequence of the 30% fall
in rCBF and of the ensuing decrease in oxygen supply to the
brain.Accordingly,a hypoxic activation of the EEG is observed,the power being mainly increased in the α-frequency
range (Fig.2).At the same time,the arterial hematocrit
decreased (Fig.3),due to the spontaneous hemodilution
occuring during the early phase of shock (Weidner et al.,
1961).This phenomenon was accentuated by the addition of the
infusion volume,thus leading to a transitory shift to the
right in the histogram.However,with the continuation of the
hypotensive state and the onset of the decompensatory phase
(mainly characterized by a re-increase in hematocrit),the
tissue becomes strongly hypoxic,whereas the EEG is markedly depressed.
Under Papaverine,rCBF almost returns to normotonic values.
However,at the end of the experiment, 2 groups of pO₂ values can be distinguished,a group of higher ones being
preserved,whereas an accummulation of lower values takes
place,similarly to the NaCl-treated cats.In spite of the
increased blood flow,the EEG remains depressed.
In contrast,administration of Dihydroergotoxine has no

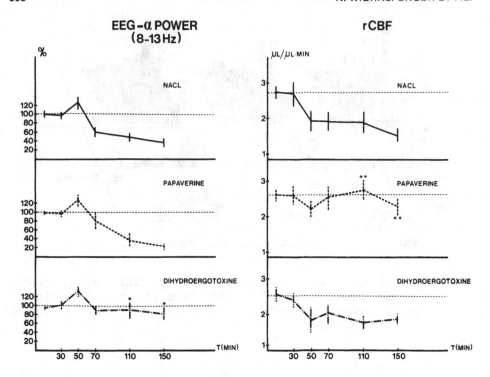

Fig.2.Drug effect on the oligemically disturbed EEG and
      rCBF.Mean values ± SEM. (p<0,05:*, p<0,01:**
      against NaCl/control).

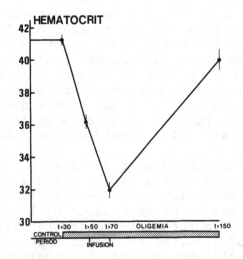

Fig.3.Variation of hematocrit during hypovolemic shock.

effect on the rCBF but the pO$_2$ distribution is clearly
improved: the histogram resembles the pre-shock profile
with a marked reegression in the incidence of lower values.
Accordingly, the decline in EEG power is prevented.

DISCUSSION

Although the major part of the pO$_2$-values were lowered
during shock,some slight increases could be observed.This
fact indicates that a redistribution of blood flow takes
place in small areas of tissue and is in agreement with
the observation of Silver (1976).In the first phase of shock,
an activation in the α-range of the EEG can already be
seen,as a consequence of the appearance of hypoxic seizures.
With the further ongoing of the hypotensive period and
particularly after the onset of the decompensatory phase,
the vasoconstriction induced by sympathetic hyperactivity
(Kovach and Sandor,1976) and the impairment of flow properties of blood (for example sludge) lead to a considerable
deterioration in tissue oxygenation.In view of the controversy about the efficiency of vasodilator therapy in treatment of shock (Regli et al.,1971),it was of particular interest to analyze the effect of Papaverine on tissue oxygena-
tion.We found that,under Papaverine,most values decreased
but the initially higher values remained at their levels,
thus leading to a dissociation in the histogram into 2 peaks
This result supports the hypothesis of a shunt perfusion,
the greater vessels being dilated and diverting the blood
away from the capillary bed (Prosenz,1972).This observation
may explain the deterioration in biochemical parameters observed in hypercapnia-induced vasodilation during reduced
cerebral perfusion (Siesjö et al.,1974).
The beneficial effect of α-blocking agents in the management
of shock has often been pointed out (Kovach and Sandor,1976).
Since cerebral microcirculation is influenced by noradrener-
gic systems (Raichle et al.,1975),a positive effect of Dihydroergotoxine was to be expected,due to its regulating
influence on catecholamine metabolism and its anti-sludge
properties (Larcan et al.,1966).Actually,the modulation of
the hypoxic disturbed metabolic turnover by Dihydroergotoxine (Enz et al.,1975) allows the blood to flow through
the capillaries (Gygax et al.,1975b) and,thus,improves the
pO$_2$-distribution in direction of the normotensive state.
Our results show that the determination of local tissue
pO$_2$ is a reliable indicator of changes in microcirculation.
It allows us to detect modifications of perfusion in very

small areas of brain tissue which could not be established
even with a blood flow measurement procedure as local as
the local hydrogen clearance technique.The above findings
demonstrate that uneven perfusion takes place in the cerebral cortex during hypovolemic shock and that this state
cannot be corrected by vasodilators as Papaverine.On the
contrary,cerebrocortical oxygenation can be improved by
drugs modulating the tissue metabolism,i.e. the site of
utilization of oxygen.

REFERENCES

1. Enz,A.,Iwangoff,P.,Markstein,R.,and Wagner,H.(1975)
      Triangel 14,90
2. Greenberg,D.A.,and Snyder,S.H.(1977) Life Sci.20,927
3. Gygax,P.,Stosseck,K.,Emmenegger,H.,and Schweizer,A.,
      (1975a) in "Blood Flow and Metabolism in the Brain"
      11.14.(Eds Harper,A.M.,Jenett,W.B.,Miller,J.D.,and
      Rowan,J.O.) Churchill,Livingstone
4. Gygax,P.,Hunziker,O.,Schulz,U.,and Schweizer,A.,(1975b)
      Triangel 14,80
5. Kovach,A.G.B.,and Sandor,P.(1976) Ann.Rev.Physiol.39,571
6. Larcan,A.,Streiff,F.,Peters,A.,and Genetet,B.(1966)
      Med.Pharmacol.Exp.15,507
7. Prosenz,P. (1972) Arch.Neurol. 26,479
8. Raichle,M.E.,Grubb,P.L.,Gado,M.H.,Eichling,J.O.,and
      Ter-Pogossian,M.M. (1976) Arch.Neurol.33,523
9. Raichle,M.E.,Hartman,B.K.,Eichling,J.O.,and Sharpe,L.G.
      (1975) Proc.Nat.Acad.Sci.USA 72,3726
10. Regli,F.,Yamaguchi,T.,and Waltz,A.G.(1971) Arch.Neurol.
      24,467
11. Siesjö,B.K.,Johannsson,H.,Ljunggren,B.,and Norberg,K.
      (1974) in "Brain Dysfunction and Metabolic Disorders"
      p.75 (Ed.Plum,F.) Raven Press,New-York.
12. Silver,I.A.,(1976) Adv.Exp.Med.Biol. 75,325
13. Sinagowitz,E.,Rahmer,H.,Rink,R.,Görnandt,L.,and Kessler,M.
      (1973) Adv.Exp.Med.Biol. 37A,505
14. Smith,R.H.,Guilbeau,E.J.,and Reneau,D.D.(1977)
      Microvasc.Res. 13,233
15. Weidner,M.G.,and Simeone,F.A.(1961) Surg.Forum 12,82
16. Wiernsperger,N.,Kunke,S.,and Gygax,P. (1976)
      Experientia 32,671

EXTRACELLULAR K$^+$ AND H$^+$ ACTIVITIES IN THE BRAIN CORTEX DURING

AND AFTER A SHORT PERIOD OF ISCHAEMIA AND ARTERIAL HYPOXIA

R. Urbanics*, E. Leniger-Follert and D.W. Lübbers

Max-Planck-Institut für Systemphysiologie

Dortmund, G.F.R.

It is well known that cerebral blood flow increases strongly after a short period of tissue anoxia. However, the exact mechanism of the regulation is still unknown. Local H$^+$ and K$^+$ activities have been assumed to play an important role in the regulation of local cerebral blood flow. But recently some evidence against H$^+$ and K$^+$ as the main factors of regulation has been published (Astrup et al., 1976). As there is little direct information available about the kinetics of these ions in the brain cortex, especially with regards to local hydrogen activity, we investigated the behaviour of these ions in the brain cortex during a short period of arterial anoxia and total cerebral ischemia. Previous data were published elsewhere (Urbanics et al., 1976). Furthermore, we tried to clarify the question as to whether the redistribution of microflow which occurs during anoxia and which was described by Leniger-Follert et al. (1976) could be caused by different local kinetics of these ions. Another problem we tried to solve was whether these ions could be responsible for the rapid decrease of oxygen consumption after a few seconds of total cerebral ischaemia (see Leniger-Follert, this symposium).

METHODS

Experiments were performed on 13 cats which were anaesthetized with Nembutal (35-40 mg/kg), immobilised with Flaxedil and artificially ventilated. Endtidal CO_2 and arterial blood pressure were monitored continuously and were in the normal range.

* Present address: Experimental Research Department, Semmelweis Medical School, Budapest, Hungary.

Arterial pH was 7.39 $\pm$ 0.048, arterial PCO_2 26 $\pm$ 3.88 Torr and PO_2 90.4 $\pm$ 11.3 Torr. Extracellular K^+ activity was measured with double-barrelled microelectrodes with a tip diameter of 1-3 μm prepared as described by Lux and Neher (1973). The sensitivity of the electrodes was 45 - 58 mV/tenfold change of potassium concentration. The second barrel, filled with 150 mM NaCl, served as the reference and as the DC-electrode against another surface reference element.

Extracellular H^+ activity was measured with H^+-sensitive glass microelectrodes according to Saito et al (1976). The tip of the electrodes was 1 to 4 μm and the sensitive length 20 to 80 μm. The sensitivity was 58 to 62 mV/pH unit at 37°C. The electrodes were mounted on a counter-balanced holder and inserted into the gyrus suprasylvius at a depth of 0.5 to 1.5 mm. The surface of the brain was covered with warmed paraffin oil to prevent the cortex from cooling and drying.

In three experiments microflow was recorded qualitatively by local hydrogen clearance (Lübbers and Stosseck, 1970). Anoxia was produced by ventilating the animals with nitrogen and total cerebral ischaemia by clamping the innominate and left subclavian arteries after ligation of both mammary arteries.

The completeness of ischaemia was ascertained by the iso-electric ECoG.

RESULTS

1. Anoxia

The results obtained during anoxia are summarized in Table 1. H^+ and K^+ activities increased are mean of about 32 sec. after the beginning of N_2 inhalation whereas the change of microflow began with a mean of about 41 sec. However, the dynamic of ionic changes was not homogeneous. The onset of changes varied in a wide range (pH between 18 and 55 sec., K^+ between 20 and 50 sec.).

In some cases, an initial alkalotic shift was observed. The maximum of the H^+ and K^+ increases was noticed always after return to air respiration. Fig. 1 shows, as an example, the reactions of K^+ and H^+ activities and of microflow during and after a short period of arterial hypoxia. In this case, K^+ activity began to increase after about 40 sec. and the H^+ activity after about 55 sec. Microflow recorded simultaneously at four sites increased at two sites during N_2 inhalation. At the third measuring site at first it decreased after some seconds and then increased, and was slightly diminished at the fourth site.

Table 1. Changes during and after a short period of anoxia

	Duration of anoxia (sec)	Initial value	Onset of changes (sec)	Maximal value	Time of max. val. (sec)	Number of measurements (n)
$[K^+]_e$ m l	63.0 ± 15	3.42 ± 0.2	32.0 ± 9 (20-50)	5.23 ± 0.74 (4-6.3)	76.8 ± 30 (4o-130)	11
pH_e	64.5 ± 14.8	7.17 ± 0.06	32.3 ± 14 (18-55)	6.89 ± 0.12 (6.62-7.0)	110.1 ± 24	8
Micro-flow	59.0 ± 7		41.5 ± 8 (25-50)		82.7 ± 22 (60-120)	11

ECoG isoelectric at 54 ± 8 sec. Activity returned at 24.5 ± 4 sec after air respiration.
The data are mean ± SD. The data in brackets indicate maximum and minimum values.

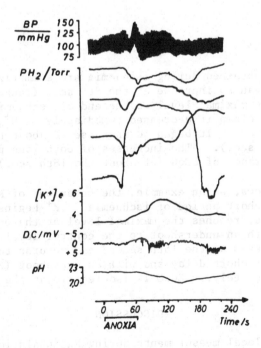

Fig. 1. Effects of 60 sec. of anoxia.

Table 2. Changes during and after a short period of cerebral ischemia

	Duration of ischemia (sec)	Initial value	Onset of changes (sec)	Maximal value	Time of max. val. (sec)	Number of measurements (n)
$[K^+]_e$	46.0	3.45	8.22	4.71	46.6.	
mM	± 3	± 0.3	± 2	± 0.74	± 2	11
			(6-12)	(4-6.3)		
pH_e	43.0	7.015	12.1	6.65	44.4	
	± 9	± 0.12	± 4	± 0.14	± 10	8
			(6-15)	(6.5-6.92)		
Microflow	40.0			103.0		7
	± 10			± 13		

ECoG isoelectric at 18,25 ± 3 sec, activity returned at 9.3 ± 2 sec after recirculation.
The data are mean ± SD. The data in brackets indicate maximum and minimum values.

2.   Ischaemia

The data obtained during ischaemia are summarized in Table 2. K^+ activity began to increase at the 8th sec. (range 6 - 12 sec.) and reached the maximal level at the end of ischaemia. After the removal of the clamp it decreased immediately. H^+ activity showed the same dynamics. It began to increase at about the 12th second (range 6 to 15 sec.). The increases of both ions preceded the total disappearance of ECoG (at about the 18th sec.).

Fig. 2 shows, as an example, the behaviour of K^+, H^+ and ECoG during a short period of ischaemia. K^+ begins to rise at the 10th second, reaches the maximal level at the end of reaction and returns with an undershoot to the control level. H^+ activity increases at the 15th second and returns to initial value sometimes after short delay and with an overshoot (Fig. 2), sometimes immediately. ECoG is isoelectric at the 16th second.

DISCUSSION

From our local measurements during N_2 inhalation it cannot be excluded that K^+ and H^+ activities play a role in the regulation

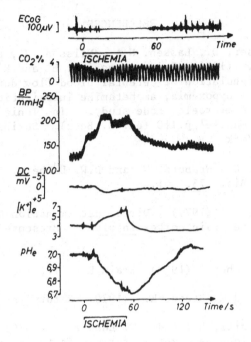

Fig. 2. Effects of 50 sec. of ischaemia.

of microflow during this situation. This is in contrast to results by Astrup et al (1976), who used rather big electrodes.

The behaviour of capillary flow is complex and does not act so uniformly as do total or regional cerebral blood flows. It is possible that the different onset of ionic changes is responsible for the inhomogeneous behaviour of microflow. However, it must be considered that the behaviour both of ions and microflow was not measured at the same location.

The question of whether the changes of extracellular H⁺ and K⁺ activities observed during the short period of ischaemia are responsible for the rapid depression of local oxygen consumption cannot be definitely answered. It remains a possibility, since the time courses of the changes of H⁺ and K⁺ agree fairly well with the time course recorded for local oxygen consumption which decreases between 5 and 15 seconds. The small changes of extra-cellular H⁺ activity may be sufficient to inhibit O_2 uptake and we can assume that the intracellular H⁺ changes are higher.

REFERENCES

Astrup, J., Heuser, D., Lassen, N.A., Nilsson, B., Norberg, K.
and B.K. Siesjö. (1976) Evidence against H^+ and K^+ as the main
factors in the regulation of cerebral blood flow during epileptic
discharges, acute hypoxemia, amphetamine intoxication, and
hypoglycemia. A microelectrode study. In 'Ionic Actions on
Vascular Smooth Muscle' p.110 (ed. E. Betz). Springer, Berlin-
Heidelberg-New York.

Leniger-Follert, E., Wrabetz, W. and D.W. Lübbers. (1976)
Adv. Expt. Med. Biol. 75, 361.

Leniger-Follert, E. (1977) Direct determination of local oxygen
consumption of the brain cortex in vivo. Presented at this
symposium.

Lux, H.D. and E.Neher. (1973) Brain Res. 17, 190.

Lübbers, D.W., and K. Stosseck. (1970) Naturwiss. 57, 311.

Saito, Y., Baumgärtl, H., and D.W. Lübbers. (1976) The RF
sputtering technique as a method for manufacturing needle-shaped
pH-microelectrodes. In 'Ion and Enzyme Electrodes in Biology
and Medicine' (eds. M. Kessler, L.C. Clark Jr., D.W. Lübbers,
I.A. Silver and W. Simon). Urban & Schwarzenberg, München.

Urbanics, R., Leniger-Follert, E., Baumgärtl, H., Shigemitsu, T.
and D.W. Lübbers. (1976) Pflügers Arch. 365, R 44.

REGIONAL HEMODYNAMIC AND METABOLIC ALTERATIONS IN FOCAL CEREBRAL

ISCHEMIA: STUDIES OF DIASCHISIS

M. Reivich, S. Jones, M. Ginsberg, R. Slater and
J. Greenberg

Cerebrovascular Research Center
University of Pennsylvania, U.S.A.

Diaschisis is thought to be due to a temporary depression of
function in areas of the brain remote from a focal cerebral injury
and to be associated with changes in cerebral metabolism and blood
flow. The phenomen of diaschisis was first described by Von-Monakow
in 1914 and was based on clinical observations.

The first report of bilateral reduction of cerebral blood flow
in patients with unilateral cerebral infarction was that of Kempinsky
et al in 1961. However, because of the method used to measure flow
(the Kety-Schmidt technique with bilateral jugular bulb sampling)
the validity of these results is open to question. Admixture of
blood from both hemispheres in the jugular bulb could have falac-
iously lowered the measured flow in the contralateral hemisphere.

Following this report, bilateral reduction of hemisphere
blood flow in patients with unilateral cerebral infarction was observed using the ^{133}Xe intracarotid injection technique which
circumvents the above problem (Hoedt-Rasmussen and Skinhoj, 1964;
and Skinhoj, 1965). It was hypothesized that a transneuronal depression of metabolism was produced by the unilateral infarct which
then resulted in reduced blood flow in both hemispheres.

Some idea of the time course of this contralateral depression
of blood flow was obtained by Meyer et al (1970). They measured
hemispheric blood flow and metabolism at various times following a
unilateral infarction and found that there was bilateral depression
of flow which persisted for two to three weeks, but thereafter, the
blood flow on the non-infarcted side gradually returned toward
normal values.

The above observations of diaschisis were limited since the
method used to measure cerebral blood flow was invasive. Since
development of the Xenon inhalation method for determining regional
cerebral blood flow, serial studies have been possible without exposing patients to risk. Using this method we have looked in detail at the flow changes occurring in the opposite hemisphere in the
immediate post stroke period (Slater et al, 1976). Studies were
performed in fifteen patients with a unilateral acute ischemic
stroke. In 12 patients, significant blood flow changes in the non-
ischemic hemisphere occurred during the period of observation.
Fig. 1 shows the time course of these changes.

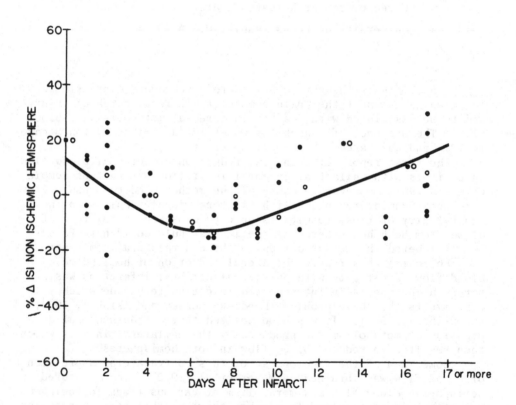

Fig. 1   Time course of change of hemispheric blood flow in the
non-ischemic hemisphere following an acute unilateral stroke. The
percent change of flow from the mean of all flows in a given patient
is plotted against time in days after the infarct. The filled
circles represent a single flow in one patient. The open circles
represent the average flow change in all patients on a given day.

It appeared, contrary to implications from prior studies which did not examine the first 10 days post stroke in detail, that diaschisis was not a phenomenon that reached its peak at the onset of stroke, but is a process that increases during the first week. These data suggest that a neuronal depression secondary to disconnection from afferent stimulation is not the only cause of diaschisis. If this were the case, the maximum decline in flow would be expected immediately and a correlation between change in flow and change in clinical status would be expected which was not found in these patients.

A similar time course of change was found in the ischemic hemisphere with the flow alterations in the two hemispheres changing in parallel to one another. The correlation coefficient of this association was .846 and was significant at the < .001 level. This correlation suggests the presence of factors affecting both hemispheres in a similar manner. The fact that the flows were not static in the nonischemic hemisphere rules out the possibility that the observed flow reductions were secondary only to pre-existing vascular disease.

In order to more closely examine the cerebral hemodynamic and metabolic alterations occurring in stroke we have examined these parameters in a cat model of middle cerebral artery occlusion. Regional cerebral glucose metabolism was studied (Ginsberg et al, 1976) in a series of cats anesthetized with sodium pentobarbital, 40 mg/kg, in which the middle cerebral artery was exposed via a modification of the transorbital approach of O'Brien and Waltz (1973). In seven animals, the left middle cerebral artery (MCA) was occluded. In four control animals, the MCA was touched but not occluded. One hour following the onset of the insult or sham insult, ^{14}C-2-deoxy-glucose 75 μc/kg, was injected intravenously as a bolus to measure regional cerebral glucose consumption by an autoradiographic technique (Sokoloff et al, 1977).

The arterial blood pressure of the ischemic animals and control animals remained stable throughout the experiment aside from a mild fall in blood pressure subsequent to extensive blood sampling. Arterial blood gases remained unchanged throughout the control, insult, or sham insult periods. Following vascular occlusion, there was a prompt reduction of the ipsilateral EEG amplitude to 25-60 percent of its pre-occlusion level in 6 of 7 animals, together with the appearance of irregular slow higher amplitude forms. In three animals, these changes persisted during ischemia, whereas in the other three the EEG improved despite the continuation of ischemia. The nonischemic hemisphere exhibited no EEG alterations.

In the autoradiograms of the ischemic animals, there was in all cases a striking derangement of metabolism visible within the basal ganglia of the ischemic hemisphere. This consisted of a central zone of decreased glucose utilization involving the caudate nucleus and in some animals parts of the internal capsule, putamen, and anterior thalamus. Surrounding this was an irregular zone of enhanced glucose metabolism. All of the ischemic animals exhibited these findings, though in some cases the affected zone was much larger than in others. In two animals, the overlying cerebral cortex at the level of the caudate nucleus and anterior thalamus was also involved in the ischemic hemisphere by patchy zones of increased and decreased glucose utilization. The areas of increased glucose metabolism are thought to represent regions in which increased anaerobic glycolysis is occurring.

In addition to the alterations in glucose metabolism observed on the side of the middle cerebral artery occlusion, there was a small but significant (p < .025) reduction in glucose utilization in the contralateral hemisphere when compared to the sham operated control animals. The average value (+ S.E.) for glucose utilization in the non-ischemic cerebral cortex in the experimental animals was 4.06 + 0.45 mg/100 gm/min compared to 5.88 + 0.71 mg/100 gm/min in the control animals or a 31% decrease. It was felt that this represented the metabolic correlate of diaschisis and if so there should be a corresponding reduction in cortical flow in the hemisphere.

In order to examine this hypothesis a further series of five cats with MCA occlusion and five sham operated control animals were studied (Reivich et al, 1977). Regional cerebral blood flow (rCBF) was measured in each middle ectosylvian gyrus by means of the hydrogen clearance technique (Pasztor et al, 1973) using platinum surface electrodes 125 μ in diameter.

After preparation of the animal a 30 min. period was allowed to elapse to ensure a steady state. Two control flow measurements were then made 30 min apart and in the experimental group of animals the left middle cerebral artery was then occluded while in an identically prepared series of cats (the sham occlusion control group) the left middle cerebral artery was gently touched. In both the experimental and control groups blood flow was then measured every 30 min for an additional 2 1/2 hours. An arterial blood sample was obtained during each flow determination and analyzed for pH, PO_2 and PCO_2 using a microelectrode system.

The control blood gas values in the sham occlusion animals (mean + S.E.) for PCO_2, PO_2 and pH were 32.6 + 0.7 mm Hg, 120.0 + 5.5 mm Hg and 7.338 + .004, respectively. In the experimental animals the control values for these same parameters were 34.0 + 1.0 mm Hg, 112.2 + 4.6 mm Hg and 7.344 + .014, respectively. There were no significant differences in the values of these parameters between the two groups and no significant changes over time.

The control mean arterial blood pressure in the sham occlusion animals was 148.2 + 10.5 mm Hg while in the experimental group it was 127.8 + 4.1 mm Hg. There was a small (approximately 10%) but significant fall in blood pressure in both groups over time (p < .01) but this time course was not significantly different in the two groups and there was no significant difference in the absolute level of blood pressure in the two groups.

In the sham occlusion series control flows in the middle ectosylvian gyri on the right and left were 73.8 ± 12.0 and 89.6 ± 18.5
ml/100 gm/min, respectively. These values were not significantly
different from each other nor was there a significant change in flow
in both sides over the next 2 1/2 hours following touching of the
left middle cerebral artery.

In the experimental series control flows in the right and left
middle ectosylvian gyri were 75.6 ± 7.0 and 73.3 ± 5.8 ml/100 gm/min
respectively. These values are not significantly different from each
other or from the sham occlusion controls values. Following occlusion of the left middle cerebral artery there was a significant
decrease in flow on both sides (p < .001) and a significant difference in the absolute value of flow between the two sides (p < .01)
being significantly lower on the side of occlusion (Fig. 2).

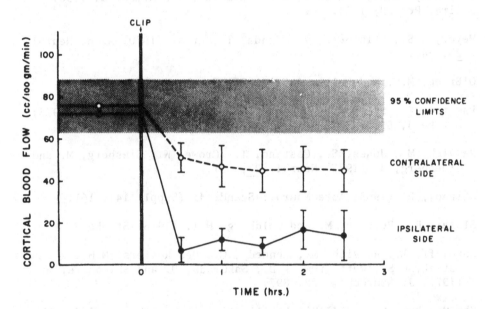

Fig. 2   Time course of change of blood flow in middle ectosylvian
gyri in ischemic (filled circles ± S.E.) and non-ischemic (open
circles ± S.E.) hemispheres following left middle cerebral artery
occlusion.

This reduction in flow in the contralateral cortex is of the
order of 38% and agrees quite well with the previously observed
depression of glucose consumption of 31% in the contralateral cortex.
We postulate that these changes are the hemodynamic and metabolic
concomitants of diaschisis and may in part be due to a transneuronal

depression of function. Further study will be necessary to
determine the exact mechanism underlying these flow and metabolic
alterations produced by a focal ischemic insult.

Supported by USPHS Grant NS-10939-05

REFERENCES

Ginsberg, M.D., Reivich, M. and Giandomenico, A. (1976) Neurol.
26, 346.

Hoedt-Rasmussen, K. and Skinhoj, E. (1964) Acta Neurol. Scand.
40, 41.

Kempinsky, W.H., Boniface, W.R., Keating, J.B.A., et al (1961)
Circ. Res. 9, 1051.

Meyer, J.S., Skinobera, Y., Kanda, T., et al (1970) Arch. Neurol.
23, 241.

O'Brien, M.D. and Waltz, A.G. (1973) Stroke 4, 201.

Pasztor, E., Symon, L., Dorsch, N.W.C. and Branston, N.M. (1973)
Stroke 4, 556.

Reivich, M., Jones, S., Castano, T., Crowe, W., Ginsberg, M. and
Greenberg, J. (1977) Neurol. 27, 381.

Skinhoj, E. (1965) Acta Neurol. Scand. 41 (Suppl. 14), 161.

Slater, R., Reivich, M. and Goldberg, H.I. (1976) Stroke 7, 7.

Sokoloff, L., Reivich, M., Kennedy, C., Des Rosiers, M.H.,
Patlak, C.S., Pettigrew, K.D., Sakurada, O. and Skinohara, M.
(1977) J. Neurochem. 28, 897.

Von Monakow, C. (1914) Die Lokalisation im Grosshirn und der Abbau
der Funktion durch kortikale Herde. Wiesbaden, Germany, J.F.
Bergmann, pp. 26-34.

OXYGEN AND CARBON DIOXIDE TENSIONS IN THE GASTROCNEMIUS

MUSCLES OF PATIENTS WITH LOWER LIMB ARTERIAL ISCHAEMIA

Erkki Jussila, Juha Niinikoski and Markku V. Inberg

Department of Surgery
University of Turku
Turku, Finland

Currently, commonly used parameters in assessing circulatory status of ischaemic limbs include peripheral pulse status, temperature and color of the extremities, type of ischaemic pain, claudication distance, capillary and venous filling, condition of the skin and nails, and arteriography. If necessary equipment and personnel are available, peripheral blood pressure measurements, pletysmography, thermography and radioactive clearance techniques may also be used to evaluate limb circulation. However, most of these parameters provide, at best, only indirect information of tissue nutrition in the ischaemic area. Recently, several investigations have demonstrated that measurements of skeletal muscle oxygen and carbon dioxide tensions provide an excellent index of peripheral tissue perfusion (Furuse et al, 1973; Brantigan et al, 1974; Wakabayashi et al, 1975).

CLINICAL MATERIAL AND METHODS

Oxygen and carbon dioxide tensions were measured in the medial head of the gastrocnemius muscle of patients submitted into the hospital for aortofemoral reconstruction with indications of obstructive arteriosclerosis (37) or·abdominal aortic aneurysm (5). Four volunteer patients showing no signs of lower limb arterial ischaemia served as controls.

Measurements of muscle PO_2 and PCO_2 were carried out by means of implanted gas-permeable Silastic tubes 16 cm long, with an external diameter of 1.4 mm and an internal diameter of 1.0 mm (Kivisaari and Niinikoski, 1973; Fig.1). Patients with lower

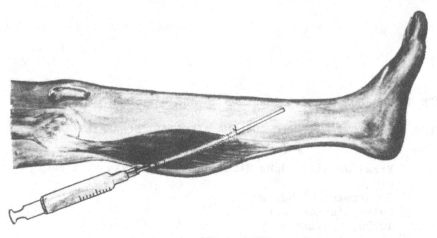

Fig.1. Measurement of tissue PO_2 and PCO_2 in the gastrocnemius muscle by means of an implanted Silastic tube and capillary sampling
technique.

limb arterial ischaemia received two tonometers, one for each leg,
whereas the control patients received only one tonometer. Implanta-
tions were carried out by means of a wide-bore needle under local
anaesthesia. The tube ends were left outside the skin and were fixed
to the dermis with polypropylene sutures which did not occlude the
tonometer lumen. The length of the tube remaining inside the gastrocnemius muscle was 14 cm.

The measurements were carried out 5-7 days after the implanta-
tions when the acute implantation trauma had subsided. The Silastic
tonometers were filled with hypoxic saline solution (PO_2 3-8 mm Hg)
whose PO_2 and PCO_2 equilibrated with the corresponding tensions of
the surrounding muscle within 2 min (Fig.1). The quilibrated fluid
was collected in an Astrup-type glass capillary tube, which was then
inserted into a microsample injector (Radiometer, Copenhagen, Denmark)
and emptied into a cuvette containing either an O_2 or CO_2 electrode.

Measurements were carried out with the patient supine during
breathing of air and 100% oxygen and immediately before and after
physical exercise on a treadmill. In parallel with these

Table I. Muscle tissue gases and ankle blood pressures in lower limb arterial ischaemia

Patient group	Extremity	Baseline conditions			O_2 breathing		Exercise		
		PO_2	PCO_2	Ankle pressure	PO_2	PCO_2	PO_2	PCO_2	Ankle pressure
I Intermittent claudication (17)	Claudication	42±1	41±1	80±9***	87±6	44±2	27±2**	46±1**	49±11***
	No symptoms	42±1	42±1	147±11**	98±9	39±3	38±3	41±2*	163±12***
II Patients with rest pain (12)	Rest pain	40±1	43±1	49±17***	68±16*	42±3	30±3**	44±1	17±14***
	Other side	41±2	41±1	90±17	70±14	42±3	37±2	42±1	72±20
III Praegangrene (8)	Praegangrene	43±3	40±1	34±11***	62±6**	41±2	29±3**	49±4	4±4***
	Other side	42±1	37±2	104±22	70±10	39±2	37±2	40±3	104±31***
IV Aortic aneurysm (5)	Claudication	46	41	40	73	44	30	46	20
	No symptoms	48±2	38±2	161±13	96±9	37±4	45±2	39±3	154±20
V Control patients (4)	No symptoms	43±2	40±2	141±15	101±6	42±3	44±2	41±3	158±14

*$p < 0.05$; **$p < 0.01$; ***$p < 0.001$. In each patient group upper symbols (stars) denote statistical significance vs. control, lower symbols denote statistical significance vs. contralateral extremity.

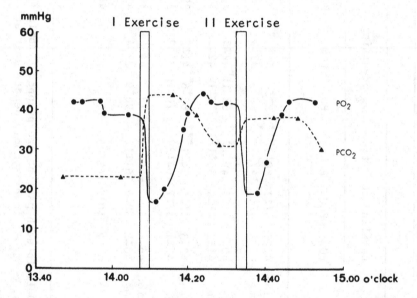

Fig.2. Response of gastrocnemius muscle PO_2 and PCO_2 to physical exercise test in a patient with obstructive arteriosclerosis and intermittent claudication.

determinations, ankle blood pressures were recorded by means of a Doppler apparatus.

RESULTS

As shown in table I baseline muscle PO_2 and PCO_2 levels showed no essential differences between various groups of patients: patients with intermittent claudication (I), with rest pain (II), praegangrene (III), abdominal aortic aneurysm (IV), and control patients (V). Neither were there any changes in tissue gas tensions between the affected and contralateral extremities under normal conditions. On the other hand, baseline ankle blood pressures were clearly decreased in extremities with arterial ischaemia and correlated well with the severity of the disease.

During breathing of pure oxygen the smallest responses of muscle oxygen tensions were observed in extremities with rest pain or praegangrene while the highest muscle PO_2 levels during systemic hyperoxia were recorded in control patients and patients with abdominal aortic aneurysm but no claudication (Table I). Overall, muscle PCO_2 values showed no marked alterations during oxygen breathing.

During physical exercise on the treadmill muscle PO_2 and PCO_2 levels as well as ankle blood pressures remained unchanged in the controls and patients with aortic aneurysm but no claudication (Table I). However, in all patients with clinical lower limb arterial ischaemia the exercise test resulted in a marked fall of muscle PO_2 and ankle blood pressure and in an increase of muscle PCO_2. Figure 2 illustrates the behavior of gastrocnemius muscle PO_2 and PCO_2 in a patient with intermittent claudication during repeated exercise.

CONCLUSIONS

This work shows that in peripheral arterial insufficiency the muscle PO_2 and PCO_2 remain normal at rest probably because the muscle energy metabolism and oxygen consumption are adapted to the reduced supply of nutrients. In physical exercise, however, the balance between oxygen supply and consumption is markedly disturbed - the tissue oxygen tension decreases and carbon dioxide is accumulated. Increased diffusion distances in tissues with obstructive arteriosclerosis are also reflected as decreased response of muscle PO_2 to systemic hyperoxia during breathing of oxygen.

REFERENCES

Brantigan, J.W., Ziegler, E.C., Hynes, K.M., Miyazawa, T.Y. and Smith, A.N. (1974) J. Appl. Physiol. 37, 117.

Furuse, A., Brawley, R.E., Struve, E. and Gott, V.L. (1973) Surgery 74, 214.

Kivisaari, J. and Niinikoski, J. (1973) Amer. J. Surg. 125, 623.

Wakabayashi, A., Nakamura, Y., Woolley, T., Mullin, P.J., Watanabe, H., Ino, T. and Connolly, J.E. (1975) Arch. Surg. 110, 802.

EFFECTS OF ISCHEMIA ON THE OXYGEN DIFFUSION COEFFICIENTS IN THE BRAIN CORTEX
(Studies on Macaca Irus)

Morawetz, R., Strong, E., Clark, D.K., Erdmann, W.

Departments of Neurosurgery, Neurology, and Anesthesiology
University of Alabama in Birmingham
Birmingham, Alabama, 35294 U.S.A.

Oxygenation of tissue is dependent both on rate and concentration of oxygen provided at the capillary level and the speed with which oxygen may diffuse from these capillaries through the tissue. Factors influencing the diffusion coefficient of oxygen in tissue include the chemical constitution of the medium, for example, protein concentration and the ratio of extracellular to intercellular volume and the density of cell membranes and other cell structures. These latter factors may be substantially modified by changes in tissue metabolism.

The present study has been designed to measure oxygen diffusion coefficients before, during and after focal cerebral ischemia. It is hoped that this will allow an assessment of the contribution of changing oxygen diffusion coefficients to the ischemic process.

METHODS

Studies were performed in waking monkeys. Three macaca irus monkeys were prepared with ketamine/barbiturate anesthesia by insertion of a hollow screw into the skull in the right posterior parietal area. A plastic cover for the hollow screw was provided to maintain sterility. An array of five platinum electrodes was placed immediately anterior to the screw and a sixth platinum electrode was placed in the opposite hemisphere to serve as a control. Using these electrodes cerebral blood flow in the area to be studied could be monitored using hydrogen washout. Seven days after placement of the screw and the electrodes the right middle cerebral artery was approached by the transorbital route and a snare ligature placed around that vessel. This vessel was brought out through a small plastic tube and the orbit sealed with acrylic. Forty-eight hours later the monkey was placed in a

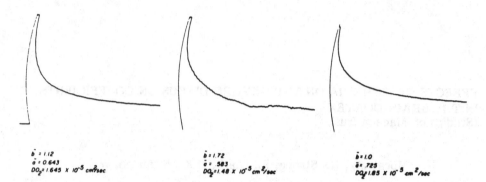

FIGURE 1: Oxygen diffusion determined curves in the brain of
macaca irus after closure of the polargraphic circuit.
    1a: Original curve in unaffected brain tissue before ligation of the
    middle cerebral aftery.
    1b: Diffusion determined curve eleven minutes following ligation.
    1c: Diffusion determined curve three hours after release of the
    ligation.

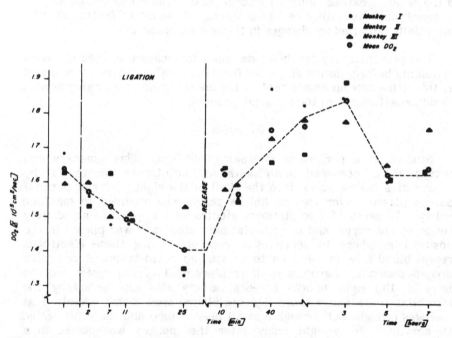

FIGURE 2: Oxygen diffusion coefficients before, during and after
ligation of the middle cerebral artery of macaca irus in the affected
hemisphere.

restraining chair and a bare noble metal electrode inserted into the cortex through the previously described hollow screw. Prior to insertion the electrode was calibrated. Baseline determinations of the oxygen diffusion coefficient were carried out. The right middle artery was then ligated by a traction on the snare ligature and occlusion confirmed by hydrogen flow measurements. Occlusion was maintained for thirty minutes and during this period multiple determination of the oxygen diffusion coefficient were made. After thirty minutes traction on the snare ligature was released and re-perfusion confirmed by hydrogen clearance. Repeated measurements of the oxygen diffusion coefficient were then made in the post ischemic period.

The methodological approach for measurement of diffusion coefficients with noble metal electrodes has been described by Clark, et al. (1977).

RESULTS

The average oxygen diffusion coefficient in the brain cortex of the monkey is calculated to be $1.634 \cdot 10^{-5}$ cm^2/sec. Following ligation of the middle cerebral artery the diffusion coefficient decreased as shown by the shape of the oxygen diffusion determined hyperbolic curve (Figure 1b) compared to the original curve obtained in normal tissue (Figure 1a). Eleven minutes following ligation a diffusion coefficient of $1.482 \cdot 10^{-5}$ cm^2/sec. was calculated. About twenty-five minutes after ligation this value had fallen to $1.402 \cdot 10^{-5}$ cm^2/sec. (Figure 2).

With release of occlusion and re-perfusion as shown by the slope of the oxygen diffusion curve (Figure 1c) the diffusion coefficient increased, reaching preocclusion levels by twelve minutes. The diffusion coefficient continues to increase, reaching a peak value at three hours following re-perfusion of $1.841 \cdot 10^{-5}$ cm^2/sec. Diffusion coefficient decreases thereafter and by five to seven hours after release has returned to preocclusion levels.

DISCUSSION

These preliminary results indicate that the ischemic process modifies tissue metabolism not only by decreasing the rate and amount of oxygen provided but by altering the diffusion coefficient as well. A hypothesis which attempts to explain this reduction in oxygen diffusion coefficient follows: The decrease of the diffusion coefficient after ligation, rendering the tissue ischemic, could be explained by reduction of water content of the tissue, by decrease of the intercellular space where oxygen has to diffuse across the cell membrane barriers and by changes of osmolality in the tissue due to anaerobic metabolism. The increase of diffusion coefficient after release could be due to an increase of fluid contents of the tissue with decrease of protein concentration, decrease of osmolality in the tissue and increase of intercellular space.

At the moment, these explanations can only be considered as vague suggestions which need further investigation.

SUMMARY

In this series of experiments changes in oxygen diffusion coefficients were measured in waking primates undergoing focal middle cerebral artery ischemia. Ligation of the middle cerebral artery is followed by a decrease of the oxygen diffusion coefficient in the areas supplied by that vessel to levels ten to twenty per cent below normal by twenty-five minutes following onset of ischemia. Following release and re-perfusion diffusion coefficient gradually increases and reaches a super normal peak value three hours after release of ligation. This is followed by a gradual reduction in diffusion coefficient with stabilization at preocclusion levels. In the three experiments described these changes following re-perfusion corresponded with clinical improvement of the neurological status of the monkeys.

REFERENCES

1. Erdmann, W., Kunke, S., and Krell, W.: Tissue-PO_2 and Cell Function. An Experimental Study with Multimicroelectrodes in the Rat Brain. In Oxygen Supply. Eds. Kessler, et al. Urban and Schwarzenberg, Muechen-Berlin-Wien, 1973.

2. Erdmann, W., and Krell, W.: Measurement of Diffusion Parameters with Noble Metal Electrodes. In: Oxygen Transport to Tissue - II. Eds. Grote, et al. Plenum Publishing Company, New York, 1976.

3. Clark, D.K., Erdmann, W., Halsey, J.H., and Strong, E.: Oxygen Diffusion, Conductivity and Solubility Coefficients in the Microarea of the Brain. International Symposium on Oxygen Transport to Tissue, Cambridge (England) 1977.

OXYGEN SUPPLY TO THE CIRRHOTIC LIVER FOLLOWING VARIOUS

PORTACAVAL SHUNT PROCEUDRES

Ch. Broelsch, J. Höper, and M. Kessler

Klinik für Abdominal- und Transplantationschirurgie
D-3ooo Hannover, Medizinische Hochschule
Max-Planck-Institut fuer Systemphysiologie
D-46oo Dortmund

Hemodynamic measurements have been of limited value in determining
the stage of liver cirrhosis and the type of.portacaval shunt to
be performed in the presence of portal hypertension and bleeding
esophageal varices (Bradley et al. 1953, Reynolds, 1974). The
effective perfusion rate and oxygen transport to the tissue, required to sustain regenerative and functional capacity of the
residual hepatocytes cannot be detected by determination of
intraoperatively obtained hemodynamic parameters such as portal
venous flow and pressure, wedged hepatic pressure and hepatic arterial flow because of the various compartments of intrahepatic
blood circulation, the severely altered   liver anatomy and an unknown portion of the hepatic inflow which is routed through func-
tionless intrahepatic anastomoses (Price et al.1967). The necessity of portal venous decompression requires the shunting of the
nutritional and oxygen enriched portal blood into the systemic
circulation, leaving the cirrhotic liver with an arterial inflow
through the hepatic artery only. In the presence of an end-to-
side shunt hepatic arterial blood cannot compensate for the lack
of sinusoidal perfusion and oxygen supply to the liver (Broelsch
et al. 1977) and leads to severe functional hepatic failure and
portal encephalopathy (Vorhees et al. 197o). Various shunting procedures have been developed in order to lower portal pressure as
well as to sustain portal blood perfusion of the liver tissue. The
benefit of these operations in respect to clinical requirements
is still a matter of controversy (Malt 1976) but it has to be
stated, that disturbances of intrahepatic microcirculation and
oxygen distribution evade determination by hemodynamic parameters.
However, experimental studies show the need for portal venous
blood to stimulate active regeneration of the liver tissue independent of portal venous blood flow (Starzl et al. 1973). Improve-

ment of liver regeneration has recently been reported by Gruen et
al.(1977) using a modified mesenterico-caval shunt, leaving the
liver with pancreatico-duodenal venous blood only. Whether this
effect is due to hepatotrophic hormones from the pancreatico venous
blood or due to improvement of intrahepatic sinusoidal perfusion
and oxygen supply needs to be determined. The application of the
Platinum multiwire electrode from Kessler et al.(1974) for diagnostic   determinations of microcirculatory disturbances in parenchymal organs provides a unique opportunity of measuring the
peripheral perfusion of the liver according to its oxygen supply
and its alterations under various intra- and extrahepatic circulatory disturbances. To investigate, whether an improvement in
hepatic microcirculation and oxygen supply to the hepatocytes can
be achieved by selection of a portacaval shunt procedure other than
an end-to-side portacaval shunt, we applied determinations of local
PO_2 by means of the oxygen electrode to an experimental animal
model with a liver cirrhosis.

Material and Methods

Five different types of portal blood diversion have been performed
in 50 male Lewis rats. Under light ether anesthesia the operations
were done using microvascular surgical techniques. An end-to-side
shunt was performed, shunting the entire portal inflow into the
systemic circulation. A side-to-side shunt was performed with a
large anastomosis of about 3 mm length. A modified mesenterico
caval shunt was performed suturing the portal vein at the junction
of splenic vein and mesenteric vein end-to-side into the inferior
vena cava, leaving only the pancreatico-duodenal venous inflow to
the liver. A splenocaval shunt was performed by suturing the splenic vein end-to-side to the inferior vena cava, leaving most of
the portal inflow unchanged. A portacaval transposition was performed by exchanging the total portal venous flow directly into
the inferior vena cava and leading the inferior vena cava into the
hepatic portion of the portal vein.

In each animal   liver cirrhosis was induced by oral application of
0.3 gm Thioacetamide (TAA) per l. drinking water over a period of 4
months. By means of the PO_2 electrode of Kessler the local PO_2 content was determined from the liver surface from various points of
the right lobe and lower left lobe. The measurements were performed
at the time of operation as a baseline, immediately following the
surgical procedure, 24 hours after the operation and after one week.
The data were digitally recorded on a magnetic tape and processed
by an IBM computer. The data accumulated are graphically presented
in a PO_2 histogram, which represents the frequency distribution of
PO_2 values determined from the liver surface.

Results

PO_2 values in the cirrhotic liver revealed an accumulation between
15 and 25 mmHg. The distribution pattern with 28% of the values
lower than 5 mmHg already demonstrates a slight degree of microcirculatory disturbance in some of the tissue areas. Following
end-to-side shunting, there was a striking shift to low oxygen

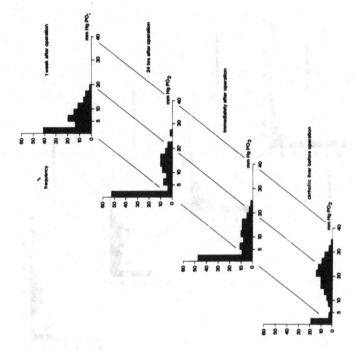

Fig. 2. Oxygen Content of the Cirrhotic Liver
Following Portacaval Side-To-Side-Shunt

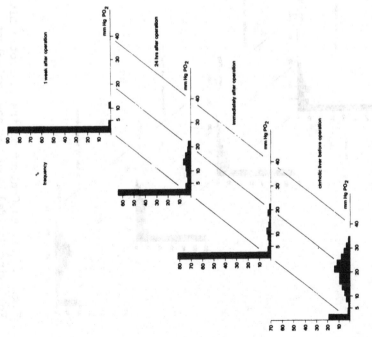

Fig. 1. Oxygen Content of the Cirrhotic Liver
Following End-To-Side Portacaval Shunt

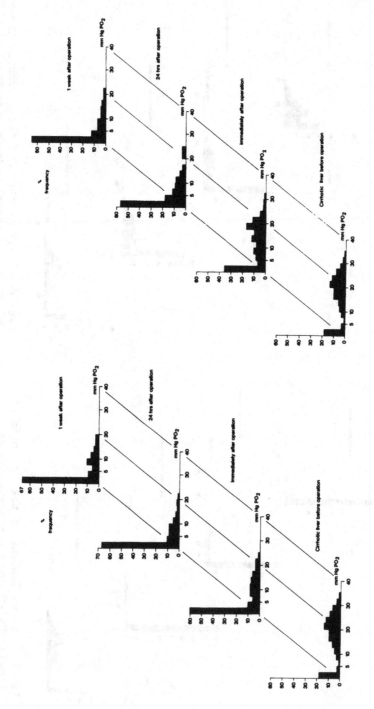

Fig. 3. Oxygen Content of the Cirrhotic Liver
Following Modifed Mesenterico-Caval-Shunt

Fig. 4. Oxygen Content of the Cirrhotic
Liver Following Spleno-Caval-Shunt

levels into the range below 5 mm Hg including 81,5% of the PO_2
values being less than 2,5 mmHg. 24 hours later only a small improvement could be observed with some peak PO_2 values between 10
and 20 mmHg. An almost anoxic stage was recorded one week after
shunting when 93% of all values were below 2.5 mmHg. After side-
to-side shunting there was only a fall of 52 % of the values into
a low PO_2 range. The distribution pattern revealed more than 34 %
PO_2 values within a normal limit. No significant alteration occured
within the first 24 hours postoperatively. After one week 49% of
the PO_2 values were above 5 mmHg indicating a sufficient oxygen
supply.

With a modified mesenterico-caval shunt (MMCS) immediately 70% of
the PO_2 values dropped to a range below 5 mmHg. But a considerable number of PO_2 values between 10 and 20 mmHg demonstrated an
improved oxygen supply to the tissue. There was no change in the
distribution pattern after 24 hours and even after one week the
portal venous blood supply coming from the pancreatico-duodenal
vein only, prevented an extreme fall of the tissue oxygen content.
Compared with the PO_2 histogram obtained after end-to-side shunting 28.4% of PO_2 values remained above 5 mmHg. The oxygen
supply following splenocaval shunting was only little changed. The
small amount of splenic blood removed from the liver circulation
did not alter the oxygen content immediately after operation. After
24 hours there was a marked drop to low oxygen levels, leaving
only 34% of the values above 5 mmHg. After one week, even in the
presence of sufficient portal blood supply, there was a lack of
oxygen. In the peripheral tissue compartments only 29% of all PO_2
values remained in an adequate range of oxygenation.

Portacaval transposition is an experimentally used method to
improve total hepatic blood flow after portal blood deprivation.
In the presence of a liver cirrhosis the peripheral local oxygen
content after this operation fell to the same low oxygen level as
was observed following end-to-side shunting. The slight attempts
at compensation after 24 hours indicated by only 17% of the PO_2
values above 5 mmHg were undetectable after one week. Despite
a large peripheral venous inflow no improvement in terms of sufficient oxygenation of the liver could be observed and no more
consideration is given to this type of portacaval shunt in the
discussion.

Discussion

Hemodynamic measurements and determinations of oxygen consumption
only reveal a 50% decrease in total hepatic blood flow (Tygstrup et
al. 1962) and almost no decrease in hepatic venous oxygen content
(Delin et al. 1977) after portacaval shunt operations. They do not
reveal more distinctive intrahepatic alterations such as critical
phases of hypoxia due to impaired microcirculation and oxygen
transport to the hepatocytes. Using direct oxygen determinations
in the liver by application of the Platinum multiwire electrode
(Broelsch et al. 1977) we have previously demonstrated that com-

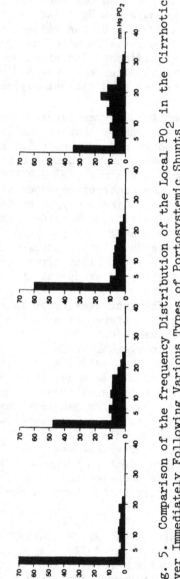

Fig. 5. Comparison of the frequency Distribution of the Local PO_2 in the Cirrhotic Liver Immediately Following Various Types of Portosystemic Shunts

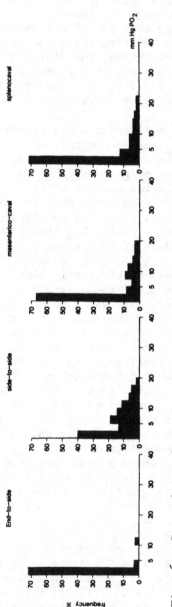

Fig. 6. Comparison of the Frequency Distribution of the Local PO_2 in the Cirrhotic Liver 7 Days Following Various Types of Portosystemic Shunts

plete diversion of portal blood from the cirrhotic rat liver leads
to a striking oxygen deficit in the liver tissue and can not be
compensated by an augmented arterial inflow. From there it seemed
reasonable to clarify the effect of other portasystemic shunt
procedures, performed to preserve portal perfusion of the liver.
Since portal blood is required for maintaining active regeneration
of the hepatocytes a sustained portal perfusion could improve
hepatocyte function and prevent postoperative hepatic failure
and other complications.
The side-to-side shunt is primarily performed to achieve hepatic
decompression in the presence of severe hepatic outflow occlusion
and reversed portal flow. However, it is performed to achieve
portal decompression and to preserve hepatic perfusion as well. In
the presence of a large vascular anastomosis and a mild hepatic
outflow occlusion it has a significant effect on maintaining sufficient oxygen supply. Total oxygen content is diminished to a
certain degree, but the follow up histogram in our experiment revealed 40.9% of the PO_2 values to be above 5 mmHG, indicating an
improved oxygenisation of the cirrhotic tissue. With a modified
mesenterico-caval shunt almost 90% of the total portal blood flow
(Liehr et al. 1976) is removed from the direct liver circulation.
However, immediately following the shunting procedures 30%
of the PO_2 values remained in a satisfactory range of tissue
oxygenisation. The most striking improvement of sufficient oxygen
supply could be demonstrated by simply shunting the splenic venous
blood into the systemic venous circulation. In this case, only 20%
of the portal inflow is removed from the liver, whereas most of
the portal blood remains for direct liver supply.
After one week following the shunt operations the microcirculatory
disturbances in our cirrhotic rat liver model became manifest as
far as they depend on the extrahepatic circulatory alterations.
We determined the oxygen supply before peritoneal and other extrahepatic collaterals could influence the liver's sinusoidal perfusion. With a side-to-side shunt, a MMCS, and a splenocaval shunt
PO_2 values in the liver tissue could be found to be convincingly
improved compared to the tissue oxygen content following end-to-
side shunting. This beneficial effect on liver oxygen supply after
side-to-side shunting may somewhat be due to our model of liver
cirrhosis and the abdominal vascular anatomy of the rat. But it
clearly demonstrates, that in the presence of an incomplete hepatic
outflow occlusion still some portal blood is perfusing the liver
directly. The almost similar effect on liver perfusion and oxygen
supply by the MMCS and the splenocaval shunt cannot be due to the
amount of portal blood supplying the liver. A vast amount is
shunted away when a MMCS is performed and only pancreatico-duodenal
venous blood directly drains into the liver. The reverse situation
in terms of blood volume supply occurs in the case of the spleno-

caval shunt. The common feature of both models is the preservation
of pancreatico-duodenal blood for the liver tissue. Since the
splenic vein drains the caudate pancreatic venous blood into the
systemic circulation in both types of shunts, only the pancreatico-
duodenal blood is accessible for the liver. If this is the case,
important hepatotrophic substances originating in the pancreas and
other gastrointestinally derived vasoactive hormones do exert
a certain stimulus on the intrahepatic blood circulation by improving the microcirculation and oxygen transport to the sinusoids
and hepatocytes and therefore need to be preserved for the liver
circulation when a portacaval shunt has to be performed. Whether
this effect is of clinical significance cannot be concluded from
our experimental model. The uniformity of the liver cirrhosis induced by TAA, the normality of the vascular anatomy, and the consistency of the surgical procedure cannot be compared with clinical
situations and exigencies. However, further experience with the
application of the PO_2 electrode in detecting microcirculatory
disturbances in liver cirrhosis, in animals as well as in patients,
may reveal some refined knowledge about alterations of intrahepatic blood perfusion and oxygen distribution before and after a
portacaval shunt operation.

Summary:

Direct measurements of local oxygen pressure by means of a platinum multiwire electrode were performed to investigate the effect of
five different portacaval shunt procedures on hepatic oxygen content in the cirrhotic rat liver. End-to-side shunt, side-to-side
shunt, mesenterico caval shunt, splenocaval shunt, and portacaval
transposition were performed and surface PO_2 was determined immediately after operation, 24 hours following operation and after
one week. Portacaval transposition and end-to-side shunt led to a
striking oxygen deficit of the liver tissue with no incidence of
compensation by the hepatic artery. Oxygen supply was improved
considerably by a side-to-side shunt and tissue hypoxia could be
prevented by a mesenterico-caval shunt and splenocaval shunt. This
improving effect is thought   to be due to the pancreatico-duodenal venous blood supply which should be carefully preserved for the liver circulation when a shunt needs to be performed.

References

Bradley, S.E., Smythe, C.M., Fitzpatrick, H.F., et al.
(1952) J. Clin. Invest. 32, 526

Broelsch, Ch.E., Strehlau, R., Boelling, B., et al.
(1977) Langenbecks Arch. Chir. Suppl. 1977, 161

Delin, N.A., Ekestrom, S., Lindahl, J. et al.
Surg., Gyn. & Obst. (1977) 144, 499

Gruen, M., Liehr, H., and Rasenach, U.
Verh. Deut. Ges. Inn. Med. (1977) 83,(in press)

Kessler, M., Hoeper, J., Schaefer, D. et al.
Klin. Anästh. Intensivth. (1974)5, 36

Liehr, H., Gruen, M., and Thiel, H.
Acta Hepato-Gastroenterolog. (1976) 23, 31

Malt,R.
New Enlg. J. Med. (1976) 295, 24

Price, J.B., Vorhees, A.B., and Britton, R.C.
Arch. Surg. (1967) 95, 843

Reynolds, T.B.
Arch. Surg. (1974) 1o8, 276

Starzl, T.E., Francavilla, A., Halgrimson, C.G. et al.
Surg., Gyn. & Obst. (1973) 137, 179

Tygstrup, N., Winkler, K., Mellemgaard, K. et al.
J. Clin. Invest. (1962) 41, 447

Vorhees, A.B., Price, J.B., Britton, R.C.
Am. J. Surg. (197o) 119, 5o1

PO$_2$ HISTOGRAMS AND EXTRACELLULAR ACTIVITY OF K$^+$ OF SKELETAL MUSCLE IN TOURNIQUET SHOCK

H. Rahmer, J. Höper, W. Heitland, J. Durst
and M. Kessler

Chirurgische Universitätsklinik Tübingen und Max-Planck-
Institut für Systemphysiologie, Dortmund, West Germany

After 4 hours of unilateral limb ischaemia rabbits develop
tourniquet shock, which is characterised by hypovolaemia, a raised
potassium level in blood and cardiac failure.   Both hypovolaemia
and accumulation of potassium indicate deterioration of the cell
membrane.   Because of the clinical importance of the tourniquet
syndrome, direct and local measurement of PO$_2$ and K$^+$ were thought
to be of interest.   Measurements of PO$_2$ histograms by means of
platinum multiwire surface electrodes (Kessler and Lübbers, 1966)
were undertaken to study tissue perfusion.   In addition extracellular activity of K$^+$ was monitored as a parameter of membrane
function with an ion selective surface electrode (Kessler, et al,
1976).

The experimental procedure was as follows:

Rabbits (n = 7) under pentobarbital anaesthesia, were subjected to a rubber tourniquet of one hind limb for 4 hours.   After a
small incision of cutis and fascia the electrodes were placed on
the surface of sartorius muscle.   Fig. 1 shows mean value measurements of PO$_2$ in five experiments.   After removal of the tourniquet
the PO$_2$ shows a fast increase in 2 experiments corresponding to the
macroscopically observed reactive hyperaemia.   Then the PO$_2$
decreases again while an interstitial oedema develops.   In 2
experiments only a slight increase of PO$_2$ is observed.   In one
experiment PO$_2$ remains near 0 showing the no reflow phenomenon
(Strock and Majno, 1969).

This finding of non homogeneous tissue perfusion is confirmed
by the histogram as shown in Fig. 2.

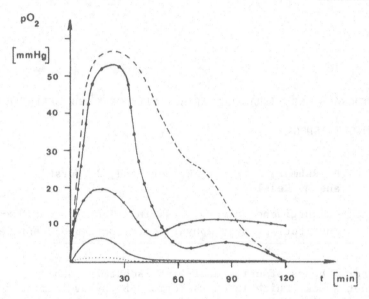

Fig. 1: This shows the mean value measurements of PO_2 in five experiments.

During the first 30 minutes of reperfusion, the PO_2 histogram is shifted to the left. In spite of the reactive hyperaemia, hypoxic and anoxic tissue areas predominate. In the following inter- val of reperfusion (up to 120 minutes), the shape of the histogram remains shifted to the left. It now reveals the developing tourni- quet shock.

Figure 3 shows the histogram of the non ischaemic muscle before and after removal of the tourniquet. PO_2 values during anaesthesia and with the tourniquet in position show the peak at 25 mmHg PO_2. The shape of the histogram is very similar to that from KUNZE (1967), obtained in non-anaesthetized humans. The general trauma of anaes- thesia and tourniquet may be responsible for more hypoxic values. Thirty minutes after removal of the tourniquet, blood pressure is still above 100 mmHg and the histogram is not changed very much. After 120 minutes, the decreasing blood pressure causes an increase of anoxic values. High values above 50 mmHg are not observed.

During four hours of ischaemia, the cellular stores of energy- rich phosphates become depleted and all energy-requiring processes come to a halt. Thus we found an increase of extracellular potas- sium activity from 5.1 ± 1.7 nM to 65.2 ± 35.1 nm during four hours of ischaemia, showing the massive efflux of potassium. It reveals changes in the biophysical properties of the membranes which cannot maintain their ionic gradients in the absence of ATP.

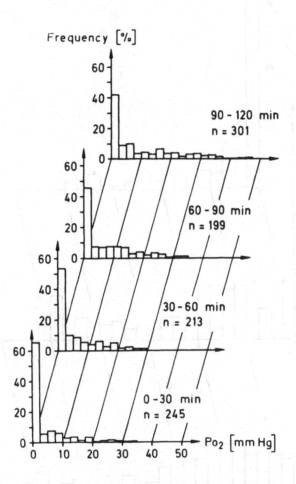

Fig.2: PO₂ histogram from skeletal muscle after 4 hours ischaemia.
It is evident that oxygenation of the muscle tissue remains
insufficient, suggesting a non homogeneous tissue perfusion.

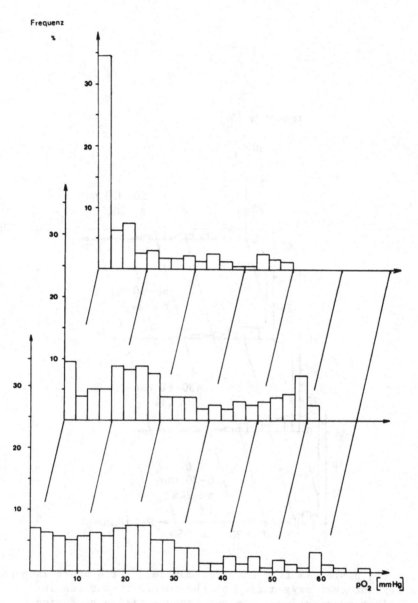

Fig. 3: PO$_2$ histogram from skeletal muscle during tourniquet:
Lower histogram - ischaemia of the contralateral limb.
Medium histogram - 30-60 minutes after removal of the contralateral
tourniquet
Upper histogram - 90-120 minutes after removal of the contralateral
tourniquet

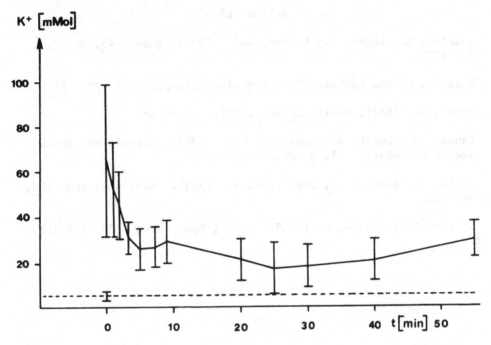

Fig. 4: Extracellular activity of potassium after 4 hours of
ischaemia. The dashed line shows the level of potassium before
ischaemia.

During reperfusion of the tissue, K^+ in muscle decreases
rapidly during the first 30 minutes, as shown in Fig. 4.

This behaviour must be attributed to the washout effect during
reactive hyperaemia. The original value could not be re-established
which confirms the exhaustion of compensatory mechanisms. During
the following shock, K^+ increased again, probably in response to
the elevated K^+ level in blood. Thus the latter flux of K^+ is of a
passive nature and accompanies, most likely, deteriorating cell
integrity. This finding is in agreement with the results of Stock
et al. (1973), who evaluated the ischaemic tolerance of rat muscle
under similar conditions and the metabolic pattern at 4 hours.

REFERENCES

Kessler, M., Höper, J., Krumme, B.A. (1976) Anaes. 45, No. 2, 184-197

Kessler, M. and Lübbers, D.W. (1966). Pflugers Arch. 291, 82.

Kunze, K. (1967), Habilitationsschrift. Giessen.

Rahmer, H., Durst, J., Schubert, G.E. (1977) Circulatory Shock (ed. A.M. Lefer), Vol. 4, No. 1, 35-40.

Stock, W., Bohn, H.J., Isselhard, W. (1973). Res. exp. med. 159, 306-320.

Strock, P.E., Majno, G. (1969) Surg., Gyn., Obst. 129, 309-318.

EFFECT OF OUABAIN ON CORTICAL POTASSIUM ACTIVITY

DURING ANOXIC DEPOLARIZATION

Eric J. Guilbeau, Daniel D. Reneau, and Charles Horton

Biomedical Engineering, Ruston, Louisiana

Louisiana Tech University, Department of

INTRODUCTION

Since the development of the ion specific liquid ion exchanger microelectrode (Walker, 1971), investigators have established that the resting potassium ion activity in the cortex of various animals (rat, cat, rabbit, guinea pig) is within the range of 2.5 mM/liter to 3.5 mM/liter (Vyskocil, et al, 1972), (Lux, et al , 1972), (Lux and Neher, 1973), (Prince, et al, 1973), (Futamachi, et al, 1973), (Mutani et al, 1973), (Morris, 1973), (Kirshner, et al, 1975), and (Dora and Zeuthen, 1975). The response of cortical potassium ion activity during hypoxia (Morris, 1974), (Kirshner, et al , 1975) and anoxia (Vyskocil, et al , 1972), (Morris, 1974), (Dora and Zeuthen, 1975) has also been well established. For the past several years our interest has been directed toward experimentally and theoretically characterizing the dynamic response of the cerebral cortex to various stimuli. These studies have been directed toward describing the response to hypoxia and anoxia in both the adult and the fetus (Guilbeau, et al , 1977), (Smith, et al , 1977), (Reneau, et al , 1977). The cortical potassium ion response to cardiac arrest (anoxia with total ischemia) is characterized by a predepolarization phase and an anoxic depolarization phase (Vyskocil, et al, 1972), (Morris, 1974), and (Dora and Zeuthen, 1975). Theoretical analyses have predicted the anoxic depolarization phase can occur following failure of the sodium potassium active transport mechanism (Reneau, 1974). Other investigators (Morris, 1974) have suggested that the potassium ion response during anoxic depolarization may be due to (a) cell membrane permeability

changes, (b) a decrease in the sodium-potassium active transport
mechanism, or (c) cell membrane permeability changes coupled with
decreased active transport of potassium.

The purpose of this investigation was to establish the
mechanism of the anoxic depolarization phase. The basic hypothesis was that the potassium response during anoxic depolarization results from decreased active transport of potassium. To
test this hypothesis, three sets of experiments were performed.
In fifteen rabbits cardiac arrest was initiated by the injection
of acetylcholine into the venous circulation. Potassium specific
liquid ion exchanger microelectrodes were used to measure the
mean time required for anoxic depolarization to occur. This
procedure was repeated in eleven additional rabbits. In these
animals, however, Ouabain was applied to the surface of the
brain one minute following the injection of acetycholine.
Ouabain specifically acts to block the sodium-potassium active
transport mechanism (Skou, 1965). Our rationale was that if it
could be shown statistically that (a) the anoxic depolarization
measured in the Ouabain experiments was of the same statistical
distribution (i.e. the same shape) as the anoxic depolarization
measured in the non-Ouabain experiments and (b) that the anoxic
depolarization in the Ouabain group occurred significantly sooner
than the anoxic depolarization in the non-Ouabain group, then
this would strongly imply that anoxic depolarization results from
the same mechanism as the potassium ion response to Ouabain,
namely the loss of sodium-potassium active transport. Finally,
if it could be shown that an increase in extracellular potassium
(like during anoxic depolarization) could be effected by simply
bathing the surface of the brain with Ouabain under normoxic
conditions (i.e. circulation normal) then this would be additional
proof that anoxic depolarization results as a consequence of
failure of the sodium-potassium active transport mechanism.

EXPERIMENTAL DESIGN

Experiments were performed on 34 New Zealand white rabbits
(12 for cardiac arrest without Ouabain, 11 for cardiac arrest
with Ouabain , 11 for Ouabain without cardiac arrest). Brain
exposure was accomplished using essentially the same procedure
as in our previous microelectrode investigations (Smith
et al., 1977) (Guilbeau, 1977).

In the experiments without Ouabain, the surgical hole was
sealed with a solution of 5% Agar in physiological saline which
had been boiled to obtain a clear solution and then cooled to
40° C. It was applied to the brain just before it jelled. This
agar controlled water and heat loss from the brain and minimized
brain movement. In the Ouabain experiments a small reservoir
was fashioned from modeling clay to hold physiological saline
which could subsequently be replaced by the Ouabain. Following

these procedures the animal was paralyzed with Flaxedil (1g/Kg)
and placed on a respirator. The animal was then shielded using
a Faraday cage, and the electrodes were placed in the upper 500
microns of the cortex with a hydraulic microdrive.

Potassium activity was measured using liquid ion-exchanger
microelectrodes (Walker, 1971). These electrodes were prepared
in the manner described by Zeuthen (Zeuthen, et al , 1974) and
exhibited similar characteristics. A Grass P-16 microelectrode
differential amplifier was used to differentially amplify the
potassium potential which was recorded on a Brush 2200 recorder.

RESULTS

Three sets of experiments were performed. In twelve rabbits
cardiac arrest was initiated by the injection of acetylcholine
into the venous circulation. In each experiment the time required
for anoxic depolarization to occur was measured. The upper curve
of Figure 1 shows a typical response. Note the presence of a
predepolarization phase and an anoxic depolarization phase.
The mean time required for the anoxic depolarization phase to
occur was calculated to be 8.3 minutes with a standard deviation
2.7 for the twelve experiments. This procedure was repeated in
eleven additional rabbits. In these animals, however, Ouabain
was applied to the surface of the brain one minute following
the injection of acetylcholine.

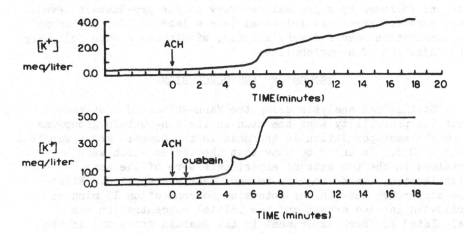

Figure 1. Potassium ion response to cardiac arrest.

The lower curve of Figure 1 shows a typical response in the
Ouabain group. In this experiment, a predepolarization phase
was also present, followed by anoxic depolarization. The anoxic
depolarization was characterized by an initial rapid increase in
potassium activity followed by a temporary decrease and a second
rapid increase. This phenonmenon was also observed in several of
the non-Ouabain responses to cardiac arrest. In the eleven
Ouabain experiments, the mean time required for anoxic depolarization to occur was reduced to 5.15 minutes with standard
deviation of 2.17.

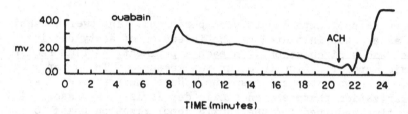

Figure 2.   Potassium ion response following Ouabain
            (flow normal).

Figure 2 shows a typical potassium ion response when Ouabain
was applied to the brain surface with flow maintained (no
cardiac arrest). Following the application of Ouabain a slight
decrease in the potassium potential was followed by a rapid
increase in extracellular potassium (like in anoxic depolarization) followed by a gradual recovery to the pre-Ouabain level.
When cardiac arrest was initiated (arrow labeled ACH) the anoxic
depolarization occurred very quickly, within one minute following
the injection of acetylcholine.

DISCUSSION AND CONCLUSIONS

Statistical analysis using the Mann-Whitney U test showed
that the probability that the mean in the non-Ouabain group was
from the same population as the mean in the Ouabain group was less
than 0.0018. In order to show that the curves which were
obtained in the two sets of experiments were of the same
distribution, the Kolmogorov-Smirnov test was applied. First
the difference between the potassium concentration 15 minutes
following cardiac arrest and the initial concentration was
calculated for each experiment in the Ouabain group and in the
non-Ouabain group. It was shown that the probability that these
two independent sets of values were from the same distribution
was 0.76. Second, the slope of the anoxic depolarization for the
Ouabain group was compared with the non-Ouabain group. The

probability that these were from the same distribution was 0.78. This statistical analysis implies that the potassium responses in the non-Ouabain and Ouabain experiments were very probably from the same distribution, but that the response occurs significantly sooner in the Ouabain group. The evidence provided by the third group of experiments that Ouabain in a normoxic animal will initiate a large increase in extra-cellular potassium ion activity coupled with the fact that (a) Ouabain specifically acts to block the sodium-potassium active transport mechanism and (b) decreases the time required for anoxic depolarization strongly implies that the failure of the sodium-potassium active transport mechanism plays a strong role in initiating anoxic depolarization.

REFERENCES

Futamachi, K., Mutani, M., and Prince, D. A. (1974) Brain Res., 75.

Guilbeau, E. J. and Reneau, D. D. (1977) Microvascular Research, 13, 241.

Kirshner, H. S., Bland, W. F., Jr., and Myers, R. E. (1975) 'Neurology' (Minneap.) 25(11).

Lux, H. D., Neher, E., and Prince, D. A. (1972) 'Pflugers Arch. Suppl.' 332, R89.

Lux, H. D., and Neher, E (1973) Brain Res., 50, 489.

Lux, H. D. and Neher, E (1973) Exp. Brain Res., 17, 190.

Morris, M. E. (1973) Can. J. Physiol. Pharmacol, 52, 372.

Mutani, R., Futamachi, K. J. and Prince, D. (1974) Brain Res., 75, 27.

Prince, D. A., Lux, H. D. and Neher, E. (1973) Brain Res., 50, 489.

Reneau, D. D. (1976) A Mathematical Analysis of Simultaneous Transport Phenomena in the Microcirculation. In 'Ion and Enzyme Electrodes in Biology and Medicine' (ed. by M. Kessler, et al).University Park Press.

Reneau, D. D., Guilbeau, E. J., and Null, R. E. (1977) Microvascular Research, 13.

Skou, J. C. (1965) Physiol. Rev. 45, 594.

Smith, R. H., Guilbeau, E. J., and Reneau, D. D. (1977)
Microvascular Research, 13, 233.

Vyskocil, F., Kriz, N. and Bures, J. (1972) Brain Res. 39, 255.

Walker, J. L. (1971) Analytical Chemistry, 43 No. 3, 89A - 93A.

Zeuthen, T., and Dora, E. (1976) Brain Metabolism and Ion
Movements in the Brain Cortex of the Rat During Anoxia. In
'Ion and Enzyme Electrodes in Biology and Medicine', p. 294,
(ed. Kessler, M., et al), Baltimore, University Park Press.

Zeuthen, T., Hiam, R. C., and Silver, I. A. (1974) Recording
of Ion Activities in the Brain. In 'Ion Selective Microelectrodes,' p. 202, (eds. H. Berman and N. Herbert).
Plenum Press, New York.

ACKNOWLEDGEMENT

This work was supported in part by NIH Grant NS-08802.

THE SIZE OF THE HYPOXIC ZONE AT THE BORDER OF AN ANOXIC REGION WITHIN THE TISSUE

U. Grossman and D.W. Lübbers

Max-Planck-Institut für Systemphysiologie

Dortmund, West Germany

To analyse the parameters which influence the state of tissue oxygenation, the anoxic zone and its volume were investigated in different tissues (Reneau et al, 1969; Blum 1960; Thews 1960). Since the critical mitochondrial oxygen pressure has been found to be rather low, the question arose whether the size of the hypoxic zone situated between normoxic and anoxic tissue has to be considered in the analysis of oxygen supply to the tissue, or whether it can be neglected.

This report describes the calculation of the width of an hypoxic zone present at the periphery of a Krogh cylinder for different kinetics of oxygen consumption.

Fig. 1 shows a drawing of the radial decrease of oxygen partial pressure (PO_2) towards the periphery of the tissue cylinder. The outer wall of the cylinder is assumed to be impermeable to oxygen, i.e. the PO_2 gradient vanishes at site R_z (see insert in Fig. 1). For PO_2 values below the critical PO_2 (p_o) a hypoxic zone develops between r_1 (PO_2 1 p_o) and R_z. To calculate the width of the zone between r_1 and R_z, Δr, we developed four models.

$$(1) \quad \frac{d^2 p(r)}{dr^2} + \frac{1}{r} \cdot \frac{dp(r)}{dr} - \frac{A}{Kp_o} \cdot p(r) = 0 \quad \text{(model I)}$$

$$(2) \quad \frac{d^2 p(r)}{dr^2} + \frac{1}{r} \cdot \frac{dp(r)}{dr} - \frac{A}{K} = 0 \quad \text{(model II)}$$

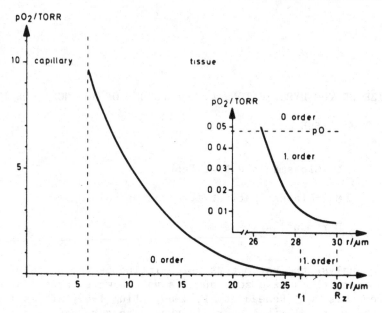

Fig. 1. Radial PO_2 decrease in a Krogh tissue cylinder
(zero and first order reaction).

$$(3) \quad \frac{d^2p(r)}{dr^2} \qquad - \frac{A}{Kp_o} \cdot p(r) = 0 \quad \text{(model III)}$$

$$(4) \quad \frac{d^2p(r)}{dr^2} \qquad - \frac{A}{K} \qquad = 0 \quad \text{(model IV)}$$

p(r) : oxygen partial pressure as a function of r

A   : oxygen consumption

K   : oxygen conductivity

p_o : critical PO_2

    Equations (1), (2), (3), (4) are the four corresponding
differential equations. Model I assumes cylindrical symmetry and
first order kinetics of oxygen consumption; model II includes
cylindrical symmetry, but kinetics of zero order. In contrast to
models I and II, models III and IV contain only a simple one-
dimensional diffusion operator. Their kinetics differ in the same
way as in models I and II. In the case of first order kinetics of
oxygen consumption p_o is the critical PO_2 value where kinetics of
zero order change to kinetics of first order.

The mathematical boundary conditions required for the solution of the differential equations are schematically drawn in Fig. 1 and explicitly given by equations (5), (6), (7).

Boundary Conditions

(5) $\quad p(r_1) = P_1 = P_0$

(6) $\quad p(R_z) = P_2$

(7) $\quad \dfrac{dp(R_z)}{dr} = 0$

Boundary condition (7) implies that the outer wall of the tissue cylinder is impermeable to oxygen.

(8) $\quad \Delta p = P_1 \cdot \left[1 - \dfrac{K_1(\lambda) \cdot I_0(\lambda) + K_0(\lambda) \cdot I_1(\lambda)}{K_1(\lambda) \cdot I_0(a\lambda) + K_0(a\lambda) \cdot I_1(\lambda)} \right]$

(9) $\quad \Delta p = \dfrac{A}{2K} R_z^2 \cdot \left[\dfrac{a^2-1}{2} - \ln a \right]$

(10) $\quad \Delta p = P_1 \cdot \left[1 - \dfrac{1}{\cosh(\lambda (1-a))} \right]$

(11) $\quad \Delta p = \dfrac{A}{2K} \cdot R_z^2 \cdot (1-a)^2$

(12) $\quad \lambda = \left[\dfrac{A}{Kp_0} \right]^{1/2} \cdot R_z$

(13) $\quad a = \dfrac{r_1}{R_z}$

(14) $\quad \Delta p = P_1 - P_2$

Equations (8), (9), (10) and (11) show the PO_2 differences obtained by the solutions of the differential equations for the different models. The equations can be used to calculate the distances Δr for given PO_2 differences (Fig. 1). To this end, values for 'a', i.e. the ratio r_1 over R_z, should be found which satisfy equations (8), (9), (10) and (11). This can readily be done with equation (11). For the other equations a solution has been found with the help of appropriate search-methods or power series expansions, respectively.

Numerical calculations using the parameters shown in Fig. 2 were carried out by computer. The calculations were done for a

critical PO_2 of 0.048 Torr.   That value corresponds to a K_M value
of 0.024 Torr (Chance et al. 1966).   In the case of first order
kinetics, the width of the hypoxic zone was obtained for a decrease
of O_2 consumption down to 10% and 1% of the maximal value.   For
the zero-order kinetics, correspondingly, a PO_2 decrease of 90% or
99% of the critical PO_2 value was assumed.

For the same kinetics, under our conditions, no distinct
differences were found between cylindrically symmetric and one-
dimensional models.   First order kinetics with a decrease to 10%
of maximal O_2 consumption resulted in a hypoxic zone of 3.85 μm in
width, and with a decrease to 1%, in a hypoxic zone of 6.78 μm.
For the corresponding models with zero-order kinetics, widths of
1.73 μm and 1.82 μm, respectively, were calculated.   With constant
O_2 consumption, the widths of the hypoxic zones differ only
marginally between the decreases to 10% and 1%.   This is due to
the fact that, in the case of constant O_2 consumption (zero-order
kinetics), the <u>difference</u> between the PO_2 values, and for first-
order kinetics, the <u>ratio</u> of the PO_2 values is decisive.   In Fig.3
the widths of the hypoxic zones are plotted against the critical
PO_2 and for decreases to both 10% and 1%.   The upper two traces
demonstrate the change of r for the first-order, the lower ones,
for the zero-order kinetics.   There is obviously a dependence on
the critical PO_2 in the case of first order kinetics.

The results obtained for zero-order kinetics are caused by the
special assumption of constant O_2 consumption down to PO_2 = zero.

Reduction of the maximal O_2 consumption with a constant
critical PO_2 increases the width of the hypoxic zone (see Fig. 4).
The volume of this zone additionally depends on the PO_2 decrease
along the capillary: a steep decrease reduces, a flat decrease
augments, the volume of the hypoxic zone.   Our results show that
within a tissue with high critical PO_2 and low maximal O_2 consump-
tions a hypoxic zone develops, the width of which has to be
considered and the volume of which depends on the PO_2 decrease in
the capillary.

data

$$V_{max} = A = 0.1 \qquad mlO_2/ml/min$$
$$K = 2.7 \times 10^{-5} \quad mlO_2/cm/min/atm$$
$$R_z = 3.0 \times 10^{-3} \quad cm$$

(Lübbers, 1973)

Fig. 2.   Parameters used for calculations.

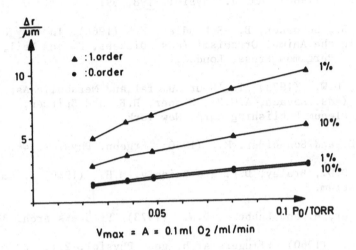

Fig. 3.   Width of the hypoxic zone vs. critical PO_2.

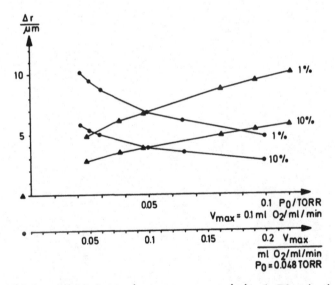

Fig. 4.   Width of the hypoxic zone vs. critical PO_2 (triangles)
and vs. maximal O_2 consumption (circles).

REFERENCES

Blum, J.J.   (1960)   Am. J. Physiol. 198, 991.

Chance, B., Schoener, B., Schindler, F.   (1966)   In 'Oxygen
Supply in the Animal Organism' (eds. Dickens, F. and Neil, E.)
p. 367.   Pergamon Press, London.

Lübbers, D.W.   (1973)   In 'Neurohumoral and Metabolic Aspects of
Injury' (eds. Kovach, A.G.B., Stoner, H.B. and Spitzer, J.J.)
p.33.   Plenum Publishing Corp. New York.

Opitz, E. and Schneider, M.   (1950)   Ergebn. Physiol. 46, 126.

Reneau, D.D., Bruley, D.F. and Knisely, M.H.   (1969) J. Am. Assoc.
Med. Instrum.

Starlinger, H. and Lübbers, D.W.   (1973)   Pflügers Arch. 341, 15.

Thews, G.   (1960)   Pflügers Arch. ges. Physiol. 271, 227.

DISCUSSION OF PAPERS IN SESSION 8

CHAIRMEN: DR. J. GROTE and DR. J. HALSEY

PAPER BY: DR. BAKER et al

Dr. Hunt: This is an intriguing and potentially valuable observation. Chronic anaemia is a real problem after severe trauma and shock in human patients. Your figures show that erythropoietin production is well below normal, even if the shock is treated by reinfusion. The known anaemia of trauma and shock may last for months. Do you have any information on the duration of depression of erythropoietin after shock?

Dr. Strauss: We have done only the short term experiments so far and have no information on the long term effects.

PAPER BY: DR. MANIL et al

Dr. Chance: Was the EEG also silent in the recovery from anoxia shown in your last slide, i.e. was there a generalised energy deficit? I ask the question because other studies in simpler models suggest complicated transients of energy metabolism during recovery from anoxia in which ATP remains low and CrP is rapidly rising (Seeley J, Radda G.K. and Chance B. unpublished observations).

Dr. Bourgain: Perhaps the first waveform in the recovery interval suggests a momentary recovery of ATP.

Dr. Leniger-Follert: We have seen a maximum increase in capillary flow in the contralateral somatomotor cortex when we stimulated the left fore paw of the cat with a frequency of 3Hz. We would, therefore, expect an increase of local tissue PO_2.

PAPER BY: DR. JI et al

Dr. Kessler: I would like to make a comment concerning extraction
of oxygen. We found that linear extraction of oxygen can be prolonged significantly by redistribution in the micro circulation
induced by infusions of norepinephrine.

Dr. Chance: 1. In your first slide, you seem to show that at the
initiation of K^+ loss there is a half maximal NAD reduction. We
would expect this result from measurements of the in vitro capacity of mitochondria to form ATP at half-maximal rate when the
NADH is half oxidized. Thus the "lag" of K^+ loss fits our
predictions.

2. Have you confirmed the heterogeneity of liver redox states
observed in our two-dimensional redox scans of freeze-trapped
liver (F_p -PN values)? Do you get different results if you move
the 80 μm light guide over the surface of the liver?

Dr. Ji: Yes, we do.

PAPER BY: DR. LASSEN

Dr. Kessler: Investigations performed with ion-selective electrodes in liver, beating heart muscle, skeletal muscle and kidney
give evidence that during the initial period of ischaemia, ion
fluxes are passing through specific channels whereas, in the later
period when massive fluxes are observed, the permeability of the
cellular membrane may be generally increased. Is the situation
in the brain comparable to that in these organs?

Dr. Lassen: We agree in principle. It is only the massive
potassium release that occurs late in ischaemia that we are led to
assume to be caused by a general permeability increase of brain
cell membranes.

Dr. Lübbers: To what level is oxygen consumption lowered in the
reduced flow area if flow falls to 10ml/100g, i.e. to a critical
flow value?

Dr. Lassen: The local PO_2 is low in the infarct with flow at the
potassium release threshold of approximately 10ml/100g/min. Histogram peaks of 3 to 4mm Hg were found. Hence, even if local
venous blood from the area still contains some 18% of oxygen, this
value is likely to represent a mixture of venous bloods with the
venous blood from the low flow area perhaps containing only 10% of
O_2 or less. We therefore conclude that one can estimate the
critical $CMRO_2$ fairly well by multiplying the ischaemia flow by the
arterial oxygen content of about 20 vol % corresponding to the
normal haemotocrit. Thus in the baboon cortex lightly anaesthetized with chloralose, control $CMRO_2$ = 60 x 1/3 x 0.20 = 4.0 ml/

$100g/min$. The critical $CMRO_2$ for K^+ release (and death?) = $10 \times 1 \times 0.20 = 2.0$ ml/$100g/min$.

PAPER BY: DR. GROOM et al

Dr. Vaupel: The results presented here concerning the intra-splenic environmental milieu agree well with the earlier results of our group. During the last few years, we have shown that in both normal and enlarged spleens of man, rabbit and rat there are no low pH values, hypoxia or glucose depletion. Therefore, these factors cannot play the important role in red cell trapping during the passage of the blood through the spleen that is suggested in many textbooks. I am happy that the results presented here by you support our previous findings.

PAPER BY: DR. HAGLIND et al

Dr. Huehns: Did you get the same results with other ways of treating shock in your experiments?

Dr. Haglind: We also tested plasma (dogs), gelatin (Haemaecel^R), dextran 70 (macrodex) and two albumins (dogs) made either by Cohns or by the PEG method. In relation to muscle oxygen tension, the gelation did not raise PO_2 above shock levels at any time during the four hours; plasma did not give any improvement either; dextran 70 raised PO_2 to control levels for at least one hour after in-fusion and maintained a moderate improvement during all four hours; albumin - PEG improved PO_2 almost to control level for the four hours, and albumin-Cohn gave a moderate improvement for one hour after infusion. I would like to point out that the method used is not to be thought of as a treatment for shock; it was merely a single infusion of plasma substitute given over a short time.

Dr. Kessler: I am surprised that your local PO_2 values, both dur-ing the control period and in shock, were so high. Under compar-able conditions we have always found a partial anoxia in the skele-tal muscle.

PAPER BY: DR. SCHÖNLEBEN et al

Dr. Goeckenjan: In clinical practice, the inspiratory oxygen con-centration is usually adjusted to a minimum value, which gives an arterial PO_2 of around 70mm Hg. Do you recommend reduction of the inspiratory oxygen concentration to hypoxic values of arterial PO_2 in order to obtain a better PO_2 histogram? What reduction of arterial PO_2 would you allow? Is there other clinical evidence that a good PO_2 histogram in tissue at a low arterial PO_2 values is more beneficial to the patient than a broader scattering of the histogram as seen with more normal arterial PO_2 values?

Dr. Schönleben: It is our intention to get both a physiological histogram and a normal arterial PO_2. Depending on the age of the patient, we tolerate for short periods values of arterial PO_2 in the lower normal range. If you have a pathological arterial PO_2, you mostly have a pathological histogram too. However, we think that the oxygen has to be applied like a drug and, therefore, it is not permissible to allow the inspiratory oxygen tension to rise in order to elevate a reasonable arterial PO_2 to a better value. With the histogram we are able to see when a dangerous "dose" of inspired oxygen is reached.

PAPER BY: DR. LUNKENHEIMER et al

Dr. Goeckenjan: What happened when you did not give dextran infusions? Did you measure cardiac output and arterial blood pressure?

Dr. Lunkenheimer: Yes, we certainly measured cardiac output. Without dextran perfusion the cardiac output decreased as much as 40 or 50%. After giving plasma expander, this was restored to 80-90% of its orginal value. However, filling up the circulation slowly with blood volume expanders is not the best way to restore venous return. We are just now combining high frequency pressure oscillation with plethysmotherapy (whole body compression). This is the most effective way to adapt the circulation to an increased intrathoracic mean pressure.

PAPER BY: DR. REVES et al

Dr. Lunkenheimer: I am not surprised by your finding of an irregular PO_2 within the myocardium after ligation of a coronary artery, but I don't follow your interpretation of the decrease in PO_2 in the vicinity of the infarcted area. We have been able to show that coronary clamping results in a distinct increase in local contraction force of the myocardium within the first ten to thirty seconds depending on the position of the force transducer relative to the clamped artery. This increase in local force can be eliminated by infiltrating the pericoronary tissue with a local anaesthetic. Thus, with clamping of the coronary artery, you probably induce a local sympathetic stimulation of the myocardium by irritating(squeezing)the nerve fibres. Your so-called "steal reaction" may be an increase in local oxygen consumption rather than a reduction in local blood supply.

Dr. Kessler: Concerning the question of a zone with high PO_2, I would like to mention investigations performed with potassium electrodes in the beating heart of a dog after occlusion of a coronary artery (in collaboration with Dr. Mecsmann of Essen).

We found different K^+ activities in different zones of ischaemic myocardium. This indicates that, depending on the amount of potassium release, there may be cells in a border zone which show depolarisation to an extent that contraction is not possible. Due to low O_2 uptake of the cells of this zone, oxygen which diffuses into it over a prolonged distance may accumulate and thus induce a zone of higher PO_2.

Tissue PO$_2$ and Cell Function

THE EFFECT OF CHRONIC HYPOXIA ON WOUND HEALING

C. W. Goodwin and R. B. Heppenstall

Departments of Surgery and Orthopedic Surgery and the
Harrison Department of Surgical Research, University
of Pennsylvania, Philadelphia, Pa. 19174 U.S.A.

In previous work, we have examined the effect of oxygen
availability on subcellular function and have established that
important oxidative reactions can adapt to changes in the oxygen environment (Mela et al, 1976). This work was extended on
the macroscopic level in a study which pointed out that a state
of moderate hypoxia resulted in decreased new bone formation and
delayed fracture healing (Heppenstall and Goodwin, 1976). In all
these studies, a state of chronic hypoxia was established by a
surgical vascular shunting procedure. This method presents certain advantages over models used by other investigators in that it
results in an unrestrained animal with normal carbon dioxide tensions and normal acid-base balance. In the present study using
this model, we examined the effects of chronic hypoxia on the
tensile strength, collagen formation, and tissue oxygen tension of
healing wounds.

METHODS

Seven adult mongrel dogs of both sexes were anesthetized with
sodium pentobarbital, 30 mg/kg, and were artificially ventilated.
Through a right thoracotomy incision the two lobes drained by the
right inferior pulmonary vein were excised. The inferior vena cava
was divided at its junction with the right atrium and was anasto-
mosed to the stump of the right inferior pulmonary vein. In addition, the azygous vein was ligated. Thus, the venous return
from the lower half of the animal was emptied directly into the
left atrium without being oxygenated. The animals tolerated the
procedure well and rapidly returned to their previous eating habits
and physical activity. In all the experiments to be described

below, one series was carried out before the shunting operation
(normoxia) and one series four weeks after the operation (hypoxia).
Therefore, each animal served as its own control.

In each series, four sterile stainless steel mesh cylinders,
2 centimeters in diameter and 5 centimeters in length, were implanted in the subcutaneous tissue of the dorsum of each dog, using
techniques previously described (Schilling et al, 1959 and Hunt et
al, 1967). At weekly intervals, fluid which had accumulated within
the chambers was aspirated aseptically and was analyzed for pO_2,
$pCO2$, and pH. At the end of the sixth week, the chambers were excised and the ingrowing tissue in the mesh was removed. The amount
of mature collagen, as reflected by hydroxyproline content, was then
measured in this tissue (Kivirikko et al, 1967). The few chambers
which became infected were eliminated from this study.

At the time of implantation of the cylinders, a standardized
7.5 centimeter long transverse skin incision was placed in the
dorsum of each dog. The edges were loosely approximated with two
stainless steel wire sutures and allowed to heal. At the end of
four weeks, the healing incision was removed for determination of
the tensile strength of the wound. The edges were attached to the
pulleys of the Instron tensometer, and breaking strength was measured directly.

Gas tensions and pH of the arterial blood and wound fluid
were determined immediately following sampling. Particular care was
given to the syringes containing the wound fluid to insure that no
air bubbles were trapped in the syringes. The measurements were
carried out on frequently calibrated commercially available gas
analyzers using standard techniques.

RESULTS AND DISCUSSION

The animals tolerated all surgical procedures, including the
shunting operation, without ill effects. Four of the 56 cylinders
became infected and were discarded; one chamber extruded. Average
arterial pO_2 preoperatively was approximately 80 torr and postoperatively was 41 torr. In the previous studies on fracture healing, all the animals undergoing the operation were kept unrestrained
on a large farm and displayed no alteration of physical activity
when compared to normal dogs. Nutrition remained unchanged, and
there was no difference in the body weights of between the normoxic
and hypoxic animals. This is particularly important because animals
made hypoxic by decreasing ambient oxygen concentration invariably
lose a major portion of normal body weight. In turn, this severe
nutritional deficit may quite well explain experimental results
found under such conditions. Finally, acid-base balance and pCO_2
remained unchanged, thus eliminating potential influences on the
results of this study.

TABLE

	PRE-SHUNT	POST-SHUNT	SIGNIFICANCE
CHAMBER pO_2 (torr)	22.9 ± 1.4	22.1 ± 1.4	N.S.
TISSUE HYDROXYPROLINE (ug/mg)	78.94 ± 5.86	41.79 ± 4.27	.01
BREAKING STRENGTH (kg-f/cm)	4.0 ± 0.5	2.4 ± 0.5	.05

Hydroxylation of proline and lysine is essential for collagen crosslinking to occur, and the necessity for molecular oxygen in this hydroxylation step has been repeatedly confirmed in the biochemical literature. In this study, mature collagen formation was markedly diminished in the hypoxic animals. Hydroxyproline content of the cylinder tissue decreased from 78.94 ± 5.86 ug/mg dry weight (± S.E.M.) in the normoxic animals to 41.79 ± 4.27 ug/mg (see Table). The means are significantly different. These data are in agreement with, but more pronounced than, those of Hunt and associates using different methods (Hunt and Pai, 1972).

The effect of arterial hypoxemia on mature collagen formation is also seen in the alteration of wound tensile strength. In the normoxic dogs, breaking strength averaged 4.0 ± 0.5 kg-f/cm, compared to 2.4 ± 0.5 kg-f/cm in the hypoxic animals. Again, the differences are statistically significant.

The most surprising data were the results of the oxygen tension in the wound chamber fluid. During the normoxic period the chamber pO_2 averaged 22.9 ± 1.4 torr and during the hypoxic period, 22.9 ± 1.4 torr. Obviously, there is no real difference between the two states. During either the normoxic or the hypoxic series, there was no systematic trend in the chamber pO_2's, and the data for each series were therefore lumped together.

The implanted cylinder method is a frequently utilized method to measure "tissue pO_2" and was used in these experiments to provide objective support to the concept that a decreased tissue level of oxygen was responsible for the defects in wound healing demonstrated

above. However, given the cylinder oxygen tensions, we can infer
either that the huge decrease in arterial pO_2 resulted in no change
in tissue oxygen supply or that the cylinder fluid tensions do not
reflect those at the cellular organelle level. The former supposition is quite unlikely, based on the other data presented here and
on the results of other methodologies (eg, oxygen microelectrodes).
On the other hand, Hunt and Pai (1972) did find a lower chamber
pO_2 using a different model of hypoxia. The control chamber oxygen tensions presented in this study are somewhat higher than the
11 to 17 torr originally reported by Hunt (Hunt et al, 1967). It
should be noted that he also reported that his experimental animals
were hypocapnic. It is therefore possible that there is some difference in the microvasculature between the two models of hypoxia
that may explain the discrepancies described above. Current investigation has been directed along those lines.

BIBLIOGRAPHY

Heppenstall, R. B. and Goodwin, C. W.   (1976) J. Bone Joint Surg.

Hunt, T. K. and Pai, M. P.   (1972) Surg. Gynecol. Obstet. 135,
561.

Hunt, T. K., Twomey, P., Zederfeldt, B., and Dunphy, J. E.   (1967)
Am. J. Surg. 114, 302.

Kivirikko, K. I., Laitinen, O., and Prockop, D. J.   (1967) Anal.
Biochem. 19, 249.

Mela, L., Goodwin, C. W., and Miller, L.D.   (1976) Am. J. Physiol.
231, 1811.

Schilling, J. A., Joel, W., and Shurley, H. M.   (1959) Surgery
46, 702.

OXYGEN AND EPIDERMAL WOUND HEALING

George D. Winter

Department of Biomedical Engineering
Institute of Orthopaedics (University of London)
Brockley Hill, Stanmore, Middlesex, England

INTRODUCTION

Healing of cutaneous wounds involves regeneration of surface epidermis and repair of connective tissues by events that are largely independent of one another. If the wound is a shallow one epidermal regeneration precedes repair in the dermis but if the injury extends the full thickness of the skin epidermal regeneration and growth of granulation tissue takes place concurrently.

In normal undamaged skin the dermis supports the epidermis mechanically and supplies it nourishment. Because the epidermis has no blood supply of its own its need for oxygen, glucose, amino-acid molecules and other metabolites are met from the dermis. These molecules diffuse through the basement membrane, a combined epidermal-dermal structure and travel in the fluid between the epidermal cells to reach the uppermost living ones in the metabolically active granular layer. If this is true for oxygen it is reasonable to expect a gradient of oxygen concentration across the epidermis and such measurements that are available confirm it. Silver (1972) reports oxygen tensions of the order of 20mm Hg at the basal layer and 7mm Hg at the surface in human forearm skin when the ambient temperature was 20°C.

Normal human epidermis and porcine epidermis have rather low oxygen permeabilities under resting conditions but a measurable fraction of the total respiratory exchange of CO_2 and O_2 takes place across the skin (Fitzgerald, 1957). The thin epidermis of mice, rats and rabbits is very permeable to oxygen and human epidermis becomes oxygen permeable if the keratin layer is stripped away. Apparently the oxygen barrier is mechanical and resides in the horny layer.

Given that human and porcine epidermis normally derives most of its oxygen from the dermis what of its situation on a wound surface when the dermal papillary layer with its rich subepidermal rete of blood vessels has been destroyed? Again we are indebted to Silver (1972) for showing that there is little oxygen available on the surface of human shallow skin wounds; measured oxygen tensions were often below 10mm Hg. The regenerating epidermis, expending energy in actively moving across the wound surface and in synthetic activities associated with making new cells is confronted with an arid, oxygen depleted, inimical environment. To make matters worse the migrating epidermal cells must compete with hosts of polymorpho-nuclear cells, macrophages and bacteria for the little oxygen available. Adapting to this altered environment the epidermal cells at the wound margins, those about to move, and this includes cells in the outer root sheaths of hair follicles too, begin to accumulate a store of glycogen. The granules can be demonstrated histo-chemically (Bradfield, 1951).

In view of the low oxygen tension on the wound surface and the observation that one of the first reactions to injury exhibited by epidermal cells is storage of the appropriate substrate it can be deduced that epidermal cells, when migrating across a wound surface, usually respire anaerobically. Support for this hypothesis comes from the work of Gibbins (1972) who showed that epidermal cell migration is inhibited by antimetabolites that block anaerobic glycolysis.

Numerous experimentalists, for more than a century past, have tried to improve the speed of wound healing with all manner of substances, to no avail. What if the epidermis were simply supplied with more oxygen, could it utilise the citric acid cycle and gain eight times more ATP? Would this increased energy production enable it to move faster and repair itself more rapidly? In other words, is the supply of oxygen the rate limiting factor in epidermal wound healing? The evidence will be reviewed.

SCAB FORMATION AND EPIDERMAL MIGRATION

The relevant observations have been made on shallow skin wounds. The base line for the study of the speed of epidermal repair is the wound exposed to the air, without a dressing, which is nature's norm, the way in which healing has evolved for land living animals. Within 24 hours the exposed dermal tissues, unprotected by an epidermis, have dehydrated to a depth of about $60\mu m$ and this desiccated tissue forms the scab together with dry blood clot, serous exudate and leucocytes. The regenerating epidermis, originating from hair follicles and the surface epidermis at the wound margins moves across the wound under the scab in an environment low in oxygen. The epidermis moves as a sheet of cells; at the moving edge the cells

roll over one another and colonise the wound surface successively
(Winter, 1962, 1964, 1972).

The speed of this migration can be measured by taking selected
serial histological sections of standard shallow wounds in young
domestic pigs at different times after wounding and measuring the
area of wound repopulated by epidermis. It is found that under a
scab, and it is the same if a cotton gauze or any similar ventilated
dressing is used, the epidermis moves one cell diameter, about 7µm,
each hour. Because cell movements do not begin until the end of the
first day by which time the scab has stabilised and because the
average distance between sources of epidermis is about 2.0mm, it is
seven days after the injury was inflicted before the entire wound
surface is covered by a new sheet of epidermis. A burst of mitotic
activity occurs in the non-migrating epidermis at the borders of the
wound and mitosis is seen in the new epidermal layer about 24 hours
after the migrating cells have implanted on the wound surface and
become static.

HYPERBARIC OXYGEN EXPERIMENTS

To investigate whether the epidermal cells can move faster if
supplied with more oxygen, Perrins and I (Winter and Perrins, 1970)
performed some experiments with hyperbaric oxygen. We chose to
study wounds at the end of the third day when under normal conditions
about 37% (37.4% $\pm$ 1.08% (S.E.); n = 26) of the surface of a
standard shallow wound is covered by new epidermis. Standard shallow
wounds were made on the backs of three young pigs which were then
treated intermittently in a 'one-man' oxygen chamber using pure
oxygen at a pressure of 7.5 lb/sq.in.(51.7kNm^{-2}), equivalent to 1.5
atmospheres absolute. The animals were in the chamber for a total
of 24 hours during the 72 hour period. It was found that an
average of 46% (45.8% $\pm$ 1.09%(S.E.); n = 18), of the wounded area
was covered by new epidermis at the end of the third day. Thus
epidermal regeneration was speeded up by about 22%. The difference
between the means of the treated and control groups was statistically
significant; t = 4.7166, p = <0.001.

A more pronounced effect was obtained when the pressure of
oxygen was doubled, (15 lb/sq.in. = 103.4 kNm^{-2}), equivalent to 2
atmospheres absolute. There was 86% more epidermis by area on the
treated wounds than the controls at the end of the third day;
(68.8% $\pm$ 1.05%(S.E.); n = 11). This is a significant difference;
t = 13.3984, p = <0.001.

It is deduced from these results that it is possible to speed
epidermal wound healing by supplying oxygen. By implication the
speed of epidermal migration on the normal wound is critically
dependent on the amount of oxygen available and this is the rate-

limiting factor. It is likely that in these hyperbaric oxygen
experiments the oxygen reached the epidermal cells directly, by
diffusion through the scab rather than via the lungs, blood plasma
and tissue fluid because it has been demonstrated that administration
of oxygen centrally is not an effective way of raising the oxygen
supply to a wound (Silver, 1969. Ehrlich et al, 1972).

OCCLUDED WOUNDS

Another way of investigating the effects of oxygen on the
speed of epidermal repair is to cover wounds with films of plastics
having widely different oxygen permeabilities and to observe the
effects on the speed of epidermal regeneration. When shallow
wounds are covered with films that restrict the loss of water
vapour from the exposed dermis, no scab forms and the superficial
fibrous tissue remains viable. Serous exudate collects on the
surface of the fibrous tissue under the dressing and the migrating
epidermis moves through this fluid layer, over the cut surface of
the dermis.

On wounds covered by thin polyester film (0.0025in., grade 0,
Melinex, I.C.I. Ltd.) having low oxygen permeability, just over
half of the total wound area was covered by new epidermis at the
end of the third day (52% $\pm$ 4.4%(S.E.); n = 19) (Winter, 1972).
Using a similar polyester film Silver (1972) found that the oxygen
tension on wound surfaces was only 4mm Hg under the epidermis and
21mm Hg above the epidermis.

When standard shallow wounds in the young domestic pig were
covered with polypropylene film (0.005in., T.R.B./5, Shorks
Metal Box Ltd.), which had 60 times greater oxygen permeability
than polyester film, 70% $\pm$ 5.1%(S.E.) (n = 7) of the wound surface
area was covered by new epidermis at the end of the third day.

Polyethylene film is highly permeable to oxygen and has a
very low water vapour permeability. When Polythene (0.0015in.,
natural grade, low density, British Cellophane Ltd.) is used to
cover standard shallow wounds the speed of epidermal movement is
increased threefold compared with that which obtains under a scab
(Polythene: 3 days, 90% $\pm$ 3.7% (S.E.); n = 12).

The differences in the speed of epidermal regeneration under
the various films are statistically significant, i.e.: polypropylene
v polyester, p = <0.005; polyethylene v polyester, p = <0.001.

The measured oxygen tensions on wounds on the human forearm
covered with polyethylene film were high; 123mm Hg above the
epidermis and 89mm Hg below it, compared with a wound with scab
formation or one covered with polyester film, confirming that

oxygen from the air had diffused through the more permeable plastics
film. A detailed study of mitosis in these shallow wounds showed
that when, as under polyethylene film, epidermal regeneration was
most rapid, there was an earlier burst of mitotic activity and more
cells entered into cell division (Winter, 1972).

The conclusions are that when wounds are covered with plastics
films preventing scab formation, the mode of epidermal regeneration
is completely altered. Under a scab the epidermis must dissolve a
pathway through bundles of collagen fibres at the interface of the
hydrated, viable dermal tissue and the overlying, dry, non-viable
scab. Under an occlusive dressing the cells move unhindered
through a moist exudate between the dressing and the wound surface.
The maintenance of hydration alone allows of more rapid epidermal
cell migration because even under polyester film there is 15% more
wound area covered by new epidermis in 72 hours. But evidently even
under these different, artificial conditions the supply of oxygen is
rate limiting because, as the data shows, the speed of regeneration
is proportional to the oxygen permeability of the plastic film
used to cover the wounds.

HYPERBARIC OXYGEN AND OCCLUDED WOUNDS

Epidermal cells under the polyethylene film moved three times
more rapidly than did the cells migrating under a scab. A
further experiment was designed to discover whether this is the
limit to which epidermis can be stimulated by oxygen or whether it
is capable of even faster regeneration. The pigs, bearing wounds
covered with polyethylene film, were put into a hyperbaric chamber.
Because over 90% of a wounded area is covered by new epidermis at
the end of the third day under polyethylene film in air at
atmospheric pressure it was appropriate in this series of
experiments to make the measurements sooner than this and so the
biopsy specimens were obtained exactly 48 hours after injury.

The mean area of wound surface covered with new epidermis in
the controls (polyethylene covered standard shallow wounds) was
$49.2\% \pm 1.05\%$ (S.E.) (n = 30) at 48 hours. When animals were
treated in the hyperbaric oxygen chamber for a total of 8 hours in
48 hours using pure oxygen at a pressure of 7.5 lb/sq.in., 53.4%
$\pm 1.17\%$ S.E. (n = 12) of the wound surface was covered by new
epidermis. The difference, + 4.2%, although small, is statistically
significant (t = 1.7588, p = <0.035). Using a pressure of 2
atmospheres absolute $79.6\% \pm 1.07\%$ S.E. (n = 5) of the wound was
covered by new epidermis at the end of the second day which
represents a 60% acceleration compared with similar wounds covered
with polyethylene film in air at atmospheric pressure. This is a
significant result; t = 10.2250, p = <0.001.

CONCLUSIONS

The conclusions are that neither the optimum rate of epidermal cell migration nor the maximum new cell production of which the epidermis is capable is expressed during normal wound healing. The reasons are that scab formation creates a physical barrier in the path of the migrating epidermal cells and damage to the superficial blood vessels causes an acute shortage of oxygen at the wound surface. The results of the various experiments reported here strongly suggest that the epidermis can utilise more oxygen if it is made available, by switching from anaerobic to aerobic metabolism of carbohydrates which results in more rapid epidermal regeneration. Nature can be improved upon by using dressings that prevent scab formation and are oxygen permeable.

REFERENCES

Bradfield, J.R. (1951) Nature, 167. 40.

Ehrlich, H.P., Grislis, G. and Hunt, T.K. (1972) Surg. 72. 578.

Fitzgerald, L.R. (1957) Physiol. Rev. 37. 325.

Gibbins, J.R. (1972) Expl. Cell Res. 71. 329.

Silver, I.A. (1969) Prog. Resp. Res. 3. 124.

Silver, I.A. (1972) Oxygen tension and epithelialization. In 'Epidermal Wound Healing' p 291 (eds. Maibach, H.I. and Rovee D.T.). Year Book Medical Publishers, Inc., Chicago.

Winter, G.D. (1962) Nature. 193. 293.

Winter, G.D. (1964) Movement of epidermal cells over the wound surface. In 'Advances in Biology of Skin' 5 p113 (eds. Montagna, W. and Billingham, R.E.). Pergamon, Oxford.

Winter, G.D. (1972) Epidermal Regeneration studied in the domestic pig. In 'Epidermal Wound Healing' p 71 (eds. Maibach, H.I. and Rovee, D.T.). Year Book Medical Publishers, Inc., Chicago.

Winter, G.D. and Perrins, D.J.D. (1970) Effects of hyperbaric oxygen treatment on epidermal regeneration. In 'Proceedings of the Fourth International Congress on Hyperbaric Medicine' p 363 (eds. Wada, J. and Iwa, T.). Igaku Shoin Ltd., Tokyo.

OXYGEN PRESSURE AND ICTAL ACTIVITY IN THE CEREBRAL CORTEX OF ARTIFICIALLY VENTILATED RATS DURING EXPOSURE TO OXYGEN HIGH PRESSURE

A. Lehmenkühler, D. Bingmann, H. Lange-Asschenfeldt[+]
and D. Berges
Physiologisches Institut der Universität, Münster, und
[+]Schiffahrtmedizinisches Institut der Marine, Kiel,
F.R.Germany

In rats breathing spontaneously, an increase in the inspiratory O_2 pressure (P_{I,O_2}) to hyperbaric values led to phasic reactions of tissue PO_2 (P_{t,O_2}) in different structures of the CNS (OGILVIE and BALENTINE, 1973; TORBATI et al., 1976). During compression, P_{t,O_2} initially rose. Then P_{t,O_2} turned over to a secondary decline. Possible mechanisms underlying this phasic PO_2 response are (i) variations of gas exchange in the lungs, (ii) changes of respiratory drive (LAMBERTSEN et al., 1953), (iii) changes of blood flow in the brain and (iv) changes of O_2-consumption in the tissue (MAYEVSKY et al., 1974). The present experiments aimed to test the question, to which extent changes of oxygen transport to tissue might contribute to the behaviour of P_{t,O_2} described above.

METHODS

The experiments were carried out on anaesthetized (40-60 mg/kg Phenobarbital), paralyzed and artificially ventilated rats weighing 400-800 g. Using a pressure regulator inside the chamber, the end inspiratory pressure remained constant above the ambient pressure under normobaric and hyperbaric conditions. The body temperature of the rats was maintained at $37\pm1^{\circ}C$ by an external heating pad. EEG was recorded with Ag/AgCl electrodes inserted into the fronto-parietal skull bone of the right hemisphere. After exposing cortical surface of the left hemisphere by a small burr hole and after slitting the dura, a double-barrelled microelectrode was inserted into the brain cortex to measure simultaneously P_{t,O_2} and local bioelectrical activity (LEHMENKÜHLER et al., 1976). The common reference electrode for the bioelectrical signals was placed

in the nasal bone. Gas exchange between the exposed cortical area
and the ambient atmosphere was widely reduced by covering the tissue with paraffin oil. Furthermore, PO_2 inside the chamber did
hardly change as the technique of artificial ventilation allowed a
compression by blowing nitrogen into the chamber. Arterial PO_2
(P_a,O_2) was measured in an arterio-venous loop by a Clark-type
oxygen electrode. Blood flow was recorded in the common carotid
artery (CCF) using an electromagnetic flowmeter. To get informa-
tions about regional cortical blood flow, cortical temperature (TC)
was registered by a thermoprobe. Furthermore, pressure, temperature
and PO_2 of the ambient atmosphere in the chamber were monitored.

RESULTS AND DISCUSSION

To understand the phasic reactions of P_t,O_2 under oxygen high
pressure (OHP), in a first series the relation between P_I,O_2 and
P_a,O_2 was investigated. The experiments demonstrated that during
artificial ventilation P_a,O_2 strictly followed P_I,O_2 in a linear
relationship up to more than 9 atmospheres (atm) as illustrated in
Fig. 1A. This relation lasted at least one hour. None the less,
after rising P_I,O_2 from 1 to 9 atm, P_t,O_2 exhibited the same phasic
reactions as found by others in spontaneously breathing animals
(Fig. 1B). The compression to 9 atm elicited an initial increase in
P_t,O_2 and a secondary decline. As shown in Fig. 1B, about 10 min
later, a further rise in P_t,O_2 was observed in parallel with the
onset of seizure discharges. As the behaviour of P_a,O_2 cannot explain the course of P_t,O_2 the question arose whether these reactions of P_t,O_2 might be due to changes in blood flow.

To analyze this question, blood flow in the common carotid artery (CCF) and cortical temperature (TC) were recorded simultaneously. In most experiments, during compression CCF increased up to
20% and remained elevated even throughout the onset of seizures
(Fig. 2). TC as well tended to rise rather than to decay, as shown
especially in Fig. 2B. The course of CCF and of TC never supported
the assumption that a marked reduction in flow causes the phasic
behaviour of P_t,O_2 following compression. As the second increase in
P_t,O_2 at the beginning of ictal activity in most experiments was
accompanied by a marked rise of TC (Fig. 1B, 2A)(c.f. BEAN et al.,
1972), one might expect that an adequate reduction of regional flow,
explaining the initial reaction of P_t,O_2, should be detected in the
TC curve. The thermoelectrical method, however, cannot exclude that
redistribution phenomena on the microcirculatory level cause this
reaction. To test the assumption that microcirculatory mechanisms
contribute to the initial phasic course of tissue PO_2, these reactions of P_t,O_2 were recorded at different ventilatory rates. Fig. 3
shows that the initial PO_2 response was prolonged in latency, reduced in steepness and amplitude, when the animal was hyperventi-
lated. Hypoventilation and the administration of a carbonic anhy-

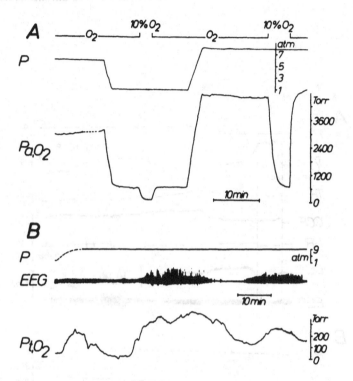

Fig. 1: A: Relation between the tracheal pressure (P), the O_2 content in the inspired gas mixture (upper line) and the arterial PO_2 (P_a,O_2). B: Reactions of tissue PO_2 (P_t,O_2) and of local EEG in the brain cortex to a rise of oxygen pressure (P) from 1 to 9 atm.

drase inhibitor (acetazolamide) elicited the opposite effects (JAMIESON and VAN DEN BRENK, 1962; BINGMANN et al., 1976).

The influence of the ventilatory rate upon the course of P_t,O_2 may also be seen in the relation between the ictal latency under OHP and the O_2-flow in the Venturi tube (Fig. 4). The graph shows that the ictal latency was prolonged with increasing hyperventilation until the generation of seizures failed. On the other hand extreme hypoventilation prevented the occurrence of seizures (c.f. CASPERS and SPECKMANN, 1972). These findings might indicate that local vaso-regulatory mechanisms markedly contribute to the phasic reactions of P_t,O_2 to OHP.

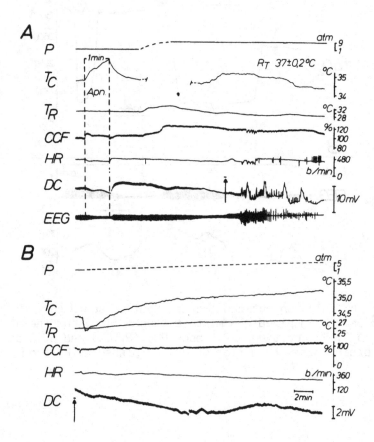

Fig. 2: A: Reactions of cortical temperature (TC) and of the common carotid blood flow (CCF) during hyperbaric oxygen exposure (P)
after a rapid compression from 1-9 atm in comparison with the reaction of these parameters to ventilatory arrest (Apn.). B: Changes
of TC and of CCF during a slow compression. TR: room temperature
inside the chamber; HR: heart rate, counted in beats per min; DC:
cortical DC-potential; EEG: electrocorticogram.

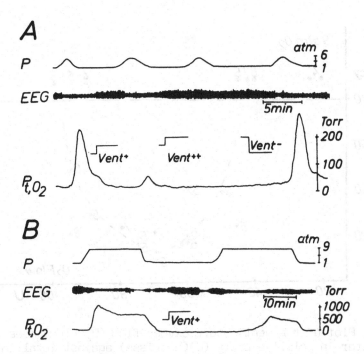

Fig. 3: Responses of tissue PO_2 (P_t,O_2) to hyperbaric exposures (P)
at different ventilatory rates (Vent.). Shortlasting exposures to
6 atm are demonstrated in A. Longlasting exposures to 9 atm are
shown in B. Note the different time scales in A and B.

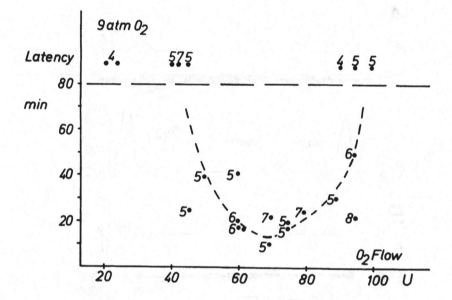

Fig. 4: Plot of the ventilatory oxygen flow (O_2 Flow) measured by a rotameter in relative units (U)(abscissa) against ictal latency (ordinate), which was determined from the beginning of compression to the onset of seizure activity. The figures in the graph denote the weight of the rats in 100 g values. The values above the broken line represent data of animals without seizures.

Provided that the poisoning effect of oxygen in CNS is a function of tissue PO_2, the course of P_t,O_2 in the brain cortex cannot explain the onset of seizure discharges, as ictal activity in some experiments preceded the reincrease of P_t,O_2. From literature, however, it is known that under OHP subcortical seizures precede ictal activity in the cortex (c.f. ZOLL, 1968). Furthermore, TORBATI et al. (1976) have observed different courses of tissue PO_2 in cortical and subcortical structures. Therefore, it is likely that cortical seizures under OHP are triggered by subcortical structures where protective mechanisms against excessive tissue PO_2 values might be exhausted earlier than in the brain cortex.

REFERENCES

Bean, J.W., Lignell, J. and Burgess, D.W. (1972) J. Appl. Physiol. 32, 650.

Bingmann, D., Lehmenkühler, A., Lange-Asschenfeldt, H. and Berges, D. (1976) Pflügers Arch. 362, R 16.

Caspers, H., Speckmann, E.-J. (1972) Epilepsia 13, 699.

Jamieson, D. and van den Brenk, H.A.S. (1963) J. Appl. Physiol. 32, 869.

Lambertsen, C.J., Kough, R.H., Cooper, D.Y., Emmel, G.L., Loeschcke, H.H. and Schmidt, C.F. (1953) J. Appl. Physiol. 5, 471.

Lehmenkühler, A., Caspers, H. and Speckmann, E.J. (1976) A method for simultaneous measurements of bioelectric activity and local tissue PO_2 in the CNS. In "Oxygen Transport to Tissue - II." Advances in Experimental Medicine and Biology, Vol. 75 p. 3 (eds. Grote, J., Reneau, D. and Thews, G.). Plenum Press, New York.

Mayevsky, A., Jamieson, D. and Chance, B. (1974) Brain Res. 76, 481.

Ogilvie, R.W. and Balentine, J.D. (1973) Oxygen tensions in the deep grey matter of rats exposed to hyperbaric oxygen. In "Oxygen Transport to Tissue." Advances in Experimental Medicine and Biology, Vol. 37A, p. 299 (eds. Bicher, H. and Bruley, D.).Plenum Press, New York.

Torbati, D., Parolla, D. and Lavy, S. (1976) Exp. Neurol. 50, 439.

Zoll, W.R. (1968) Dissertation, Univ. Münster, F.R.Germany.

SIMULTANEOUS MEASUREMENT OF PO_2 AND FLOW AT THE SAME LOCUS DURING SEIZURES AND BARBITURATE SUPPRESSION OF EEG

R. S. McFarland, J. H. Halsey, Jr., and D. D. Reneau

University of Alabama Medical Center

Birmingham, Alabama 35294, U.S.A.

This is a progress report of our effort to measure local blood flow by the hydrogen clearance method and PO_2 at the same point in tissue with the objective of gaining information about oxygen consumption rate. In initial trials we followed Lübber's example that platinum electrodes polarized at -600 mV were responsive to both O_2 and H_2. We have found that bare palladium works equally well. This method has the effect of superimposing a H_2 saturation and clearance curve on the PO_2 as a baseline. While this is satisfactory in such organs as the carotid body where flow is extremely fast, in the brain, particularly in the presence of ishemic injury, a 10 to 20 minute H_2 clearance is difficult to define accurately because of lack of constancy of the PO_2 baseline.

The second approach has been to switch the polarity of the electrodes from +200 mV when it is relatively selectively sensitive to hydrogen to -600 mV when it is relatively selectively sensitive to oxygen. A palladinized palladium electrode was found to have this character. Initial attempts with this method were frustrated by the relatively long time required after initially applying the polarization voltage to obtain a stable H_2 oxidation or O_2 reduction current.

The final development, which we describe here, has been to utilize automatic short constant interval switching of polarization voltage at approximately 30 second intervals. A one second short circuit between recording electrode and Ag-AgCl reference was placed between the two polarization voltages to eliminate whatever contribution to polarization artifact might be due to capacitance of the electrode. Despite this a substantial artifact remained, consisting of an initially high but rapidly declining current which after

several minutes would asymptotically approach a stable level.
Part of this we believe is due to establishment of the diffusion
field around the electrode, as described elsewhere in this symposium
by Dr. Erdmann. The H_2 and O_2 measurements were taken as the current
levels just prior to the voltage switch, as shown in figure 1. The
effect of this recording method is to add a constant artifact to the
PO_2 level. This can be approximately calibrated _invivo_ by comparing
it with the true PO_2 level when the electrode was continuously
polarized while the animal was in the same steady state physiologic
condition. Calibration of the PH_2 level was not necessary since the
flow calculation depends only on the rate of H_2 clearance, assuming
only that the electrode sensitivity and diffusion rate do not change
during the duration of the H_2 saturation and clearance curve.

Experiments were performed in cerebral cortex of 7 gerbils.
The electrodes used in these experiments were slightly recessed-tip
25 micron diameter palladinized palladium insulated in glass. The
animals were paralyzed and ventilated. EEG was continuously monitored by scalp electrodes. Rectal temperature was monitored and
maintained at 37° C. with a heat lamp. The brain metabolism was
alternately stimulated to produce continuous epileptic EEG discharge
with Pentylene Tetrazole, and suppressed with deep barbiturate anesthesia.

During pentobarbital-induced EEG silence, the mean cortical
PO_2 was 14.2 mm Hg, and the flow 23.3 cc/100 gm/min. During seizure
activity the PO_2 was 20.6 mm Hg and the flow 50.3 cc/100 gm/min.
These PO_2 and flow differences between barbiturate suppression and
seizures were highly significant ($p < .001$). The measurements
demonstrate that tissue hypoxia not only does not occur as a
consequence of epileptic seizure activity, but the PO_2 is actually
increased if arterial PO_2 is maintained, due to the associated flow
increase. A typical experiment is illustrated in figure 2.

Based on the Krogh cylinder geometry of the micro-circulation,
a distributed parameter mathematical model equation has been used to
enable computations of quantitative changes in O_2 consumption rate.
The model accounts for capillary blood flow non-linear release of
oxygen from oxyhemoglobin as blood flows through the capillary, the
diffusion of O_2 throughout the tissue region, and homogenous metabolic consumption of all tissue sites. Following standardization of
all circulatory, diffusional, and metabolic parameters for normal
conditions, the model was used to determine changes in metabolism
during seizure and depression by using the experimentally measured
values for local flow and tissue PO_2 . Oxygen metabolism was
predicted to decrease to approximately 70% of normal for cases of
severe barbiturate anesthesia but was found to increase as much as
1.5 to 3.0 times greater than normal for epileptic activity. The
increased rate of oxygen delivery was greater than the increased

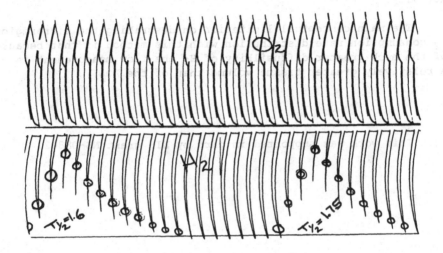

Fig. 1

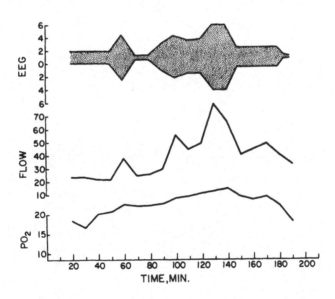

Fig. 2

demand for oxygen, accounting for the increased PO_2 during seizure activity.

The main conceptual limitation on describing the microregional O_2 consumption rate distribution with this method is that because of the much greater diffusilbity of H_2 the flow measurement is of a relatively greater tissue volume than of the PO_2.

This work was supported in part by NIH grant NS-08802.

THE SENSITIVITY OF APLYSIA GIANT NEURONS TO CHANGES IN EXTRACELLULAR AND INTRACELLULAR PO$_2$

Chun-fan Chen, Wilhelm Erdmann, and James H. Halsey

Department of Biological Sciences, Florida International University, Miami, Florida; Departments of Anesthesiology and Neurology, University of Alabama, Birmingham, Alabama

INTRODUCTION

The effects of oxygen on the excitability of neurons have been studied in various groups of animals (Chalazonitis and Sugaya, 1958; Eccles et al, 1966; Chalazonitis, 1968; Kerkut and York, 1969; Steefin, 1975). However, the difficulty in recording intracellular PO$_2$ (I·PO$_2$) has prevented gathering of essential information concerning the effects of I·PO$_2$ on oxidative processes and on the bioelectric phenomena of neurons. Since many giant neurons in the Aplysia abdominal ganglion are easily identifiable, stable for several days and can be penetrated with newly improved PO$_2$ microelectrodes, we have employed them in a study of neuronal oxygen sensitivity. Chalazonitis has shown the effects of oxygen on the properties of the neuronal membrane in Aplysia by recording simultaneously, their bioelectrical properties and their I·PO$_2$ by spectrophotometry. In the present study, we have confirmed his results of hypoxic effects on change in membrane potential and spontaneous activity. In addition, our observations reveal oxygen profiles in Aplysia neurons by recording extracellular PO$_2$ (E·PO$_2$) and I·PO$_2$ from very small points at various depths in the cell. This allows us to correlate more closely the local oxygen level, metabolic processes and active pump with the bioelectric activities of the neurons.

METHODS

Specimens of the opisthobranch mollusc, <u>Aplysia</u>
<u>californica</u>, were maintained in a well-aerated aquarium
containing artificial sea water.   The abdominal ganglion
dissected from the animal was pinned to a recording
chamber filled with saline.   Identification of individual neurons employed the criteria and nomenclature of
Frazier et al (1967).

KCl-filled glass microelectrodes with a resistance
of 1-10 $\mu\Omega$ were used for recording bioelectric function.
The recording and reference Ag-AgCl electrodes were connected through a high impedance electrometer (WPI M4-A)
to a Mark 220 penwriter.   Both $E \cdot PO_2$ and $I \cdot PO_2$ were recorded polarographically by employing gold PO_2 microelectrodes with tip diameters of 1 μ and resistances of
100 MΩ to 1000 MΩ. PO_2 electrodes were constructed by
stripping the initial 20-200 μ glass coat from gold-
glass wires with 10 μ diameter and then electrochemically
etching the tips to less than 1 μ in diameters with
tapering suitable for recordings at various depths (Fig.
1).   Each etched tip was cleaned and coated with 5-7
layers of Insul-X and Epoxylite, resulting in a high
impedance electrode.   Some PO_2 microelectrodes required
a final coat of collodion to minimize erratic electrode
response.   Only the electrodes with oxygen sensitive
areas of less than 10 μ from the tip were selected for
recording to minimize the effects of depth recording.
The gold PO_2 electrode was polarized with -700 mV against
the reference Ag-AgCl anode and connected via a polarographic oxygen sensor to a penwriter for recording PO_2.
The $I \cdot PO_2$ was recorded by inserting both the gold PO_2
microelectrode and the reference KCl filled glass microelectrode into the neuron to avoid interference of the
applied voltage with neuronal electric potential.

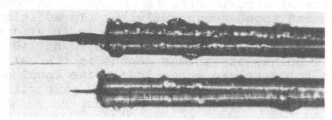

Fig. 1.   Gold PO_2 microelectrodes with various shapes
for different depth recordings.   1000X.

RESULTS

Oxygen Profiles. The PO_2 recorded from the chamber containing stagnate saline and the abdominal ganglion showed a typical PO_2 profile. When the PO_2 microelectrode was lowered from the bath surface toward the ganglion, a marked reduction from 150 to 40 mmHg in PO_2 was recorded in the vicinity of the ganglion. As the electrode penetrated the neuronal membrane, PO_2 rapidly dropped to approximately 10-15 mmHg and then leveled off at 0.5-1 mmHg deep in the neuron. Once the electrode penetrated the entire neuron and entered the extracellular space in the core of the ganglion, PO_2 increased by a few mmHg. Withdrawal of the electrode revealed a similar oxygen profile.

Oxygen Dependent Bioelectric Parameters. In the majority of silent neurons examined, increasing PO_2 hyperpolarized the membrane potential (MP) while decreasing PO_2 caused depolarization. Raising the I·PO_2 from 3 mmHg to 15 mmHg in the silent neuron R2 with an initial MP of -52 mV, induced hyperpolarization of 6 mV. Lowering I·PO_2 below 3 mmHg frequently depolarized the MP beyond the firing level and induced spike activity for a short period of time. Prolonged hypoxic condition led to a gradual repolarization, suggesting a strong adaptability of Aplysia neurons to hypoxia.

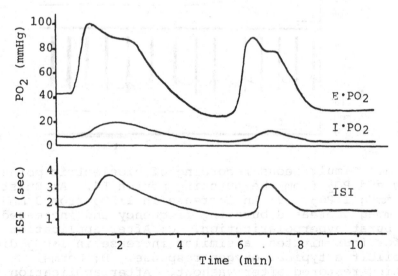

Fig. 2. Simultaneous recording of extracellular PO_2 (E·PO_2), intracellular PO_2 (I·PO_2) and spikes from R6.

Many beating pacemaker neurons (R3-R8) spontaneously discharge spikes at a regular rate under a constant environment. However, the discharge rate and
pattern are also oxygen dependent. Hyperoxia hyperpolarized the MP and flattened the pacemaker potential

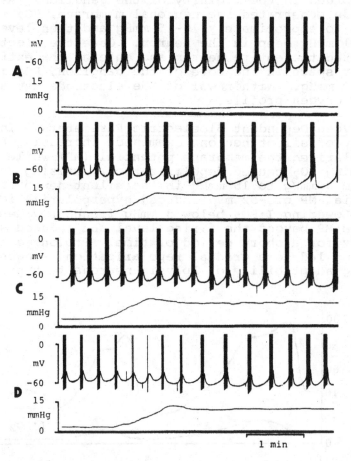

Fig. 3. Simultaneous recording of bioelectric potentials and PO_2 from the bursting neuron L4. A: Bursting
at 3 mmHg I·PO_2. B: An increase in I·PO_2 from 3 mmHg
to 13 mmHg decreased bursting frequency and increased
post-burst hyperpolarization. C: After application of
DNP for four minutes, a similar increase in I·PO_2 did
not elicit a typical oxygen response. D: Normal
bursting restored after washout. After application
of ouabain for four minutes, typical oxygen response
diminished.

thus decreasing the firing frequency in beating
neurons. Hypoxia led to the opposite effects. Fig. 2
shows the simultaneous recording of E·PO$_2$, I·PO$_2$ and
bioelectric activity from a beating neuron R6. The
firing frequency expressed in terms of inter-spike
intervals (ISI) corresponded better to the changes in
I·PO$_2$ than in E·PO$_2$. Consequently, attempts were made
to correlate I·PO$_2$ to bioelectric parameters. Many
unidentifiable beating neurons were found to be very
sensitive to changes in PO$_2$. Increasing I·PO$_2$ from 5
to 18 mmHg completely abolished their spike activities
within 3 minutes. In the bursting neurons (L2-4, L6,
R15), hyperoxia decreased burst frequency, increased
post-burst hyperpolarization and flattened inter-burst
pacemaker potential (Fig. 3).

        Oxygen Dependent Electrogenic Pump. The above-
mentioned changes in oxygen induced bioelectric
potential were decreased by the treatment of neurons
with metabolic blockers such as 2-4-dinitrophenol
(DNP 10^{-4}M) or ouabain (4 x 10^{-4}). After treatment of
neurons with DNP or ouabain for 4 minutes, typical
oxygen responses such as hyperoxic hyperpolarization,
post-burst hyperpolarization and increased spike interval, started to diminish. Complete abolition of
oxygen responses required at least 20 minutes of DNP
or ouabain treatment (Fig. 3).

                        DISCUSSION

        The results of these experiments show that bio-
electric responses to changes in PO$_2$ correspond better
to the I·PO$_2$ where the oxygen is actually utilized than
to the E·PO$_2$ where the oxygen has to diffuse into the
cell for oxidative metabolism. It is possible that the
mitochondrial activity is higher near the inner neuromembrane than deep in the neuron since the rate of oxygen decrease is higher in the former.

        Increase in the I·PO$_2$ hyperpolarizes membrane
potential, enhances post-spike and post-burst hyperpolarization and flattens pacemaker potential, thus
decreasing the excitability of the neurons. It is of
special interest that these oxygen responses can be
abolished by metabolic blockers, DNP and ouabain. DNP
is known to uncouple oxidative phosphorylation and consequently prevents   synthesis   of ATP. Ouabain is a
Na$^+$-K$^+$ membrane ATPase inhibitor and thus blocks ATP
hydrolysis.Both DNP and ouabain affect cellular energy
levels.

In many <u>Aplysia</u> neurons, the active Na^+-K^+ transport system which requires ATP, pumps more Na^+ out than K^+ in (Carpenter and Alving, 1969; Pinsker and Kandel, 1969; Carpenter, 1973; Cooke, 1974). This excessive outflow of Na^+ causes membrane hyperpolarization which is called the electrogenic pump. Blockage of the Na^+-K^+-ATPase suppresses energy supply for the active transport of these ions. The contribution of the electrogenic Na^+-K^+ pump to the membrane potential is therefore dependent on the availability of oxygen in the neurons. Hypoxia impedes the process of oxidative phosphorylation, thus depleting ATP for the electrogenic pump and results in membrane depolarization. The magnitude of the hypoxic depolarization varies in different <u>Aplysia</u> neurons. However, irrespective of firing patterns, silent, beating, and bursting neurons all show oxygen responses to some extent. The different oxygen sensitivities in different neurons may well be related to the size of their electrogenic pump.

Obviously, our study leaves many questions still open. Further tests are needed to clarify the availability of ATP, the precise rate of ATP hydrolysis, substrate phosphorylation and other oxidative metabolic processes.

REFERENCES

Carpenter, D. O. (1973) in Symposium Neurobiol. Invert., Tihany pp. 35.

Carpenter, D. O. and Alving, B. O. (1968) J. Gen. physiol. 52:1.

Chalazonitis, N. (1968) Ann. N. Y. Acad. Sci. 147: 421.

Chalazonitis, N. and Sugaya, E. (1958) C. R. Acad. Sci. 247:1495.

Cooke, I. K. <u>et al</u>. (1974) Nature 251:254.

Eccles, R. M. <u>et al</u>. (1966) J. Neurophysiol. 29:315.

Frazier, W. T. <u>et al</u>. (1967) J. Neurophysiology 30:1288.

Kerkut, G. A. and York, B. (1969) Comp. Biochem. Physiol. 28:1125.

Pinsker, H. and Kandel, E. R. (1969) Science 163:931.

Steefin, M. (1975) Comp. Biochem. Physiol. 52A:691.

OXYGEN DIFFUSION, CONDUCTIVITY AND SOLUBILITY COEFFICIENTS IN THE MICROAREA OF THE BRAIN
(Measurements with Noble Metal Microelectrodes)

Clark, D.K., Erdmann, W., Halsey, J.H., Strong, E.

Departments of Anesthesiology and Neurology
University of Alabama in Birmingham
Birmingham, Alabama 35294, U.S.A.

Oxygen transport to the cells occurs in three major steps: Oxygen uptake in the lungs, oxygen transport via the blood and oxygen diffusion from blood to tissue. So far, oxygen diffusion in tissue could only be determined indirectly by using slices of tissue on thin layers of medium taken out of their context. It had been assumed that these tissues had the same characteristics for oxygen diffusion as normal tissue. It had not been taken into account that the diffusion coefficient of oxygen very much depends on the constitution of the medium, the protein concentration, the size of intercellular space and the density of cellular net work.

The development of oxygen microelectrodes (Silver, 1965) made the studies of oxygen supply mechanisms accessible in the microarea. However, oxygen diffusion parameters have merely been subject to biomathematical consideration based on rather indirect measurements since the works of Krogh (1918/19), Kreuzer (1950, 1970), Niesel and Thews (1959), and Thews (1960) e.g.

A recently developed microelectrode system for direct measurement of oxygen diffusion (DO_2) and oxygen conductivity (KO_2) coefficients (Erdmann & Krell, 1976) has been employed for determination of DO_2, KO_2, and solubility coefficient ($\alpha\, O_2$) in the different layers of the mammalian brain in gerbils.

METHODS

Mongolian gerbils of 70 gm body weight were anesthetized by intraperitoneal injection of 6 mg sodium pentobarbital. Injection of barbital was repeated with 1 mg during the procedure as needed. The

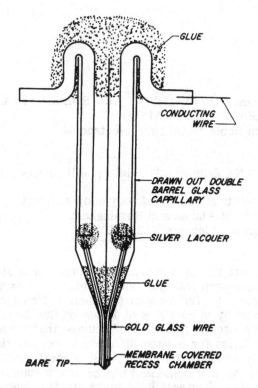

FIGURE 1: Schematic of double barrelled microelectrode for oxygen diffusion and oxygen conductivity measurements in the tissue.

gerbil was positioned on a heating mattress feedback controlled to a body temperature of 37° C.

The skull bone was prepared free and fenestrated on both sides above the frontal brain by 2 x 2 mm. The head of the gerbil was fixed in a stereotactic micromanipulator system and the electrodes inserted into the tissue through small incisions in the dura. Measurements of PO_2 and KO_2 were performed at the brain surface, in steps of 50 μ down to a depth of 1000 μ and at 1500 μ depth in the white matter of the brain.

Electrode System: The measuring device consists of a double barrelled O_2 microelectrode: A bare O_2 concentration measuring electrode and a membrane covered recessed tip PO_2 measuring electrode. (Figure 1)

Glass covered gold wires of 10 μ in diameter are connected to a conducting wire by means of silver lacqer. For production of the recessed electrode tip, the gold glass conducting wire system is

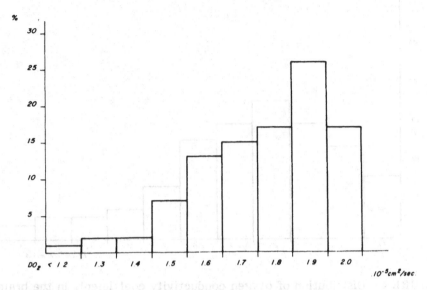

FIGURE 2: Distribution of oxygen diffusion coefficients in the brain. A peak in distribution is between 1.8 and $1.9 \cdot 10^{-5}$ cm^2/sec.

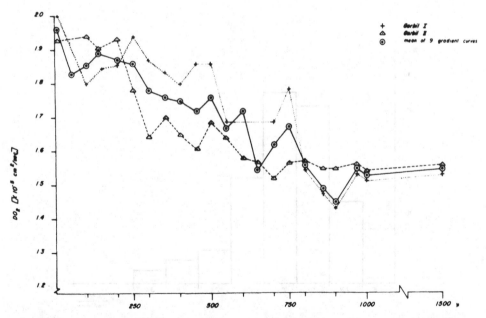

FIGURE 3: Oxygen diffusion coefficient in different layers of the brain. The PO$_2$ in the white matter is decisively lower than in the grey matter.

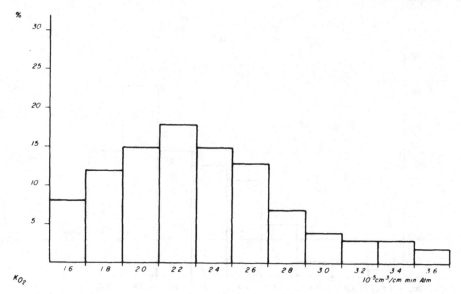

FIGURE 4: Distribution of oxygen conductivity coefficients in the brain of mongolian gerbils with a peak between 2.3 and 2.4 • 10^{-5} cm^2 O$_2$/ cm min.

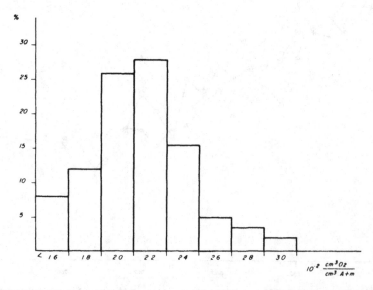

FIGURE 5: Distribution of oxygen solubility coefficients in the brain of mongolian gerbils calculated out of PO$_2$ and KO$_2$.

connected to a 9 volt battery supplied electric circuit and introduced into HCl The HCl is vibrating as it is positioned on a loud speaker. A horizontally adjusted microscope permits control of the recessed chamber size. After this process, the recessed microelectrode tips are kept in distilled water for 2 hours to permit trapped HCl to diffuse out of the recessed chambers. The electrode tip is then inserted into Rhoplex solution for 5 hrs. to allow it to fill the recessed chamber. An eight hour drying period of the electrode tip follows whereafter the membrane covered tip is soaked in 0.2 molar KCl solution until tested in the polarographic circuit in 25% albumin at 150 mmHg compared to 0.2 molar KCl at 150 mmHg. Only electrode tips which proved to measure the same current in both solutions were used for the further process.

A membrane covered and a bare electrode are inserted into a double barrelled drawn out glass capillary. Both electrode tips protrude with the same length and a drop of glue is brought to the opening of the glass capillary meticulously gluing the two tips together to abolish the possibility that one of the electrode tips might be covered with glue. The conducting wires at the other side of the double barrelled glass capillary are bent along the glass capillaries and glued.

A circuit breaker is introduced into the polarographic circuit which disconnects the bare gold microelectrode from the polarization voltage while grounding it to the indifferent electrodes. After reapplication of the polarization voltage, the diffusion (DO_2) determined curve is recorded.

Determination of DO_2: the hyperbollic function was taken for mathematical analysis of the time course of the adjustment curve: $Y = \frac{a}{x} + b$ (x = time passed from the beginning of the curve, Y = current values registered). b can be calculated according to: $b = \frac{X1\,Y1 - X2\,Y2}{X1 - X2}$.

Starting at 0.25 sec. after closure of the circuit six Y values were read from the diffusion curve in intervals of 0.25 sec.

Thus, $\overline{b} = \frac{X1\,Y1 - X6\,Y6}{5\,(X1-X2)}$

a can be calculated with known b according to:

$a = (y - \overline{b}) \cdot X$

Thus, $\overline{a}$ can be calculated as:

$\overline{a} = \frac{X1\,Y1 + X2\,Y2 + \text{through} + X6\,Y6 - 5.25 \times b}{6}$

For calculation of the unknown DO_2 of a medium $\overline{a}$ is measured in 0.2 molar KCl with $DO_2 = 2.0 \times 10^{-5}$ cm^2/sec (Goldstick, 1966). $\overline{a}$ of the medium with unknown DO_2 is measured and DO_2 is calculated according:

$DO_2 = \frac{2.0 \times 10^{-5}}{\overline{a}\,(0.2\ \text{mol. KCl})} \times \overline{a}\ (\text{medium})$

Determination of KO_2: Bare and membrane covered electrode tip are calibrated in a 0.2 molar KCl concentration with known KO_2 of 3.7×10^{-5} cm^3 O_2/cm x min x Atm and the output voltage of the two amplifiers is adjusted to the same value. At a constant partial pressure the registered current of a bare noble metal electrode is proportional to the KO_2 of the investigated medium. Thus, the KO_2 of the medium with unknown diffusion parameters can be determined according to the equation

$$KO_2 \text{ (medium)} = \frac{KO_2 \text{ (0.2 mol. KCl)}}{\bar{b} \text{ (0.2 mol. KCl)}} \text{ x } \bar{b} \text{ (medium)}$$

* if PO_2 is constant

(b = registered current). If the PO_2 of the medium in which the KO_2 is to be determined does not correspond to the PO_2 during the calibration process correction has to be introduced according to the quotient of PO_2 during calibration and actual PO_2 in the investigated medium which is recorded with the membrane covered PO_2 measuring electrode. The KO_2 of the medium to be analyzed is thus calculated accordingly by:

$$KO_2 \text{ (medium)} = \frac{KO_2 \text{ (0.2 mol KCl)}}{\bar{b} \text{ (0.2 mol KCl)}} \text{ x } \bar{b} \text{ (medium) x } \frac{\text{cal } PO_2}{PO_2 \text{ (medium)}}$$

*cal PO_2 = PO_2 during calibration

In order to get correct values, main emphasis has to be put on:

1)   Exact partial pressure measuring membrane covered electrode tip

2)   Calibration has to be performed in a temperaturized calibration chamber (37° C.).

If DO_2 and KO_2 are known, the solubility coefficient α can be calculated according to:

$$\alpha O_2 = \frac{KO_2}{DO_2 \text{ x } 60}$$

RESULTS

The oxygen diffusion coefficient in the brain tissue of gerbils shows steep gradients with a range between 1.2 and 2.0 x 10^{-5} cm^2/sec. The peak distribution is found between 1.8 and 1.9 x 10^{-5} cm^2/sec. During insertion of the electrodes into the tissue from the surface, low diffusion coefficients might be registered in the region of the dura. The values in the cortex are rather high and decrease slowly towards deeper regions. At depths between 400 and 800 μ a sudden drop of the oxygen diffusion coefficient is seen and stays then at this lower level of DO_2 (Figure 3).

The respective KO_2 values were ranging from 1.6 x 10^{-5} to 3.3 x 10^{-}

5 cm^3 O$_2$/ cm min. Atm, with a peak distribution between 2.3 and 2.4·10$^-$ 5 cm^3 O$_2$/cm min. Atm. Significant differences of KO$_2$ values in more superficial parts of the brain tissue (brain cortex) as compared to the KO$_2$ values in the deeper parts of the brain (white matter) could so far not be stated. (Figure 4)

The oxygen solubility coefficient ranged from 1.5 to 3.0·10^{-2} cm^3 O$_2$/cm^3 Atm. More than 50% of the values were between 1.8 and 2.2·10^{-2} cm^3 O$_2$/ cm^3 Atm. (Figure 5)

An attempt to prove a correlation of DO$_2$, KO$_2$ and αO$_2$ to the local PO$_2$ was not significant.

DISCUSSION

The described experiments have shown that the brain tissue has inhomogenous gradient pattern of oxygen diffusion coefficients, oxygen conductivity coefficients and oxygen solubility coefficients. Thus, the assumption of homogenous distribution of these values in the brain tissue which was the basis for biomathematical modeling of the brain O$_2$ supply is questionable. The diffusion coefficient in the brain cortex are higher than in the white matter of the brain and significantly above the oxygen diffusion coefficient so far assumed (DO$_2$ = 1.7 x 10^{-5} cm^2/sec, Thews, 1960). For the white matter of the brain, however, this so far assumed oxygen diffusion coefficient value seems to be in the right range.

The KO$_2$ values showed a broad range but could not be correlated to the area (grey matter vs white matter) in which they were measured. The average value was a little lower than so far assumed (KO$_2$ = 2.3 x 10$^-$ 5 cm^3 O$_2$/cm min Atm. Thews, 1969). It is also interesting that the KO$_2$ showed bigger variables from step-to-step measurements then the DO$_2$.

The oxygen solubility coefficients were pretty much in accordance with the so far stated values (αO$_2$ = 2.2 x 10^{-2} cm^3 O$_2$/cm^3 Atm, Thews, 1960). The peak distribution was a little broader and more than 50% of the values were measured to be in between 1.8 and 2.2 x 10^{-2} cm^3 O$_2$/cm^3 Atm.

It is concluded that the assumption of a homogenious distribution of DO$_2$, KO$_2$ and α O$_2$ in brain tissue is questionable in biomathematical modeling of the brain O$_2$ supply. Furthermore, it has to be taken into account that the oxygen diffusion coefficient values in the grey matter of the brain are different from the oxygen diffusion coefficients in the white matter of the brain which are about 10% lower.

REFERENCES

1.   Erdmann, W., and Krell, W.: Measurement of Diffusion Parameters with Noble Metal Electrodes. In: Oxygen Transport to Tissue - II, Eds, Grote et al., Plenum Publishing Company, New York, 1976.

2.   Goldstick, T.K.: Diffusion of Oxygen in Protein Solutions. Ph.D. Thesis, University of California. Berkeley, 1966.

3.   Gmelins Handbuch der anorganischen Chemie. Hrsg. Deutsche Chemische Gesellschaft, Weinheim/Bergstr.: Chemie, Nr. 3,446-495.

4.   Kolthoff, J.M., and Lingane, J.J.: Polarographie. New York and London: Interscience Publishers, 1952.

5.   Krell,   W.:   Die   Polarographische   Messung   des Sauerstoffpartialdruckes mit Mikroelektroclen Untersuchungen der Methodischen Voraussetnungen fuer die Anwandung in VIVO. Med. Diss., Mainz, 1972.

6.   Kreuzer, F.:   Ueber die Diffusion von Sauerstoff in Serumeiweisslesungen verschiedener Konzentration. Acta Helvet. physiol. 8, 505-521 (1950.

7.   Kreuzer, F.:   Facilitated Diffusion of Oxygen and Its Possible Significance. A Review Respiration Physiol. 9, 1-30 (1970).

8.   Krogh, A.: The Rate of Diffusion of Gases through Animal Tissues, With Some Remarks on the Coefficient of Invasion. J. Physiol. (London) 52, 391-408 (1918/19).

9.   Niesel, W., and Thews, G.: Diffusion in Medien. Pfluegers Arch. ges. Physiol. 269, 282 (1959).

10.   Thews, G.:   Ein Verfahren zur   Bestimmung des O_2 - Diffusions koeffizienten, der O_2 - Leitfaehigkeit und des O_2 - Loeslichkeitskoeffizienten im Gehirngewebe. Pfluegers Arch. ges. Physiol. 271, 227-244 (1960).

11.   Thews, G.: Sauerstoffdiffusion im Gehirn (Ein Beitrag zur Frage der Sauerstoffversorgung der Organe).   Pfluegers Arch. ges. Physiol. 271, 197-226 (1960).

TRANSIENT METABOLIC AND VASCULAR VOLUME CHANGES FOLLOWING RAPID BLOOD PRESSURE ALTERATIONS WHICH PRECEDE THE AUTOREGULATORY VASODILATION OF CEREBROCORTICAL VESSELS

A.G.B. Kovách, E. Dóra, J. Hamar,
A. Eke, and L. Szabó
Semmelweis Medical University
Budapest, Hungary

INTRODUCTION

Cerebral blood flow (CBF) is autoregulated which means that the flow does not change significantly in the range of arterial blood pressure of 50-200 mmHg (Harper 1966). Although great efforts have been devoted to understanding CBF autoregulation, its exact mechanism is till unknown. Fog (1937) showed that the diameter of the pial arteries first decreases and later increases after a transient decrease of arterial blood pressure. Since this initial observation not much attention has been devoted to the biphasic nature of the alterations in diameter of the pial vessels evoked by a rapid drop in arterial blood pressure. The present study was mainly focused on the transitory changes of cerebro-cortical vascular volume and NAD-NADH redox state during a rapid decrease of arterial blood pressure. The other aim of our study was to investigate the effect of phenoxybenzamine on these vascular and metabolic changes.

METHODS

The experiments were performed on cats anaesthetised with 60 mg/kg α-D glucochlorolose, immobilised by 2-4 mg/kg Flaxedil and artificially respired. The ventilation was adjusted to keep the arterial PO_2 and PCO_2 around 100 and 35 mmHg respectively. The cerebro-cortical reflectance and NADH fluorescence was measured by the modified microfluoro-reflectometer of Chance. To avoid movement artefacts and to close the skull a glass window was implanted into the parietal bone. The correction of the NADH fluorescence reading was made by the method of Harbig et al (1976).

In the untreated animals after a 30-40 minute control period the arterial blood pressure was decreased in a stepwise fashion to

80, 60 and 40 mmHg by means of a buffer reservoir system connected
to the femoral artery.   Each hypotensive step was maintained for
25-30 min.   After the bleeding period the arterial blood pressure
was restored by reinfusing the shed blood.   Tests involving 40
sec. electrical stimulation of the cerebral cortex and 1 - 1.5 min.
nitrogen inhalation were applied in the control period, during each
step of the bleeding phase and after reinfusion.   In the second
series of animals prepared as already described, the effect of
phenoxybenzamine (1 mg/kg by intracarotid injection) was tested on
the cerebro-cortical NAD-NADH redox state and vascular volume.
Before the phenoxybenzamine administration the animals were
connected to the buffer reservoir system to prevent the arterial
blood pressure decrease which normally accompanies the α-receptor
blockade.   One hour after phenoxybenzamine administration the
experimental protocol was the same as in the untreated experimental
group.

RESULTS

    In Fig. 1 the effect of bleeding on cerebrocortical reflectance
and arterial blood pressure is demonstrated.   It can be seen that
the new level of MABP was reached within 30 secs.   The cerebrocortical reflectance shows an inverse relationship to the blood
content. Thus if the blood content decreases the reflectance increases.

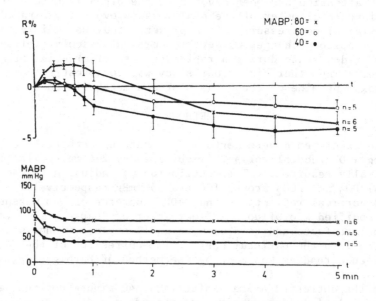

Fig. 1. The effect of graded arterial blood pressure decrease
(GABPD) on cerebrocortical reflectance (R%) and on the mean
arterial blood pressure (MABP).

Where arterial blood pressure is constant one can infer vascular
volume changes from the reflectance changes. As was shown by Fog
(1937) rapid arterial blood pressure decrease induced by vagal
stimulation evokes a biphasic vascular volume change. Our results
after lowering the arterial pressure shows that cerebrocortical
vascular volume first decreases and later increases. The most
pronounced vascular volume decrease was obtained when the arterial
blood pressure was decreased from the control level to 80 mmHg.
It is remarkable that the vasodilatation in this group starts much
later than in any other groups.

In Figs. 2 and 3 the cerebrocortical corrected NADH fluorescence changes are shown in the same experimental group. As can be
seen in Fig. 2 NADH reduction starts parallel to the vascular volume
decrease in both groups but interestingly enough the NADH reduction
continues after the onset of vasodilatation. In Fig. 3 one can see
that the rate of NADH reduction during the first 30 sec. of arterial
hypotension is nearly equal in the three groups. Later there is
a less steep reduction at 80 mmHg MABP and finally (after 5 min.
arterial hypotension) the cerebrocortical NAD-NADH redox state
shifts towards reduction with almost the same rate in both groups.

On Fig. 4 the sum of cerebrocortical corrected NADH fluorescence, NADH fluorescence, and reflectance changes is shown during
graded arterial hypotension and after reinfusion. One can see
that inspite of the considerable vasodilatation a significant NADH
reduction occurred at the end of each hypotensive step and furthermore the restoration of the MABP near to the prebleeding level
caused only a slight reoxidation of the NADH. These results
suggest that the NADH reduction obtained before the autoregulatory

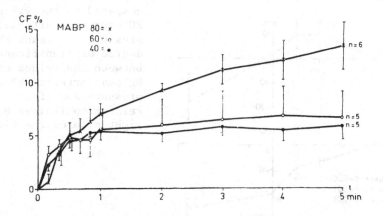

Fig. 2. Effect of GABPD on the cerebrocortical corrected NADH
fluorescence (CF%).

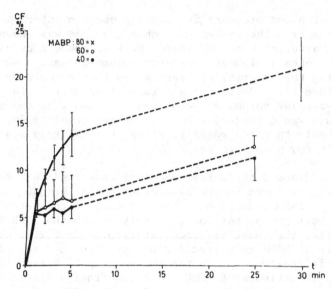

Fig. 3. Effect of GABPD on cerebrocortical NADH fluorescence (CF%).

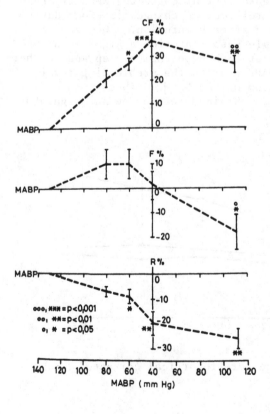

Fig. 4. Maximal corrected NADH fluorescence (CF%), NADH fluorescence (F%) and reflectance (R%) changes during GABPD after reinfusion. *means the degree of significance of changes compared to the values at 80 mmHg mean arterial blood pressure. o means the degree of significance between the values at 40 mm Hg mean arterial blood pressure and after reinfusion (values on the right side of the figure).

threshold of CBF and after reinfusion is not a sign of mitochondrial hypoxia but probably an indicator of increased substrate mobilisation and of reduction of cytoplasmic NADH.   However the steepest NADH reduction which occurs during the first 30 sec. of arterial hypotension might have been caused by cerebrocortical hypoxia due to the transient decrease in the cortical volume flow.   The vaso-dilatation appearing subsequent to arterial blood pressure decrease could be explained by accumulation of anaerobic tissue metabolites or by some unknown mechanism connected to cerebrocortical NADH reduction.   Whether the initial vasoconstriction is a passive phenomenon related to the arterial blood pressure drop or is the result of activation of the sympathetico-adrenal system is an open question.   To clarify the mechanism of this vasoconstriction and the role of NADH reduction in the CBF autoregulatory vasodilatation, in the second group of experiments an α-receptor blocker, phenoxy-benzamine was injected prior to arterial hypotension.

     In Fig. 5 the effect of an intracarotid injection of phenoxy-benzamine on cerebrocortical reflectance and corrected NADH fluor-escence is demonstrated in a single experiment.   The phenoxybenz-amine administration decreased the reflectance by about 20% and increased the NADH fluorescence by about 15%.   The arterial blood

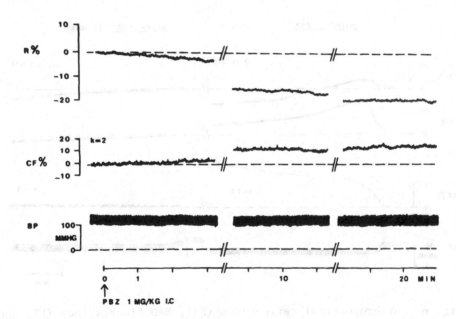

Fig. 5. The effect of intracarotid (i.c.) administration of phenoxy-benzamine (PBZ) on the cerebrocortical reflectance (R), corrected NADH fluorescence (CF%) and on MABP in a single experiment.

pressure was kept constant by the buffer system and was unchanged
after phenoxybenzamine administration.   Since the cerebral
perfusion pressure did not change but the reflectance decreased,
a significant CBF increase must have occurred after the phenoxybenzamine injection.   The increase of CBF excludes the possibility of
brain hypoxia and consequent mitochondrial NADH reduction.   The
most probable explanation is that PBZ increased the rate of
cerebral substrate mobilisation and shifted the cytosolic NAD/NADH
redox state towards reduction.   Besides this one cannot exclude
the possibility that the PBZ treatment decreased the rate of
mitochondrial electron transport.   Neither of these possible
explanations can be confirmed by the surface fluoro-reflectrometric
method.   However the NADH reduction and the vasodilatation seem
to be coupled.

The most obvious differences between PBZ treated and untreated
experimental groups with respect to the cortical reflectance and
corrected NADH fluorescence changes in response to graded arterial
hypotension are as follows:-

(1) After PBZ treatment there is no reflectance increased during
the first 30-60 secs. of arterial hypotension.

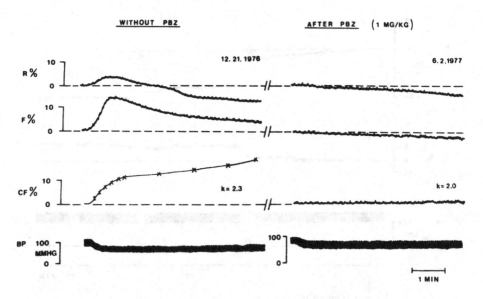

Fig. 6. Cerebrocortical reflectance (R%), NAD fluorescence (F%) and
corrected NADH fluorescence (CF%) changes evoked by decreasing the
arterial blood pressure (BP) from the control level to 80 mmHg in
a PBZ untreated and a PBZ treated animal.

(2) The steepest NADH reduction is lacking in the treated groups and at 80 and 60 MABP after an initial NAD reduction, NADH is reoxidised after a period of about 5 minutes of hypotension.

Fig. 6 shows the effect of arterial blood pressure drop from the control level to 80 mmHg on the cortical reflectance, NADH fluorescence and corrected NADH fluorescence in single experiments. It can be seen that PBZ treatment prevents the vasoconstriction and the considerable NADH reduction following the fall of arterial blood pressure.

SUMMARY

It has been shown by surface fluoro-reflectometry that step-wise decrease of arterial blood pressure causes a biphasic cerebro-cortical vascular volume response. After the arterial blood pressure decrease the vascular volume first decreased and later increased. In both parts of the biphasic reflectance change, the cerebrocortical NAD-NADH redox state shifted considerably towards reduction and there was no reoxidation after the onset of cortical vasodilatation. Since a very rapid NADH reduction occurred during the first 30 secs. of the arterial hypotension in parallel with the vascular volume decrease, it is suggested that in the transient phase of arterial hypotension cerebral hypoxia may occur. Furthermore it is suggested that anaerobic tissue metabolites or some unknown NAD-NADH dependent process might dilate the cerebrocortical arterial network during the autoregulatory adjustment of CBF. The participation of the sympathetico-adrenal system in transient brain hypoxia caused by bleeding is a possibility since both the early vasoconstriction and the steep NADH reduction were prevented by the administration of phenoxybenzamine (1 mg/kg) before bleeding.

REFERENCES

Fog, M. (1937) Archs. Neurol. Psychiat. 37, 351.

Harbig, K., Chance, B., Kovách, A.G.B. and Reivich, M. (1976) J. appl. Physiol. 41, 480.

Harper, A.M. (1966) J. Neurol. Neurosurg. Psychiat. 29, 398.

THE INFLUENCE OF ELECTRICAL STIMULATION ON CORTEX PO$_2$ LEVEL IN THE RAT BRAIN

Hermann Metzger

Dept. of Physiology, Med. School Hannover

Hannover, Fed. Rep. of Germany

INTRODUCTION

Oxygen consumption rate of small brain tissue slices is considerably increased if the tissue is stimulated by means of electrical impulses. This has been demonstrated in vitro by use of the Warburg apparatus (McIlwain, 1951; Klaus, 1967; among others). Until now the effect of artificial stimulation on oxygen consumption in vivo has not been analysed. In order to investigate the influence of electrical stimulation on the O$_2$ consumption rate, we used bipolar platinum microelelectrodes to excite a defined tissue volume of the rat brain cortex. Both the field potentials and the local PO$_2$ were measured at the same point in the cortex. The aim of our study was to produce local hypoxia or anoxia by increasing the local oxygen consumption rate and to analyse any regional cerebral blood flow reactions which may be caused by small areas of hypoxic tissue.

METHODS

Electrodes

Local PO$_2$ and action potential measurements were performed by means of gold microelectrodes. Electrode construction and calibration have been described in detail earlier (Metzger, 1971; 1973). As electrode material gold has better qualities than platinum resulting in a pronounced, al-

most flat polarogram, excellent longterm stability
(drift of less than 1 mmHg/h), reproducibility and a low
noise level (about 0.5 µV).   The electrical stimulation of the cortex tissue was induced with bipolar
platinum microelectrodes with tip diameter of 15   µm and
a tip distance of 5 - 10 mm.

Electronic Equipment

An improved version of the device described before was
used (Metzger et al, 1970;   Kunze et al, 1972).
Principally, the local PO_2 and action potentials could
be measured by means of the same gold microelectrode
because the frequency content of both signals differed
significantly.

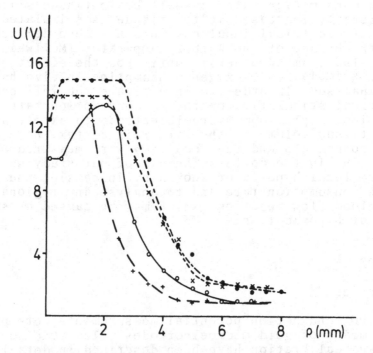

Fig. 1: Radial space dependence of the field potential
        distribution. An almost exponential potential de-
        crease occurs with increasing distances from the
        stimulation electrode. Preamplification = 600
        times.

The APs were filtered by means of a high pass filter (corner frequency 7o Hz), the PO_2 signal by a low pass filter
(corner frequency 1o Hz). Spontaneous activity was registered as extracellular action potentials which were characterized by a triphasic shape; we measured amplitudes of
1oo μV to 2 mV depending upon the size and distance of
the individual cells from the microelectrode tip. During
electrical stimulation a field potential was originated
and a large number of cells were depolarized. This is an
energy consuming process and consequently should influence
the rate of O_2 consumption. In order to prevent any leakage of current between the two different electrodes it
was necessary to isolate the stimulation unit completely
with the aid of an optocoupling device.

Animal Preparation and Experimental Procedure

Male white Albino rats (type Louis, free from pathogens,
18o-25o g body weight) were anaesthetized by means of
Urethane (75o mg/kg b. w.) injected intraperitoneally and
then tracheotomized. PO_2 and stimulation electrodes were
inserted into the skull through a small window with an
area of 4x7 mm. The open tissue was kept moist by use of
artificial liquor and warmed paraffin kept at 37°C. During the experiments the animals were held in stereotaxic
equipment.

RESULTS

Analysis of the Field Potential Distribution

Stimulation impulses of o.5 to 1 V, 1 msec duration and
of 1oo msec intervals were applied. The size of the field
potentials induced,decreased almost exponentially with
increasing distance from the stimulation electrodes (Fig.
1). In order to compare the experimental and theoretical
results (Metzger, 1977) two-dimensional cable theory was
used to calculate the potential distribution and to evaluate the electrical parameters. The following values were
obtained from the theoretical analysis: resistance r_m =
4ooo Ohm cm, capacitance c_m = o.1 μF/cm^2, time-constant
of the potential propagation = o.1 msec. These values
correspond very closely with those obtained for other excitable tissues. From the data above, the volume of the
stimulated tissue area was roughly calculated to be a
sphere approximately 5 mm in diameter.

Changes in PO_2 Response to Stimulation

A continuous PO_2 decrease was observed in 216 stimulation experiments performed with 22 rats (Fig. 2). The rate of PO_2 decrease was found to be dependent upon the stimulation strength and duration as well as the distance between the stimulating and measuring microelectrodes. In 3 rats a PO_2 decrease was detected at some points (19 stimulation experiments) whereas at others there was a PO_2 increase (39 stimulation experiments). In all the stimulation experiments the PO_2 decrease was completely reversible at the end of the stimulation period. It is interesting to note that the initial PO_2 was regained within a matter of seconds if the animals were in good condition. In

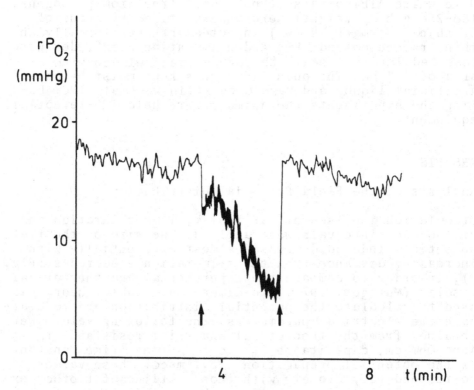

Fig. 2: PO_2 decrease during electrical stimulation. Stimulus amplitude 5 V, duration 1 msec, interval 1oo msec. Note the rapid reoxygenation after the cessation of stimulation.

hypoxic rats however, especially at the end of the four hour experiment the local PO_2 values in some of the rats tended to oscillate and the reoxygenation of the excited tissue after phases of stimulation was delayed.

In a second group of experiments, local PO_2 values were increased by the inspiration of a hypercapnic gas mixture of 15% CO_2, 2o.8% O_2, 64.2% N_2 in order to balance the O_2 deficiency caused through stimulation. Stimulation was started when the hypercapnic PO_2 plateau had been reached. Local PO_2 values were only minimally af-

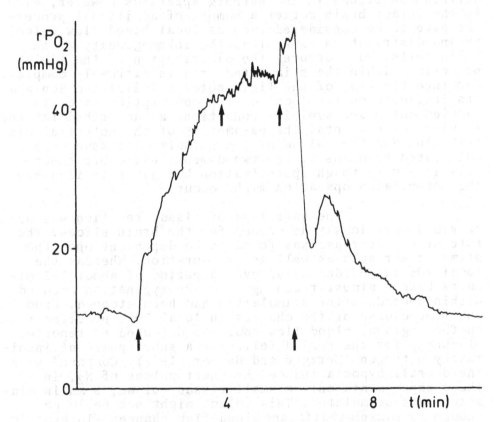

Fig. 3: PO_2 time-course during respiratory hypercapnia and additional electrical stimulation. First arrow: start respiratory hypercapnia; second arrow: start stimulation (parameter see Fig. 2); third arrow: stop stimulation; fourth arrow: stop hypercapnia. Note the almost constant PO_2 during stimulation and the small increase after stimulation was stopped.

fected by stimulation, remaining almost constant in 32 stimulation experiments with 7 animals; in only two cases was there a small PO_2 decrease and in one case a pronounced PO_2 decrease was observed. After a stimulation and hypercapnic period of 5 minutes, the original PO_2 levels were regained within 1-2 minutes (Fig. 3).

DISCUSSION

An increase in the oxygen consumption rate of brain slices is observed under in vitro conditions. Compared with the defined conditions in the Warburg apparatus however, within the intact brain cortex a number of additional processes have to be considered such as local blood flow velocity and distribution as well as the inhomogeneity of the brain cells. Furthermore, the distribution of the field potential within the stimulated area is extremely complex. Our investigation of the field potential distribution and its influence on the local oxygen consumption rate was carried out under similiar conditions as described for the in vitro experiments. The parameters of the potential distribution and the volume of the stimulated tissue were calculated by means of the two-dimensional cable theory. This is a very rough approximation but gives an idea how the potential propagation might occur.

The same type of tissue reaction was observed as previously described for the brain slices. The rate of PO_2 decrease was found to be dependent upon the stimulus strength as well as its duration. Whereas the local PO_2 values decreased over a period of about 1-3 minutes before almost reaching zero, reoxygenation occured within seconds after stimulation had been stopped. From the time-course of the changes in local PO_2, no effects on the regional blood flow could be detected as reported elsewhere for the period following a short pulse of inspiratory nitrogen (Metzger and Heuber, 1977). Compared with the overall hypoxia induced by short pulses of N_2, in these experiments only a small tissue volume, 5 mm in diameter, was stimulated. This volume might not be large enough to cause significant blood flow changes. In hypoxic animals however, oscillatory PO_2 fluctuations were observed which were probably due to changes in blood flow. Reoxygenation in these animals after the stimulation period was delayed.

In some animals spontaneous activity was observed. Stimulation in such cases resulted in a decrease in activity after 1-2 minutes probably due to lack of energy and

O_2 deficiency.At the end of the stimulation period, local PO_2 returned to normal causing a restoration of
activity to approximately the initial level within one
to two minutes.

The experimental results lead to the conclusion that
local blood flow reactions can not be detected from the
PO_2 time-course if a tissue sphere of 5 mm in diameter is
stimulated. General hypoxia observed in response to a
pulse of inspiratory N_2 is more effective in causing an
overshoot-undershoot phenomenon. Nevertheless, in experiments with spontaneous activity a decrease of action potential frequency has been measured during electrical
stimulation. We assume that local hypoxia and anoxia is
followed by a decrease in energy stores which causes depolarization of the membrane potential of a group of
cells and leads to a decrease of spontaneous activity as
it is described for in vitro experiments by many authors.

SUMMARY

Local oxygen consumption of the rat brain cortex was artificially increased through local electrical stimulation
of a small tissue sphere 5 mm in diameter. Measurements
of the local PO_2 distribution within the stimulated tissue
as well as the induced field potential were performed with
the same gold microelectrode. During stimulation the oxygen consumption increased significantly giving rise to local hypoxia and after 1-3 minutes to local anoxia depending upon the stimulus strength and duration.If however
pronounced respiratory hypercapnia was applied the increased demand for oxygen was met by an increase in cerebral blood flow resulting in an almost constant PO_2 level.
According to these results it is concluded that the
anoxic tissue sphere was not large enough to cause changes
in the local blood flow. On the other hand recovery from
local hypoxia and anoxia as well as reoxygenation of the
stimulated tissue were delayed if a general hypoxia
already existed.

REFERENCES

Klaus, W. (1967) Anaesthesiology and Resuscitation Ser.
11 (eds. Frey, R., Kern, F. and Mayrhofer, O.). Springer
Berlin, Heidelberg and New York.

Kunke, S., Erdmann, W. and Metzger, H. (1972) J. Appl.
Physiol. 32, 436.

McIlwain, H. (1951) Biochem. J. <u>49</u>, 382.

Metzger, H., Kunke, S. and Erdmann, W. (1970) Pflügers Arch. <u>319</u>, R 68.

Metzger, H. (1971) Habilitationsschrift, Mainz.

Metzger, H. (1973) In "Oxygen Supply" p. 164 (eds. Kessler, M., Bruley, D.F., Clark, L.C., Lübbers, D.W., Silver, I.A. and Strauss, J.). Urban & Schwarzenberg, München.

Metzger, H. and Heuber, S. (in press) Pflügers Arch.

LOCAL TISSUE PO$_2$ IN KIDNEY SURGERY AND TRANSPLANTATION

E. Sinagowitz, M. Golsong, and H.J.Halbfaß*

Urologische Universitätsklinik and *Chirurgische Universitätsklinik Freiburg, West-
Germany

In recent years polarographic measurements of
local oxygen tension in tissue has been developed as
a most reliable method for evaluation of oxygen supply
to tissue and microcirculation (Bicher and Bruley,
1973, Grote et al., 1976, Kessler et al., 1973).
Apart from its high experimental value this method
seems to be of great clinical importance for measurements in patients as shown recently for human skeletal muscle (Kunze, 1967, Schönleben et al., 1976) and
the kidney (Sinagowitz et al., 1976, Sinagowitz and
Golsong, 1977). This paper deals with further expe-
riences in measuring local tissue PO$_2$ in patients.

MATERIAL AND METHODS

Measurements of local tissue PO$_2$ in the human
kidney were performed in 13 patients with various
urologic diseases (renal cell carcinoma, carcinoma of
the renal pelvis, renal shrinkage, hydronephrosis) and
in 3 transplanted kidneys.
Tissue oxygenation was studied by means of the multiwire PO$_2$ surface electrode, designed by Kessler and
Lübbers (Kessler et al., 1976). This electrode contains 8 platinum wires each one with a diameter of
15 µ. This electrode makes it possible to measure the
real local tissue PO$_2$ simultaneously and continuously
at different places on the surface of the kidney. By
changing the position of the electrode on the surface

of the kidney a histogram can be obtained in a relatively short period of time. The electrode was steri-
lized by gas sterilisation, and mounted under sterile
conditions, at least one hour before starting measurements.
All monitoring was performed within at least 20 min.
With respect to the most valuable information for
further surgical treatment this seems to be a justi-
fiable period of time.

RESULTS

The PO_2 histogram gives a detailed analysis of
tissue oxygenation by demonstrating the distribution
of local oxygen tension in the tissue. Fig. 1 shows
the histogram of normal human renal parenchyma as
compared with a histogram of the rat kidney (Sinagowitz and Reinehr, 1977). The ranges of both are quite
equal: in the rat from 10 - 55 mm Hg and in the human
kidney from 10 - 50 mm Hg. Also similar is the shape
of the histogram. Due to the high number of values
the histogram of the rat kidney is nearly bellshaped,
whereas the histogram of the human kidney is more inclined to the left-hand side. The maximum frequency
in the human kidney is in the column 30 - 35 mm Hg
with 30.2 % as compared to 35/40 mm Hg with 36 % in
the rat kidney.

Fig. 2 shows the comparison between the normal
histogram and a "pathological" histogram, both in the
cumulative form. The "pathological" histogram was obtained from a kidney with malignant glomerulosclero-
sis. Whereas the normal curve shows a sigmoid shape
the "pathological" curve is straighter and shifted
distinctly to the left. All the values of the latter
are below 25 mm Hg, 25 % are in the hypoxic and
anoxic range below 5 mm Hg.

The increase of local oxygen tension after a
short artificial ischemic period shows varying types
of response. Fig. 3 shows the comparison between normal and pathological responses. Whereas the decrease
of local PO_2 after clamping is similar, the increase
is very different. The increase in healthy kidneys is
instant and rises to control-values within 30 to 40
seconds as shown in the lower part of the figure. In
the upper part the local tissue PO_2 in a kidney with
pyelonephrotic renal shrinkage is demonstrated. After

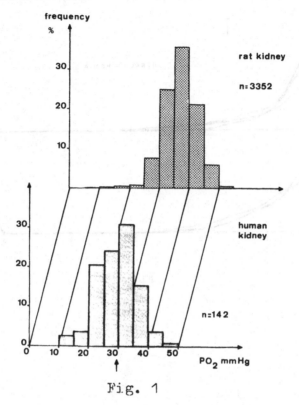

Fig. 1

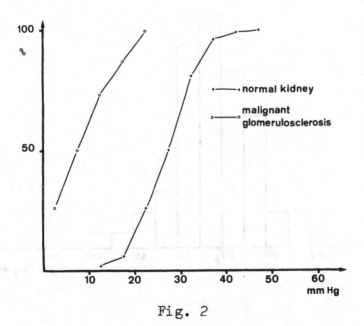

Fig. 2

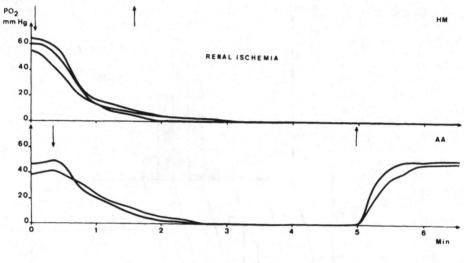

Fig. 3

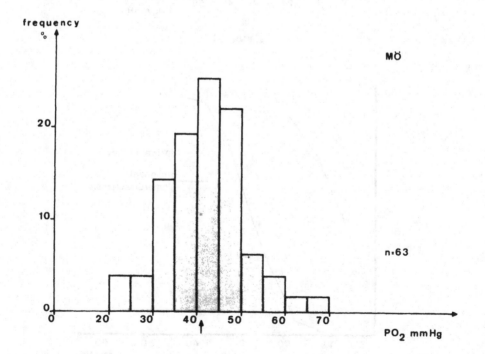

Fig. 4

only 1 min of ischemia there is no increase of tissue PO_2. Even after 5 min the PO_2 is zero. This same type of postischemic PO_2 response was observed in a kidney with normal macroscopic appearance but with severe pyelonephritis, confirmed by subsequent histological examination. Thus, microcirculatory disturbances were detected before histological examination.

Fig. 4 shows the PO_2 histogram of a transplanted kidney in the first 20 min after revascularization. The range is from 20 to 70 mm Hg and the maximum frequency is in the column 40 to 45 mm Hg. The curve is rather bellshaped. The period of warm ischemia was 4 min and the hypothermic storage time 2.5 hours.

DISCUSSION

Local oxygen tension is influenced mainly by 3 factors: arterial oxygen delivery, microcirculation, and cellular oxygen uptake. In considering these factors a three dimensional oxygen tension field in tissue with low and high PO_2 values physiologically was assumed (Krogh, 1919). Graphically this is best demonstrated by the PO_2 histogram - the frequency distribution curve of focal oxygen tension in tissue. A bellshaped histogram indicates that there are no disturbances of microcirculation and oxygen supply to tissue. The PO_2 histogram of the normal human kidney, as measured in the outer cortex with multiwire electrodes is very similar to histograms of animals as shown in fig. 1 (Sinagowitz and Reinehr, 1977). Changes in the shape and the location of the PO_2 histogram such as appearance of more than one peak and an increasing percentage of hypoxic and anoxic PO_2 values indicate microcirculatory disturbances (Kessler et al., 1976). This increase is best shown in the cumulative form of the histogram which is obtained by successive addition of the frequency of the classified PO_2 values. The marked disturbances of microcirculation as indicated by the distinct left shift of the curve (Fig. 2) were confirmed by the histological diagnosis of malignant glomeruloclerosis which is characterized by sclerosis of the smallest vessels.

Experiments on renal ischemia in different animals have shown that the postischemic PO_2 increase in healthy animals is immediate, rapid, and very uniform, but varies to a great extent in animals with hemodynamic disturbances or renal disorders such as hydro-

nephrosis (Kessler et al., 1977, Sinagowitz et al.,
1976, 1977). The non-appearance of postischemic PO_2
increases in pathologically altered kidneys may be
due to disturbed microcirculation and/or increased
oxygen uptake. This pathological response of local PO_2
to ischemia was observed even in kidneys which had a
normal macroscopic appearance but histologically showed
renal parenchyma severely damaged by interstitial
pyelonephritis.

The PO_2 histogram of the transplanted kidney
immediately after revascularization corresponds to the
histogram shown in fig. 1 and therefore would suggest
an undisturbed microcirculation. Consequently kidney
function after transplantation was sufficient and improving. However, at present we cannot state whether
or not the PO_2 histogram will predict the fate of the
transplanted kidney.

CONCLUSIONS

Our measurements of local tissue PO_2 on the human
kidney show a close correspondance with animal experiments. Moreover, PO_2 histograms and postischemic PO_2
responses may give valuable information for evaluating
the actual state of microcirculation and oxygen supply
in the renal cortex before results of histological
examination are available to the surgeon. Thus, this
method may serve as diagnostic aid in cases where the
decision has to be taken intraoperatively whether to
nephrectomize or to perform reconstructive surgery.
In addition, it may be of prognostic value in kidney
transplantation and of significance in further kidney
research.

REFERENCES

Bicher, H. I. and Bruley, D. F. (eds) (1973) Oxygen
transport to tissue.
Adv. Exp. Med. Biol. 37 A + B, Plenum Press, New York,
London

Grote, J., Reneau, D., Thews, D. (eds) (1976) Oxygen
transport to tissue II.
Adv. Exp. Med. Biol. 75, Plenum Press, New York,
London

Kessler, M., Bruley, D. F., Clark jr., L. C., Lübbers, D. W., Silver, I. A., Strauss, J. (eds) (1973) Oxygen supply.
Urban & Schwarzenberg, München, Berlin, Wien

Kessler, M., Höper, J., Krumme, B. (1976) Anesthesiology 45, 184

Kessler, M., Höper, J., Messmer, K., Sinagowitz, E., Lübbers, D. W., Chance, B., Barlow, C., Goodwin, C. (1977) (submitted) Microvasc. Res.

Krogh, A. (1919) J. Physiol (Lond.) 52, 391

Kunze, K. (1967) Habil.-Schrift, Marburg

Sinagowitz, E., Höper, J., Krumme, B., Kessler, M. (1976) Bibl. anat. 15, 399

Sinagowitz, E., Höper, J., Krumme, B., Kessler, M. (1977) Urol. Res. 5, 39

Sinagowitz, E. and Reinehr, L. (1977) (in press) Microvasc. Res.

Sinagowitz, E. (1977) Habil.-Schrift, Freiburg

Sinagowitz, E. and Golsong, M. (1977) Helv. chir. Acta 44, 359

Schönleben, K., Krumme, B., Bünte, H., Kessler, M. (1976) Langenbecks Arch. Chir. Suppl. Chir. 72

MEASUREMENTS OF OXYGEN PARTIAL PRESSURE AND SINGLE-UNIT ACTION

POTENTIALS IN THE PARIETO-VISCERAL GANGLION OF Aplysia californica

P. E. Coyer, E. R. Strong, and J. H. Halsey

Department of Neurology
University of Alabama Medical Center
Birmingham, Alabama 35294, U. S. A.

INTRODUCTION

Repeatable microelectrode recording from identifiable neurons within the isolated parieto-visceral ganglion of the sea hare Aplysia californica has been accomplished because the somatic positions and axonal projections into either hemisphere of these cells have been demonstrated both anatomically and electrophysiologically (Rosenbluth, 1963; Coggeshall, 1967; and Frazier et al, 1967). Only reference has been made to the metabolic dependence of these neurons (Chalazonitis and Arvanitaki, 1970) although interruption of the burst pattern in isolated pacemaker neurons exposed to metabolic blocking agents occurs (Chen et al, 1973). However, the direct measurement of the cytosolic oxygen levels and activity levels of specific neurons has not been attempted through multi-electrode recording of simultaneous action potentials and oxygen partial pressure.

It is known that the neurons occupying the outer-margins and inner layers of the ganglion are indirectly supplied by branches of the aorta coursing over the ganglionic connective sheath and emptying into its interstitial regions, but current thought, in opposition to Eales' observation (Eales, 1921), is that the neurons are not bathed in hemolymph and that the internal core is avascular (Coggeshall, 1967). Measurements of the in vivo oxygen partial pressure values of Aplysia hemolymph are reported to be low (A PO_2 of 25 mm Hg according to Chalazonitis, 1976). Moreover, diffusion of oxygen into the cells is limited by the existing barriers due to neuroglia and other supporting tissue. Chalazonitis (1976) has shown that the specific membrane potential of some pigmented cells (for example Br using his terminology) can vary with respect to intracellular PO_2 levels. This procedure was adapted for pigmented neurons as he compared intra-cellular pigment absorption measurements during administered periods of hyperoxia and hypoxia to the percentage hemoglobin absorbance, thus inferring the PO_2 from oxygen saturation curves for hemoglobin constructed in vitro.

Therefore, in order to better understand neuronal functioning under hypoxia and hyperoxia, an initial measurement of its activity and conjoint PO_2 should be established in situ at a stable temperature to which the ganglion has been acclimated. As a first step, the membrane potential, PO_2, and repetitive firing frequency or bursting rate must be determined for these neurons. Then, alteration in the internal PO_2 can be made experimentally to determine the role of oxygen on the neuron's activity and its effect on diffusion into the cell. Thus, some insight concerning the following questions may initially become known.

1.   What is the trans-membrane PO_2 differential?
2.   Does a change in cell membrane potential produce an artifact in the recorded PO_2 values?
3.   How much does PO_2 vary between cells?
4.   Does intracellular PO_2 vary between those cells with characteristically different firing patterns? Furthermore, as a corollary, does PO_2 affect cell activity?

METHODS AND MATERIALS

Specifically, the protocol is to isolate neurons within the parieto-visceral ganglion by careful dissection after desheathing the ganglion, identifying the neuron by its patterns of activity and established membrane potential through intracellular glass micropipette recording (filled with 3 M KCl; impedances ranging between 1 and 3 MΩ), and then to record the intrasomatic PO_2 with a Whalen-type electrode (Whalen, 1973) manufactured by Transidyne General Corporation, Ann Arbor, Michigan. Double microelectrode recording with a passive micropipette and a polarographic measuring PO_2 electrode can be made in a Corning 35 mm dish at 18° C. with continuously flowing air - equilibrated Aplysia saline whose composition is contained in Smith et al (1975). The intracellular oxygen electrodes are calibrated under 100% air saturation conditions and in nitrogen-equilibrated saline to establish the full-scale and zero positions, and finally under 5.2% oxygen conditions to increase sensitivity of the DC recording preamplifier (Grass 7P 1) for the expected lower PO_2 values; being less than 35 mm Hg. Calibrations were made pre- and post-experimentally at 18° C.

RESULTS

Microelectrode recording of oxygen partial pressure and single-unit action potentials from three cells (R_{15} and L_7; L_8 in Fig. 1) are preliminary but show that the intracellular PO_2 can be measured without influencing the membrane potential. Since this value does not vary, there is no artificially-induced somatic stimulation appearing in Fig. 1.

Conversely, noted changes in the membrane potential in a normally beating cell as in Fig. 2 do not artifactually affect the PO_2 levels. Overlapping standard deviations for the PO_2 values at the various membrane potential levels demonstrate that there is no apparent relation between the membrane potential shift and intracellular oxygen levels. Membrane potentials are subject to extrinsic alterations by temperature (Carpenter, 1967), but slight changes during the experiment might reflect chronic hyperpolarization by the oxygen measuring electrode, cell injury, or presynaptic inhibition or excitation. In these experiments the value for the membrane potential R_{15} averaged -72.5 ± 3.3 (S.D.) and -70.4 ± 3.0 for L_8 with PO_2 values remaining relatively invariant during the measurements; 2.4 ± 1.3 and 4.0 ± 1.1 respectively.

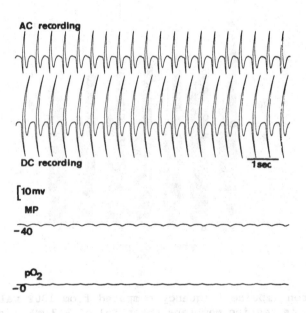

Figure 1
Top; Simultaneous AC recording of action potentials from Whalen-type and glass microelectrodes within L_8.
Bottom; Corresponding DC potentials-both membrane potential level and PO_2.

Figure 2 summarizes the preliminary baseline data for another
cell L_7. It represents the procedure for gathering and analyzing
data in the future and for cataloging cell activity and intracellular
PO_2. L_7 is one such neuron referred to above in the discussion of
synaptic influences on the beating properties of neurons. It is both
synaptically excited and inhibited by an interneuron L_{10}.
(Blankenship et al, 1971). The cell's mean PO_2 at $18°$ C. is 4.0 ± 1.1
throughout a range of membrane potentials of -45.3 to -57.3. Taken
as 100% its normally beating rate, the average calculated repetitive
firing rate at its peculiar but predictable membrane potential of -45
mV (Blankenship et al, 1971) is 0.93 ± 0.13 Hz. (Fig. 2). Alterations
in the membrane potential (range being from -45 to -57 mV, Fig. 2),

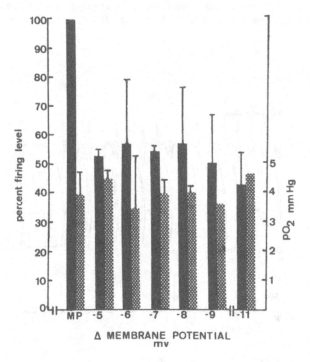

Figure 2
Percent neuron impulse frequency computed from 100% value of $0.93 \pm$
.13 Hz. at L_7's resting membrane potential of -43 mV (right ordinate
scale). Left ordinate scale; PO_2 value - (mm Hg) represented at each
of the occurring membrane potential changes. Vertical bars
represent standard deviations calculated as percentage of mean
firing rates and deviations from absolute PO_2 means. Only one PO_2
observation was made at -9 and -11 mV hyperpolarization.

however, do not reflect chronologically-occurring cell behavior so that more negative values do not precess one another. Changes in the membrane potential occurred while the PO_2 was not experimentally manipulated but varied slightly between 3.3 and 4.3 mm Hg. (right ordinate scale, Fig. 2). L_7 maintained its repetitive firing rate at 40-60% its normal rate (left ordinate scale, Fig. 2) under these conditions of membrane potential change and somewhat variable oxygen conditions throughout double intracellular recording.

DISCUSSION AND SUMMARY

Once measurements of critical oxygen partial pressure within characteristically-spiking neurons have been established for many cells within the parieto-visceral ganglion, the effects of imposed hypoxia or hyperoxia conditions on the cells' activities can be taken into account. Then, we will be able to answer questions pursuant to those raised in the introduction. In earlier experiments apart from those described for R_{15}, L_7, and L_8 there was an abrupt change in the oxygen partial pressure as the electrode penetrated single neurons within the ganglion and elicited action potentials. In 2 cases, the transmembrane PO_2 differential in these cells ranged from 12 - 18 mm Hg PO_2 (16 - 4 and 27 - 9 mm Hg PO_2; extracellular to intracellular respectively). Secondly, we have demonstrated that measurements of cell membrane potential and oxygen partial pressure are discrete, individual processes with no interaction of the membrane potential on the polarographic oxygen measurement or vice-versa. In response to questions 3 & 4 there is a continuing research effort to categorize these neurons intracellular oxygen levels while investigating their spiking - both frequency and bursting responses. Chalazonitis and Arvanitaki (1970) demonstrated chemoreceptor function of specific neurons within this ganglion by showing that many cells depolarize and increase spiking activity at PO_2 levels below 8 mm Hg. However, only a systematic intracellular study of oxygen levels and neuronal activity in those pigmented and these unpigmented neurons investigated in this paper can reveal the mechanisms by which cells are inhibited or excited by directional changes in oxygen levels compared to their normal values. As stated earlier, the results of these experiments are preliminary because of the limited number of observations and can only be interpreted as an initial contribution towards understanding how cellular activity is affected by or contributes to diffusion limited processes of oxygen delivery into nervous tissue.

REFERENCES

Blankenship, J.E., Wachtel, H., and Kandel, E.R. (1971) J. of Neurophysiol. 34, 76.

Carpenter, D.O. (1967) J. Gen. Physiol. 50, 1469.

Chalazonitis, N. (1976) Chemoreception and Transduction on Neuronal Models. In 'Tissue Hypoxia and Ischemia: Advances in Experimental Medicine and Biology' (eds. Reivich, M; Coburn, R; Sukhamay, L, and B. Chance) p. 85. Plenum, New York and London

Chalazonitis, N. and Arvanitaki, A. (1970) Neuromembrane Electrogenesis During Changes in PO_2, PCO_2, and pH. In 'Biochemistry of Simple Neuronal Models: Advances in Biochemical Psychoparmacology' (eds. Costa, E. & Giacobini, E.). Raven, New York.

Chen, C.F., von Baumgarten, R., and Harth, O. (1973) Pflugers Arch. 345, 179.

Coggeshall, R. E. (1967) J. Neurophysiol. 30, 1263.

Eales, N.B. (1921) Proc. Trans. Liverpool. Biol. Soc. 35, 183.

Frazier, W.T., Kandel,E.R., Kupferman, I, Waziri, R., and Coggeshall, R.E. (1967) J. Neurophysiol. 30, 1288.

Rosenbluth, J. (1963) Zeitschrift Fur Zellforschung 60, 213.

Smith, T.G., Barker, J.L., Gainer, H. (1975) Nature 253, 450.

Whalen, W. J. (1973) Intracellular Oxygen Microelectrodes. In 'Oxygen Transport to Tissue (Instrumentation, Methods, & Physiology): Advances in Experimental Medicine & Biology' p. 17 (eds. Bicher, H.I. and Bruley, D.F.) Plenum, New York and London.

THE RESPONSES OF AN AWAKE BRAIN TO HPO UNDER INCREASED CO_2 CONCENTRATIONS

A. Mayevsky

Dept. of Life Sciences, Bar-Ilan University

Ramat-Gan, Israel

The interrelations between convulsive activity, and CO_2 concentration under hyperbaric oxygen conditions were investigated by few investigators. It was shown in mice (Marshall and Lambertsen, 1961) and in cats (Taylor, 1949) that small elevation of CO_2 under HPO, potentiated the toxicity phenomenon while higher levels of CO_2 inhibited convulsions. Other investigators (Levy and Richards, 1962) came to the conclusion that addition of CO_2 to the HPO chamber provided the animal with protection against toxicity. In our previous communication (Mayevsky et al., 1974) we found that 1.5% CO_2 in oxygen potentiates the toxicity under pressure of 6 ATA. In order to understand the effects of CO_2 on the response of the brain to HPO we measured the effects of various concentrations of CO_2 on the electrical activity as well as the metabolic activity of the awake brain.

METHOD

Male Wistar rats (180-220 gr) were used. The animal was anesthetized and operated on using the same techniques as described previously (Mayevsky and Chance, 1975). The measurement of NADH was done from the right hemisphere while electrical activity (ECoG) was monitored bilaterally.

A time-sharing fluorometer/reflectometer was used for measurements of NADH oxidation reduction state as well as reflected light at the excitation wavelength (Chance et al., 1975). Each animal was located in the hyperbaric chamber 30 minutes after the operation and the common part of the light guide was connected to the cannula

to make a contact with the brain. Figure 1 shows the experimental
setup including the rat in the hyperbaric chamber. The compression
to 6 ATP was done 3-4 hours after the operation.

RESULTS AND DISCUSSION

A typical response of the awake cerebral cortex to oxygen was
published previously (Mayevsky et al., 1974). In the present study
we exposed a total number of 30 rats to HPO with various concentrations of CO_2 (as shown in Table 1). Figure 2 shows a record taken
from a rat exposed to 2% CO_2 in pure oxygen. As the compression
started the reflected light (upper trace) decreased, probably due
to vasodilatation of blood vessels. The uncorrected trace shows
the same decrease, so the corrected trace of this animal did not
show the classical oxidation of NADH as we described previously.
Several minutes later the electrical activity increased, namely,
spiking activity was recorded.

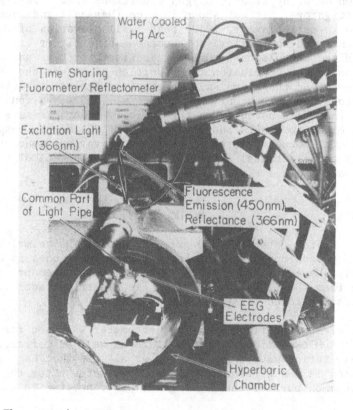

Fig. 1: The experimental setup by which the interrelation between
HPO and CO_2 concentration was measured.

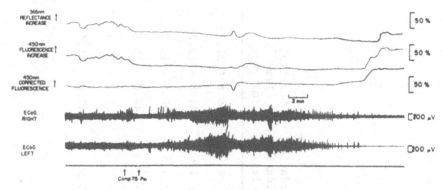

Fig. 2:   The response of the awake brain to 2% CO_2 in pure oxygen
          under 6 ATA.

Following this activity an oxidation-reduction cycle of NADH
was measured.   The termination of the experiment was when respiration stopped, ECoG activity decreased to almost 0 and NADH showed
a large increase.   Figure 3 shows the response of the brain to
3.1% CO_2 in oxygen.   Here again the same vasodilatation response
and a small oxidation was measured.   The typical convulsive
activity was not recorded and probably was blocked.   Only one
oxidation cycle was measured from this animal.

In order to understand the effect of CO_2 in detail, each
record was analyzed and the results are shown in Table 1.   The

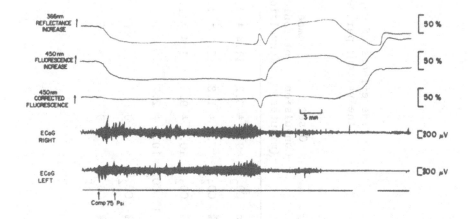

Fig. 3:   The effects of 3.1% CO_2 on the metabolic and electrical
          response of an awake brain.

TABLE 1

The effects of various CO_2 concentration in oxygen on the various parameters calculated from the records.

	Onset Convulsion (minutes)	Number of tonic Convulsions	Onset of Oxidation Cycles (min)	Number of Oxidation Cycles	PN Oxidation of Oxidation Cycles	Survival Time (minutes)
No CO_2	9.4 ± 3.2	11.4 ± 4.2	12.7 ± 4.1	4.8 ± 1.3	17.8 ± 4.0	69.6 ± 31.7
1% CO_2	7.4 ± 1.8	3.8 ± 1.6	11.6 ± 2.1	2.6 ± 0.9	17.2 ± 2.6	41.8 ± 12.3
2% CO_2	10.6 ± 9.4	1.4 ± 1.1	15.6 ± 12.3	1.4 ± 0.5	18.0 ± 4.5	40.0 ± 13.9
3.1% CO_2	10.2 ± 2.2	0	-	0.4 ± 0.5	-	48.0 ± 19.8
4% CO_2	0	0	-	0.2 ± 0.4	-	51.2 ± 25.4
5% CO_2	0	0	0	0	0	41.8 ± 11.4

initial oxidation of NADH was calculated (not shown in the Table) and appeared in 19 out of 30 rats used and was in the range of 5-15% of the initial fluorescence level in the normoxic brain. One can see from the Table that 4% CO_2 and 5% CO_2 blocked all the metabolic and electrical responses of the cortex to HPO. The survival time was shorter in all the CO_2 groups but was not statistically significant due to high variability between the animals. The number of tonic convulsions decreased as CO_2 went up and disappeared at 3.1% CO_2. The time to the onset of oxidation cycle was longer than that for the convulsion and it suggests that perhaps these cycles are the spreading depression type response after the convulsion, as was previously suggested (Mayevsky et al., 1974).

The oxidation of NADH during the cycles was the same in all groups found to show this response, suggesting that whenever extracellular potassium elevates, energy utilization will go up. All the results show that increase in CO_2 concentration in oxygen toxicity may block the convulsive activity but does not protect the animal against the toxicity process and the animal may die earlier than the control animals (Chapin, 1955).

ACKNOWLEDGEMENT

This work was supported by a grant from the United States-Israel Binational Science Foundation (BSF), Jerusalem, Israel, by a portion of the Program Project Grant NINDS 10939-05 and by the Research Committee at Bar-Ilan University, Ramat-Gan, Israel.

REFERENCES

Chance, B., Legallais, V., Sorge, J., and Graham, N. (1975) Anal. Biochem. 66, 498.

Chapin, J.L. (1955) Proc. Soc. Exp. Biol. Med. 90, 663.

Levy, J.V., and Richards, V. (1962) Proc. Soc. Exp. Biol. Med. 109, 941.

Marshall, J.R., and Lambertsen, C.J. (1961) J. Appl. Physiol. 16, 1.

Mayevsky, A., and Chance, B. (1975) Brain Res. 98, 149.

Mayevsky, A., Jamieson, D., and Chance, B. (1974) Brain Res. 76,481.

Taylor, H.J. (1949) J. Physiol. 109, 272.

OXYGEN TRANSPORT TO THE INNER EAR

C. Morgenstern and M. Kessler

HNO-Klinik der Universität Düsseldorf, and
Max-Planck-Institut für Systemphysiologie
Dortmund, West Germany

INTRODUCTION

Maass, Baumgärtl and Lübbers showed in 1976, that oxygen is
being transported from the tympanic cavity to the inner ear through
the membrane of the round window. So far there has been a paucity
of studies done on the quantitative and functional significance
of this way of oxygen transport.

This mode of oxygen transport may play an important role in
the treatment of sudden deafness or in the influence of high tone
damage after middle ear diseases especially chronic middle ear
effusion. The influence of high pO_2 in the middle ear cavity on
the endolymphatic potential is still unknown. In the present
study both the quantitative and functional role of oxygen diffusion
through the fenestra membranes were investigated.

METHODS

70 coloured guinea pigs weighing from 170 to 210 g were
anaesthetized intraperitoneally with Pentobarbital (30 mm/kg) or
urethane (1 g/kg). Bulla tympanica were opened from the ventral
or the retroauricular side, and pO_2-micro-electrodes (tip diameter
less than 1 micron) were inserted through the round window membrane
or through the cochlear wall in a drilled hole. The microelectrodes were prepared according to the technique of Lübbers and
Baumgärtl (1967, 1973) which were described in detail by
Sinagowitz and Kessler (1973).

RESULTS

Measurements of the oxygen partial pressure (PO_2), performed
in the surface layers of the inner ear yielded values of about
135 mm Hg; i.e. values that were distinctly higher than the PO_2
level measured in blood.

With increasing depth of penetration of microelectrodes into
the inner ear the PO_2 falls from the values of the perilymph to
the values of the endolymph (Fig. 1).

N_2-breathing causes the PO_2 in the layer about 20 μ below the
surface to decrease to zero, but not in the surface layers.

The velocity of PO_2 decrease caused by N_2-breathing is high in
the stria vascularis area, lower near the REISSNER-membrane and
very low in the middle of the endolymph space (see Fig. 2).

High pO_2 in the middle ear cavity gives rise to an increase in
PO_2 in the first turn of cochlea by diffusion and possibly
convection.   Pure oxygen breathing has a little effect on the PO_2
values in cochlear fluids. (Mean value 12.5 mm Hg). See Fig. 3.

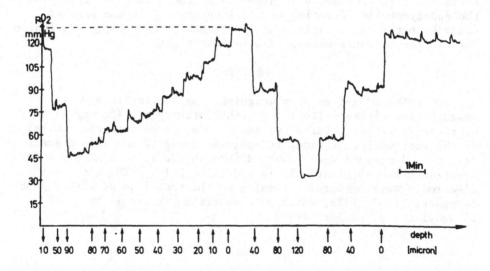

Fig. 1

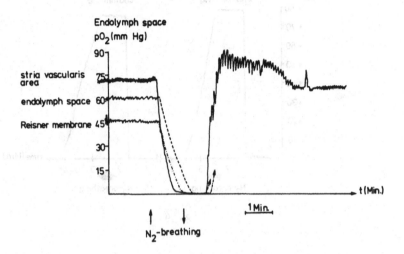

Fig. 2

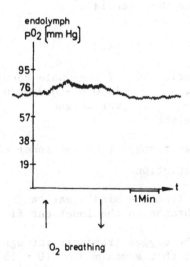

Fig. 3

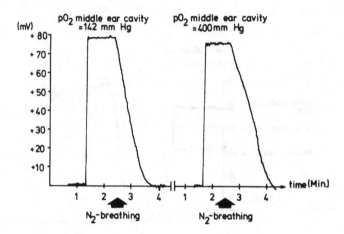

Fig. 4.

The endocochlear potential is normally + 80 mV.   After N_2-breathing it falls to 0.   The high PO_2 in the middle ear cannot prevent this fall of the DC-potential.

SUMMARY

1.   The oxygen consumption VO_2 of the whole cochlea
      $$VO_2 = \frac{AVDO_2 \times flow}{100 \text{ g wet weight}}$$ is 0.6 - 0.8 ml O_2/Min x 100 g wet weight.

2.   Two forms of oxygen transport to the inner ear exist:

      (a) by blood circulation

      (b) by diffusion from the middle ear cavity through
           fenestra-membranes to the inner ear fluids.

3.   Calculations of the oxygen transport through the fenestra
      membranes indicate that a maximum of 10 - 15% of the oxygen
      consumption of the first turn - representing the high tones
      area is based by diffusion at high levels of PO_2 in the
      middle ear cavity (400 mm Hg).

4.   This oxygen transport by diffusion alone is not sufficient to prevent the disappearance of DC-potential induced by systemic anoxia during N_2-breathing.

REFERENCES

Baumgärtl, H., and D.W. Lübbers. (1973) Platinum needle electrodes for polarographic measurement of oxygen and hydrogen. In 'Oxygen supply, theoretical and practical aspects of oxygen supply and microcirculation of tissue' (ed. M. Kessler et al). Urban & Schwarzenberg, München.

Lübbers, D.W. and H. Baumgärtl. (1967) Pflügers Arch. 294, R 39.

Maass, B., Baumgärtl, H. and D.W. Lübbers. (1976) Arch. Oto-Rhino-Laryng. 214, 109-124.

Sinagowitz, E. and M. Kessler. (1973) Adv. Exper. Med. Biol. 37A, 23.

KINETICS OF CHANGES IN PO_2 AND EXTRACELLULAR POTASSIUM ACTIVITY IN STIMULATED RAT SYMPATHETIC GANGLIA

C. Friedli

(Present address) Department of Physiology
School of Medicine
University of Geneva, Switzerland

Increase in metabolic rate during electrical activity has been recorded in various nervous tissue preparations yet measurements of oxygen uptake by isolated tissues have so far suffered from important time lags (Larrabee, 1958; Lipton, 1973) and therefore have not permitted analysis of transients. This paper describes PO_2 changes recorded within tissue with fast responding microelectrodes. A perfused preparation with relatively simple geometry was chosen to facilitate the interpretation in terms of oxygen consumption per unit volume (Q).

METHODS

Superior cervical ganglia from Wistar rats 120-180 g b.w. were excised under urethane anaesthesia (1.5 g/kg i.p.), mounted in a closed chamber and perfused at $26 \pm 2°C$ with a modified Krebs-bicarbonate HEPES solution gassed with 95% O_2 + 5% CO_2. Electrical stimuli, slightly supramaximal in intensity, were applied to the preganglionic nerve at 6 Hz. Compound action potentials were recorded from the postganglionic nerve. PO_2 was measured with gold plated recessed microelectrodes (Whalen et al, 1967). The electrodes were kept constantly polarized at 0.85 - 0.95 V against an Ag-AgCl reference. Then sensitivity varied by less than 10% during the penetration and by less than 15% over a week of experiments. Extracellular potassium activity (a_K^e) was followed within the ganglion with single barrelled microelectrodes siliconised and filled with K-sensitive resin (Corning 477317) (Zeuthen et al, 1974). Control measurements with saline filled microelectrodes showed that changes in extracellular DC potential induced by stimulation were small compared to the potential changes recorded by K-electrodes. K-electrodes were calibrated in the bath. Movement artifacts did

not allow continuous determination of changes in a_K during penetration of tissue but resting ganglia **were assumed to have the same**
a_K **as that of the perfusion fluid.**

The PO_2 transients recorded were compared to curves predicted
by a simple model.   The ganglion was considered as an homogeneous
solid, laid on an O_2 impermeable support, consuming O_2 at a uniform
rate.   Oxygen was assumed to be supplied by diffusion from the
bulk medium, through the upper exposed surface and the surrounding
stagnant layer.   A hemicylindrical model was chosen as a good
approximation to the actual shape of the ganglion.   Planar and
hemispherical models were also considered to assess limiting cases.
The diffusion equation:

$$\nabla^2_p = \dot{Q}/DS + 1/D \ (\partial p/\partial t)$$

was solved for a square-waved increase in $\dot{Q}$ according to Carslaw
and Jaeger (1959) (Eq. 7.9.3.)   The necessary parameters, namely
the diffusional conductance of the stagnant layer normalized to
that of the tissue thickness (G) and the O_2 diffusion coefficient
in the tissue (D), were determined experimentally by comparing
steady state gradients within and around each ganglion (Carslaw and
Jaeger, 1959;   Ganfield et al, 1970;   Friedli 1977) O_2 solubility
in tissue (S) was assumed to be 95% of that in 0.15M NaCl when
calculating D from experimental DS.   The tissue 'thickness' or
radius R_0 at the point of penetration was evaluated by measuring
the height of the top of the ganglion above its support.

As enlargement of an anoxic core at the onset of stimulation
would modify the kinetics of the PO_2 responses by reducing the
equilibration space, steady state $P\bar{O}_2$ distribution in resting and
stimulated ganglia was checked for possible hypoxia.   Hypoxia was
assumed and data were discarded whenever the relative PO_2 decrease
observed while penetrating radially 100 μm below the surface
exceeded by more than 5% the decrease expected if the O_2 flux from
the surface was just sufficient to reach the centre of the ganglion
of radius R_0:

$$1 - P_{100}/P_0 \ > \ 1.05 \ (1 - R^2_{o\,100}/R^2_o).$$

This study had thus to be limited to responses obtained at a
relatively low temperature (26 °C) with a moderate stimulation
frequency (6Hz).

RESULTS AND DISCUSSION

Changes in PO_2

The solid lines in Fig. 1A and 1B are recordings of PO_2 at
100 μm depth in two different ganglia.   During a 10 minute stimulation at 6 Hz, PO_2 fell to a new steady state level.   The onset

and initial recovery phase of another PO_2 response are shown with
an expanded time scale in Fig. 2. The amplitude of the PO_2 fall
and the time course of the onset were reproducible in a given penetration but the off phase was less reproducible.

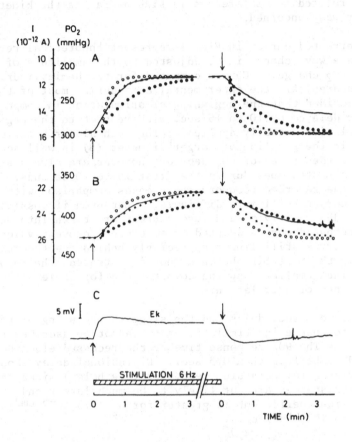

Fig. 1 : (A, B) : Tissue PO_2 decrease in response to a 10 min.
stimulation at 28°C. Solid lines, recordings in two ganglia of
different sizes. Symbols, curves predicted for a square-wave
increase in $\dot{Q}$ in planar (open circles), hemicylindrical (crosses)
and hemispherical (filled circles) models. Parameters used were:

	R (μm)	G	D (10^{-5} cm²/sec)
(A)	370	3.38	0.153
(B)	650	6.01	0.149

A typical E_K record (C) is shown to allow comparison of the time
courses. The peak increase in E_K at the beginning of the stimulation represents a 45% increase in a_K (+ 2.5 mM).

Table 1 (left part) summarises kinetics parameters from 12 records
in 5 different ganglia without anoxic cores. $T^{0.5}$ and $T^{0.9}$ are
given as mean $\pm$ SD between ganglia and other parameters as limit
estimates.   The corresponding changes in PO_2 level are reported in
Table 2.   Variability between ganglia was rather large, and
appeared related to differences in size as far as the kinetic
behaviour was concerned.

Interrupted curves in Fig. 1 represent theoretical responses
to a square wave change in $\dot{Q}$, adjusted to the amplitude of the
recorded PO_2 change.   Curves computed for the hemicylindrical
model (squares) fit the experimental data during most of the onset
phase, provided that the beginning of stimulation in computing the
curves is delayed by 10 to 15 sec. with respect to the beginning of
the stimulation actually applied.   The much slower kinetics
observed in the ganglion of larger diameter (B) is well accounted
for.   Recorded rates of PO_2 decrease however, are always smaller
than the computed ones during the first 15 to 20 seconds.   Variability in the recorded recovery phase makes comparison with the
computed curves still more difficult.   But even if possible drifts
in electrode sensitivity and zero current are taken into account
and the computed curves adapted to a reduced recovery value, the
recorded curves still linger appreciably behind the theoretical
ones.   In the best fit obtained (not illustrated) the recovery
rate remained smaller than the computed one for at least 30 sec.
after the end of stimulation.

The 1 to 3 sec. delay and the sluggish beginning of the PO_2
response to change in stimulation rate cannot be ascribed to
artifacts.   The 90% response time of the recessed electrodes used
was found to be less than 0.5 sec.   Diffusional delay should not
be longer than for potassium responses (see below) since the
diffusion distances are not likely to be much larger and the apparent diffusion coefficient is greater for O_2 (1.5 10^{-5} cm2/sec) than
for K^+ (3-5 10^{-6} cm2/sec.).

Changes in a_K

Fig. 1C shows a typical recording from experiments conducted
on 3 different ganglia with K-electrodes.   Another example is
shown in an expanded time scale in Fig. 2.   During stimulation a_K
rose and quickly attained a ceiling level.   Responses were reproducible in a given location but varied considerably between ganglia.
Limit values are given in Table 1 for kinetics data and in Table 2
for maximal a_K changes.   The shape of the observed a_K response was
similar to that described for perfused nervous tissue (Krnjevic and
Morris 1974; Kriz et al, 1975).   A slow recovery from ceiling
levels during stimulation and an undershoot after the arrest were
generally noted.   Both were found to increase with frequency and

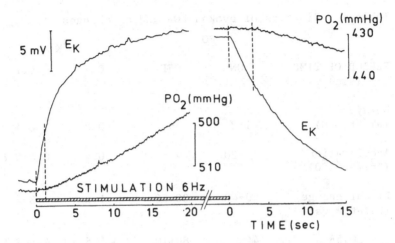

Fig. 2. Early PO_2 and E_K changes recorded at the onset and arrest of stimulation in similar preparations. Full responses attained - 87 mmHg for PO_2 and + 150% (+ 8.4 mM) for a_K.

duration of the stimulus. In spite of the difference in equilibration distances expected for diffusional wash-out between capillaries in vivo (50-100 μm) and superfusion medium in vitro (400-800 μm), the half response time for a_K increase is of the same order in superfused ganglia (3-5 sec.) and in perfused nervous tissues (2-4 sec.) following stimulation (Krnjevic and Morris 1974; Kriz et al, 1975). The time to peak of 0.7 - 0.9 sec. observed for single pulses in this study (not illustrated) would suggest an apparent diffusion radius of only 35-45 μm when interpreted with an instantaneous point source model (Krnjevic and Morris 1974). Reuptake thus seems to be more important than diffusional wash-out in controlling the equilibration process for a_K. Potassium loss into the perfusion medium has been found to be negligible in ganglia stimulated for a long period of time (20') (Brinley 1967).

Relationship between PO_2 and a_K changes

Steady-state increases in a_K similar to those observed here (2.5 - 8.5 mM) have been reported to activate the rate of sodium extrusion by 10-25% (Brown and Scholfield 1974) but the same authors showed the rate of intracellular Na accumulation is very close to the rate of intracellular K loss during the first minutes of carbachol exposure. Taking a volume fraction of 0.5 for the extracellular space, and admitting that water shift towards the intracellular space may compensate for a small K diffusional loss, one may tentatively equate the increase in intracellular Na activity (a_{Na}^i) to that in a_K^e.

Table 1 : Kinetics of evoked PO_2 and a_K changes

PERIOD OF TIME (sec)	PO_2 ON	PO_2 OFF	a_K ON	a_K OFF
Delay $(\partial Y/\partial t = 0)$	1-2	3-4	<0.2	0.4
Acceleration $(\partial^2 Y/\partial t^2 \lesssim 0)$	10-20	>15	0.4	0.4-0.6
Linear change $(\partial Y/\partial t \cong Cst)$	20-40	30-50	1-2	3-4
$T^{0.5}$*	44±8	80±10	3-5.5	4.5-8.5
$T^{0.9}$*	113±28	>240	10-18	14-20

*From the beginning or arrest of stimulation i.e. including delay and acceleration phases.

Table 2 : Amplitude of evoked PO_2 and a_K changes

Δp (mmHg)	$\Delta \dot{Q}$ (%)	Δa_K (%)	Δa_K (mM)
-100 ± 30	40 ± 16	$45 - 150$	$2.5 - 8.5$

This may account for a further 25-85% increase in pumping rate if one assumes a resting a_{Na}^l of 10 mM and first order kinetics for Na extrusion (Brown and Scholfield 1974). If ion pumping does account for about 40% of basal $\dot{Q}$ as indicated by ouabain inhibition in nerve tissue, such a concomitant increase in a_K^e and a_{Na}^l may increase basal $\dot{Q}$ by 16-52%. This is in good agreement with the mean $\dot{Q}$ of 40 + 16% (n = 5) calculated from the stimulated increase of tissue PO_2 gradients between 0 and 100 μm depth (Table 2). Other experiments showed that increase in calculated $\dot{Q}$ with stimulation frequency, even when corrected for an anoxic core, became saturated at 10-20 Hz like the increase in a_K response. This may be attributed to failure in transmitter release (Birks and MacIntosh 1961).

Time courses of a_K and PO_2 responses may be compared in Fig.2 and Table 1. In the onset one sees that (a) the abrupt initial rise in a_K takes place during the absolute delay of the PO_2

response, and begins to slow somewhat when the PO_2 response starts; (b) the progressive rise in the rate of PO_2 change (and in $\dot{Q}$ as inferred from comparison with square wave model of Q change) follows with a small delay (1-2 sec) the a_K rise and attains its full development at a time when a_K is close to the ceiling level. This temporal relationship may result from (a) progressive limitation of extracellular K accumulation by accelerated reuptake and (b) progressive increase of the respiratory rate under increasing energy demand from the Na-K pump. In the recovery phase, the early steep decline in a_K is also concomitant with the delay in PO_2 response. Yet recovery in $\dot{Q}$ is generally far from complete at the time when a_K attains its lowest level.

CONCLUSIONS

1. The time course of onset of the PO_2 response is largely in agreement with that predicted for establishment of a new steady rate of diffusion from the surface.

2. The time course of onset of the K^+ response is more rapid and suggests that equilibration involves diffusion over shorter distances than for O_2.

3. Comparison of time courses for K^+ and O_2 consumption are compatible with the hypothesis that at 26°C increase in pumping rate at the onset of stimulation stimulates O_2 consumption within 1-2 sec.

4. Steady state increases in a_K^e can account for the increase in $\dot{Q}$ calculated from PO_2 data, if a concomitant and equal rise in a_{Na}^i is postulated.

REFERENCES

Birks, R. and MacIntosh, F.C. (1961) Can.J.Biochem.Physiol.39,787.

Brinley, F.J. (1967) J.Neurophysiol. 30, 1531.

Brown, D.A. and Scholfield, C.N. (1974) J.Physiol. 242, 307.

Carslaw, H.S. and Jaeger, J.C. (1959) Conduction of Heat. Oxford Univ. Press, London.

Friedli, C. Thesis. Manuscript in preparation.

Ganfield, R.A., Nair, P. and Whalen, W.J. (1970) Am.J.Physiol. 219, 814.

Kriz, N., Sykova, E. and Vyklicky, L. (1975) J.Physiol., Lond., 249, 167.

Krnjevic, K. and Morris, M.E.   (1974)   Can.J.Physiol.Pharmacol.
52, 852.

Larrabee, G.   (1958)   J.Neurochem. 2, 81.

Lipton, P.   (1973)   Biochem.J. 136, 999.

Whalen, W.J., Riley, J. and Nair, P.   (1967)   J.appl.Physiol.23,798.

Zeuthen, T., Hiam, R.C. and Silver, I.A.   (1974)   Adv.exp.Biol.Med.
50, 145.

ACKNOWLEDGEMENT

The author would like to thank Professor I.A. Silver at
Bristol for continuous help and encouragement, and for allowing her
to perform the K^+ measurements in his laboratory.

The part of this work performed in Switzerland was supported
by SNSF Grant No. 3.457.70, and in Bristol by NINCDS Program
Project NS 10939.

EVIDENCE FOR EXISTENCE OF INTRAMYOCARDIAL STEAL

J. G. Reves, Wilhelm Erdmann, M. Mardis, Robert B. Karp
M. King and William A. Lell
University of Alabama, School of Medicine
University Station
Birmingham, Alabama 35294

Intramyocardial steal is defined as a process in which blood flow is diverted away from one area of the myocardium to another or away from the heart altogether. There are three potential causes of coronary steal syndrome: 1) congenital or acquired anatomic coronary malformations, 2) coronary atherosclerotic obstructive disease, and 3) vasoactive pharmacologic interventions. There is angiographic and physiologic data to support the existence of coronary steals in patients with congenital coronary artery disease, (Talner et al, 1965) as well as iatrogenic coronary steals (Pierach et al, 1971 and Barman et al, 1973). Evidence for the presence of coronary steals in exercised patients with ischemic heart disease (IHD) (Maseri et al, 1974 and Robertson et al, 1976) or pharmacologically induced steals in patients with IHD (Wilcken et al, 1971 and Utley et al, 1975) is scant and controversial (Rowe 1970). A reason for the controversy in this area is that indirect methods have been used to demonstrate coronary steals. The present report documents changes in directly measured myocardial oxygen tension that can be explained by the existence of a coronary steal phenomena.

METHODS

Fasted dogs of each sex weighing 18-26 kg were used in the study. Anesthesia was induced with sodium pentobarbital, 30 mg/kg, intravenously and maintained with nitrous oxide and oxygen in a concentration such that the PO_2 of arterial blood was kept constant in a range between 100 to 150 mm Hg. Supplemental anesthesia was administered by adding small amounts of methoxyflurane to the inspired oxygen/nitrous oxide to maintain the heart rate $\leq$ 130 beats per minute and systolic blood pressure $\leq$ 140 mmHg. Ventilation was controlled with a mechanical ventilator via a cuffed endotracheal tube at a minute volume adjusted to maintain the

755

arterial PCO_2 within the range of 35 to 45 mm Hg. Rectal temperature was maintained at 36 to 38 degrees C with a warming blanket. Fluid was administered at a rate of 3-5 ml/kg/hr with a pH 7.4 electrolyte solution.

The operative procedure consisted of a left lateral thoracotomy with placement of catheters for measurement of central aortic blood pressure (BP), right atrial pressure (RAP), and left atrial pressure (LAP). The left anterior descending (LAD) coronary artery was dissected at the first septal branch and a ligature placed around the first diagonal branch of the LAD or the LAD itself at that site. Oxygen microelectrodes were fixed to a plastic plate 1 cm by cm and sutured in the distribution of the artery to be ligated and in normal area of the heart (Fig. 1).

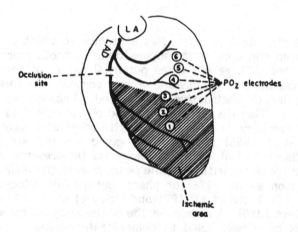

Fig. 1: Placement of PO_2 microelectrodes in the canine left ventricle.

The microelectrodes are constructed from glass insulated gold wires with a total diameter of 25 μ. The gold glass wire is cut and obliquely ground exposing the inner gold core at the tip. On the opposite side the glass is dissolved from the gold core by dipping the gold glass into flourocarbonic acid. The gold wire is connected to a conducting wire by means of silver lacquer. In a further step the gold core is electrolytically ground back into the glass coat and a recessed chamber formed in front of the measuring gold surface. Rhoplex, an acrylic polymer, which is permeable to oxygen serves as a membrane and separates the electrode chamber from the medium. To ensure mechanical stability microelectrodes are inserted into 30 gauge steel cannulas and fixed with epoxy glue slightly protruding at the tip by 1 to 2 mm (Fig. 2). The electronics of the electrode are similar to those used previously (Kunke et al, 1972).

Prior to electrode use, calibration procedure included:
1. Calibration of the electrodes in 0.2 molar K Cl solution at three different PO_2 values obtained by equilibration of the K Cl solution in a perfusion chamber heated to 38° C with known oxygen gas mixtures. 2. Comparison of the stability of the measured values between 0.2 molar K^+ Cl and 45% glycerin in 0.2 molar K Cl at the same oxygen partial pressure to ensure PO_2 measurement and independence from changes of O_2 diffusion coefficients. 3. Absence of stirring effects during gas perfusion to ensure independence from convection.

All electrodes were recalibrated after the experiment and tracings from electrodes which showed deviations from the original calibration of more than 10% were discarded. Indifferent electrodes were freshly chlorided silver-silver chloride electrodes. During the experiment, the indifferent electrode was brought into electrolyte contact with the tissue via a saline soaked sponge.

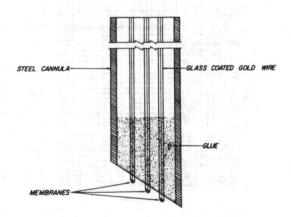

STEEL CANNULA

GLASS COATED GOLD WIRE

GLUE

MEMBRANES

Fig. 2: Schematic drawing of the PO_2 microelectrode encased in a 300 micron cannula.

Control measurements were made thirty minutes after any adjustment in the basal anesthesia and after stable hemodynamic measurements for a period of at least ten minutes. There were no further changes in basal anesthesia during the experiment. The BP, LAP and myocardial PO_2 (PMO_2) were continuously measured during interventions designed to totally occlude the ligated coronary artery. Various pharmacologic interventions were made to assess the affects of ketamine 4 mg/kg, halothane 1%, phenylephrine (↑BP 25%) and nitroprusside (↓ BP 30%) on PMO_2.

RESULTS

The results of the different pharmacologic interventions have been reported elsewhere (Reves et al, 1977). Total occlusion results in significant decrease of PMO_2 in electrodes well within the area of ischemia that is little affected by administration of ketamine and halothane. In several experiments, changes in PMO_2 in electrodes placed at the border zone of the ischemic area (electrode #3 in figure 1) reflected changes consistent with an intramyocardial steal. Figure 3 shows such a case where there are significant drops in PMO_2 of 38% and 41% in the 2 electrodes in the area of ischemia, but a 65% increased PMO_2 in the border area adjacent to the ischemic zone and a 24% decrease in the normal area.

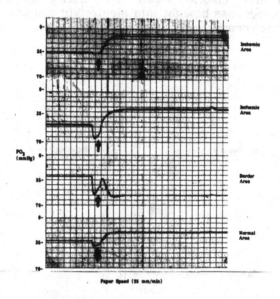

Fig. 3: Continuous PO_2 recording from areas of canine heart. Arrows indicate occlusion artifact.

Figure 4 (upper panel) shows the composite results of 5 experiments illustrating the PMO_2 changes in three myocardial areas. There was an average peak increase of 65% in border areas, 91% decrease in ischemic areas and 22% decrease in normal areas adjacent to the border areas. With release of the total occlusion there is almost immediate reoxygenation of the ischemic areas and a rebound hyperoxia. Simultaneous to the rebound increased hyperoxia in the former ischemic zone, there is a reduction in PMO_2 in the steal area - "reverse steal". The rebound effects last 5-10 minutes after an occlusion of 25 minutes and PMO_2 returned to control levels in all experiments.

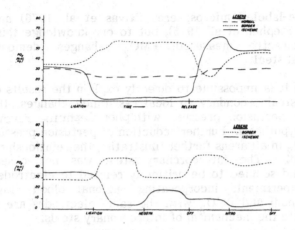

Fig. 4: Composite PO₂ changes in 5 experiments showing: Upper panel:
acute coronary ligation and release of occlusion. Lower panel:
influence of BP increase with neosynephrine and decrease with
nitroprusside.

The lower panel of figure 4 shows the effects of changing perfusion
pressure on the changes in PMO_2 in ischemic and border areas. Increasing
BP with neosynephrine resulted in an increase in PMO_2 in the ischemic
zone and a decrease in the border zone. Decreasing BP with sodium nitroprusside resulted in slight decrease in PMO_2 in both areas.

DISCUSSION

Intramyocardial steals may result from shunting of blood from one
coronary to another (intercoronary) , from one location in a coronary to
another location of the same coronary through collateral flow (intra-
coronary) and from a coronary artery to a venous connection
(arteriovenous).   The present data was obtained in acute canine
experiments amd demonstrates changes in PMO_2 consistent with an
intercoronary steal. Microelectrodes in the ischemic area consistently
documented significant drops in PMO_2 with acute coronary occlusion. In a
few electrodes placed in areas bordering the ischemic area, the PMO_2
increased while the PMO_2 in neighboring "normal" areas decreased. This
can be explained as an example of intercoronary steal resulting in an increased myocardial blood flow (with resultant increased tissue PO_2) to an
area of the myocardium in which decreased coronary artery resistance
occurred presumably as a function of autoregulation (Berne & Rubio, 1969)
causing an increased flow.   The increased flow apparently was at the
expense of the neighboring normal area where the PMO_2 slightly decreased.

Previous   acute   animal   experiments   have   demonstrated
intramyocardial steals primarily from endocardium to epicardium by means

of radioisotope-labeled microspheres (Rivas et al, 1976) and epicardial electrograms (Stephan et al, 1975); but to our knowledge this is the first report of directly measured PMO_2 changes demonstrating an intramyocardial steal.

Although it is impossible to directly explain the results of the PMO_2 changes as a steal secondary to local resistance changes, the fact that increasing the perfusion pressure with phenylephrine reversed the steal supports this hypothesis. Further reduction of perfusion pressure tended to lower the PMO_2 in all areas further illustrating the relationship of PMO_2 to blood pressure. The intercoronary steal was not observed in all experiments and seemed to be critically related to electrode placement. Subsequent experiments incorporating regional blood flow (hydrogen clearance method) and PMO_2 with the same electrodes are underway to further elucidate the mechanism of intercoronary steals.

REFERENCES

Barman, P.C., Geraci, A.R. and McAlpine, W.A. (1973) J. Thorac. Cardiovasc. Surg. 65, 152.

Berne, R.M. and Rubio R. (1969) Amer. J. Cardiol. 24, 776.

Kunke, S., Erdmann, W. and Metzger, H. (1972) J. Appl. Physiol. 32, 436.

Pierach, C.A., Siruno, E.S. and Jensen, N.K. (1971) J. Amer. Med. Ass. 218, 880.

Reves, J.D., Erdmann, W., Lell, W.A., Karp, R., and King, M. (1977) Abstracts. Scientific Program International Anes. Res. Soc. 51, 52.

Rivas, F. Cobb, F.R., Bache, R.J. and Greenfield, J.C. (1976) Circ. Res. 38, 439.

Robertson, D., Kostuk, W.J. and Ahuja, S.P. (1976) Am. Heart J. 91, 437.

Rowe, G.G. (1970) Circulation 42, 193.

Stephan, K., Mresmann, W. and Sadony, V. (1975) Cardiovasc. Res. 9, 640.

Talner, N.S., Halloran, K.H., Mahdary, M., Gardner, T.H. and Hipona, F. (1965) Amer. J. Cardiol. 15, 689.

Utley, J.R., Michalsky, G.B., Treat, R.C., Mobin-Uddin, K. and Parlin, A.R. (1975) Circulation, Suppl. 51 and 52, I-9.

Wilcken, DEL, Paoloni, H.J., and Eikens, E. (1971) Aust. N.Z. J. Med. 1, 8.

THE INTERRELATION BETWEEN CBF, ENERGY METABOLISM AND ECoG IN A NEW AWAKE BRAIN MODEL

A. Mayevsky and D. Bar-Sagie

Dept. of Life Sciences, Bar-Ilan University

Ramat-Gan, Israel

The measurement of intramitochondrial NADH oxidation-reduction state from the brain of an awake animal is a well established technique and is in use for the last few years. We had used this animal model in studying the effects of hypoxia, spreading depression, epileptiform activity (Mayevsky and Chance, 1975) or ischemia (Mayevsky, 1977) on the metabolic activity. In all of the studies made by our group or other groups, only one site or side of the brain was monitored fluorometrically. In the ischemia studies we found that under certain experimental conditions it is very important to measure metabolic activity from the "experimental" site as compared to the "control" site or side simultaneously. In our awake model we used a topical application technique to study the effects of drugs on the cortical tissue without any effects on the rest of the brain. This model also requires a bilateral measurement technique. We present in this presentation a new type of fluorometer/ reflectometer by which NADH fluorescence, as well as reflected light, can be measured simultaneously from two points of an awake brain model. This model was exposed to anoxia, spreading depression or ischemia and the results are presented. In another group of rats the effects of topical application of 2-Deoxyglucose were tested.

METHOD

A four-channel DC fluorometer/reflectometer was build according to the principles described earlier (Chance et al., 1975) and is shown in Figure 1. The excitation light (366 nm) from a 100 watt Hg arc is divided equally by a special light guide (Schott Co., Mainz, Germany) into the two spots of the measurements (2 mm diameter active fibers). The emitted light from each side of the brain was split by

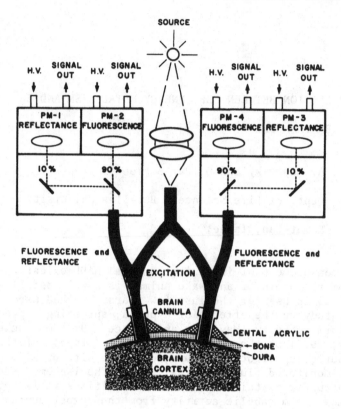

Fig. 1: Four-channel DC fluorometer-reflectometer for simultaneous
        measurement of NADH from two points of an awake brain.

a special mirror so that 90% was used for fluorescence measurements
and 10% for reflectance. Appropriate filters were located in front
of the photomultipliers. Measurements were recorded by a multi-
channel Grass polygraph.

    Wistar male rats were used in our studies (100-200 gr). After
anesthesia with Equi-thesin the animal was mounted to a head holder
during the operation. Two holes of 5 mm diameter were drilled in
the middle of the right and left parietal bone. In each hole a
plexiglass cannula was screwed epidurally. Two pairs of stainless
steel screws were implanted for ECoG measurements from both hemispheres. Two push-pull cannulas were also implanted for topical
application of KCl solution in order to elicit cortical spreading
depression. The cannulas and screws were cemented to the skull by
dental acrylic. The common parts of the light guide were inserted
through the cannulas and measurements were started 30 min after the
operation.

RESULTS AND DISCUSSION

In order to test the new instrument we used the N_2-O_2 breathing cycle and a typical result is shown in Figure 2. The upper three traces were measured from the right hemisphere and the lower three from the left hemisphere. The response to nitrogen was identical from the two hemispheres as one expected, and was similar to those described previously using the time-sharing technique (Mayevsky and Chance, 1975).

Figure 3 shows a typical response of the brain to spreading depression elicited by 0.5M KCl solution. One can see that the two hemispheres show the typical oxidation cycles due to increase in energy utilization in order to pump the large amount of K$^+$ ions

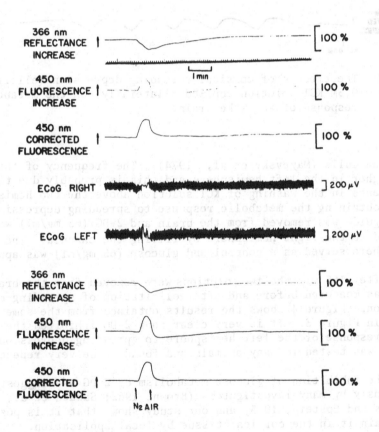

Fig. 2: The response of the brain to 1 min anoxia measured from the right and left hemispheres.

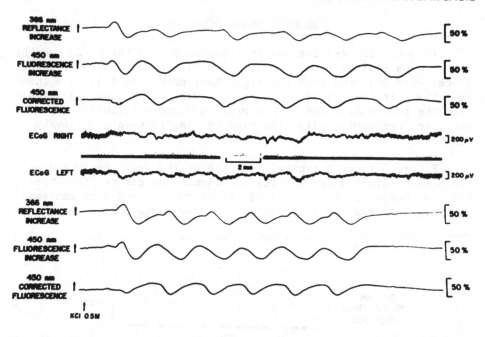

Fig. 3:   The effects of cortical spreading depression (elicited by
          0.5M KCl solution applied bilaterally) on the metabolic
          response of an awake brain.

into the cells (Mayevsky et al, 1974). The frequency of the cycles
was higher in the left hemisphere and this is probably due to
difference in the washing of KCl solution above the two hemispheres.
After obtaining the metabolic response to spreading depression the
light guide was removed from the brain and 2-DG (65 mg/ml) was
applied to the right hemisphere by filling the cannula. The left
hemisphere served as a control and glucose (65 mg/ml) was applied.

     After 165 min the two solutions were removed from the brain and
NADH was measured before and after elicitation of spreading depression. Figure 4 shows the results obtained from the same brain
shown in Figure 3. It is very clear that 2-DG inhibited the metabolic response of the left hemisphere to spreading depression. This
effect was tested in many animals and found to be very repeatable.

     The inhibition of glucose metabolism by 2-DG was suggested
previously by many investigators (Brown, 1962; Sakate et al, 1963;
Miselis and Epstein, 1975) and our study shows that it is possible
to obtain it in the cortical tissue by local application.

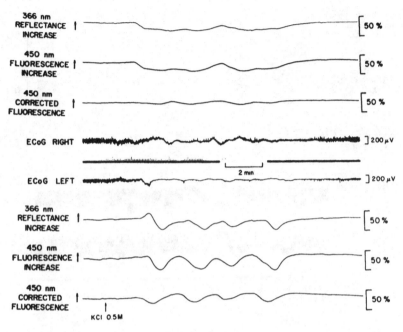

Fig. 4:   The metabolic response of an awake brain to spreading
          depression after application of glucose (left side) and
          2-Deoxyglucose (right side) for 165 min.

          In order to test the effects of ischemia we used the best model
for unilateral carotid artery occlusion, the gerbil model (Meriones
tristami).   This model is now in use by various investigators for
ischemia studies (for example, Levy and Duffy, 1977).   The gerbil
was anesthetized and operated on in the same way as the rat, and
ischemia was induced by occlusion of the common carotid artery.   In
preliminary experiments we found that there is a large variability
between the various individual gerbils which were tested.   Figure 5
shows the response of the gerbil's brain to unilateral or bilateral
carotid artery occlusion, while NADH was measured only from one
hemisphere, the right hemisphere.   After occlusion of the left
carotid artery a transient increase of NADH was recorded which
quickly returns to the baseline level.   When the right artery was
occluded (while the left remained closed) a large increase in NADH
was found and only after release of the arteries did the NADH return
to normal values.   After the recovery of the NADH to normal, an
oxidation cycle was recorded and we interpret it as an increase in
metabolic activity due to spreading depression elicited by high extracellular K^+ accumulated during the ischemia (Mayevsky et al, 1974).

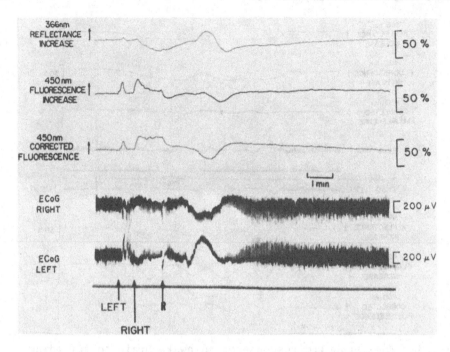

Fig. 5: The effects of unilateral or bilateral occlusion of the
carotid artery on the metabolic and electrical response
of the gerbil's brain.

In summary, the new fluorometer/reflectometer presented in this
communication opens up new possibilities to study brain energy
metabolism in the awake animal exposed to various physiological or
pathological situations.

ACKNOWLEDGEMENT

We wish to thank Mr. Victor Legallias and Mr. Eli Zimmerman
for their help in developing the instrument. This work was supported
by a grant from the United States-Israel Binational Science
Foundation (BSF), Jerusalem, Israel, by a portion of the Program
Project Grant NINDS 10939-05 and by the Research Committee at Bar-
Ilan University, Ramat-Gan, Israel.

REFERENCES

Brown, J. (1962) Metabolism 11, 1098.

Chance, B., Legallais, V., Sorge, J., and Graham, N. (1975) Anal. Biochem. 66, 498.

Levy, D.E., and Duffy, T.E. (1977) J. Neurochem. 28, 63.

Mayevsky, A. (1977) Brain Res. (in press).

Mayevsky, A., and Chance, B. (1975) Brain Res. 98, 149.

Mayevsky, A., Zeuthen, T., and Chance, B. (1974) Brain Res. 76, 347.

Miselis, R.R., and Epstein, A.N. (1975) Am. J. Physiol. 229, 1438.

Sakata, K., Hayano, S., and Sloviter, H.A. (1963) Am. J. Physiol. 204, 1127.

TISSUE PO$_2$ CHANGES IN ACUTE INFLAMMATION

I.A. Silver

Department of Pathology
University of Bristol Medical School
Bristol, England

The acute inflammatory response is a relatively stereotyped
reaction of vascularised tissue to almost any kind of physical,
chemical or biological irritant. The response is characterised
by a primary "vascular" phase, which is followed by a "cellular"
phase. The two phases are not discrete in that the vascular
changes continue during the initial period of cellular infiltra-
tion and neither are they of constant duration or intensity. Some
forms of insult provoke chiefly a vascular reaction e.g. ionising
radiation or thermal burns; others stimulate especially obvious
accumulations of inflamatory cells e.g. staphylococcal infection.
The time course of the response depends on the nature of the insult;
for instance whether it is short lived or persistent or if it
causes cell death or involves a major immunological component.

Trauma leading to skin wounds inevitably provokes local
inflammation and the biological sequence of cellular activity in
the inflamed area forms the basis of wound repair (Ross and
Oldland, 1969). These local changes in the tissues in terms of
blood flow, cellular accumulation and increased metabolism
considerably affect oxygen supply and uptake. Several previous
studies (see Hunt et al 1977) have shown that oxygen availability
plays an important part in the healing of both the connective
tissue and epidermal components of a wound, while it is also
general knowledge that wounds that have been contaminated with
either inert or irritant foreign material tend to show prolonged
inflammation and heal more slowly than clean wounds.

This report concerns a series of observations on changes of PO_2 during inflammatory responses to experimental wounding and introduction of foreign bodies into tissues grown in rabbit ear chambers.

MATERIALS AND METHODS

Transparent chambers turned from a single piece of 2 cm diameter polycarbonate rod and modified from the designs of Wood et al (1966) and Silver (1968) were inserted into the ears of half-lop rabbits where they were left until the dead space had become filled with new connective tissue. When the new tissue was established a fine needle was introduced on a micromanipulator into the chamber through the full thickness of the tissue (100 μm) and then advanced horizontally 250 μm to produce a standard lesion. In some cases the wound was either :
  a) implanted with a sterile, non-irritant, foreign body
     (a flake of dental prosthetic porcelain approximately
     50 μm³)
  b) implanted with a similar flake infected with Staphy-
     lococcus aureus,
  c) infected with Staph. aureus alone.

Oxygen tension in the vicinity of the lesions was followed continuously with a Pt-Ir needle electrode (tip size approximately 1 μm) (Silver, 1965) for two hours after the insult; at half hour intervals thereafter for the next 7 hours and hourly for the next 10 hours. The animals were very lightly sedated with a neuro-leptanalgesic ("Hypnorm"; Janssen S.A., Antwerp, Belgium). Simultaneous control measurements were made in non-injured tissue in the same chamber or in another chamber on the same rabbit to ensure that any changes of PO_2 at the experimental sites were not merely reflections of systemic events. As a control for the possible effects of "Hypnorm" trained rabbits were used that would remain passive for long periods without sedation. This was possible because the ear chamber tissue did not develop a somatic sensory innervation initially, although autonomic nerves could be demonstrated in association with small blood vessels.

The cellular events in the chambers were followed by direct microscopic observation, and at the same time relative changes in the diameter of small blood vessels could be measured.

RESULTS

The immediate response to simple injury was a very transient arteriolar spasm lasting 15-45 sec which was accompanied by a sharp, small drop in PO_2 as shown in figs. 1 and 2. This was followed by vasodilatation and a prolonged rise of oxygen tension which reached

a peak after 1-2 hours. At around 2 hours the accumulation of
inflammatory cells (in this case almost all were neutrophil polymorphs) became obvious. In some sterile wounds many more cells
appeared than in others and the numbers of cells aggregating in
the area had a marked effect on the local PO$_2$.

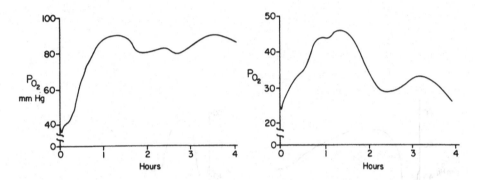

Figure 1. (left) PO$_2$ changes in early acute inflammation with a
minimal, late cellular component.
Figure 2. (right) PO$_2$ changes in the presence of a marked cellular
response.
Figs. 1 and 2 contrast the PO$_2$ changes in a wound with minimal,
late cellular accumulation with those in one which rapidly became
infiltrated with a large number of polymorphs. In general, the
larger the cellular response the more rapidly did the local PO$_2$
fall from its maximum at about 2 hours after wounding.

In lesions into which pyogenic organisms had been deliberately
introduced a PO$_2$ profile similar to that of fig. 2 developed except
that the secondary fall continued and reached almost zero by 16
hours after infection. In these cases the whole chamber content
eventually became necrotic and sloughed.

The pattern of changes in oxygen tension that followed the
insertion of a small foreign body, whether infected or not, were
different from those in a simple wound in that the initial fall of
PO$_2$ was much more profound and longer lasting. This seemed to be
due to compression of local capillaries, or to vascular spasm in
the immediate vicinity of the implant. After 20-40 min. the PO$_2$

increased (figs. 3 and 4) and reached a peak at 2 to 4 hours.
Thereafter, PO_2 fell either slowly and continuously if the material
was sterile or relatively rapidly and more erratically if it was
infected; in either case it eventually reached zero. This appeared
to be caused by the metabolic activity of the large numbers of
macrophages which surrounded the foreign substance. If infection
was present the predominant cells were polymorphs and tended to
obscure the macrophage involvement.

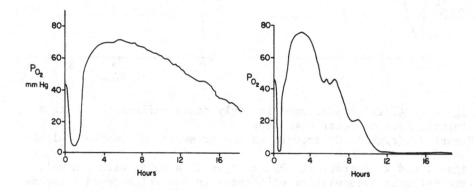

Figure 3. (left) Tissue PO_2 changes in the vicinity of a small,
sterile foreign body.
Figure 4. (right) Tissue PO_2 changes around a small infected
foreign body.

        In a few experiments involving sterile porcelain, measurements
were continued at irregular intervals for up to 14 days. After
approximately 72 hours the "wound" had completely healed and PO_2
rose in the neighbourhood of the implant. By 7 days there was no
interference with the normal tissue-PO_2 profile. This contrasts
with what happened in the vicinity of sterile, but non-biocompa-
tible implants where an accumulation of macrophages and lymphocytes
persisted together with a very low PO_2 and eventually gave rise
either to a sterile abscess or to fibrous encapsulation.

DISCUSSION

Local environmental changes are probably important in trigger-
ing the healing process and in determining whether it gives a
biologically satisfactory repair. Oxygen is known to have a role
in promoting efficient phagocytosis (Hunt and Pai 1972; Leibovich
and Ross 1975) and is essential in the formation of collagen, but
there are probably several factors, for instance pH, ionic balance,
tissue tension etc. which are also vital in the restoration of
tissue integrity.

A number of points have emerged from this study which require
comment. The relatively prolonged rise of PO$_2$ during the early
phase of inflammation seems to be at odds with the rather rapid
rise in blood flow that accompanies the "histamine release" period
of vasodilatation which primarily affects venules. This may be
explained partly by the increase in vessel wall permeability which
causes "inflammatory oedema", and thus increases diffusion distance
distances between capillaries and cells, and partly by the increase
in local temperature which increases O$_2$ uptake. Polymorph accumulation begins almost immediately after injury, due to surface
changes in the endothelium and to chemotaxis caused by various
elements in the complement cascade. These cells, although capable
of anaerobic respiration, metabolise oxygen actively and appear to
be a major factor in stopping the rise of oxygen tension. If the
polymorph population is depleted by the administration of nitrogen
mustards or anti-PMN serum the PO$_2$ rise is much greater in the
first hours after wounding (Silver; unpublished observation).

The second point of interest is that the initial rise of PO$_2$
after injury is very rapid even in the absence of a sensory innervation which makes the theory of the sensory "axon-reflex" difficult
to maintain in spite of its popularity in physiological and
pathological textbooks.

Finally, the accumulation of macrophages around inert foreign
bodies whether infected or sterile produces conditions which
greatly favour anaerobic organisms. However, the finding that
reduced oxygen availability lasts only about 72 hours around
biocompatible materials as compared to a much more persistent
reduction near non-compatible implants suggests the basis for a
relatively quick, simple method of screening potential prosthetic
products.

REFERENCES

Hunt, T.K. and Pai, M.P. (1972) Surg. Gynec. Obstet. <u>135</u>, 561.

Hunt, T.K., Niinikoski, J., Zederfeldt, B. and Silver, I.A. (1977)
In "Hyperbaric Oxygen Therapy" (eds. J.C. Davis and T.K. Hunt),
Year Book Medical   Publishers, Chicago, Illinois

Leibovich, S. J. and Ross, R. (1975) Amer. J. Path. <u>78</u>, 71.

Ross, R. and Oldland, G. (1969) In "Repair and Regeneration "
(Eds. Dunphy, J.E. and Van Winkle, W.) McGraw Hill N.Y.

Silver, I.A. (1965) Med. Electron Biol Engng. <u>3</u>, 377.

Silver, I.A. (1968) Prog. Resp. Res. <u>3</u>, 124.

Wood , S., Lewis, R., Mulholland, J. H. and Knaack, J. (1966)
Bull. Johns Hopkins Hosp. <u>119</u>, 1.

THRESHOLDS OF ISCHAEMIA IN BRAIN CORTEX

L. Symon, N.A. Lassen,* J. Astrup,** and N.M. Branston
Institute of Neurology, Univ. of London, Dept. of
Neurological Surgery, The National Hosp., London, U.K.
*Bispebjerg Hosp., 2400 Copenhagen, Denmark
**Fredensvej 17, 2900 Charlottenlund, Denmark

The effects of ischaemia on the central nervous system have been
the subject of much experimental and clinical investigation.
Occlusion of the middle cerebral artery in baboons simulates the
production of an acute clinical stroke (Harvey and Rasmussen,1951,
Symon, 1961, Symon et al, 1974, Symon et al, 1972, Yagamuchi et
al, 1971) and produces an ischaemic lesion whose extent is
restricted to known regions of the cerebral hemisphere and which
therefore interferes only selectively with the neural pathways.
We have shown (Symon et al, 1974) that the density of ischaemia
produced by occlusion of the middle cerebral artery is graded
over the surface of the hemisphere, and, for example, that areas
of the sensori-motor strip, show varying levels of residual blood
flow. Since the thalamic nuclei are not significantly affected by
occlusion of the middle cerebral artery (Kaplan and Ford, 1966,
Lazorthes and Campan, 1964) the electrical activity of the sensori-
motor strip assessed as the somatosensory evoked response may be
measured in relation to regional changes in tissue blood flow.
The creation of ischaemia which middle cerebral occlusion produces
also enables the relationships between regional cerebral blood
flow (rCBF) and extracellular potassium concentration (Ke) to be
determined. Examination of animals maintained for some years after
an acute stroke enables determination of the ultimate extent of
infarction resulting from a similar ischaemic insult (occlusion of
the middle cerebral artery).

METHODS

A standard technique of middle cerebral occlusion in baboons has
been used to produce ischaemic stroke. In acute experiments,
animals are anaesthetized with α chloralose after a sleep dose of

thiopentone (Symon et al, 1974). A cortical evoked response (EP)
to stimulation of the contralateral third division of the trigem-
inal nerve, is recorded from the somatosensory cortex, blood flow
over a wide area of the lateral aspect of the cerebral hemisphere
is recorded by hydrogen clearance electrodes (Pasztor et al, 1973)
and Ke measured by liquid ion exchanger microelectrodes (Astrup,
1976, Astrup and Norberg, 1976). A standard technique of transorbital occlusion of the middle cerebral artery is performed using
in acute experiments a light spring clip, which may subsequently
be removed, and in chronic experiments double occlusion between
tantalum clips with division of the artery immediately after its
origin from the internal carotid artery, thus sparing the
perforating bearing segment. Where indicated, in acute
experiments, blood flow in the cortex may be further reduced by
controlled exsanguination, since autoregulation in the ischaemic
zone is abolished (Symon et al, 1976). After a variable period
of reduction in perfusion, perfusion may be restored by removal of
the middle cerebral clip. The experiments reported have been
performed in a total of 12 chronic animals, and 40 acute
preparations.

RESULTS

Patterns of blood flow reduction over the hemisphere
The reduction of regional cerebral blood flow over the lateral
aspect of the baboon hemisphere induced by such preparations is
shown in Fig. I. It can be seen that the most densely ischaemic
area in the opercula has a blood flow of around 10-12mls/100g/min.
(20% of basal rCBF).

The threshold of blood flow for electrical function
The characteristic behaviour of evoked response in the period
immediately following middle cerebral occlusion is for a rapid and
progressive decline in the amplitude of the evoked response, the
rapidity with which the amplitude decreases being related to the
level of blood flow permanently established following the occlusion. This is shown in Fig. II, the variables being highly and
significantly correlated (R = -0.95, p < 0.001). Shortly following
occlusion a stable level of evoked response is obtained and under
these circumstances the amplitude of the evoked response is related
to the local flow in an apparent threshold fashion. This is shown
in Fig. III, thus, the level of ischaemia sufficient to reduce local
blood flow to a level below 12mls/100g/min. results in virtual
disappearance of the evoked response. Maintainance of a flow
greater than about 18mls/100g/min substantially sustained the
evoked potential. The 50% reduction in the evoked response is at
16mls/100g/min. It appears therefore that there is a threshold
level of blood flow between 14 and 18mls/100g/min., at which
metabolic activity in the cortex becomes insufficient to sustain

BLOOD FLOW IMMEDIATELY FOLLOWING M.C.A.
OCCLUSION
(ml/100g/min.)

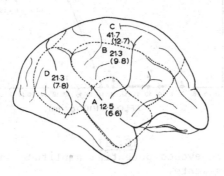

FIG. I

Reduction of regional blood flow produced by middle cerebral artery
occlusion. The figures are mean and S.D. of flow over the indicated
regions of the hemisphere.

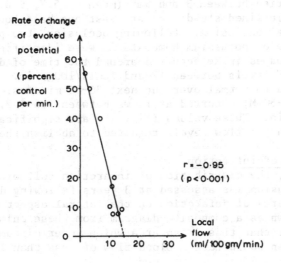

FIG. II

Relationships between rate of decrease of evoked potential amplitude
and local blood flow, following middle cerebral artery occlusion.

E.P(% of CONTROL)

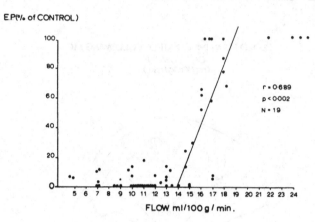

FLOW ml/100 g / min.

FIG. III

Relationship between evoked potential amplitude and local blood flow, in the steady state.

electrical function.

Potassium Thresholds

Control Ke varied between 3 and 9mM (mean = 5.7, S.D. 1.5) and was invariably maintained steady for at least one half hour before middle cerebral occlusion. Following occlusion, two principal types of disturbance of potassium homeostasis were identified. Small self-limiting increases in Ke occurred around the time of disappearance of EP, at rCBF levels between 12 and 16mls/100g/min. These invariably reverted to normal over the next 30-60 minutes. Massive increases, 30-60mM, occurred at flows between 7.6 $\pm$ 2.2 and 11 $\pm$ 2.6mls/100g/min. These values (Fig. IV) are significantly lower (p< 0.01) than the flow levels required to abolish the EP.

The occurence of infarction

In 10 animals, the distribution of infarction following middle cerebral occlusion was assessed at 3 years following division of the artery. The area of infarction on the lateral aspect of the hemi-sphere is shown as a composite diagram from these animals in Fig. V. It is apparent that this is an area which under circumstances of acute occlusion would have a blood flow of less than 12mls/100g/min.

DISCUSSION

A recent discussion by Marshall et al has summarised current thinking relating causation of electrical failure to ischaemia. Possible factors are primary depletion of high energy phosphates, synaptic

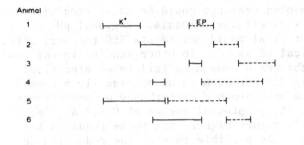

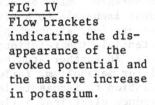

FIG. IV
Flow brackets
indicating the dis-
appearance of the
evoked potential and
the massive increase
in potassium.

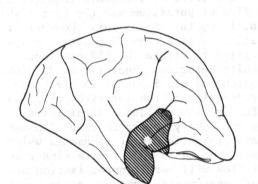

FIG. V
Distribution of
infarction at 3
years following
division of middle
cerebral artery.

depolarisation by release of intracellular potassium, severe lactacidosis and impaired neurotransmitter metabolism. Our results were,
we felt initially, consistent with the hypothesis of synaptic depolarisation subsequent to release of cellular potassium. However, the
clear separation of potassium thresholds from the evoked response
thresholds, demonstrate that massive potassium release does not occur
until a level well below the level of flow at which failure of the
evoked response occurs. Only slight elevation in local potassium was
found at levels of ischaemia which produced complete electrical
failure. We consider that these elevations in potassium are too
small to produce inexcitability, since full electrical activity is
seen at potassium values as high as 10-12mM per litre during epileptic discharges (Astrup et al, 1977, Futamachi et al, 1974) and
following electrical stimulation (Lux and Neher, 1973). It is clear
therefore that the association of massive potassium release with
electrical failure in ischaemia cannot be sustained by the present
study. The relationship between tissue lactacidosis and complete
electrical failure has not been directly assessed in our experimental
model. It is, however, shown that neither abolition of evoked

response nor recovery of evoked response could be associated with a
critical level of tissue extracellular acidosis. Regional pH
measurements made by Heuser et al could not relate EEG recovery after
total ischaemia to a critical pH value. In other studies in our own
preparation, although pH changes accompanied failure of electrical
potential, the relationship did not seem to us necessarily a causal
one. In further studies we have shown a disturbance of neurotransmitter metabolism, failure of synaptosmal uptake of G.A.B.A., in
relation to ischaemic levels rather higher than those required to
produce electrical failure. The possible role of the reduction in
glutamate and disordered G.A.B.A. metabolism for electrical function
has been emphasised by several investigators (Folbergrova et al,1974,
Duffy et al, 1972, Kobayashi et al, 1975, Marshall et al, 1975).

The close correspondence between the level of ischaemia required in
acute experiments to produce efflux of potassium and the levels which
subsequently produce infarction, is worthy of comment. However, in
our experiments, occlusion duration of less than 70 minutes always
resulted in restoration of potassium to within the 95% confidence
band of controlled potassium, while durations greater than 70 minutes
produced normalisation of potassium in only 8 out of 25 electrode
sites. Calculation of linear regression of the logarithm of potassium recovery on maximum reperfusion flow yielded a significant
inverse correlation, and it appears likely therefore that although
massive release of potassium may betoken levels of ischaemia which if
sustained lead to death of tissue, yet there is a finite time interval during which restoration of flow will permit normalisation of
extracellular potassium. In our experiments, however, normalisation
of potassium from massive efflux has not been associated with recovery of the evoked response, although the time circumstances of an
acute experiment do not permit us to state that such recovery of
electrical activity could not necessarily occur after a prolonged
period of time. From comparison of the distribution of electrode
sites and of the subsequent extent of infarction, it is clear that
efflux of potassium during acute ischaemia occurs over a wider area
that will subsequently infarct in normal animals, in line with the
demonstration that such flux is reversible provided flow is restored
within a finite time. It appears likely therefore that collateral
flow will normally reverse significant impairment of membrane permeability and restrict the area of infarct to an area smaller than
that originally affected by massive K^+ efflux. The linear relationship of blood flow to systemic arterial pressure in the ischaemic
zone has profound clinical implications. A drop in blood pressure in
the stroke patient may result in the conversion of zones with spared
electrical function into a state of electrical failure, and the conversion of areas in which electrical failure has already occurred
into a state in which massive cellular potassium release occurs with
a potentially lethal outcome. Such extensions of areas of impaired
brain function produced by hypotension may be reversed with subsequent clinical improvement simply by the re-establishment of normoten-
sion, or as has been shown in recent neurosurgical paractice (Hope et

et al, 1977, Kosnig and Hunt, 1976) by the induction of hypertension
following transient ischaemic neurological disturbance after aneurysm
surgery.

REFERENCES

1. Astrup, J: A double barrelled K+ selective liquid ion exchanger
    microelectrode designed for a continuous measurement of the local
    extracellular K+ activity in brain cortex in animals. (1976)
    Scand. J. Clin. Lab. Invest. (in press).
2. Astrup, J., Norberg, K. (1976) Potassium activity in cerebral
    cortex in rats during progressive severe hypoglycaemia. Brain
    Res. 103: 418-423.
3. Astrup, J., Heuser, D., Nilsson, B., et al: Epileptic discharges
    and extracellular K+ and H+ in rat cortex at critical levels of
    ischaemia. (in preparation).
4. Duffy, T.E., Nelson, S.R., Lowry, O.H.: Cerebral carbohydrate
    metabolism during acute hypoxia and recovery. J. Neurochem 19:
    959-977, 1972.
5. Folbergrova, J., Ljunggren, B., Norberg, K. et al: Influence of
    complete ischaemia on glycolytic metabolites, citric acid cycle
    intermediates and associated amino acids in the rat cerebral
    cortex. Brain Res. 80: 265-279, 1974.
6. Futamachi, K.J., Mutani, R., Prince, D.A.: Potassium activity
    in rabbit cortex. Brain Res. 75: 5-25, 1974.
7. Harvey, J., and T. Rasmussen. 1951. Occlusion of the middle
    cerebral artery. Arch. Neurol. (Chicago) 66: 20-29.
8. Heuser, D., Schindler, U., Hossmann, K.A. et al: The significance
    of cerebral extracellular H+- and K+- activities, brain volume
    and metabolism for recovery after prolonged cerebral ischaemia.
    In Harper, A.M., Jennett, W.B., Miller, J.D. et al (eds): Blood
    flow and metabolism in the brain. Edinburgh, Churchill and
    Livingstone p10:10, 1975.
9. Hope, D.T., Symon, L., and Branston, N.M.: Proceedings of the
    Copenhagen Meeting.
10. Kaplan, H.A., and D.H. Ford: 1966. "The Brain Vascular System".
    Elsevier, London.
11. Kobayashi, K., Kwakima, S., Hossmann, K.A. et al: Free amino acid
    levels in the cat brain during cerebral ischaemia and subsequent
    recirculation. In Harper, A.M., Jennett, W.B., Miller, J.D.
    et al (eds): Blood flow and metabolism in the brain. Edinburgh,
    Churchill and Livingstone, p10:3, 1975.
12. Kosnig and Hunt, Journal of Neurosurgery.
13. Lazorthes, G., and L. Campan. 1964. "La Circulation Cerebrale".
    Editions Sandoz, Paris.
14. Lux, H.D., Neher, E: The equilibrium time course of (K+) in cat
    cortex. Exp. Brain Res. 17: 190-205, 1973.
15. Marshall, L.F., Welsh, F., Durity, F, et al: Experimental
    cerebral oligemia and ischaemia produced by intracranial hyper-
    tension. Part 3: Brain energy metabolism. J. Neurosurg. 43:
    323-328, 1975.

16. Pasztor, E., Symon, L., Dorsch, N.W.C., and N.M. Branston: 1973. The hydrogen clearance method in assessment of blood flow in cortex, white matter and deep nuclei of baboons. Stroke 4: 556-567.

17. Symon, L., 1961. Studies of leptomeningeal collateral circulation in macacus rhesus. J. Physiol. (London) 159: 68-86.

18. Symon, L., N.W.C. Dorsch, and J.C. Ganz. 1972. Lactic acid efflux from ischaemic brain. J. Neurol. Sc. 17: 411-418.

19. Symon, L., Pasztor, E., and N.M. Branston. 1974. The distribution and density of reduced cerebral blood flow following acute middle cerebral artery occlusion: An experimental study by the technique of hydrogen clearance in baboons. Stroke 5: 355-364.

20. Symon, L., Branston, N.M., and Strong, A.J.: Autoregulation in acute focal ischaemia - An experimental study. 1976. Stroke 7: 547-554.

DISCUSSION OF PAPERS IN SESSION 9

CHAIRMEN: DR. C. HONIG and DR. J. STRAUSS

PAPER BY: DRS: GOODWIN and HEPPENSTALL

Dr. Hunt: A number of investigators have measured the wound fluid PO_2 in the same model. All have seen low PO_2 values. Why are yours higher? Was wound fluid PCO_2 measured? We have shown, using Antimycin A injected into the chamber, that hypoxia reduces the gradient from capillary to wound space. Although we saw small PO_2 decrements in hypoxia, it is true that the wound fluid PO_2 does not indicate fully the degree of the hypoxia which may occur. We obtained the same decrement of collagen synthesis in simple hypoxia without producing a cardiac lesion.

Dr. Goodwin: Our PO_2's (around 22 torr) are not much different from yours reported in 1967 (12 to 17 torr). We did not, as you did, notice any systematic differences with time. We measured PCO_2 and found an average around 70 torr. We were surprised that the chamber PO_2 was not lower in the hypoxaemic animal. We are currently using the silastic tissue tonometer familiar to you in an attempt to document a decreased tissue PO_2. We are convinced that it should be lower, based on the above work, and on mitochondrial studies carried out with Mela.

PAPER BY: DR. CHEN et al

Dr. Chance: What is the profile of PO_2 versus distance in the presence of dinitrophenol? These data seem an essential control on the hypothesis of hypermetabolic mitochondria near the cell membrane.

Dr. Chen: We have not recorded the PO_2 profile in the presence of dinitrophenol. I agree that such data are essential. We hope we will shortly be able to compare carefully these profiles by using a more precise depth recorder.

Dr. Lübbers: 1. Is the oxygen pressure decrease in the neighbourhood of the cell membrane caused by a stagnant layer?

2. Did you compare the intracellular PO_2 you measured, with the observed electrical changes? The intracellular PO_2 values are well above the critical mitochondrial PO_2 value of approximately 0.05 torr. I therefore don't understand in what direct way the oxygen pressure can be involved in this reaction.

Dr. Chen: 1. The PO_2 values were recorded in a completely stagnant saline environment.

2. Yes, we did. We suggest that a great change in intracellular PO_2 well above 0.05 mm Hg affects the rate of mitochondrial oxidation, thus changing the energy supply for the sodium-potassium electrogenic pump which in turn changes the membrane potential.

Dr. Silver: 1. What was the coating on the gold micro electrode tips that made them stiff enough to insert?

2. Dr. Cater and I some years ago, saw a similar fall in PO_2 close to the membrane in large plant cells, which was not apparently associated with large numbers of mitochondria.

Dr. Chen: The insulation was epoxylite and Insl-x. These electrodes were quite stiff if they were inserted absolutely straight and were of the right shape but of course, they bent easily in response to any shearing force.

Dr. Metzger: Dr. Metzger was concerned that equipment might have been affected by capacitance currents picked up both by the apparatus and by the electrode tip but was reassured by Dr. Erdmann that this had been taken into account and elimated.

PAPER BY: DR. METZGER

Dr. Lutz: The metabolic response of the brain to electrical stimulation is quite different from that in other organs for instance the intestine whose response is widely influenced by the behaviour of the vasculature. There we see under electrical stimulation a large decrease of O_2 consumption, even if we keep the blood supply constant by perfusion. We suggest that what is happening is that there is a redistribution of blood away from the nutritive vessels. Have you also seen responses of brain vessels which limited oxygen supply and thus induced a reduction of O_2 consumption?

<u>Dr. Metzger:</u> In principle, an influence on the cerebral vessels
cannot be excluded. Unfortunately, the deep vessels cannot be
observed and we have certainly never placed the stimulating electrodes in the neighbourhood of superficial vessels.

INDEX